BASIC
DENTAL
MATERIALS

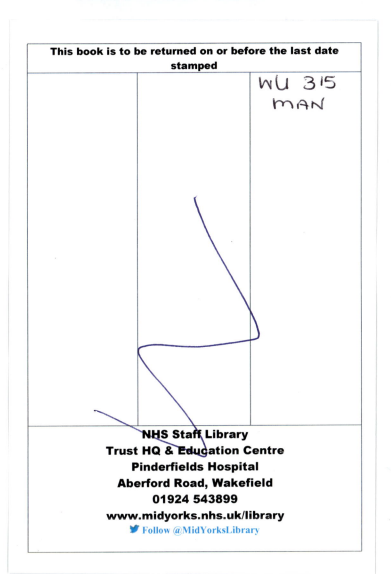

BASIC
DENTAL
MATERIALS

Fourth Edition

JOHN J MANAPPALLIL MDS

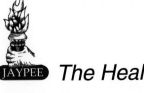

The Health Sciences Publisher

New Delhi | London | Philadelphia | Panama

Jaypee Brothers Medical Publishers (P) Ltd

Headquarters

Jaypee Brothers Medical Publishers (P) Ltd
4838/24, Ansari Road, Daryaganj
New Delhi 110 002, India
Phone: +91-11-43574357
Fax: +91-11-43574314
Email: jaypee@jaypeebrothers.com

Overseas Offices

J.P. Medical Ltd
83 Victoria Street, London
SW1H 0HW (UK)
Phone: +44 20 3170 8910
Fax: +44 (0)20 3008 6180
Email: info@jpmedpub.com

Jaypee Brothers Medical Publishers (P) Ltd
17/1-B Babar Road, Block-B, Shaymali
Mohammadpur, Dhaka-1207
Bangladesh
Mobile: +08801912003485
Email: jaypeedhaka@gmail.com

Jaypee Brothers Medical Publishers (P) Ltd
Bhotahity, Kathmandu
Nepal
Phone: +977-9741283608
Email: kathmandu@jaypeebrothers.com

Jaypee-Highlights Medical Publishers Inc
City of Knowledge, Bld. 237, Clayton
Panama City, Panama
Phone: +1 507-301-0496
Fax: +1 507-301-0499
Email: cservice@jphmedical.com

Jaypee Medical Inc
325 Chestnut Street
Suite 412, Philadelphia, PA 19106, USA
Phone: +1 267-519-9789
Email: jpmed.us@gmail.com

Website: www.jaypeebrothers.com
Website: www.jaypeedigital.com

Inquiries for bulk sales may be solicited at: jaypee@jaypeebrothers.com

Basic Dental Materials

First Edition: 1998

Second Edition: 2003

Reprint: 2004, 2007, 2008

Third Edition: 2010

Fourth Edition: **2016**

ISBN: 978-93-5250-048-2

Printed at Replika Press Pvt. Ltd.

Dedicated to

The teachers
who have inspired us

Contributors

Akshay Bhargava

Dean
Faculty of Dental Sciences
Shree Guru Gobind Singh Tricentenary (SGT)
University, Gurgaon
Haryana, India

G Vinaya Kumar

Professor and Head
Department of Prosthodontics
College of Dental Sciences
Davangere, Karnataka, India

Jacob Kurien

Professor and Head
Department of Conservative
Dentistry and Endodontics
Kannur Dental College
Kannur, Kerala, India

Rajashekar Sangur

Professor and Head
Department of Prosthodontics
Rama Dental College
Hospital and Research Centre
Kanpur, Uttar Pradesh, India

Preface

A successful dentist has to combine technical skills along with sound clinical knowledge. Knowledge of dental materials is one of the keys to a successful dental practice. To the beginner, the task may appear formidable because of the wide array of materials available. This is quite normal and fortunately disappears with use and familiarity. Intimate knowledge of dental materials is required throughout one's career for a successful practice. As with dentistry in general, the science of dental materials combines a wide array of disciplines, including chemistry, physics, mechanics, and biology with clinical sciences.

Format

Basic Dental Materials, first published in 1998, is now in its 18th year. Its publication was inspired by the desire to help students navigate the complex field of dental materials from the very first year of the course. Being the first published book on dental materials in India, it had set new standards, including moving away from traditional format. Its unique student-friendly format has contributed much to its popularity particularly among dental students from India and around the world and has made the understanding of this subject within the grasp of the novice. Over the years, readers have contributed valuable information as well as suggestions, many of which have been incorporated in the current edition. Comments and suggestions are welcomed and readers are encouraged to send their feedback via e-mail (jonsbin@yahoo.com).

Challenges

With each new edition, the challenges continue to grow, and revising the previous edition had certainly no exception. Dental material is a vibrant subject as new products and technology are constantly appearing in the market. A few of the materials have been eliminated from the book or have just briefly been mentioned as they are no longer marketed. Knowledge of the history of dental materials is useful to understand the evolution of materials and why newer materials were developed. Over the past decade, the field of ceramics has seen vast improvements. Current developments in CAD/CAM and 3D printing are opening new frontiers. Knowledge of values helps improve depth of understanding and is useful for making comparisons. Actual values of the various materials have been presented wherever possible. However, one must remember that values are not necessarily absolute, variations can occur over time, between brands and methods of testing. Climatic differences affect properties like working and setting times.

New chapters

Another challenge is defining dental materials. Traditionally, the subject of dental materials primarily included materials used in restorative dentistry and related auxiliary materials. Currently, there is a trend to be more inclusive of materials from other specialties, which have traditionally been excluded. This has been partly addressed in this edition by including two chapters on endodontic materials. With succeeding editions, it is hoped to be even more inclusive and cover the entire spectrum of materials used in dentistry, including surgical and orthodontic materials. Materials, such as anesthetics and drugs are not within the scope of this book. Metallurgy which was not included earlier has been included in the current edition (Structure and Properties of

Metals and Alloys). Another new chapter is in the field of 'additive manufacturing', popularly known as 3D printing. Biomaterials is another exciting area of development with an explosion of new materials and technology.

Differences in information

One of the challenges faced by the readers is the wide variation in information between different books. Differences do exist between different books and the reader is often in a dilemma as to which information to follow. The best source is the original source which includes original studies, information from the manufacturers and publications of the International Standards Organization (ISO). The 'International Standards Organization' is a significant reference source for manufacturers as well as authors and researchers. The technical committees in-charge of the specification constantly strive to keep pace with changes in knowledge and technology, through publication of new editions of the specifications periodically. The edition is indicated by the year attached to the specification. Most dental product manufacturers strive to keep pace with changes in standards. Significant changes have taken place in the specifications and classifications of many products. The fourth edition of *Basic Dental Materials* too has reflected these changes and, therefore, differences will exist between the current edition and previous editions as well as other textbooks on the subjects, particularly in the area of classifications and technical details. Readers and teaching staff in particular are requested to look out for these changes and refer to the source wherever provided. Explanatory footnotes have been provided wherever needed.

International Standards Organization (ISO)

Many nations, including India and the US are members of the ISO. Founded in 1947 with just 26 members, its membership has grown to 162, including 119 full members, 38 correspondent members and 5 subscriber members. India has not only been a full member since its inception, but has also assumed council positions and has been a part of technical committees at various times. Current ADA specifications have been adopted from the ISO. In its website, the ADA has stated that their specifications are identical to the relevant ISO standards. Therefore, use of both specifications for the same product is repetitive. The fourth and subsequent editions of the book will therefore gradually phase out the ADA specifications and replace them with those of the ISO wherever relevant. Other specifications, including the ADA will be used only if ISO standards are not available for the particular product.

Organization of the book

Other changes include the reorganization of the book into segments. The 30 chapters in the book have been organized into 7 parts for ease of reference. Another new feature is the chapter outline at the beginning of each chapter as requested by some readers. Many materials adversely affect the other's property, and therefore, material interactions have been introduced where information is available. A familiar one to most readers is the effect of eugenol from ZOE-based products on composites. Another relatively less familiar one is that between provisional composites and elastomeric impression materials.

Critical assessment of new products

Today's dentists in India are fortunate to have a wide choice of materials. The economic liberalization of the late 1980s saw the opening of the market to a range of high quality international products. Dental practitioners should have a good understanding of basic dental materials science to enable them to select and critically assess the plethora of new materials that are constantly being introduced and aggressively marketed. It is also advisable to request long-term *in vitro* and *in vivo* independently acquired evidence of the performance of a material before deciding to use it. It is not possible to cover every material in the book; therefore, the operator should read the information which comes with a particular product whenever available.

Information exchange and update

Students are encouraged to read from a wide source of materials for greater understanding and depth of knowledge. Thanks to journals, scientific conferences and the internet, there is exchange of information between individuals, transcending geographical barriers. Concepts are constantly changing with improved understanding and new research. It is encouraging to see a lot of new publications within the country and abroad. Encouragement, from professional publishing houses and new regulations by the DCI have in no small measure, contributed to this increase. Indian professionals are now contributing significantly to international research literature and education world over.

Educational challenges

Dental institutions today are facing innumerable challenges, and constant adaptation is required to reflect changing curricula around the world and higher expectations among the student community. The challenge now is in reorganizing and streamlining the courses to changing times. It is encouraging to see some leading institutions take bold new initiatives in instituting improved learning techniques and investing in infrastructure to raise standards of education. In this regard, the roles of regulatory bodies, including the Dental Council of India and various Dental Associations are critical to ensure that the profession continues to develop. It is my fervent hope that a new generation of young, highly trained and motivated dentists will emerge providing improved patient care and upholding the dignity of the profession.

John J Manappallil

Acknowledgments

Every book has its share of contributors and influences, and this book is certainly no exception. I am deeply indebted to professors Akshay Bhargava, Jacob Kurien, G Vinaya Kumar and Rajashekar Sangur who over the years have contributed their knowledge and experience to the various chapters in the book. It is my honor and privilege to have you all associated with this book.

My deepest gratitude goes to all those who helped with the proofreading and corrections of the manuscripts. In this regard, I thank Dr Rajanikant AV and Preeti Pachauri from Rama Dental College, Hospital and Research Centre, Kanpur, Uttar Pradesh, India; Ginu Philip, Vijayasree Sreekumar and Jojen Thomas from Bneid Al Gar Dental Center, Kuwait; and my wife Dr Divya Susan.

The countless hours I have spent on the project meant I remained hours away from my family. My deep appreciation goes to my family especially my wife Divya and kids Reuben and Jordan and my parents. Without their encouragement, support and tolerance, this project would not have been possible.

This edition is dedicated to our respected teachers who have influenced all of us. This includes not only the professors and clinicians who taught us at dental school, but also those who shared their information at the continuing education programs and conferences. I wish to acknowledge the significant influence of the genius authors from around the world whose books have been a source of so much knowledge and inspiration. I pay tribute to these great individuals who have inspired all of us.

I wish to express my appreciation to those who contributed to the previous editions in particular my former colleagues Shubha Rao and Atley George from BDCH, Davangere. In spite of the significant modifications many of the chapters contain portions created by them.

I also take this occasion to once again renew bonds of friendship and affection with all my students and readers. I thank all the readers who have given their feedback and suggestions. Your support is what gives me the inspiration to continue this book. It is a privilege to have you all on board.

Last but not least, a special thanks to Shri Jitendar P Vij (Group Chairman), Mr Ankit Vij (Group President), Mr Tarun Duneja (Director-Publishing) and staff of M/s Jaypee Brothers Medical Publishers (P) Ltd, New Delhi, India, for their great expertise in creating a truly remarkable book.

Contents

Part 2: Direct Restorative Materials

Part 5: Dental Laboratory—Materials and Processes

Part 7: Indirect Restorative and Prosthetic Materials

PART-1

Structure and Properties of Dental Materials

Overview of Dentistry and Dental Materials

Dentistry over the years has evolved into a highly complex field and materials play a crucial role in every aspect of treatment. Dental treatment not only includes the practice of medicine and surgery but also restoration of missing or lost structures. Besides restorations, appliances for various functions are also constructed for use in the mouth. The oral cavity is a challenging environment and materials placed in the mouth have to withstand high masticatory forces as well as corrosion. Besides direct use in the oral cavity, many materials are also used in the laboratory to aid in the fabrication of appliances or prostheses. Thus dentistry incorporates the knowledge of various materials as well as principles of engineering.

DENTAL TREATMENT

For convenience of description, dental care may be divided into various phases. These include preventive, disease control and elimination, restorative, rehabilitative and maintenance phases.

PREVENTIVE

The preventive phase is very important. It includes *educating* the patient on how to maintain his oral hygiene through regular *brushing*, *flossing* and *periodic checkup* at the dental office. Regular brushing with a suitable brush and paste has been shown to be very effective at controlling caries as well as gum (periodontal) problems. The role of *fluorides* and fluoride therapy in the control of dental caries has been known to us for a long time. Fluoridation of drinking water and fluoride therapy at the dental office has played a significant role in reducing dental caries especially in children. Caries often begins in deep fissures in teeth. Fissure sealants is another preventive measure especially in children to prevent caries.

DISEASE CONTROL AND ELIMINATION

The next stage in the progress of dental disease is the actual development of dental caries and periodontal disease. This phase of treatment focuses on eliminating or controlling diseases of the mouth to halt their destruction. Commonly, patients will come to a dental office because of pain caused by cavities or infection. This phase focuses on treating cavities (by placing fillings), eliminating infection (by root canal or tooth removal), and managing gum health (oral prophylaxis and other periodontal procedures).

Caries involves the demineralization and destruction of tooth structure. The focus is to arrest the caries process. This involves removing the carious tooth structure and restoring the cavity with a suitable temporary or permanent filling material. The famous *silver filling* has been in use for more than a century and is currently the most widely used filling material. The silver amalgam restoration would certainly look unpleasant if used for the front (anterior) teeth. Therefore anterior teeth are restored with an esthetic (tooth colored) material. Other ways to restore teeth involve the use of gold inlays and ceramic inlays.

As caries progresses, it gets closer to the pulp, which can lead to pain (pulpitis) and infection of the pulp. If the pulp is only mildly affected, pulp therapy is started using materials which have a therapeutic effect on the pulp. These materials can be soothing and promote healing by forming a new layer of dentin (secondary dentin).

If the pulp is infected, it is removed (pulpectomy) and *root canal treatment* popularly known as RCT is initiated. After removing the pulp, the canal is made sterile and sealed using root canal filling materials. The root canal treated tooth is weak and is prone to fracture if not protected with a crown or onlay.

RESTORATIVE

This phase of treatment focuses on restoring the function and/or form of the teeth and mouth following the destruction caused by the original disease process. Common treatments during this phase include prosthesis (implants, bridges, partials, and dentures) to replace missing teeth and crowns to protect teeth.

Before the discovery of tooth colored crown materials, metallic crowns were given (the famous gold tooth). Modern dentists are able to provide crowns that are *natural looking* and pleasing. Many of these structures are processed outside the mouth, in the laboratory. The dental technician uses an accurate *model* of the teeth to fabricate these restorations. Models are made from a *negative record* of the mouth called an *impression*. This is sent to the laboratory where the technician pours a mix of plaster or stone into the impression. When the mix hardens, we obtain a model.

If the coronal tooth structure is entirely gone or destructed, even a crown would not stay. In this case, the dentist has to place a *post and core*. The part placed into the root canal is known as post and the rest of it is known as the core. The crown is then constructed and cemented onto the core.

Following extraction of teeth, the patient often desires that it be replaced with an *artificial tooth*. There are many ways of replacing the tooth. Today implants have become very popular. A *titanium screw* can be implanted into the jaw surgically followed by an artificial crown.

Another next choice is the *fixed partial denture* (bridge). Usually the teeth by the side of the missing tooth is reduced in size (prepared) in order to receive the bridge. The bridge is then cemented onto these teeth.

If too many teeth are missing, we might have to consider the *removable partial denture* which replaces the missing teeth but is not fixed in the mouth. It can be removed by the patient for cleaning and hygiene. The ideal removable partial denture is usually made of a combination of metal and plastic (cast partial denture). Interim or temporary partial dentures are made entirely of plastic also and are often referred to as *treatment partial dentures.*

The final stage is when all the teeth have to be replaced. One is, of course, familiar with the *complete denture* which is often seen in elderly individuals. These artificial teeth replace the entire dentition and are usually of the removable type (*fixed complete dentures* are also available which are supported and retained by implants). The complete denture is usually made of a type of plastic called acrylic. The teeth used in the denture can be made of acrylic or porcelain.

Besides all the materials mentioned above, different specialties in dentistry have their special materials. Some of these are not covered in this book. For example, endodontists use root canal files along with various irrigants to clean and debride the root canal. A variety of root canal sealing pastes and medicaments are also available. The periodontists use different types of graft material to restore lost periodontal bone and tissue. Unfortunately, not all the materials used in dentistry are within the scope of this book.

MAINTENANCE PHASE

Once the treatment is completed, a maintenance phase focuses on keeping the dental work in functioning order through periodic recalls, maintaining health (oral prophylaxis), and screening for oral cancer at each six-month exam.

THE DENTAL SPECIALTIES

Currently nine specialties are recognized by the Dental Council of India.

1. Conservative Dentistry and Endodontics
2. Periodontics
3. Prosthodontics
4. Public Health Dentistry
5. Oral Medicine and Radiology
6. Oral and Maxillofacial Surgery
7. Orthodontics and Dentofacial Orthopedics
8. Oral and Maxillofacial Pathology
9. Pedodontics and Preventive Dentistry

Conservative dentistry   That phase of dentistry concerned with restoration of parts of the teeth that are defective through disease, trauma, or abnormal development to a state of normal function, health, and esthetics, including preventive, diagnostic, biologic, mechanical, and therapeutic techniques, as well as material and instrument science and application.[1]

Endodontics   Endodontics is the branch of dentistry which is concerned with the morphology, physiology and pathology of the human dental pulp and periradicular tissues. Its study and practice encompass the basic and clinical sciences including biology of the normal pulp, the etiology, diagnosis, prevention and treatment of diseases and injuries of the pulp and associated periradicular conditions.[1]

Periodontics   Periodontics is that specialty of dentistry which encompasses the prevention, diagnosis and treatment of diseases of the supporting and surrounding tissues of the teeth or their substitutes and the maintenance of the health, function and esthetics of these structures and tissues.

Prosthodontics   Prosthodontics is the dental specialty pertaining to the diagnosis, treatment planning, rehabilitation and maintenance of the oral function, comfort, appearance and health of patients with clinical conditions associated with missing or deficient teeth and/or oral and maxillofacial tissues using biocompatible substitutes.[2]

[1] Free Dictionary
[2] Adapted from the Council on Dental Education and Licensure, American Dental Association

Public health dentistry   Dental Public Health is the science and art of preventing and controlling dental diseases and promoting dental health through organized community efforts. It is that form of dental practice which serves the community as a patient rather than the individual. It is concerned with the dental health education of the public, with applied dental research, and with the administration of group dental care programs as well as the prevention and control of dental diseases on a community basis.[*2]

Oral medicine and radiology
- ***Oral medicine*** is concerned with clinical diagnosis and nonsurgical management of nondental pathologies affecting the orofacial region (the mouth and the lower face).
- ***Oral and maxillofacial radiology*** is the specialty of dentistry and discipline of radiology concerned with the production and interpretation of images and data produced by all modalities of radiant energy that are used for the diagnosis and management of diseases, disorders and conditions of the oral and maxillofacial region.[*2]

Oral and maxillofacial surgery   Oral and Maxillofacial Surgery is the specialty of dentistry which includes the diagnosis, surgical and adjunctive treatment of diseases, injuries and defects involving both the functional and esthetic aspects of the hard and soft tissues of the oral and maxillofacial region.[*2]

Orthodontics and dentofacial orthopedics   Orthodontics and dentofacial orthopedics is the dental specialty that includes the diagnosis, prevention, interception, and correction of malocclusion, as well as neuromuscular and skeletal abnormalities of the developing or mature orofacial structures.[*2]

Oral and maxillofacial pathology   Oral Pathology is the specialty of dentistry and discipline of pathology that deals with the nature, identification, and management of diseases affecting the oral and maxillofacial regions. It is a science that investigates the causes, processes, and effects of these diseases. The practice of oral pathology includes research and diagnosis of diseases using clinical, radiographic, microscopic, biochemical, or other examinations.[*2]

Pedodontics and preventive dentistry   Pediatric Dentistry is an age-defined specialty that provides both primary and comprehensive preventive and therapeutic oral health care for infants and children through adolescence, including those with special health care needs.[*2]

THE DENTAL LABORATORY

Many materials are used in the dental laboratory to aid in the fabrication of stents, prostheses, appliances and other structures used in and around the mouth. These include cutting, abrading and polishing materials. Investment materials are used in the creation of moulds in the casting of metal structures. Waxes are used in various stages of construction of different structures. Gypsum products are used to make casts, models, molds and to secure articulators.

CLASSIFICATION OF DENTAL MATERIALS

Traditionally the subject of dental materials primarily included materials used in Restorative Dentistry including related auxiliary material. Currently, there is a trend to be more inclusive and include materials from specialties, which have traditionally been excluded like the Endodontic and Surgical specialties.

There is no classification that satisfactorily categorizes all materials used in dentistry. This is because many of the materials have multiple utilities and overlapping functions.

[*1] Free Dictionary
[*2] Adapted from the Council on Dental Education and Licensure, American Dental Association

General classification of all materials

All materials can be classified into four classes

1. Metals
2. Ceramics
3. Polymers
4. Composites

Classification of dental materials

1. Preventive materials	5. Appliance materials
2. Restorative materials	6. Biomaterials
3. Auxiliary materials	7. Therapeutic agents
4. Prosthetic materials	

Preventive materials include pit and fissure sealants and other materials used to prevent the onset of dental diseases.

Restorative materials include materials used to repair or replace tooth structure. This includes materials like amalgam, composites, ceramics, cast metal structures and denture materials.

Auxiliary materials are substances that aid in the fabrication process but do not actually become part of the restoration, appliance or prosthesis. This includes materials like gypsum products, impression materials, casting investments, waxes, etching gels, custom tray materials, etc.

Prosthetic materials are materials used to replace missing teeth and oral and maxillofacial structures. These include the alloys, ceramics and polymers used in fixed and removable partial denture construction and maxillofacial prostheses.

A biomaterial is a biological or synthetic substance which can be introduced into body tissue as part of an implanted medical device or used to replace an organ, bodily function. Although many traditional materials qualify as biomaterials, this term has been introduced to include bone and tissue grafts.

Therapeutic agents include various chemicals, medicaments, antimicrobials and other locally applied agents that are capable of producing a specific effect in the area to which it is applied.

In reality, many materials have dual or multiple uses and so the above categorization is difficult to strictly apply.

INTERNATIONAL STANDARDS ORGANIZATION (ISO)

The Federation Dentaire Internationale (FDI) and the International Organizations for Standardization (ISO) are two organizations working for the development of specifications and terminology on an international level. The FDI is restricted to dental products whereas the ISO covers all products. The ISO is a nongovernmental body composed of the national organizations of more than 80 countries including India (Bureau of Indian Standards). The ISO standards **(Fig. 1.1A)** (see also appendix) are formulated by a 'technical committee' (TC). Dental products are covered by TC 106. Various subgroups known as 'subcommittees' (SC) cater to specific areas. The subcommittees are further divided into 'working groups' (WG) to cover individual products or items. For example, TC 106/SC 1: WG 7 covers dental amalgam and mercury.

Considering the worldwide supply and demand for dental products the benefits from the ISO are invaluable. Suppliers and consumers can be assured of impartial reliable data to assess the quality of products and equipment regardless of its country of origin and use. Standards are constantly revised; therefore, it is imperative for manufacturers and researchers alike to refer to the latest edition of the ISO specifications to stay abreast of changes in requirements and classifications.

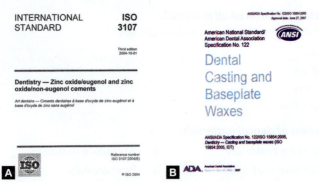

FIGURES 1.1A AND B Examples of standards: **(A)** International Standards Organization's specification for zinc oxide eugenol cement (ISO). **(B)** ANSI/ ADA specification No. 122 for dental waxes.

US STANDARDS FOR DENTAL MATERIALS

Standards are specifications by which the quality of a product can be gauged. Standards identify the requirements of physical and chemical properties of a material which ensures satisfactory performance for the function for which it is intended.

The earliest standards in the US were developed by the National Bureau of Standards in 1919 on the request of the US Army for the purchase and use of dental amalgam. The task was assigned to a team led by Wilmer Souder. Souder's report and testing methods were well received by the dental profession and test data were requested for other dental materials. By 1928, the responsibility for continued research into standards was assumed by the ADA.

ADA CERTIFICATION

Currently the ADA under direction of the ANSI (American National Standards Institute) sponsors two committees. The ADA Standards Committee for Dental Products develops specifications for all dental products, instruments and equipment (excluding drugs and X-ray films). The ADA's Council on Scientific Affairs is responsible for the evaluation of drugs, teeth cleaning agents, teeth whitening agents, therapeutic agents used in dentistry and dental X-ray films. After formulation of the specifications by the ADA, it is submitted to the ANSI. On approval, it becomes a national standard *(Fig. 1.1B)*.

Manufacturers can submit their product for the ADA seal of approval. This falls into three categories – Accepted, Provisionally Accepted, and Unaccepted. ADA certification is an important symbol of a dental product safety and effectiveness. ADA acceptance is effective for a period of 5 years.

Currently, the ADA have adopted the ISO specifications. The ADA specification for a particular product is *identical* to its ISO counterpart.

SUMMARY

Materials used for dentistry are highly specialized. Each one is designed with a specific set of properties depending on what it is intended for. For example, materials used as tooth restorations should be able to withstand occlusal forces as well as bond to tooth structure. Impression materials should be highly accurate and stable in order to duplicate the original structure. Modern science, research and technology has provided dentistry with an ever-expanding selection of unique combinations of materials and techniques to serve dental treatment needs.

Structure and Properties of Dental Materials

CHAPTER OUTLINE

- Structure of Matter
- Forms of Matter
- Change of State
- Interatomic Bonds
  - Primary Bonds
  - Secondary Bonds
- Thermal Expansion
- Crystal Structure
- Noncrystalline Structure
- Stress and Strain
- Diffusion
- Surface Tension
- Wetting
- Contact Angle
- Physical Properties of Dental Materials
- Stress
- Complex Stresses
- Poisson's Ratio
- Proportional Limit
- Elastic Limit
- Yield Strength
- Modulus of Elasticity
- Flexibility
- Resilience
- Impact
- Impact Strength
- Permanent Deformation

- Strength
  - Tensile Strength
  - Compressive Strength
  - Shear Strength
  - Transverse or Flexural Strength
- Fatigue
  - Static Fatigue
- Toughness
- Brittleness
- Ductility
- Malleability
- Hardness
  - Brinell
  - Rockwell Hardness Number (RHN)
  - Vickers Hardness Test (VHN)
  - Knoop Hardness Test (KHN)
  - The Shore and the Barcol
- Rheology
  - Viscosity
  - Creep
  - Flow
  - Thixotropic
  - Relaxation
  - Shear Stress and Shear Strain Rate

- Newtonian
- Pseudoplastic
- Dilatant
- Physical Properties
- Forms of Matter
- Melting Point
- Boiling Point
- Density
- Glass Transition Temperature (Tg)
- Solubility
- Thermal Properties
  - Thermal Conductivity
  - Thermal Diffusivity
  - Thermal Expansion
  - Coefficient of Thermal Expansion (CTE)
- Optical Properties and Color
- Dimensions of Color
- Measurement of Color
- Metamerism
- Translucence, Transparence and Opacity
- Fluorescence
- Radiopacity and Radiolucency
  - Measurement of Radiopacity
- Magnetic Properties

All materials are made up of atoms. If the reaction of a material and its properties are to be predicted, a basic knowledge of matter is essential. All dental restorations, whether they be ceramic, plastic or metal, are built from atoms.

STRUCTURE OF MATTER

Atom An atom is the smallest unit of matter that defines the chemical elements. Atoms are very small. The size of atoms is measured in picometers, which is trillionths (10^{-12}) of a meter. Every atom is composed of a nucleus and one or more electrons that orbit the nucleus (***Fig. 2.1***).

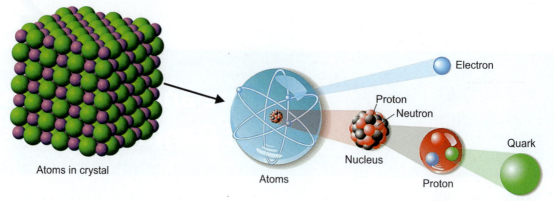

FIGURE 2.1 Building blocks of matter.

Protons, neutrons and electrons The nucleus is made of one or more protons and neutrons. Over 99.94% of the atom's mass is in the nucleus. The protons have a positive electric charge, the electrons have a negative electric charge, and the neutrons have no electric charge. If the number of protons and electrons are equal, that atom is electrically neutral. If an atom has in excess or lesser number of electrons relative to protons, then it has an overall positive or negative charge, and is called an ion.

Electrons of an atom are attracted to the protons in an atomic nucleus by the electromagnetic force. The protons and neutrons in the nucleus are attracted to each other by a different force, the nuclear force, which is usually stronger than the electromagnetic force repelling the positively-charged protons from one another. The number of protons in the nucleus defines to what chemical element the atom belongs, for example, all copper atoms contain 29 protons.

Quarks Protons and neutrons are made up of subatomic particles called quarks. Quarks are believed to be the basic building blocks of matter.

INTERATOMIC BONDS

Atoms are held together by some force. These interatomic bonding forces that hold atoms together are cohesive forces.

Interatomic bonds may be classified as

1. Primary bonds, or
2. Secondary bonds

PRIMARY BONDS

These are chemical in nature.

1. Ionic   2. Covalent   3. Metallic

Ionic Bonds These are simple chemical bonds, resulting from mutual attraction of positive and negative charges. The classic example is sodium chloride $Na^+ Cl^-$.

Covalent Bonds In many chemical compounds, two valence electrons are shared. The hydrogen molecule (H_2) is an example of covalent bonding. Another example is methane. The carbon atom has 4 valence electrons that can be stabilized by joining with hydrogen.

$$4H + \overset{..}{\underset{..}{C}} \longrightarrow H : \overset{\overset{H}{..}}{\underset{\underset{H}{..}}{C}} : H$$

Metallic Bonds   One of the chief characteristics of a metal is its ability to conduct heat and electricity. Such conduction is due to the mobility of the so-called free electrons present in the metals. The outer shield valence electrons can be removed easily from the metallic atom leaving the balance of the electrons tied to the nucleus, thus forming a positive ion.

The free valence electrons are able to move about in the metal space lattice to form what is, sometimes, described as an electron 'cloud' or 'gas'. The electrostatic attraction between this electron 'cloud' and the positive ions in the lattice bonds the metal atoms together as a solid.

SECONDARY BONDS (VAN DER WAALS FORCES)

A second type of bond between molecules may be seen. They are also known as van der Waals forces (named after Dutch scientist Johannes Diderik van der Waals. They differ from covalent and ionic bonding in that they are caused by correlations in the fluctuating polarizations (dipole) of nearby particles. They are defined as weak, short-range electrostatic attractive forces between uncharged molecules, arising from the interaction of permanent or transient electric dipole moments.

Dipole van der Waals Forces are due to the formation of dipole. A dipole is formed when electrons shift to one side of the atoms or molecules resulting in the formation of a negative polarity on the side and on the other half a positive polarity. This attracts other similar dipoles.

There are three kinds of van der Waals forces – 1. Keesom force (between two permanent dipoles), 2. Debye force (between a permanent dipole and an induced dipole) 3. London dispersion force (between two instantaneously induced dipoles).

Van der Waals forces are relatively weak compared to covalent bonds, but play a fundamental role in fields as diverse as supramolecular chemistry, structural biology, polymer science, nanotechnology, surface science, and condensed matter physics. Van der Waals forces define many properties of organic compounds. In nature geckos and spiders utilize van der Waals forces to climb and cling on to smooth surfaces *(Fig. 2.2)*.

CRYSTAL STRUCTURE

Space lattice or crystal can be defined as any arrangement of atoms in space such that every atom is situated similar to every atom. Space lattice may be the result of primary or secondary bonds.

There are 14 possible lattice type forms, but many of the metals used in dentistry belong to the cubic system. The simplest cubic space lattice is shown in *Figs. 2.3A to C.* The solid circles represent the position of the atoms. Their positions are located at the points of intersection of three sets of parallel planes, each set being perpendicular to other planes. These planes are often referred to as *crystal planes.*

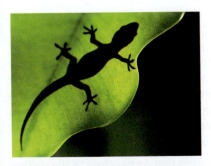

FIGURE 2.2 Geckos can stick to walls and ceilings because of van der Waals forces.

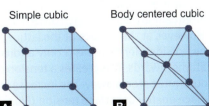

Simple cubic   Body centered cubic   Face centered cubic

A   B   C

FIGURES 2.3A TO C Crystal structure.

NONCRYSTALLINE STRUCTURE

In a crystalline structure, the arrangement of atoms in the lattice is orderly and follows a particular pattern. In noncrystalline structures or amorphous structures, e.g. waxes, the arrangement of atoms in the lattice is disorderly and distributed at random.

There is, however, a tendency for the arrangement of atoms or molecules to be regular, for example, glass is considered to be a noncrystalline solid, yet its atoms bind to form a short range order rather than long range order lattice. In other words, the ordered arrangement of glass is localized with large number of disordered units between the ordered units. Since such an arrangement is also typical of liquids, such solids are, sometimes, called *supercooled liquids*.

STRESS AND STRAIN

The distance between two atoms is known as interatomic distance. This interatomic distance depends upon the electrostatic fields of the electrons. If the atoms come too close to each other, they are repelled from each other by their electrons charges. On the other hand, forces of attraction keep them from separating. Thus the atoms are kept together at a position where these forces of repulsion and attraction become equal in magnitude (but opposite in direction). This is the normal equilibrium position of the atoms.

The normal position of the atoms can be changed by application of mechanical force. For example, the interatomic distance can be increased by a force pulling them apart. If the displacing force is measured across a given area it is known as a *stress* and the change in dimension is called a *strain*. In simple words, stress is the force applied and strain is the resulting change in shape.

Theoretically, a stress and a strain exist whenever the interatomic distance is changed from the equilibrium position. If the stress pulling the atoms apart exceeds the resultant force of attraction, the atoms may separate completely, and the bonds holding them together are broken.

Strain can also occur under compression. However, in this case, the strain produced is limited because when the atoms come closer than their normal interatomic distance, a sudden increase in energy is seen.

DIFFUSION

The diffusion of molecules in gases and liquids is well known. However, molecules or atoms diffuse in the solid state as well. Diffusion rates depend mainly on the temperature. The higher the temperature, the greater will be the rate of diffusion. The diffusion rate will, however, vary with the atom size, interatomic or intermolecular bonding lattice imperfections. Thus every material has its own diffusion rate. The diffusion rate in noncrystalline materials may occur at a rapid rate and often may be seen.

SURFACE TENSION

Energy at the surface of a solid is greater than in its interior. For example, inside a lattice, all the atoms are equally attracted to each other. The interatomic distances are equal, and energy is minimal. However, at the surface of the lattice, the energy is greater because there are no atoms on the outside. Hence there is only a force from the inside of the lattice pulling the outermost atoms inwards. This creates a tension on the outer surface and energy is needed to pull the outermost atoms away. The increase in energy per unit area of surface is referred to as the surface energy or surface tension *(Figs. 2.4A and B)*.

The surface atoms of a solid tend to form bonds to any atom that comes close to the surface in order to reduce the surface energy of the solid. This attraction across the interface for unlike

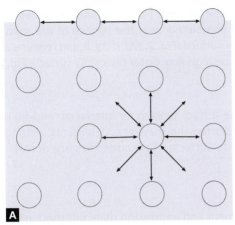

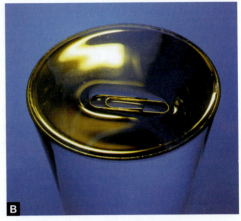

FIGURES 2.4A AND B **(A)** Schematic representation of molecular view of surface tension. **(B)** Surface tension causes a paper clip to float on water despite the fact that metal in the paper clip has a higher density than water.

molecules is called adhesion. In summary, the greater the surface energy, the greater will be the capacity for adhesion.

WETTING

It is very difficult to force two solid surfaces to adhere. However smooth their surfaces may appear, they are likely to be very rough at the atomic or molecular level. When they are placed together, only the 'hills' or high spots are in contact. Since these areas form only a small percentage of the total surface, no adhesion takes place. For proper adhesion, the distance between the surface molecules should not be greater than 0.0007 micrometer or micron (μm).

One method of overcoming this difficulty is to use a fluid that will flow into these irregularities and thus provide contact over a great part of the surface of the solid. For example, when two glass plates are placed one on top of the other, they do not usually adhere. However, if a film of water is placed in between them, it becomes difficult to separate the two plates.

To produce adhesion in this manner, the liquid must flow easily over the entire surface and adhere to the solid. This characteristic is referred to as *wetting*. The degree of wetting is indicated by the contact angle of the adhesive to the adherend.

Contact angle

The contact angle is the angle formed by the adhesive (e.g. water) and the adherend (e.g. glass) at their interface. The extent to which an adhesive will wet the surface of an adherend may be determined by measuring the *contact angle* between the adhesive and the adherend.

Based on the contact angle there are four classes of wetting *(Figs. 2.5A to D)*:

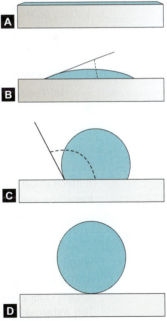

FIGURES 2.5A TO D Four classes of wetting based on the contact angles.

Contact Angle = 0	Perfect wetting
Contact Angle = 0 < <90°	High wettability
Contact Angle = 90° ≤< 180°	Low wettability
Contact Angle = 180°	Perfect non-wetting

If the forces of adhesion are stronger than the cohesive forces holding the molecules of the adhesive together, the liquid will spread completely over the surface of the solid and no angle will be formed (e.g. water on a soapy surface *(Fig. 2.5A)*. If the liquid remains as a drop without spreading, the contact angle will be high (e.g. water on an oily surface, *Fig. 2.5C*).

Surfactant

Surfactants are compounds that lower the surface tension (or interfacial tension) between two liquids or between a liquid and a solid. Surfactants may act as detergents, wetting agents, emulsifiers, foaming agents, and dispersants. Surfactants are added to some dental materials to improve wetting.

Significance

1. The mouth is a highly moist environment and impression materials used in the mouth should be hydrophilic in order to record details even under moist conditions.
2. Good wettability is again desired in the laboratory for products contacting gypsum products like dental stone and plaster which have a high moisture content. While pouring casts the stone should be able to wet the impression well in order to minimize voids.
3. Good wetting is important in soldering in order to produce a good strong joint.

PROPERTIES OF DENTAL MATERIALS

To select and use a dental material one must understand its properties. Knowledge of the properties of the material predicts its behavior, functioning in the mouth and longevity. Accordingly one can optimize design and techniques in order to get the best out of a particular material.

Various properties important to dental materials are

1. Physical properties
2. Mechanical properties
3. Chemical properties
4. Thermal properties
5. Optical properties

MECHANICAL PROPERTIES

A mechanical property is the behavior of the material when it's linked to the application of force. The mechanical properties of a material describe how it will react to physical forces.

STRESS

When a force acts on the body, tending to produce deformation, a resistance is developed within the body to this external force. The internal resistance of the body to the external force is called stress. Stress is equal and opposite in direction to the force (external) applied. This external force is also known as load. Since both applied force and internal resistance (stress) are distributed over a given area of the body, the stress in a structure is designated as a force per unit area.

$$\text{Stress} = \frac{\text{Force}}{\text{Area}} = \frac{F}{A}$$

The internal resistance to force (stress) is impractical to measure. The convenient way is to measure the external force applied to the cross-sectional area.

Area over which the force acts is an important factor especially in dental restorations in which areas over which the forces applied often are extremely small. Stress at a constant force is inversely proportional to the area—the smaller the area, the larger the stress and *vice versa*.

TYPES OF STRESSES

- Tensile stress
- Compressive stress
- Shear stress

Tensile stress

Results in a body when it is subjected to two sets of forces that are directed away from each other in the same straight line. The load tends to stretch or elongate a body.

Compressive stress

Results when the body is subjected to two sets of forces in the same straight line but directed towards each other. The load tends to or shortens a body.

Shear stress

Shear stress is a result of two forces directed parallel to each other. A stress that tends to resist a twisting motion, or a sliding of one portion of a body over another is a shear or shearing stress.

STRAIN

If the stress (internal resistance) produced is not sufficient to withstand the external force (load) the body undergoes a change in shape (deformation). Each type of stress is capable of producing a corresponding deformation in the body. The deformation resulting from a tension, or pulling force, produces an elongation of a body, whereas a compression, or pushing force, causes compression or shortening of the body.

$$\text{Strain} = \frac{\text{Deformation or change in length}}{\text{Original length}} = \frac{E}{L}$$

Strain is expressed as change in length per unit length of the body when a stress is applied. It is a dimensionless quantity and may be elastic or plastic or a combination of the two.

COMPLEX STRESSES

It is difficult to induce just a single type of stress in a body. Whenever force is applied over a body, complex or multiple stresses are produced. These may be a combination of tensile, shear or compressive stresses *(Fig. 2.6)*. These multiple stresses are called complex stresses. For example, when a wire is stretched, the predominant stress is tensile, but shearing and compressive stresses will also be present because the wire is getting thinner (compressed in cross-section) as it elongates.

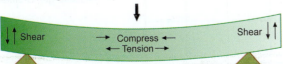

FIGURE 2.6 Complex stresses produced by a three-point loading of a beam.

POISSON'S RATIO

If we take a cylinder and subject it to a tensile stress or compressive stress, there is simultaneous axial and lateral strain. Within the *elastic range,* the ratio of the lateral to the axial strain is called Poisson's ratio.

PROPORTIONAL LIMIT

A tensile load is applied to a wire in small increments until it breaks. If each stress is plotted on a vertical coordinate and the corresponding strain (change in length) is plotted on the horizontal coordinate, a curve is obtained. This is known as *stress-strain curve* **(Fig. 2.7)**. It is useful to study some of the mechanical properties. The stress-strain curve is a straight line up to point 'P' after which it curves.

The point 'P' is the proportional limit, i.e., up to point 'P' the stress is proportional to strain (Hooke's Law). Beyond 'P' the strain is no longer elastic and so stress is no longer proportional to strain. Thus proportional stress can be defined as the greatest stress that may be produced in a material such that the stress is directly proportional to strain.

ELASTIC LIMIT

Below the proportional limit (point 'P'), a material is elastic in nature, that is, if the load is removed, the material will return to its original shape. Thus elastic limit may be defined as the maximum stress that a material will withstand without permanent deformation (change in shape). For all practical purposes, the elastic limit and the proportional limit represent the same stress. However the fundamental concept is different, one describes the elastic behavior of the material whereas the other deals with proportionality of strain to stress in the structure.

YIELD STRENGTH

Very few materials follow Hooke's law perfectly and some permanent change may be seen in the tested material. A small amount of permanent strain is tolerable. The limit of tolerable permanent strain is the yield strength. Thus yield strength is defined as the stress at which a material exhibits a specified limiting deviation from proportionality of stress to strain.

Determination of yield strength

How much of permanent deformation can be tolerated? This varies from material to material and is determined by selecting an offset. An *offset* is an arbitrary value put for a material. It represents the percent of total permanent deformation that is acceptable for the material. In

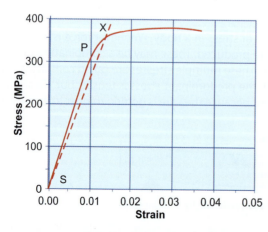

FIGURE 2.7 Stress-strain curve. P-proportional limit, X-yield strength, S-offset.

dentistry 0.1% (1% offset) and 0.2% (2% offset) are most commonly used. The yield strength is determined by selecting the desired offset and drawing a line parallel to the linear region of the stress-strain curve *(Fig. 2.7)*. The point on the stress-strain curve where the offset meets is the yield strength (point X).

MODULUS OF ELASTICITY

It is also referred to as 'elastic modulus' or 'Young's modulus'. It represents the relative stiffness or rigidity of the material within the elastic range.

Young's modulus is the ratio of stress to strain. Since stress is proportional to strain (up to the proportional limit), the stress to strain ratio would be constant.

$$\text{Modulus of elasticity} \atop \text{or} \atop \text{Young's modulus} \qquad E = \frac{\text{Stress}}{\text{Strain}} = \frac{F/A}{E/L} = \frac{FL}{EA}$$

It, therefore, follows that the less the strain for a given stress, the greater will be the stiffness, e.g. if a wire is difficult to bend, considerable stress must be placed before a notable strain or deformation results. Such a material would possess a comparatively high modulus of elasticity.

Application

The metal frame of a metal-ceramic bridge should have a high stiffness. If the metal flexes, the porcelain veneer on it might crack or separate.

FLEXIBILITY

Generally in dental practice, the material used as a restoration should withstand high stresses and show minimum deformation. However, there are instances where a large strain is needed with a moderate or slight stress. For example, in an orthodontic appliance, a spring is often bent at a large distance with a small stress. In such a case the material is said to be flexible. The 'maximal flexibility' is defined as the strain that occurs when the material is stressed to its proportional limit. The relation between the maximum flexibility, the proportional limit and the modulus of elasticity may be expressed as

$$\text{Maximum flexibility (EM)} = \frac{\text{Proportional limit (P)}}{\text{Modulus of elasticity (E)}}$$

Application

It is useful to know the flexibility of elastic impression materials to determine how easily they may be withdrawn over undercuts in the mouth.

RESILIENCE

Popularly, the term resilience is associated with 'springiness'. Resilience can be defined as the amount of energy absorbed by a structure when it is stressed not to exceed its proportional limit. For example, when an acrobat falls on a trapeze net the energy of his fall is absorbed by the resilience of the net, and when this energy is released, the acrobat is again thrown into the air.

The resilience of a material is measured in terms of its *modulus of resilience*, which is the amount of energy stored in a body, when a unit volume of a material is stressed to its proportional limit. It is expressed mathematically as

$$R \text{ (Modulus of Resilience)} = \frac{P^2 \text{ (Proportional limit)}}{2E \text{ (Modulus of elasticity)}}$$

Resilience is also measured by the area under the straight line portion of the stress-strain curve **(Fig. 2.8)**.

IMPACT

It is the reaction of a stationary object to a collision with a moving object. Depending upon the resilience of the object, energy is stored in the body without causing deformation or with deformation.

The ability of a body to resist impact without permanent deformation is represented by the formula—*KVR*

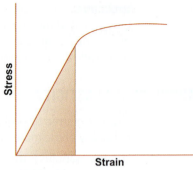

FIGURE 2.8 Area of resilience in a stress-strain curve.

where, K = Constant of proportionality

V = Volume

R = Modulus of resilience

But we know $R = P^2/2E$

Therefore, impact resistance $= \dfrac{KVP^2}{2E}$

From the above formula, we can conclude

Impact resistance will be *decreased* with an increase in the modulus of elasticity, which means that stiffer materials will have less impact resistance. Resilient materials will have better impact resistance (however, a high stiffness is also necessary to provide rigidity to a material under static loads, e.g. a cement base should be able to support an amalgam restoration). Increase in volume leads to an increase in impact resistance.

IMPACT STRENGTH

It is the energy required to fracture a material under an impact force. A *Charpy* type impact tester is used **(Figs. 2.9A and B)**. It has a heavy pendulum which swings down to fracture the specimen. Another instrument called Izod impact tester can also be used.

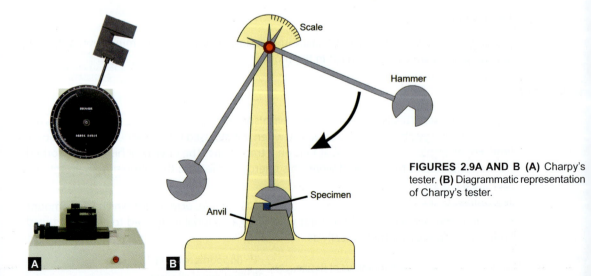

FIGURES 2.9A AND B (A) Charpy's tester. **(B)** Diagrammatic representation of Charpy's tester.

Application

Dentures should have a high impact strength to prevent it from breaking if accidentally dropped by the patient.

PERMANENT DEFORMATION

Once the elastic limit of a material is crossed by a specific amount of stress, the further increase in strain is called permanent deformation, i.e., the resulting change in dimension is permanent.

Application

An elastic impression material deforms as it is removed from the mouth. However due to its elastic nature, it recovers its shape and little permanent deformation occurs. Some materials are more elastic than others. Thus permanent deformation is higher in hydrocolloids than in elastomers.

STRENGTH

Strength of a material is its resistance to fracture. It is measured by measuring the maximal stress required to fracture a structure.

The three types of strength are

- Tensile strength
- Compressive strength
- Shear strength

TENSILE STRENGTH

Tensile strength is determined by subjecting a rod, wire or dumbbell shaped specimen to a tensile loading (a unilateral tension test). Tensile strength is defined as the maximal stress the structure will withstand before rupture.

Tensile strength of brittle materials

Brittle materials are difficult to test using the unilateral tension test. Instead, an indirect tensile test called 'diametral compression test' (or Brazilian test) is used **(Fig. 2.10)**. In this method, a compressive load is placed on the diameter of a short cylindrical specimen. The tensile stress is directly proportional to the load applied as shown in the formula.

$$\text{Tensile-stress} = \frac{2P}{\pi \times D \times T} = \frac{(\text{load})}{\pi(\text{diameter} \times \text{thickness})}$$

COMPRESSIVE STRENGTH

Compressive strength or 'crushing strength' is determined by subjecting a cylindrical specimen to a compressive load. The strength value is obtained from the cross-sectional area and force applied. Though the load is compressive in nature, the failure is due to complex stresses.

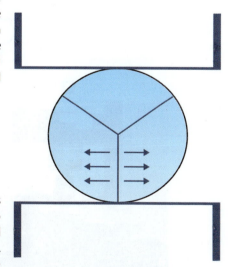

FIGURE 2.10 Diametral compression test.

SHEAR STRENGTH

Shear strength is the maximum stress that a material can withstand before failure in a shear mode of loading. It is tested using the punch or pushout method. The formula is as follows.

$$\text{Shear Strength} = \frac{F}{\pi DH}$$

Where, F is the force
D is punch diameter
H is the thickness of the specimen

Application

Used to study the interface between two materials, e.g. porcelain fused to metal.

TRANSVERSE OR FLEXURAL STRENGTH

Transverse strength or modulus of rupture, or bend strength, or fracture strength is obtained when a load is applied in the middle of a beam supported at each end.

Three types of flexural tests are used

1. Three-point flexural test
2. Four-point flexural test
3. Biaxial flexural test

Three-point flexural test

This test is also called a *three-point bending test* (3PB) **(Figs. 2.11A to C)**.

The flexure strength may be represented by the formula below.

$$\text{Flexural Strength } \alpha f = \frac{3PL}{2wt^2}$$

where, P = fracture load in Newtons
L = distance between supports
w = width of the speciment
t = thickness of the specimen

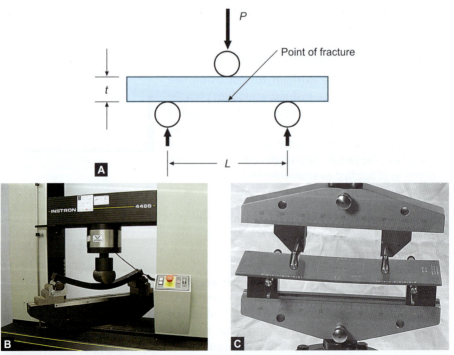

FIGURES 2.11A TO C Flexural testing. **(A)** Representation of 3-point flexure testing. **(B)** 3-point flexure tester. **(C)** 4-point flexure tester.

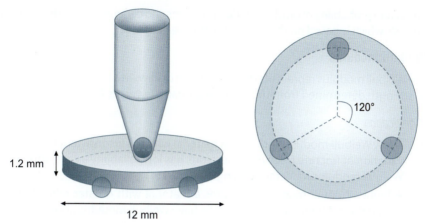

FIGURE 2.12 Biaxial flexural test.

Four-point flexural test

The addition of a 4th bearing brings a much larger portion of the beam to the maximum stress, as opposed to only the material right under the central bearing. This difference is of prime importance when studying brittle materials, where the number and severity of flaws exposed to the maximum stress is directly related to the flexural strength and crack initiation. Formula for the four-point flexural test is shown below.

$$\text{Flexural Strength } \alpha f = \frac{3PL}{4wt^2}$$

Biaxial flexural test

This test is used to avoid the problem of edge fractures which can occur with the other flexural tests. Disc-shaped specimens are used of 12 mm diameter and 1.2 mm thickness *(Fig. 2.12)*. The disc is supported by 3 balls (3.2 mm diameter). The load is applied by a round ended piston.

Application

Used to test materials like porcelain.

WEIBULL STATISTICS

Weibull analysis

Waloddi Weibull invented the Weibull distribution in 1937 and delivered his hallmark paper on this subject in 1951. It is also known as 'life data analysis'. The primary advantage of Weibull analysis is the ability to provide reasonably accurate failure analysis and failure forecasts. Thus it is used to estimate important life characteristics of a product such as reliability or probability of failure at a specific time, the mean life for the product and failure rate.

Although manufacturers provide data on strength values. This typically represents the mean value of a specific test. This may not correlate with its strength and survival probability under clinical situations because in the mouth the restorations experience cyclic loading conditions. It would be more useful to know the 95% stress level. This is the stress level below which 95% of the specimens would survive the stress test.

Dental application   Many restorative materials in dentistry are brittle materials like resins and ceramics. These materials do not exhibit a normal or symmetric distribution of strength values.

The failure probability of brittle materials like resins and ceramics is best described using Weibull analysis which is based on the concept of the weakest link.

Weibull modulus

The Weibull modulus represents the distribution of flaws in a brittle material or the distribution of strength determined from the fracture probability versus failure test.

Significance

1. A low Weibull modulus indicates a material which is inconsistent in strength, has a wide variation of fracture force and, therefore, has low reliability as a restorative material, e.g. Weibull modulus for ceramics range from 5-15.
2. A higher Weibull modulus indicates a material with greater reliability as a structural material, e.g. Metals which are ductile have Weibull modulus above 20.

STRESS CONCENTRATION

A stress concentration (often called stress raisers) is a location in an object where stress is concentrated.

Causes of stress concentration

Knowledge of the causes and effects of stress concentration is important in dental restorations to prevent early failure.

Stress concentrations occur due to

1. Structural defects
2. Improper design

Structural defects   An object is strongest when force is evenly distributed over its area, so a reduction in area, e.g. caused by a crack, results in a localized increase in stress. A material can fail, via a propagating crack, when a concentrated stress exceeds the material's theoretical cohesive strength. The real fracture strength of a material is always lower than the theoretical value because most materials contain small cracks or contaminants (especially foreign particles) that concentrate stress.

Design defects   A structure should be designed in such a way that stress is evenly distributed. An example of a stress concentration design is a narrow post with supporting a large core. The weakest point of this structure is at the junction of the post and core. When occlusal forces are applied stress concentration at this point can lead to a fracture. Slight alteration of design can reduce stress concentration. In this case increasing the diameter of the post and increasing the bulk of the metal at the junction of the post to the core so that the transition is gradual rather than abrupt.

FATIGUE

A structure subjected to repeated or cyclic stresses below its proportional limit can produce abrupt failure of the structure. This type of failure is called fatigue. Fatigue behavior is determined by subjecting a material to a *cyclic stress* of a known value and determining the number of cycles that are required to produce failure. The stresses used in fatigue testing are usually very low. However, the repeated application causes failure.

Application

Restorations in the mouth are often subjected to cyclic forces of mastication. In order to last, these restorations should be able to resist fatigue.

STATIC FATIGUE

It is a phenomenon exhibited by some ceramic materials. These materials support a high static load for a long period of time and then fail *abruptly*. This type of failure occurs only when the materials are stored in a wet environment and this property is related to the effect of water on the highly stressed surface of the material.

TOUGHNESS

It is defined as the energy required to fracture a material. It is a property of the material which describes how difficult the material would be to break. Toughness is also measured as the total area under the stress-strain curve *(Fig. 2.13)*.

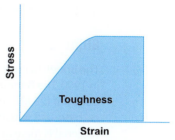

FIGURE 2.13 Area of toughness in the stress-strain curve.

BRITTLENESS

A brittle material *fractures at or near its proportional limit*. Brittleness is the opposite of toughness, e.g. glass is brittle at room temperature. It will not bend appreciably without breaking. It should not be wrongly understood that a brittle material lacks strength. From the above example of glass, we see that its shear strength is low, but its tensile strength is very high. If glass is drawn into a fiber, its tensile strength may be as high as 2800 MPa.

Application

Many dental materials are brittle, e.g. porcelain, cements, dental stone, etc.

DUCTILITY

It is the ability of a material to withstand permanent deformation under a tensile load without rupture. A metal that can be drawn readily into a wire is said to be ductile. Ductility is dependent on tensile strength. Ductility decreases as the temperature is raised.

Ductility may be measured by three methods

○ By measuring the percentage elongation after fracture.
○ By measuring reduction in cross-sectional area of fractured ends in comparison to the original area of the wire or rod and the method is called *reduction in area method*.
○ By using the cold bend test.

MALLEABILITY

It is the ability of the material to *withstand rupture under compression*, as in hammering or rolling into a sheet. It is *not* dependent on strength as is ductility. Malleability increases with rise in temperature.

Toughness of a material is dependent upon the ductility (or malleability) of the material than upon the flexibility or elastic modulus.

Application of malleability and ductility

Gold is the most ductile and malleable metal. This property enables manufacturers to beat it into thin foils. Silver is second. Among other metals, platinum ranks third in ductility and copper ranks third in malleability.

HARDNESS

Hardness is difficult to define specifically. There are numerous factors which influence the hardness of a material such as strength, proportional limit, ductility, malleability, etc. In mineralogy the hardness is described as the ability of a material to resist scratching. In metallurgy and in most other fields, the resistance to indentation is taken as the measure of hardness. There are many surface hardness tests **(Figs. 2.14A and B)**.

BRINELL

The Brinell hardness scale was developed by a Swedish engineer named Johan August Brinell in 1900. The Brinell test utilizes a 10 mm diameter steel ball as an indenter, applying a uniform 3000 kgf (29 kN) force. A smaller amount of force is used on softer materials and a tungsten carbide ball is used for harder materials. The diameter of the indentation left in the test material is measured with a low powered microscope. The load is divided by the area of the surface of the indentation and the quotient is referred to as Brinell Hardness Number (BHN).

Application

Used for measuring hardness of metals and metallic materials.

ROCKWELL HARDNESS NUMBER (RHN)

Like the BH test, a steel ball or a conical diamond point is used. However, instead of measuring the diameter of the impression, the *depth* is measured directly by a dial gauge on the instrument.

Application

The Rockwell test has a wider application for materials, since Brinell test is unsuitable for brittle materials as well as plastic materials.

VICKERS HARDNESS TEST (VHN)

This is also similar to the Brinell test, however, instead of a steel ball, a *diamond* in the shape of a square pyramid is used **(Fig. 2.14A)**. Although the impression is square instead of round. The load is divided by the area of indentation. The length of the diagonals of the indentation (sides of the diamond) are measured and averaged.

Application

Vickers test is used in the ADA for dental casting golds. This test is suitable for brittle materials and so is used for measuring hardness of tooth structure.

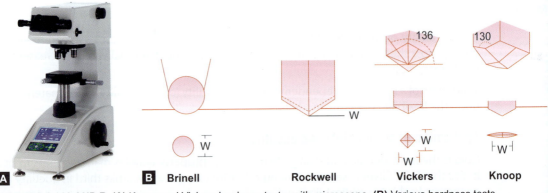

FIGRUES 2.14A AND B (A) Knoop and Vickers hardness tester with microscope. **(B)** Various hardness tests.

KNOOP HARDNESS TEST (KHN)

A diamond indenting tool *(Fig. 2.14B)* is used of a different shape from that of Vickers. The indentation is more narrower and elongated. Knoop hardness value is independent of the ductility of the material and values for both exceedingly hard and soft materials can be obtained from this test.

The Knoop and Vickers tests are classified as *microhardness tests*. The Brinell and Rockwell tests are classified as *macrohardness tests*.

THE SHORE AND THE BARCOL

These are less sophisticated tests. They are compact portable units *(Figs. 2.15A and B)*. A metal indenter that is spring loaded is used. The hardness number is based on depth of penetration and is read directly from a gauge.

Applications

Used for measuring the hardness of rubber and plastics.

ABRASION RESISTANCE

Like hardness, abrasion is influenced by a number of factors. Hardness has often been used to indicate the ability of a material to resist abrasion.

Applications

It is useful for comparing materials in the same class, e.g. one brand of cement is compared to another and their abrasion resistance is quoted in comparison to one another. However, it may not be useful for comparing materials of different classes like metals and plastics.

The only reliable test for abrasion is a test procedure which simulates the conditions which the material will eventually be subjected to, e.g. *toothbrush abrasion tests*.

RHEOLOGY

Rheology is the study of flow of matter. In dentistry, study of rheology is necessary because many dental materials are liquids at some stage of their use, e.g. molten alloy and freshly mixed impression materials and cements. Other materials appear to be solids but flow over a period of time.

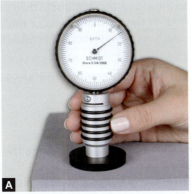 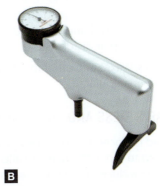

FIGURES 2.15A AND B (A) Shore tester. **(B)** Barcol tester.

TERMS AND PROPERTIES IN RHEOLOGY

VISCOSITY

Viscosity is the resistance offered by a liquid when placed in motion, e.g. honey is more viscous than water. It is measured in poise or centipoise (1 cp = 100 p).

CREEP

Time dependent plastic deformation or change of shape that occurs when a metal is subjected to a constant load near its melting point is known as creep. This may be static or dynamic in nature.

Static creep is a time dependent deformation produced in a completely set solid subjected to a constant stress.

Dynamic creep produced when the applied stress is fluctuating, such as in fatigue type test.

Importance

Dental amalgam has components with melting points that are slightly above room temperature and the creep produced can be very destructive to the restoration, e.g. glass tube fractures under a sudden blow but bends gradually if leaned against a wall.

FLOW

It is somewhat similar to creep. In dentistry, the term flow is used instead of creep to describe rheology of amorphous substances, e.g. waxes. Although creep or flow may be measured under any type of stress, compression is usually employed for testing of dental materials.

THIXOTROPIC

These materials exhibit a different viscosity after it is deformed, e.g. latex paints for ceilings show lower viscosity after it is stirred vigorously. Zinc oxide eugenol cements show reduced viscosity after vigorous mixing. Dental prophy paste is another example.

RELAXATION

Every element in nature makes an attempt to remain in a stable form. If an element is changed from its equilibrium or stable form by either physical or chemical means, it tries to come back to its original form.

When substances are deformed, internal stresses get trapped because of the displacement of the atoms. The condition is unstable and the atoms try to return to their original positions. This results in a change in shape or contour in the solid as atoms or molecules rearrange themselves. This change in shape due to release of stresses is known as *relaxation*. The material is said to warp or distort.

Examples, Waxes and other thermoplastic materials like compound undergo relaxation after they are manipulated.

SHEAR STRESS AND SHEAR STRAIN RATE

A liquid is placed between two plates and the upper plate is moved to the right. The stress required to move the plate is called shear stress (= F/A or force applied/ area of plate). The change produced is called shear strain rate (= V/d or velocity of plate/distance covered).

NEWTONIAN

Shear stress and shear strain rate can be plotted. An ideal fluid shows a shear strain rate that is proportional to shear stress. This behavior is called Newtonian *(Fig. 2.16)*.

PSEUDOPLASTIC

If a material viscosity decreases with increase in shear rate, it is said to exhibit pseudoplastic behavior, e.g. elastomeric impression materials when loaded into a tray shows a higher viscosity, whereas the same material when extruded under pressure through a syringe tip shows more fluidity *(Fig. 2.16)*.

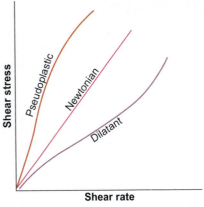

FIGURE 2.16 Shear diagrams of pseudo-plastic, Newtonian and dilatant liquids.

DILATANT

These are liquids that show higher viscosity as shear rate increases, e.g. fluid denture base resins *(Fig. 2.16)*.

PHYSICAL PROPERTIES

Physical properties can be observed or measured without changing the composition of matter. Physical properties are used to observe and describe matter. Physical properties of importance in dentistry include appearance, texture, color, optical properties, odor, glass transition, temperature, melting point, boiling point, density, solubility, polarity, etc.

FORMS OF MATTER

CHANGE OF STATE

Matter exists in the forms—solid, liquid and gas *(Fig. 2.17)*. The difference in form is mainly due to difference in energy. Matter is made up of atoms and for these atoms to be held together there must be a force, e.g. when 1 gram of water is to be changed into gaseous state at 100° C, 540 calories of heat are needed (known as heat of vaporization). Thus the gaseous state has more energy than the liquid state. Although the molecules in a gas have a certain amount of mutual attraction, they can diffuse readily and need to be confined in order to keep the gas intact. Energy of the liquid is decreased by reducing the temperature sufficiently, a second transformation in state occurs and energy is released in the form of heat (latent heat of fusion). This decrease in energy state changes the liquid to a solid or *freezes* it.

The reverse is true when solid is changed to liquid, i.e., heat is required. The temperature at which it occurs is called *fusion temperature.*

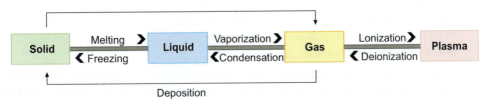

FIGURE 2.17 The 4 states of matter.

MELTING POINT

The melting point (or liquefaction point) of a solid is the temperature at which it changes state from solid to liquid at atmospheric pressure. At the melting point the solid and liquid phase exist in equilibrium.

BOILING POINT

The boiling point of a substance is the temperature at which the vapor pressure of the liquid equals the pressure surrounding the liquid and the liquid changes into a vapor. The boiling point of a liquid varies depending upon the surrounding environmental pressure.

DENSITY

The density, or more precisely, the volumetric mass density, of a substance is its mass per unit volume. The symbol most often used for density is ρ (the lower case Greek letter rho). Mathematically, density is defined as mass divided by volume–

$$\rho = \frac{m}{V}$$

where ρ is the density, m is the mass, and V is the volume.

In some cases (for instance, in the United States oil and gas industry), density is loosely defined as its weight per unit volume, although this is scientifically inaccurate—this quantity is more specifically called specific weight.

For a pure substance, the density has the same numerical value as its mass concentration. Different materials usually have different densities. Osmium and iridium are the densest known elements at standard conditions for temperature and pressure.

To simplify comparisons of density across different systems of units, it is sometimes replaced by the dimensionless quantity "relative density" or "specific gravity", i.e. the ratio of the density of the material to that of a standard material, usually water. Thus a relative density less than one means that the substance floats in water.

The density of a material varies with temperature and pressure. This variation is typically small for solids and liquids but much greater for gases. Increasing the pressure on an object decreases the volume of the object and thus increases its density. Increasing the temperature of a substance (with a few exceptions) decreases its density by increasing its volume.

GLASS TRANSITION TEMPERATURE (TG)

The glass transition temperature (Tg) is the temperature at which an amorphous solid becomes soft upon heating or brittle upon cooling. The Tg is one of the most important properties of any epoxy and is the temperature region where the polymer transitions from a hard, glassy material to a soft, rubbery material. The glass transition temperature is always lower than the melting temperature (Tm) of the crystalline state of the material, if one exists.

Glass transition temperature is the most important property of a polymer. The value of the glass transition temperature is directly related to the mechanical properties (strength, hardness, brittleness, elongation, etc.).

The glass transition temperature is more important in plastics applications than is the melting point, because it tells a lot about how the polymer behaves under ambient conditions. If a polymer's glass transition temperature is well above ambient room temperature, the material behaves like a brittle glassy polymer (it is stiff with low impact resistance). Conversely, if the

Tg is well below room temperature, the material is what is commonly termed a rubber or elastomer (soft and easily stretched). Those materials whose Tg is reasonably close to the ambient temperature exhibit plastic material behavior (strong and tough with good impact resistance). There are chemical compounds known as plasticizers that are used to decrease the glass transition temperature.

SOLUBILITY

Solubility is the property of a solid, liquid, or gaseous chemical substance called solute to dissolve in a solid, liquid, or gaseous solvent to form a homogeneous solution of the solute in the solvent.

Restorations placed in the oral cavity require to be insoluble in oral fluids. The tendency of cements to dissolve in the oral fluids can lead to marginal ditching, microleakage, recurrent caries, and ultimately failure of the restoration.

THERMAL PROPERTIES

Thermal properties are the response of a material to the application of heat.

THERMAL CONDUCTIVITY

Thermal conductivity is defined as the property of a material that indicates its ability to conduct heat through its body under a steady state condition. It is measured in watts per meter per degree Kelvin (W/(mK)). In Imperial units, thermal conductivity is measured in BTU/(hr.ft.°F)

It is defined as the quantity of heat in calories per second passing through a material 1 cm thick with a cross-section of 1 cm² having a temperature difference of 1 K (1°C) and is measured under a steady-state condition in which the temperature gradient does not change.

Thermal conductivity depends on many properties of a material, its structure and temperature. The transfer of heat within a material takes place by conduction; in this process the materials do not move as a whole but the energy flows through the body of the material by the transfer of the molecular kinetic energy. Various materials exhibit varying degrees of thermal conductivity (*Fig. 2.18*).

The divided bar method (steady-state method) is the most common way of measuring thermal conductivity. The sample to be measured is placed between two samples of known conductivity (usually brass plates). The sample

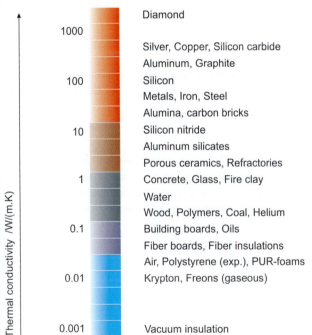

(Thermal conductivity at RT)

FIGURE 2.18 Thermal conductivity of various materials.

is placed at the top of the vertical setup and the known conductivity brass bars are kept at the bottom. To stop any convection within the sample, heat is supplied at the top and moved downwards. After approximately 10 minutes, the measurements are taken after the whole sample becomes equally hot.

THERMAL DIFFUSIVITY

Thermal diffusivity measures the ability of a material to conduct thermal energy relative to its ability to store thermal energy. Thermal diffusivity is the thermal conductivity divided by density and specific heat capacity at constant pressure. It has the SI unit of m^2/s. Thermal diffusivity is usually denoted by α but a, κ, K, and D are also used. The formula is

$$\alpha = \frac{\kappa}{\rho \times C_p}$$

κ is thermal conductivity (W/(mK))

ρ is density (kg/m^3)

C_p is specific heat capacity (J/(kgK))

THERMAL EXPANSION

Thermal energy is due to the kinetic energy (internal energy) of the atoms or molecules at a given temperature. At temperatures above absolute zero, atoms are in a constant state of vibration. The average amplitude of vibration depends upon the temperature; the higher the temperature, the greater will be the kinetic energy and amplitude of the atomic (or molecular) vibration increases. As the amplitude and internal energy of the atoms increase, the interatomic spacing increases as well. The gross effect is an expansion known as thermal expansion. If the temperature continues to increase, the interatomic spacing will increase and eventually a change of state will occur (e.g. solid to liquid).

COEFFICIENT OF THERMAL EXPANSION (CTE)

When a substance is heated, the kinetic energy of its molecules increases. This usually results in an expansion called thermal expansion.

The coefficient of thermal expansion describes how the size of an object changes with a change in temperature. Specifically, it measures the fractional change in size per degree change in temperature at a constant pressure.

Measurement of CTE

Several types of coefficients have been developed—volumetric, area, and linear. Which is used depends on the particular application. For solids, one might only be concerned with the change along a length, or area. The volumetric thermal expansion coefficient is commonly used for fluids and gases. It is normally quoted in parts per million per degree Celsius rise in temperature (ppm/K).

$$\alpha = \frac{\Delta L}{L \times \Delta T}$$

α (alpha) is CTE

L is original length of material

ΔL (delta L) is change in length

ΔT (delta T) is change in temperature

Negative thermal expansion

A number of materials contract on heating within certain temperature ranges; this is usually called negative thermal expansion. For example, the coefficient of thermal expansion of water drops to zero as it is cooled to 3.983°C and then becomes negative below this temperature;

this means that water has a maximum density at this temperature, and this leads to bodies of water maintaining this temperature at their lower depths during extended periods of sub-zero weather. Another example is pure silicon. It has a negative coefficient of thermal expansion for temperatures between about 18 and 120 Kelvin.

Significance of CTE

1. The mismatch of thermal expansion and contraction between restorative materials and tooth may cause stresses at their interface, which may lead to microleakage.
2. Metal ceramics restorations require a close match between the CTE of the alloy and porcelain in order to reduce stresses in the porcelain. These stresses can cause immediate or delayed cracking in the ceramic.
3. An inlay wax pattern created in the mouth may contract when transferred to the colder room.
4. Denture teeth set in wax may shift slightly when room temperature changes.

OPTICAL PROPERTIES AND COLOR

Light is a form of electromagnetic radiant energy within a certain portion of the electromagnetic spectrum that can be detected by the human eye. The eye is sensitive to wavelengths from approximately 400 nm (violet) to 700 nm (dark red). The combined intensities of the wavelengths present in a beam of light determine the property called *color.*

In order for an object to be visible, either it must emit light or it must reflect or transmit light falling upon it from an external source. Objects of dental interest generally transmit light. The incident light is usually polychromatic (mixed light of various wavelengths). The reaction of an object to the incident light is to selectively absorb and/or scatter certain wavelengths. The spectral distribution of the transmitted or reflected light will resemble that of the incident light although certain wavelengths will be reduced in magnitude.

Cone-shaped cells in the retina are responsible for color vision in humans. The eye is most sensitive to light in the green-yellow region and least sensitive at either extremes (i.e., red or blue).

DIMENSIONS OF COLOR

The three dimensions of color are — hue, value and chroma.

HUE

Refers to the basic color of an object, e.g. whether it is red, green or blue.

VALUE

Colors can be separated into 'light' and 'dark' shades. Value represents the amount of lightness or darkness in the color. This lightness which can be measured independently of the hue is called value.

CHROMA

A particular color may be dull or more 'vivid', this difference in color intensity or strength is called chroma. Chroma represents the degree of saturation of a particular hue (color). In other words, the higher the chroma, the more intense is the color. Chroma cannot exist by itself and is always associated with hue and value. The three dimensions of color is represented in *Figs. 2.19 and 2.20.*

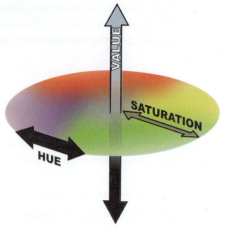

FIGURE 2.19 Illustration representing the three dimensions of color.

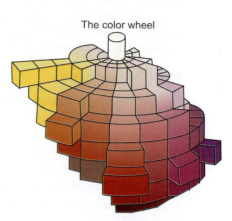

FIGURE 2.20 Munsell color solid is also used to demonstrate the three dimensions of color.

MEASUREMENT OF COLOR

One of the most commonly used method to define and measure color quantitatively is the *Munsell System*. It is a coordinate system which can be viewed as a cylinder. The lines are arranged sequentially around the perimeter of the cylinder, while the *chroma increases along a radius* from the axis. The *value coordinate varies along the length* of the cylinder from black at the bottom to *neutral* grey at the center to white at the top.

METAMERISM

The appearance of an object depends on the type of the light by which the object is viewed. Daylight, incandescent lamps and fluorescent lamps are all common sources of light in the dental operatory. Objects that appear to be color matched under one type of light may appear very different under another light source. This phenomenon is called *metamerism*.

TOOTH ESTHETICS

Reproducing a tooth—both art and science. The esthetics of a dental restoration is determined by

1. Shape
2. Color
3. Texture

The shade and color of a tooth is a complex interplay of many factors. The color of the tooth is determined by the shade, thickness and composition of the enamel and dentin, the pulp chamber, extrinsic stains, color reflections from the gum and adjacent teeth and the incident light itself. Light is a form of energy and must obey the basic law of conservation of energy which states that energy cannot be created or destroyed but only changed from one form into another or transferred from one object to another.

Light Incident	=	Light Reflected	+	Light Scattered	+	Light Transmitted	+	Light Absorbed	+	Light Fluoresced	+	Light changed to heat

TRANSPARENCE, TRANSLUCENCE, AND OPACITY

A transparent object allows all the light to pass through an object, whereas a translucent object allows only partial passage of light. For example, plain glass is transparent, whereas frosted glass is translucent. An object which does not allow any passage of light is said to be opaque.

Relevance

Teeth and oral tissue are translucent and allow passage of some of the incident light. In some individuals, the enamel may be translucent or in rare circumstances transparent. This may be particularly evident in the incisal edges of upper or lower incisors. Metal-ceramic restorations are opaque unlike natural teeth which are translucent *(Fig. 2.21)*. One of the reasons for improved esthetics with all-ceramic restorations is the improved translucency.

FLUORESCENCE

Natural tooth structure also absorbs light of wavelengths which are too short to be visible to the human eye. These wavelengths between 300 to 400 nm are referred as *near ultraviolet*. Natural sunlight, photoflash lamps, certain types of vapor lamps and the ultraviolet lights used in decorative lighting are all sources containing substantial amounts of near U-V radiation and invisible U-V light (also called black light).

This energy that the tooth absorbs is converted into light with larger wavelengths, in which case the tooth actually becomes a light source. The phenomenon is called fluorescence *(Fig. 2.22)*. The emitted light is primarily in 400-450 nm range, having blue white color. Improved fluorescence adds esthetic value to artificial restorations.

Relevance

In UV light a natural tooth emits a weak whitish-blue fluorescence. This should be taken into account when selecting restoratives. If restorative materials do not offer this property of fluorescence, they will look dark in UV light *(Fig. 2.23)*, and the restored tooth will stand out against the other teeth in the mouth. Some patients want their restorations to match natural tooth under fluorescent light conditions, e.g. in stage shows and discotheques. Some porcelain restorations are able to match the natural teeth under fluorescent lighting.

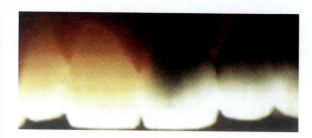

FIGURE 2.21 Poor translucency exhibited by the metal-ceramic restoration on the right when compared to the natural teeth (left).

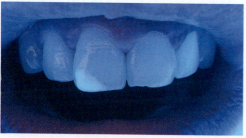

FIGURE 2.22 Composite restoration (on right central incisor) showing greater fluorescence.

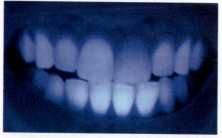

FIGURE 2.23 Artificial crown on left central appears dark under UV light because of insufficient fluorescence.

CLINICAL CONSIDERATIONS

Esthetics play a very important role in modern dental treatment. The ideal restorative material should match the color of the tooth it restores. In maxillofacial prosthetics the color of the gums, external skin and the eyes have to be duplicated.

Clinically in the operatory or dental lab, color selection is usually done by the use of *shade guides (Fig. 2.24)*. These are used in much the same way as paint chips are used to select the color for house paint. The process of selection is described in *(Figs. 2.25A to C)*.

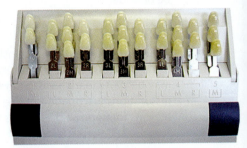

FIGURE 2.24 The Vitapan 3D Master is used as a guide for selecting tooth color.

Digital shade guides are also available *(Figs. 2.26A to C)*. The probe is simply placed against the tooth and on the press of a button the reading is displayed on the screen. The device is also useful to measure the progress of bleaching.

RADIOLOGICAL PROPERTIES

RADIOPACITY AND RADIOLUCENCY

Radiopacity may be defined as the quality or property of a material to obstruct the passage of radiant energy, such as X-rays. Thus materials that inhibit the passage of electromagnetic

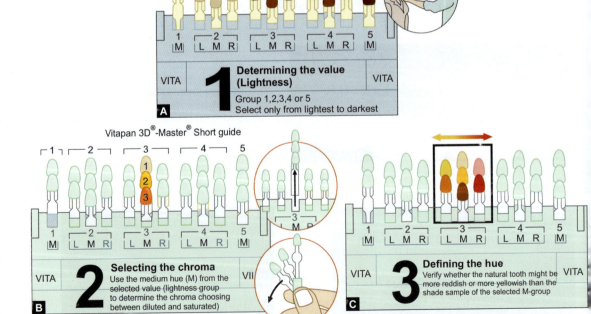

FIGURES 2.25A TO C Selecting the color using the Vitapan system. The color is determined in 3 steps. Step 1 determines the value. Step 2 determines the chroma (basic saturation). Step 3 determines the hue (basic color). The figure shows step 1. The guide is held along the patient's face at arm's length.

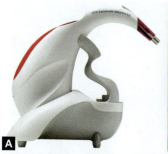
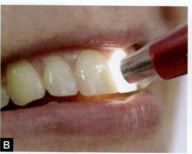
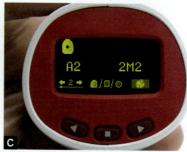

FIGURES 2.26A TO C (A) Digital shade guide - VITA Easyshade Advance 4. **(B)** The shade is selected by placing the probe against the tooth. **(C)** The reading is displayed on the screen.

radiation are called *radiopaque*. On the other hand those that allow radiation to pass more freely are referred to as *radiolucent*.

Significance in dentistry

Radiography plays a significant role in dentistry. It is very useful as a diagnostic tool. Radiographs help to detect problems within the restorations, teeth, bone, etc. Manufacturers add certain elements in many dental materials in order to make them radiopaque. Commonly used elements are heavy metal glasses (strontium or barium glasses) and compounds (barium sulphate) and metal oxides (zirconium dioxide and ytterbium oxide. Pure polymers like acrylic resins and bis-GMA are radiolucent. Composites, ceramics and metals are radiopaque, with metals showing the highest radiopacity.

Measurement of radiopacity

Human tissues like teeth, bone and soft tissue have varying levels of radiopacity. Within the tooth, the enamel is more radiopaque that dentin. Radiopacity similar to hard tissues of the body provide an optimal contrast for diagnosis. If the radiopacity of material is too low, it will not be visible. Generally, a restorative material should have radiopacity slightly greater than that of enamel in order to present a contrast. The thickness of the material also affects its radiographic properties. Radiopacity increases with increase in thickness.

Aluminum is used as a standard to measure radiopacity. The radiopacity of a material is expressed as equivalent thickness of aluminum (millimetres of aluminum). Typically an aluminum step wedge *(Fig. 2.27A)* is used for comparative studies. Specimens of specified thickness are radiographed together with the step wedge for comparison *(Fig. 2.27B)*.

Ingredient	Al equivalent (mm) approx.
Enamel	4–4.3
Dentin	2.2–2.5
Composites	1.5–6.2
ZOE endodontic sealer (Kerr)	8.9
Pro-Root MTA	2.5
Compoglass	4
Zinc phosphate cement (Hoffman)	6.5
Zinc polycarboxylate cement (Hoffman)	3.6
Cercon (core ceramic)	8.73
Cercon ceram S (veneering ceramic)	1.71

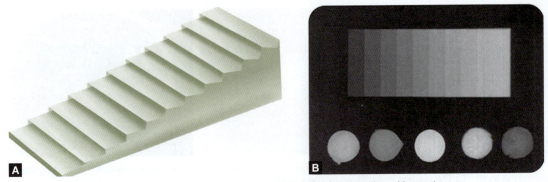

FIGURES 2.27A AND B **(A)** Aluminum step wedge. **(B)** Radiograph of step wedge with specimens.

MAGNETIC PROPERTIES OF MATTER

Magnetism is a class of physical phenomena that are mediated by magnetic fields. Electric currents and the fundamental magnetic moments of elementary particles give rise to a magnetic field. All matter exhibits magnetic properties when placed in an external magnetic field.

Aristotle attributed the first of what could be called a scientific discussion on magnetism to Thales of Miletus, who lived from about 625 BCE to about 545 BCE. Around the same time, in ancient India, the Indian surgeon, Sushruta, was the first to make use of the magnet for surgical purposes. The Chinese were believed to be using the compass for navigation prior to the Europeans. Alexander Neckam, by 1187, was the first in Europe to describe the compass and its use for navigation.

CLASSIFICATION

Depending on whether there is an attraction or repulsion by the pole of a magnet, matter is classified as being either

1. Paramagnetic—attracted to a magnetic field
2. Diamagnetic—repulsed by a magnetic field

TERMS

Magnetic field A magnetic field is the magnetic effect of electric currents and magnetic materials ***(Fig. 2.28)***. The magnetic field at any given point is specified by both a direction and a magnitude (or strength).

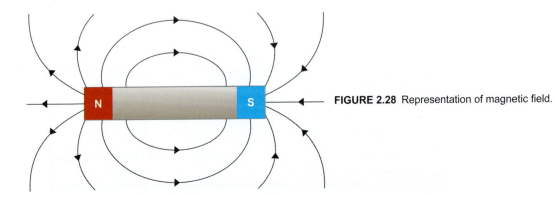

FIGURE 2.28 Representation of magnetic field.

Magnetic moment The magnetic moment (or magnetic dipole moment) of an object is a measure of the object's tendency to align with a magnetic field. It is a vector quantity. The object will tend to align itself so that its magnetic moment vector is parallel to the magnetic field lines. Some materials like iron (ferromagnets) have permanent magnetic moments. Most materials do not have permanent moments.

Ferromagnetism It is the basic mechanism by which certain materials can retain their magnetization when the external field is removed. Examples of ferromagnetic substances include iron, nickel, cobalt and some of the rare earth elements, such as gadolinium and dysprosium.

Nonmagnetic substances Substances that are negligibly affected by magnetic fields are known as nonmagnetic substances. They include copper, aluminium, gases, and plastic. Pure oxygen exhibits magnetic properties when cooled to a liquid state.

Magnetocrystalline anisotropy Magnets are capable of producing high forces relative to their size due to the property of magnetocrystalline anisotropy. Samarium-cobalt ($SmCo_5$) and neodymium-iron-boron magnets ($Nd_2Fe_{14}B$) magnets not only have the property of magnetocrystalline anisotropy, but they also have high coercivity.

Coercivity It is the ability of the magnet to resist demagnetization. Materials with high magnetic anisotropy usually have high coercivity.

TYPES

1. *Ceramic magnets* are used in refrigerators and elementary-school science experiments, contain iron oxide in a ceramic composite. Most ceramic magnets, sometimes known as ferric magnets, aren't particularly strong.
2. *Alnico magnets* are made from aluminium, nickel and cobalt. They're stronger than ceramic magnets, but not as strong as the ones that incorporate a class of elements known as rare-earth metals.
3. *Neodymium magnets* contain iron, boron and the rare-earth element neodymium. Compared to other available magnets, neodymium magnets are the strongest permanent magnets available. Today they are used in computer hard drives, speakers, electric motors, wind turbines, etc.
4. *Samarium cobalt* magnets combine cobalt with the rare-earth element samarium.
5. *Others* In the past few years, scientists have also discovered magnetic polymers, or plastic magnets. Some of these are flexible and mouldable. However, some work only at extremely low temperatures, and others pick up only very lightweight materials, like iron filings.

USES

Magnetic resonance imaging

Magnetic resonance imaging (MRI), nuclear magnetic resonance imaging (NMRI), or magnetic resonance tomography (MRT) is a medical imaging technique used in radiology to investigate the anatomy and physiology of the body in both health and disease. MRI scanners use strong magnetic fields and radiowaves to form images of the body. The technique is widely used in hospitals for medical diagnosis.

In dentistry

Magnets have generated great interest within dentistry. They have been used for various applications in orthodontics and prosthodontics. Earlier use of magnets was limited due to the unavailability of small size magnets, but after the introduction of rare earth magnets and

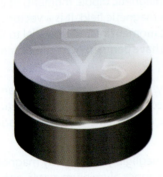

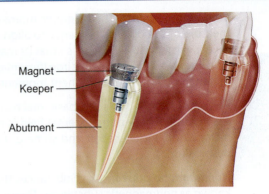

Magnet —

Keeper —

Abutment —

FIGURE 2.29 Dental magnet.　　　　　　**FIGURE 2.30** Dental magnet.

their availability in smaller sizes, their use has increased considerably. They can be placed within prostheses without being obtrusive.

In orthodontics Their main use in orthodontics has been for tooth movement

In prosthodontics They are primarily used as retentive aids in maxillofacial prosthesis and in tooth and implant supported ***(Figs. 2.29 and 2.30).***

Structure and Properties of Metals and Alloys

CHAPTER OUTLINE

All matter can be classified as either *metals, nonmetals or metalloids.*

A metal can be defined as a substance with high thermal and electrical conductivity, lustre, and malleability, which readily loses electrons to form positive ions (cations). They yield basic oxides and hydroxides. Roughly 80 percent of the periodic table are metals (*Fig. 3.1*).

Metalloids are borderline elements showing both metallic and nonmetallic properties. Examples are carbon and silica.

USES IN DENTISTRY

Metals and their alloys are used extensively in dentistry. They are used in restorations, prostheses, etc. They are used in orthodontics in the form of wires and various appliances for the movement of teeth. Various instruments and appliances used in clinics and laboratory dentistry are fabricated from metals.

In dentistry, metals or their alloys are used in three capacities

1. Dental restorations
   a. Direct intracoronal restorations, e.g. direct filling gold (DFG)
   b. Indirect (cast) coronal and extracoronal restorations like inlays and crowns, e.g. alloys of gold, platinum, chrome, cobalt, etc.
2. Prosthetic uses, e.g. implants, intra and extraoral prostheses like dentures and maxillofacial prostheses using cast alloy frames.

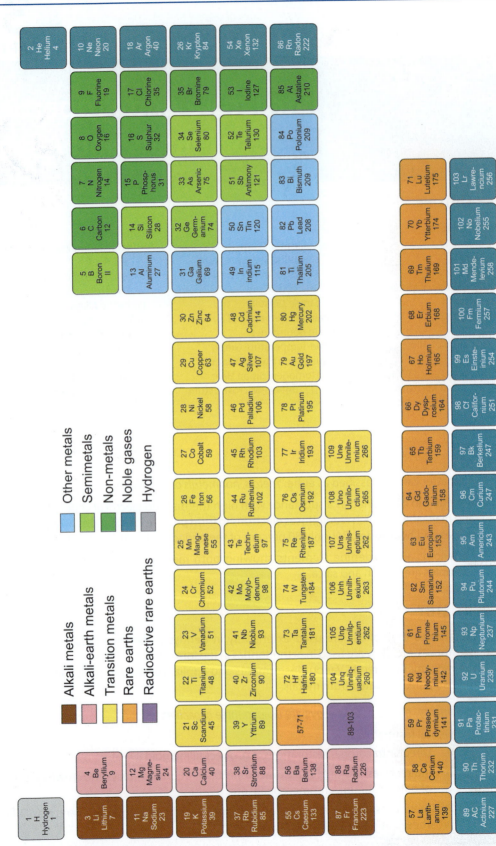

FIGURE 3.1 Periodic table of elements.

BOX 3.1 | History of metals

Metallurgy is one of the oldest applied sciences. Its history can be traced back to 6000 BCE. The earliest metals known to man were Gold (6000 BCE), Copper (4200 BC), Silver (4000 BCE), Lead 3500 BCE, Tin (1750 BCE), Iron 1500 (BCE) and mercury 750 BCE. Collectively these were called the *seven metals of antiquity*. Over time more and more metals were discovered, it greatly revolutionized human evolution and culture. Zinc was known to the Chinese in 1400s. Platinum was discovered in Mexico by the Spaniards. Aluminium was first produced by Christian Oersted in 1825.

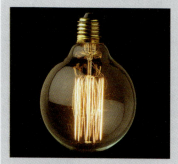

Tungsten Pure tungsten has some unique properties including the highest melting point (3695 K), lowest vapor pressure, and greatest tensile strength out of all the metals. For this reason it is commonly used for light bulb filaments. Tungsten carbide burs are used in dentistry.

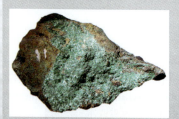

Copper Natural Copper ore has a blue-green hue.

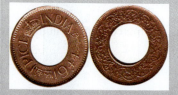

Copper coins from India - 1944

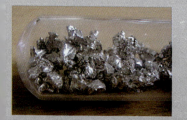

Calcium metal

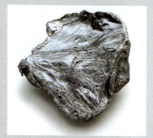

Molybdenum Molybdenum is used in base metal casting alloys.

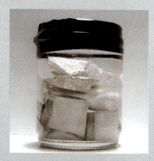

Sodium metal

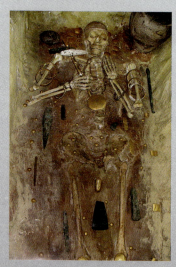

Burial site at Varna, Bulgaria, circa 4600 BCE, containing some of the oldest sophisticated examples of ancient copper and gold metallurgy. (*Courtesy:* I, Yelkrokoyade.)

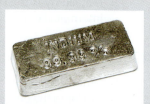

Indium

The Metalloids
These exhibit both metallic and nonmetallic properties.

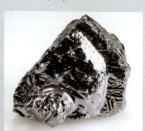

Silicon

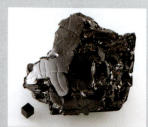

Carbon

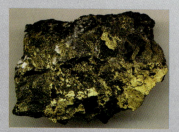

Gold ore

3. Functional appliances and splints, e.g.
    a. Orthodontic therapy, e.g. wires and appliances for tooth movement
    b. Surgical uses, e.g. titanium plates
4. Auxiliary uses, e.g. clinical and laboratory instruments and materials

METALLURGY

Metallurgy is the study of the physical and chemical behavior of metallic elements, their intermetallic compounds, and their mixtures, which are called alloys.

PERIODIC TABLE

Dmitri Mendeleev was the first scientist to create a periodic table of the elements (1869) similar to the one we use today. This table showed that when the elements were ordered by increasing atomic weight, a pattern appeared where properties of the elements repeated periodically. Thus the periodic table is a chart that groups the elements according to their similar properties.

Features

The periodic table helps predict some properties of the elements compared to each other. Atom size decreases as you move from left to right across the table and increases as you move down a column. Energy required to remove an electron from an atom increases as you move from left to right and decreases as you move down a column. The ability to form a chemical bond increases as you move from left to right and decreases as you move down a column.

There are 118 elements in the periodic table. Roughly 80 percent (94) of these elements are classified as metals.

Groups

Columns of elements help define element groups. Elements within a group share several common properties. Groups of elements have the same outer electron arrangement. The outer electrons are called valence electrons. Because they have the same number of valence electrons, elements in a group share similar chemical properties.

GENERAL PROPERTIES OF METALS

General properties of metals are

1. Most metals are solid except for hydrogen which is a gas, and mercury and gallium which is liquid at room temperature.
2. Good thermal and electrical conductivity.
3. Hard, strong and dense.
4. Generally malleable and ductile, deforming under stress without cleaving.
5. Optical properties, metals are shiny and lustrous.
6. They make a metallic sound when struck.
7. Forms positive ions in solutions during electrolysis.

VALENCE ELECTRON

The outer-most electrons of the atom are known as valence electrons *(Fig. 3.2)*. Metals have outer valence electrons that are highly mobile. These are readily given up and are responsible for most of their properties.

Valence electrons are such an essential part of the atom's stability. For the most part, eight valence electrons are necessary for an atom to be stable. A valence electron participates in the formation of a chemical bond with other elements.

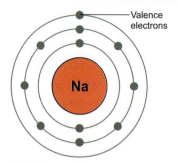

FIGURE 3.2 Valence electron of the sodium atom.

METALLIC BONDING

Metals are tough because atoms of the metals are held together by means of metallic bonds. Metallic bond is the bonding between molecules within metals (also called alkali reactive force).

In metals, valence electrons are shared by all the atoms of the metal and so are not considered to be associated with any one atom. This is very different from ionic or covalent bonds, where electrons are held by one or two atoms. The sea of shared 'delocalised electrons' amongst a lattice of positive ions acts as a kind of "electron glue" giving the substance a definite structure.

The metallic bond is, therefore, strong and uniform. Since electrons are attracted to many atoms, they have considerable mobility to be good conductors of heat and electricity.

Metallic bonds, though strong, also allow movement of the individual atoms. This property allows metals to be hammered into sheets or drawn into wires.

ALLOYS

Most metals used in dentistry are used in the alloyed form. Examples of alloys in dentistry are steel, chrome-cobalt, nickel-chrome, gold-palladium, etc.

One of the first alloys made by humans was bronze, which is made by mixing the metals tin and copper.

Definition

An alloy is a material composed of two more elements; at least one of which should be a metal. Thus an alloy is made by fusing two or more metals, or a metal and a nonmetal.

An alloy may be a solid solution of the elements (*a single phase*), a *mixture of metallic phases* (two or more solutions) or an *intermetallic compound* with no distinct boundary between the phases.

Solid solution alloys give a single solid phase microstructure, while partial solutions exhibit two or more phases that may or may not be homogeneous in distribution, depending on the thermal (heat treatment) history of the material. An inter-metallic compound has one other alloy or pure metal embedded within another pure metal.

Alloys are used in some applications, where their properties are superior to those of the pure component elements for a given application.

Why do we need to alloy?

An alloy has properties which are beneficial over that of the parent materials. A metal that is normally very soft and malleable, such as aluminium, can be altered by alloying it with another soft metal, like copper. Although both metals are very soft and ductile, the resulting aluminium alloy will be much harder and stronger. Adding a small amount of nonmetallic carbon to iron produces an alloy called steel. Due to its very-high strength and toughness (which is much higher than pure iron), and its ability to be greatly altered by heat treatment, steel is one of the most common alloys in modern use. By adding chromium to steel, its resistance to corrosion can be enhanced, creating stainless steel, while adding silicon will alter its electrical characteristics, producing silicon steel.

Classification of alloys

Alloys are usually classified as *substitutional* or *interstitial alloys*, depending on the atomic arrangement that forms the alloy.

They can further be classified based on solubility as

1. Homogeneous (consisting of a single phase)
2. Heterogeneous (consisting of two or more phases)
3. Intermetallic (where there is no distinct boundary between phases)

During the fabrication of a restoration, the alloy is melted and the liquid metal forced into a mold to create the particular restoration. Thus a knowledge of the behavior of alloys during melting and solidification is beneficial.

Manufacture of alloys

Alloys may be prepared by different technological methods: melting, sintering of a powder mixture, high temperature diffusion of an alloying element into the base metal, plasma and vapor deposition of different elements, electroplating, etc.

PHASE

A phase is a uniform part of an alloy, having a certain chemical composition and structure, and which is separated from other alloy constituents by a phase boundary.

An alloy phase may be in the form of a compound (substance formed from two or more elements), with a fixed ratio determining the composition) or in form of solid solution.

SOLID SOLUTIONS

Can one metal dissolve in another?
Two or more metals can dissolve to form solutions. This usually occurs at high temperatures and the product formed is called an alloy. Some metals can also be dissolved at room temperatures, e.g. mercury-tin *(Box 3.2)*. This property is used in the creation of dental amalgam.

Solid solution

A solid solution is a solid-state solution of one or more solutes in a solvent. Such a mixture is considered a solution rather than a compound when the crystal structure of the solvent remains unchanged by addition of the solutes, and when the mixture remains in a single homogeneous phase. This often happens when the two elements (generally metals) involved are close together on the periodic table; conversely, a chemical compound generally results when two metals involved are not near each other on the periodic table.

The solid solution needs to be distinguished from a mechanical mixture of powdered solids like two salts, sugar and salt, etc. The mechanical mixtures have total or partial miscibility gap in solid state.

Examples of solid solutions include crystallized salts from their liquid mixture, metal alloys, moist solids. In the case of metal alloys intermetallic compounds occur frequently.

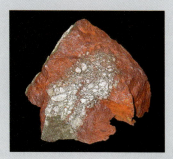

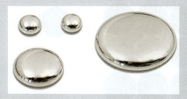

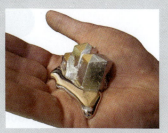

Mercury ore Mercury ore is produced from its ore called Cinnabar. Cinnabar is a toxic mercury sulfide mineral with a chemical composition of HgS. It was used extensively as a pigment for thousands of years in many parts of the world.

Mercury Mercury is the only known metal which is *liquid* at room temperature. Mercury dissolves many metals such as gold and silver to form amalgams. This unique property is used in dentistry to form the filling material 'Dental Amalgam'. Iron and platinum are exceptions, and iron flasks have been traditionally used to trade mercury. Other metals which dissolve in mercury are manganese, copper and zinc.

Gallium Gallium melts at 29.76 °C which is near room temperature. Thus one is able to melt a block of Gallium simply by holding it in one's hands. Our body temperature of 37 °C is sufficient for melting this unique metal.

Types of solid solutions

Depending on the ratio of the solvent (matrix) metal atom size and solute element atom size, two types of solid solutions may be formed.

1. Substitutional
2. Interstitial

Substitution solid solution

If the atoms of the solvent metal and solute element are of similar sizes (not more than 15% difference), they form substitution solid solution, where part of the solvent atoms are substituted by atoms of the alloying element *(Fig. 3.3)*.

Examples are brass (copper with zinc) and palladium-silver.

Interstitial solid solution

If the atoms of the alloying elements are considerably smaller than the atoms of the matrix metal, interstitial solid solution forms, where the matrix solute atoms are located in the spaces between large solvent atoms *(Fig. 3.4)*.

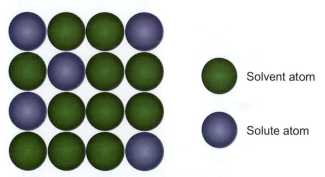

Solvent atom

Solute atom

FIGURE 3.3 Substitution solid solutions.

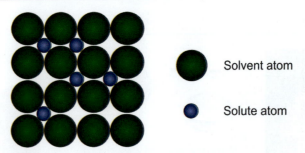

FIGURE 3.4 Interstitial solid solutions.

Steel is an example of an interstitial alloy in which a relatively small number of carbon atoms slip in the gaps between the huge iron atoms in a crystalline lattice of iron. Titanium (CPTi) used in dental implants is another example (99% titanium with oxygen, carbon, nitrogen and hydrogen as interstitial substitutes).

DENTAL APPLICATIONS

Most noble alloys used in dentistry are based on solid solutions. In case of Pd-Ag both metals are mutually soluble in each other in the solid state regardless of the proportion of each.

SOLIDIFICATION AND MICROSTRUCTURE OF METALS AND ALLOYS

Microstructure is defined as the structure of a prepared surface or thin foil of material as revealed by a microscope. The microstructure of a material can strongly influence physical properties such as strength, toughness, ductility, hardness, corrosion resistance, high/low temperature behavior, wear resistance, and so on, which in turn, govern the application of these materials in laboratory and clinical practice. Microstructure at scales smaller than can be viewed with optical microscopes is often called ultrastructure or nanostructure.

GRAINS

Solidification occurs by a process of crystallization *(Fig. 3.5)*. Crystallization begins around a nucleus. Crystals are also known as grains as they seldom show the customary crystal shapes because of interference from neighboring crystals. Crystallization process results in various types of microstructures depending on the type of metal or alloy and the cooling process.

The crystals are otherwise known as grains since they seldom exhibit the customary geometric forms due to interference from adjacent crystals during the change of state.

Nuclei of crystallization

Surface tension of liquid metal is 10 times higher than that of water. When molten alloy cools, the solidification process begins with the formation of atom clusters called 'embryos' or 'nuclei of crystallization'.

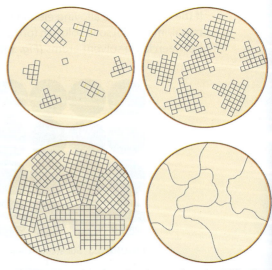

FIGURE 3.5 Illustration of grain growth and solidification.

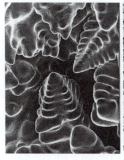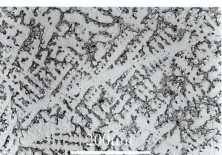

FIGURE 3.6 Photomicrograph showing dendritic structure.

CRYSTALLIZATION FORMS

Metals solidify in roughly three predominant crystal forms *(Figs. 3.6 and 3.7)*

1. Dendritic microstructure
2. Polycrystalline microstructure
   a. Equiaxed grains
   b. Columnar grains
3. Monocrystalline or Single crystal

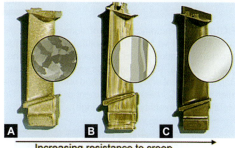

Increasing resistance to creep

FIGURES 3.7A TO C Illustration of different grain structures in a turbine blade. **(A)** Equiaxed grains. **(B)** Columnar grains. **(C)** Monocrystalline or Single crystal.

Dendritic microstructure

In the dendritic form, the crystals that form in the liquid during freezing generally follow a pattern consisting of a main branch with many appendages. A crystal with this morphology slightly resembles a pine tree and is called a dendrite, which means branching. The formation of dendrites occurs because crystals grow in defined planes due to the crystal lattice they create. Secondary dendrite arms branch off the primary arm, and tertiary arms off the secondary arms, etc., resulting in a three-dimensional dendritic structure *(Fig. 3.6)*.

Dental base metal alloys and titanium based casting alloys in which nickel (N), cobalt (Co), iron (Fe), and titanium (Ti) are the main elements generally have a dendritic as cast microstructure.

Equiaxed polycrystalline microstructure

Equiaxed grains *(Figs. 3.7A and 3.8)* are crystals that have axes of approximately the same length. The crystal grows from multiple nucleation points. The expanding crystals continue to grow until they impinge on adjacent growing crystals at grain boundaries. The final sizes of the individual crystals depend on the number of nucleation points. Most noble metal casting alloys solidify with this type of microstructure.

Dental noble metal alloys generally have equiaxed fine-grain microstructures because of certain grain refining elements added into the composition.

Columnar polycrystalline alloys

Columnar grain structured castings *(Figs. 3.7B and 3.9)* are created using a special casting technique called 'directional solidification'. They have grains parallel to the major stress axes. They are less prone to creep deformation compared to equiaxed grain structured metal components.

Single crystal

Normally when a material begins to solidify, multiple crystals begin to grow in the liquid and a polycrystalline (more than one crystal) solid forms. However, it is possible

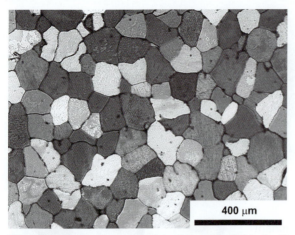

400 μm

FIGURE 3.8 Photomicrograph of aluminium alloy (Al-Mg-Fe-Si containing < 1 wt.% of each solute) showing equiaxed grain structure. Addition of TiB2 particles facilitates fine, equiaxed grain structure. (Specimen was electrolytically etched using Barker's reagent and photographed under cross-polarised light microscopy. (*Courtesy:* Department of Materials Science and Metallurgy, University of Cambridge).

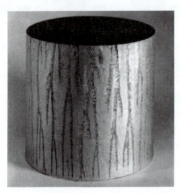

FIGURE 3.9 Columnar grained ingot through directional solidification.

to produce a single large crystal, so there are no grain boundaries in the material *(Fig. 3.7 C)*. Single crystals are produced under carefully controlled conditions. The expense of producing single crystal materials is only justified for special applications, such as turbine engine blades, solar cells, and piezoelectric materials.

Jet engine turbine blades must endure tremendous forces at extremely high temperatures for prolonged periods of time. Under such conditions, metals with a grain structure tend to "creep," or slowly deform, along grain boundaries. Because single-crystal alloy parts have no grain boundaries they are highly resistant to creep.

Forming single-crystal metal objects requires both special alloys and special casting techniques (modified version of the directional solidification technique). The alloys are almost always nickel-based, with as many as nine minor metal components including chromium, cobalt, tungsten, tantalum, aluminium, and/or rhenium.

GRAIN BOUNDARIES

As mentioned previously, the grains meet at grain boundaries *(Fig. 3.8)* which are regions of transition between differently oriented crystals.

These are regions of importance

1. Less resistance to corrosion
2. High internal energy
3. Collection of impurities
4. Barriers for dislocations

GRAIN REFINEMENT AND GRAIN SIZE

Control of grain morphology and size are important in order to predict the properties of the cast metal. Generally alloys with fine grains have superior properties including corrosion resistance.

Control of Grain Size

Grain size can be controlled by

1. Addition of small quantities of grain refining elements like iridium (Ir), ruthenium ((Ru), rhenium ((Re), etc.
2. Use of different casting techniques.
3. Heat treatment, namely annealing.

TIME-TEMPERATURE GRAPH

In order to understand the solidification of alloys, one has to understand the solidification of a pure metal. This can be understood by melting a pure metal and then cooling it back to room temperature. As it cools, a time-temperature graph is plotted *(Fig. 3.10)*.

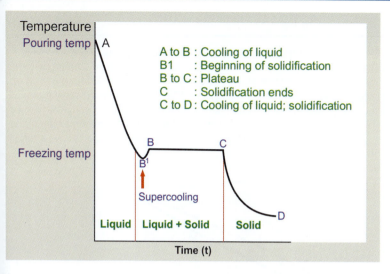

A to B : Cooling of liquid
B1   : Beginning of solidification
B to C : Plateau
C   : Solidification ends
C to D : Cooling of liquid; solidification

FIGURE 3.10 A time temperature cooling curve for a pure metal.

The molten metal starts cooling from A to point B¹, this is called *supercooling*. During the supercooling process crystals of metal begin to form. Crystallization releases latent heat of fusion causing a rise in temperature (B¹ to B).

Completion of crystallization occurs at point C. Between B and C the metal has both liquid and solid phases. The temperature remains steady (plateau) until crystallization is completed. Point D indicates cooling to room temperature.

EQUILIBRIUM PHASE DIAGRAMS

A phase diagram is also known as a constitutional diagram. It helps to identify the phases present in an alloy at different compositions and temperatures. The phase diagram may be explained using the example of the palladium-silver alloy. The two metals exhibit complete solubility in liquid and solid states. The equilibrium phase diagram of Pd-Ag at a composition of 65% Pd and 35% Ag is presented in *Figure 3.11*.

HOMOGENIZATION HEAT TREATMENT - MICROSTRUCTURE

From the phase diagram of the palladium-silver alloy, it is evident that the composition of the structure is not uniform. The grains that form early on during solidification have a higher palladium content compared to the layers that solidify later. Thus the core contains dendrites of varying or nonuniform composition.

Heat treatments can be used to homogenize cast metal alloys to improve their hot workability, to soften metals prior to, and during hot and cold processing operations, or to alter their microstructure in such a way as to achieve the desired mechanical properties.

Definition

Homogenization heat treatment can be defined as a combination of heating and cooling operations applied to a metal or alloy in its solid state to eliminate as cast nonuniform compositional variations (coring effect) to a more uniform equiaxed grain structure through atomic diffusion.

Procedure

The heat treatment of metals involves raising the temperature of an alloy to a defined temperature, usually near its solidus. The material is then held at this temperature for a period

Equilibrium Phase Diagrams

Consider the cooling of Pd-Ag alloy at 65% and 35% composition respectively. This is represented by the line PO. At 'P' the alloy is in liquid state. At 'R' the alloy begins to solidify. However the first crystals have a higher Pd content than the expected 65 %. To determine the exact percentage composition of the first crystals a line is extended from 'R' to 'M' on the solidus line. Point 'M' determines the composition of the first solids which is 77% Pd. At 'S' it is midway through its solidification. Here the composition of the solid is determined as 71% Pd (Point W). The liquid composition is 57% Pd (Point Y). As it cools to the solidus line (1340 °C) Point 'T' the solid phase has 65 % palladium and the remainder of the liquid solidifies at a composition of only 52% Pd. Thus it can be seen from this phase diagram that grains have a varied composition within the structure, though the overall composition is 65% palladium

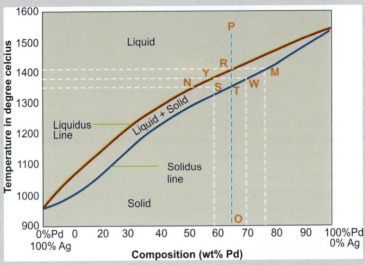

FIGURE 3.11 Equilibrium phase diagram for the palladium-silver system.

of time (up to 6 hours) before being cooled either at a prescribed rate or under rapid quenching conditions to a fixed temperature. Heat treatment is carried out in furnaces and ovens.

EUTECTIC ALLOYS

Eutectic is a 'term' used to describe two components which are 'completely soluble' in each other in the liquid or molten state, but only partially soluble in the solid state. Therefore these alloys do not form solid solutions. Rather, eutectic alloys upon cooling, convert from liquids to intimately mixed solids.

In an eutectic system, the "eutectic alloy" composition has the lowest melting point in the system. It is lower than the melting points of either of the pure components.

Applications

1. Pb-Sn alloy is a good example of an eutectic alloy system.
2. In Dentistry, the Au-Cu eutectic alloy is used in the silver amalgam system.
3. Gold-iridium system is eutectic at iridium concentration of 0.005%.

Equilibrium-phase diagrams of Ag-Cu

In the phase diagram **(Fig. 3.12)**, at three different concentrations, the material will be solid until it is heated to its melting point, and then (after adding the heat of fusion) becomes liquid at that same temperature.

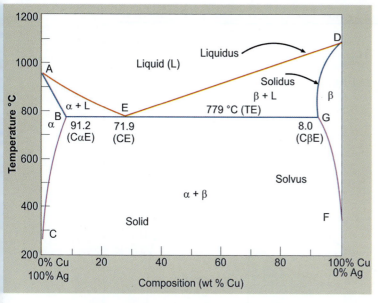

FIGURE 3.12 Equilibrium phase diagram for the silver-copper system

α - Silver-rich substitutional solid solution

β - Copper-rich substitutional solid solution

L - Liquid phase

AED - Liquidus line

ABEGD - Solidus line

Solidus and Liquidus lines meet at E rather than at the pure metal composition seen in the earlier phase diagram. This composition of 72% Ag and 28% Cu is called as the Eutectic. Eutectic means lowest melting. The Eutectic composition melts at a temperature of 779 °C which is lower than either of the pure parent metals.

1. The unalloyed extreme left
2. The unalloyed extreme right
3. The dip in the center E (the eutectic composition).

At other compositions, the material will enter a mushy or pasty phase until it warms up to its melting temperature.

The mixture at the dip point (E) of the diagram is called an *eutectic alloy*.

Features of the eutectic system

1. The eutectic composition melts at a temperature of 779 °C which is lower than either of the pure parent metals. This property is useful in solders.
2. Solidus and liquidus lines meet at the Eutectic temperature. Thus there is no solidification range at the eutectic temperature of 779 °C.

Hypoeutectic and hypereutectic alloys

Alloys with compositions less than that of the eutectic are called hypoeutectic alloys and those with a composition greater than the eutectic are known as hypereutectic alloys.

PERITECTIC ALLOYS

Peritectic transformations are also similar to eutectic reactions. Here, a liquid and solid phase of fixed proportions react at a fixed temperature to yield a single solid phase *(Fig. 3.13)*.

The peritectic reaction during the cooling phase can be written as

Liquid + β Solid solution → α Solid solution

Peritectic alloys are susceptible to coring during rapid cooling. This cored structure is more brittle and has lower corrosion resistance than a homogeneous solid solution.

Examples

1. The dental amalgam alloy silver-tin is based on the peritectic system.
2. Dental casting alloy gold-platinum.
3. Palladium-ruthenium alloy at 16.5% has a peritectic reaction.

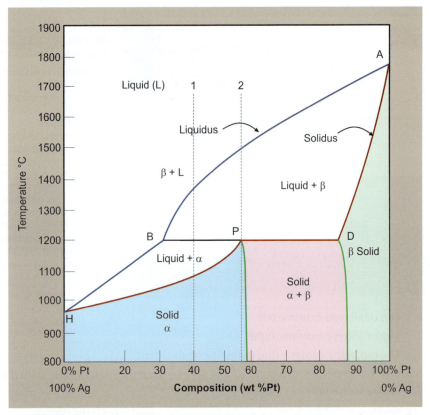

FIGURE 3.13 Equilibrium phase diagram for the platinum-silver system demonstrating peritectic reaction

α - Silver rich phase
β - Platinum rich phase
P - Peritectic transformation point
A - Platinum melting point (1768 °C)
H - Silver melting point (961.8 °C)
A peritectic reaction is a reaction where a solid phase (β) and liquid phase will together form a second solid phase (α) at a particular temperature and composition.
In this case, it occurs at a composition of 56% Pt.

SOLID STATE REACTIONS

Knowledge of solid-state reactions is important to understand strengthening mechanisms in Type III and IV gold alloys like age hardening. Solid state reactions can be explained through the gold-copper phase diagram.

GOLD-COPPER PHASE DIAGRAM

Gold and copper are completely soluble in each other in the liquid state. The gold-copper equilibrium phase diagram is presented in **(Fig. 3.14)**. The difference between the liquidus and solidus is small at all compositions. The two curves meet at 80.1%. This composition marks the lowest temperature at which a gold-copper alloy can melt. At temperatures between the solidus and 410 °C the gold and copper are mutually soluble and form a *disordered solid solution* (α). The atoms are in random arrangement in an FCC structure. However, as the alloy cools down further, certain solid state transformations are seen. The various phases on cooling at various compositions are summed up in **Table 3.1**.

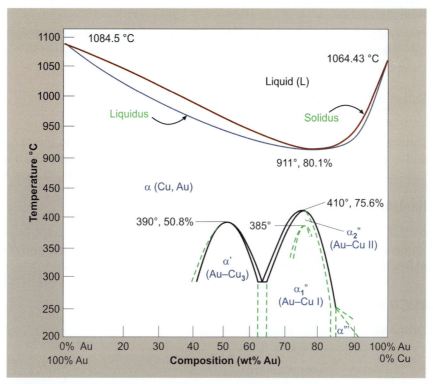

FIGURE 3.14 Equilibrium phase diagram for the gold-copper system.

TABLE 3.1 Phases formed at various temperature and composition range

Phase	Temperature	Composition range
Disordered α phase (Au-Cu)	Between solidus and 410 °C	40–65%
Ordered α′ phase (Au-Cu₃)	Below 390 °C	40–65%
Ordered α″₂ phase (Au-Cu II)	Below 410 °C	65–85%
Ordered α″₁ phase (Au-Cu I)	Below 410 °C	65–85%

HEAT TREATMENT OF GOLD ALLOYS

The ordered phases (α′, α″2 , and α″1) have superior mechanical properties. The disordered phase (α phase) on the other hand is relatively soft and ductile. This soft ductile phase is convenient for laboratory finishing and grinding procedures. The disordered phase which exists at the higher temperatures can be preserved by *rapid quenching*. Rapid cooling prevents atomic movement to the more ordered lower temperature phases. Following adjustments of the crown, the alloy is again *age hardened* by holding it at specified temperature for a specified period. This permits the solid state reactions to take place (through atomic fusion) and convert the alloy to its mechanically superior ordered phases (α′, α″2 , and α″1). The alloys can be restored to its softened condition by again raising it to a temperature just below its solidus (700 °C) and holding it at this temperature for 10 minutes and then rapidly quenching. Thus essentially, gold alloys can be both softened and hardened through heat treatment.

TYPES OF HEAT TREATMENT

From the above, it is clear that a variety of heat treatments are available for various purposes. The various heat treatments are summarized below.

Homogenization

This treatment is used prior to hot working processes and is performed to equalize temperatures throughout an alloy or to reduce the coring effect caused by the nonuniform chemical composition.

Softening heat treatment

Synonyms Solution heat treatment, annealing.

Softening heat treatment covers a variety of heat treatment processes used to soften alloys and increase their ductility as an aid to cold working. It is also performed to remove internal stresses within components following cold working, welding, casting or rapid cooling.

Hardening heat treatment

Synonyms Precipitation hardening, age hardening

Hardening heat treatment is a heat treatment technique used to increase the strength of malleable materials, including most structural alloys of nickel, titanium, and some stainless steels.

CLASSIFICATION OF ALLOYS

Dental alloys can be classified in many ways.

1. Based on the number of alloying elements
   a. Binary (two constituents)
   b. Ternary (three constituents)
   c. Quaternary (four constituents)
   d. Quinary (five constituents)
2. Based on noble metal content
   a. High Noble
   b. Noble
   c. Predominantly base

FUNCTIONS OF ALLOYING ELEMENTS

Elements are added into the alloy in various proportions to modify its properties. Most elements affect the properties of the metal in multiple ways. The various properties and the effect of the modifiers are described.

Grain refinement

Grain refinement is the process by which the grain size is restricted during solidification. Smaller grain sizes block dislocation movements within the structure. This improves the yield strength of the alloy.

Metals that refine grain sizes are

○ Iridium
○ Rhenium
○ Ruthenium

Mechanical properties

Alloys like palladium, platinum, copper and iron improve mechanical properties like strength, hardness and modulus of elasticity in gold-based alloys.

Color modification

The alloying metals have varying effects on the color of the alloy. Metals like gold and copper impart a gold and reddish hue to the alloy. White metals like palladium and silver tend to whiten the alloy. Silver-rich alloys tend to have a greening hue.

CTE (TEC) modification

The thermal expansion coefficient (TEC) (also called coefficient of thermal expansion-CTE) of an alloy used to construct porcelain-fused to metal crowns (PFM) requires to be closely matched to that of the veneering porcelain. TEC mismatch can cause fracture or separation of the veneer from the metal. Silver increases CTE whereas palladium lowers the CTE in the alloy.

Melting range modification

Generally metals with higher melting points raise the melting range, whereas metals with lower melting point tend to lower the melting range of the corresponding alloys. Example, silver reduces the melting range of palladium and gold alloys. Palladium and platinum raise the melting range of gold-based alloys.

Castability

The castability of a material is the ease with which a casting can be produced with minimal energy and defects. Generally castability is related to the density of a material. Denser metals improve the castability of the alloy. Noble alloys are generally more easy to cast because of their greater density when compared to base metal alloys like cobalt-chromium.

Oxygen scavenger

Zinc is added to remove oxygen during the casting process, thereby reducing porosity.

Tarnish and corrosion resistance

Tarnish and corrosion resistance is a desirable property especially in the oral environment. Improving the concentration of noble metals improve the tarnish and corrosion resistance of an alloy.

In base metal alloys, the mechanism for tarnish and corrosion resistance is different. In chrome-based alloys, a surface oxide is readily formed. The surface oxide forms a protective layer which protects the metal from further corrosion. This property is called 'passivation'. Other metals which use a similar mechanism is stainless steel and titanium.

Density and specific gravity

In certain instances like large cast removable partial dentures, a light weight framework is preferable to a more heavier frame in terms of patient comfort and appliance retention. Base metal alloys are popular as RPD alloys because of their low density. Palladium being lighter than gold lowers the density and weight of gold-palladium-based alloys. The density of a palladium based alloy is midway between that of base metal and of high noble alloys.

Oxide formation

Metals used for porcelain fused to metal restorations have the additional requirement of facilitating porcelain attachment. Porcelain does not bond readily to noble metal alloys. Certain elements like tin, indium and iron oxide are added to noble metal alloys to form oxides which aid in the bonding of porcelain to the alloy. Base metal alloys form oxides quickly.

4
CHAPTER

Electrochemical Properties of Materials

Except for a few, pure metals do not occur naturally. They occur in the form of minerals such as oxides and sulfides and these have to be refined to produce the pure metal. Most pure metals attempt to reconvert to the combined state. The process by which this takes place is called corrosion.

One of the primary requisites of any metal that is to be used in the mouth is that it must not produce corrosion products that will be harmful to the body. The mouth is moist and continually subjected to fluctuations in temperature. The foods and liquids ingested have wide range of pH. All these factors make the mouth an extremely favorable environment for corrosion.

DEFINITIONS

TARNISH

Tarnish is a surface discoloration on a metal or even a slight loss or alteration of the surface finish or lustre.

Tarnish generally occurs in the oral cavity due to

1. Formation of hard and soft deposits on the surface of the restoration, e.g. calculus, mucin and plaque.
2. Pigment producing bacteria, produce stains.
3. Formation of thin films of oxides, sulfides or chlorides.

Tarnish is often the forerunner of corrosion.

PASSIVATION

In certain cases, the oxide film can also be protective in nature. For example, chromium alloys (used in dental castings) are protected from corrosion by the formation of an oxide layer on its surface which protects the metal against any further corrosion. This is known as passivation. Another example is titanium.

CORROSION

It is not a surface discoloration but actual deterioration of a metal by reaction with the environment. It can be defined as the deterioration of metals by chemical interaction with their environment.

Most metals exist in their stable oxide state in nature except for some of the noble metals like gold. Metals are refined from these natural ores to produce the pure metals and alloys. However, the pure state of metals is unstable. Corrosion is a natural process, which converts refined metal to their more stable forms.

In the most common use of the word, this means electrochemical oxidation of metal in reaction with an oxidant such as oxygen. Rusting, the formation of iron oxides, is a well-known example of electrochemical corrosion. This type of damage typically produces oxides or salts of the original metal.

However element other than oxygen also can cause corrosion particularly in the oral environment. Water, oxygen, chloride ions, sulfides like hydrogen sulfide or ammonium sulfide contribute to corrosion attack in the oral cavity. Various acids such as phosphoric, acetic and lactic are also present. Among the specific ions responsible for corrosion, oxygen and chloride have been implicated in amalgam corrosion both at the tooth interface and within the body of amalgam. Sulfide has been implicated in the corrosion of silver containing casting alloys.

Corrosion degrades the useful properties of materials and structures including strength and appearance. In due course, it may lead to rapid mechanical failure of the structure.

ELECTROMOTIVE FORCE SERIES (EMF)

The EMF series is a classification of elements in the order of their dissolution tendencies. That is, if two metals are immersed in an electrolyte and are connected by an electrical conductor, an electric couple is formed. The metal that gives up its electrons and ionizes is called the anode. In the EMF series, hydrogen has been used as the standard electrode to which other metals have been compared. Hydrogen has been given the value zero in the EMF series *(Table 4.1)*.

TABLE 4.1 Electromotive force values		
Metal	*Ion*	*Electrode potential*
Gold	Au	+ 1.50
Platinum	Pt	+ 0.86
Silver	Ag	+ 0.88
Copper	Cu	+ 0.47
Hydrogen	H$^+$	0.00
Cobalt	Co	−0.28
Iron	Fe	−0.44
Zinc	Zn	−0.76

The metal with lowest electrode potential corrodes. Also the more active metal corrodes (anode) and the more noble metal becomes the cathode.

CLASSIFICATION OF CORROSION

Corrosion can be classified as

1. Chemical or dry corrosion
2. Electrochemical or wet corrosion

CHEMICAL OR DRY CORROSION

The metal reacts to form oxides and sulfides in the absence of electrolytes.

Example　　Formation of Ag_2S in dental alloys containing silver.

　　　　　　Oxidation of alloy particles in dental amalgam.

ELECTROLYTIC OR ELECTROCHEMICAL OR WET CORROSION

This requires the presence of water or other fluid electrolytes. There is formation of free electrons and the electrolyte provides the pathway for the transport of electrons. An electrolytic cell is as follows:

$$M^0 \rightarrow M^+ + e^-$$

The anode is the surface where positive ions are formed. This metal surface corrodes since there is loss of electrons. This reaction is sometimes referred to as *oxidation reaction*.

$$M^+ + e^- \rightarrow M^0$$

$$2H^+ + 2e^- \rightarrow H_2$$

$$2H_2O + O_2 + 4e^- \rightarrow 4(OH)^-$$

At the cathode a reaction must occur that will consume the free electrons produced at the anode. The reactions 2, 3 and 4 occur at the cathode and are referred to as *reduction reactions*. Hence, the anode loses electrons and the cathode consumes. The surface of the anode corrodes due to loss of electrons.

TYPES OF ELECTROLYTIC CORROSION

GALVANIC CORROSION

Saliva with its salts provides a weak electrolyte. Galvanic corrosion occurs when dissimilar metals lie in direct physical contact with each other *(Fig. 4.1)*.

If a gold restoration comes in contact with an amalgam restoration, the amalgam forms the anode and starts corroding. The electric couple (500 millivolts) created when the two restorations touch, causes sharp pain called *'galvanic shock'*. It usually occurs immediately after insertion and can be minimized by painting a varnish on the surface of the amalgam restoration. However, the best precaution is to *avoid dissimilar metals* in contact. Another variation of galvanic corrosion can occur even in a lone standing restoration *(Fig. 4.2)*.

Note　Seldom there is any one type of corrosion found alone, generally two or more act simultaneously and thus aggravate the problem.

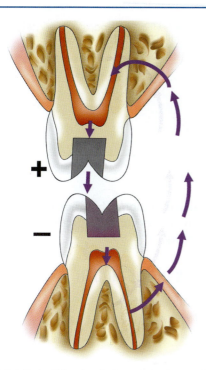

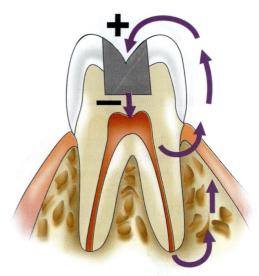

FIGURE 4.2 A current pathway may exist even in a single metallic restoration. In this case the tissue fluid behaves like a cathode (because of the higher concentration of Cl^- ions in tissue fluid when compared to saliva) whereas saliva behaves like an anode. This current is usually less intense.

FIGURE 4.1 Potential galvanic current pathway when dissimilar metals contact. The tissue fluid and saliva behaves like an electrolyte.

HETEROGENEOUS COMPOSITIONS

This kind of corrosion occurs *within* the structure of the restoration itself. Heterogeneous (mixed) compositions can cause galvanic corrosion.

- ❍ When an alloy containing eutectic is immersed in an electrolyte the metallic grains with the lower electrode potential are attacked and corrosion results.
- ❍ In a cored structure differences in the composition within the alloy grains are found. Thus a part of a grain can be anode and a part, cathode. Homogenization improves the corrosion resistance of the alloy.
- ❍ In metals or alloys the grain boundaries may act as anodes and the interior of the grain as the cathode.
- ❍ Solder joints may also corrode due to the nonhomogeneous composition.
- ❍ Impurities in any alloy enhance corrosion.

STRESS CORROSION

A metal which has been stressed by cold working, becomes more reactive at the site of maximum stress. If stressed and unstressed metals are in contact in an electrolyte, the stressed metal will become the anode of a galvanic cell and will corrode. For example, if an orthodontic wire has been cold worked, stress corrosion may occur and cause the wire to break.

CONCENTRATION CELL CORROSION OR CREVICE CORROSION (FIG. 4.3)

- ❍ *Electrolyte concentration cell* In a metallic restoration which is partly covered by food debris, the composition of the electrolyte under the debris will differ from that of saliva and this can contribute to the corrosion of the restoration.

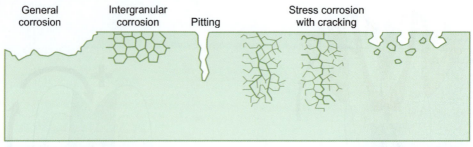

FIGURE 4.3 Different types of corrosion.

○ *Oxygen concentration cell* Differences in oxygen tension in between parts of the same restoration causes corrosion of the restoration. Greater corrosion occurs in the part of the restoration having a lower concentration of oxygen.

FACTORS AFFECTING CORROSION OF RESTORATIONS IN THE MOUTH

Corrosion of dental restorations in the mouth is influenced by

1. Diet
2. Drug
3. Smoking
4. Bacterial activity
5. Oral hygiene and habits

PROTECTION AGAINST CORROSION

PASSIVATION

Certain metals readily form strong adherent oxide film on their surface which protects them from corrosion. Such metals are said to be passive. *Chromium, titanium,* and *aluminium* are examples of such metals.

Adding more than 12% Cr to iron or cobalt produces a chromic oxide layer on the surface of stainless steel or cobalt chromium alloys which is highly corrosion resistant. Since this film is passive to oxidative chemical attack, their formation is called passivation.

INCREASING NOBLE METAL CONTENT

Alloys with a noble metal content below 65% may tarnish. So it has been suggested that at least 50% of the atoms in a dental alloy should be gold, platinum or palladium to ensure against corrosion. Noble metals resist corrosion because their EMF is positive with regard to any of the common reduction reactions found in the oral environment.

POLISHING

Polishing metallic restorations like amalgam and cast metal to a high luster minimizes corrosion. The patient should also maintain good oral hygiene.

OTHER METHODS

Dissimilar metal restorations should be avoided. Avoid using a high mercury containing amalgam as it is more susceptible to corrosion. Mercury tarnishes gold, thus, care must be taken to protect gold ornaments worn by the operator, assistant or patient.

Biological Properties of Dental Materials

The science of dental materials must include a knowledge and appreciation of the biological considerations that are associated with selection and use of materials designed for the oral cavity. Strength and resistance to corrosion are unimportant if the material irritates or injures the pulp or soft tissue. The biological characteristics of dental materials cannot be isolated from their physical properties. In the early days of dentistry, the patient's mouth was often the testing ground of dental materials. Modern dentistry, however, involves extensive testing before the material is certified for human use.

BIOMATERIALS

Many materials used in the mouth are classed as 'biomaterials'.

A *biomaterial* can be defined as any substance other than a drug that can be used for any period of time as a part of a system that treats, augments, or replaces any tissue, organ or function of the body.

BIOLOGICAL REQUIREMENTS OF DENTAL MATERIALS

A dental material should

1. Be nontoxic to the body
2. Be nonirritant to the oral or other tissues
3. Not produce allergic reactions
4. Not be mutagenic or carcinogenic

CLASSIFICATION OF MATERIALS FROM A BIOLOGICAL PERSPECTIVE

A. Those which contact the soft tissues within the mouth
B. Those which could affect the health of the dental pulp, e.g. restorative materials and luting cements.
C. Those which could affect the periapical areas of the tooth such as root-canal medicaments, filling materials, etc.
D. Those which affect the hard tissues of the teeth.
E. Those used in the dental clinics and laboratory which when handled may be accidentally ingested or inhaled, e.g. alginate dust, mercury vapors, alloy dust containing beryllium formed while cutting metal.

BIOHAZARDS RELATED TO THE DENTAL MATERIALS

❍ Some dental cements are acidic and may cause pulp irritation.
❍ Polymer based filling materials may contain irritating chemicals such as unreacted monomers, which can irritate the pulp.
❍ Phosphoric acid is used as an etchant for enamel.
❍ Mercury is used in dental amalgam, mercury vapor is toxic.
❍ Dust from alginate impression materials may be inhaled, some products contain lead compounds.
❍ Monomer in denture base materials is a potential irritant.
❍ Some people are allergic to alloys containing nickel *(Fig. 5.1)*. Dental applications of nickel alloys include orthodontic wires, fixed and removable partial dentures, etc. Allergies are confirmed using the *patch test (Figs. 5.6A and B)*.
❍ The frequency of titanium allergy seems to be very rare. Titanium allergies are similar to other metal allergies. They show symptoms adjacent to the area where it is placed *(Fig. 5.2)*. Some patients report worsening of health after placement of titanium implants.
❍ During grinding of beryllium containing casting alloys, inhalation of beryllium dust can cause berylliosis.
❍ Some dental porcelain powders contain uranium.
❍ Metallic compounds (e.g. of lead, tin etc.) are used in elastomeric materials.
❍ Eugenol in materials like restorations and impressions can cause irritation and burning in some patients.
❍ Laboratory materials have their hazards, such as cyanide solution for electroplating, vapors from low fusing metal dies, siliceous particles in investment materials, fluxes containing fluorides asbestos, etc.
❍ Some periodontal dressing materials have contained asbestos fibers.

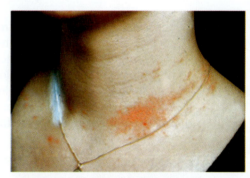

FIGURE 5.1 Nickel allergy from a necklace.

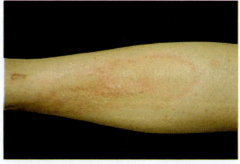

FIGURE 5.2 Titanium allergy. The shin of a woman with dermatitis adjacent to implanted titanium orthopedic device.

BIOLOGICAL CONSIDERATIONS OF RESTORATION DESIGN

Besides material considerations, the design of the restoration plays an important part in biological response and function. Faulty design is a major cause of recurrent caries, gingival inflammation, periodontal disease and tooth loss or damage. Every year countless restorations and teeth are lost due to faulty design *(Fig. 5.3A)*.

Biological requirements of restoration design

The restoration should be designed such that

1. It should not impede natural cleansing mechanisms of the mouth (crevicular fluid *(Fig. 5.4)* and saliva).
2. It does not provide a habitat for bacterial colonization.
3. It should not trap food *(Fig. 5.5B)*.
4. It should not trap defoliating epithelial cells lining the gingival sulcus.

In short, a restoration design should avoid *'biotraps'* and allow natural cleansing mechanisms.

Biotraps in the oral environment

Many restorations serve as biotraps because of improper design or poor clinical skills.

1. Amalgams overhang in the proximal regions *(Fig. 5.5A)*.
2. Overhanging crown margins especially those which are subgingival or in close proximity to the *biological width*.

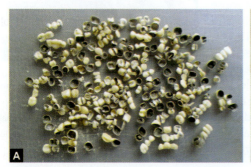 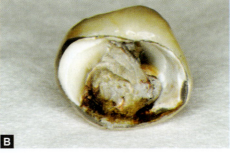

FIGURES 5.3A AND B (A) Every year hundreds of crowns fail due to various reasons including poor technique and material selection. **(B)** Microleakage under a crown.

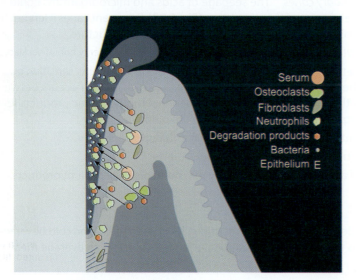

Serum ●
Osteoclasts ●
Fibroblasts ●
Neutrophils ●
Degradation products ●
Bacteria ●
Epithelium E

FIGURE 5.4 Biotraps in the gingival sulcus can trap defoliated epithelial cells and degradation products by preventing the natural exit and cleansing activity of the crevicular fluid. Biotraps provide a habitat for bacterial colonization and potential infection.

3. Microleakage due to improper restoration adaptation or bonding *(Fig. 5.3B)*.
4. Cracked teeth or roots.
5. Cracked restorations in the interproximal or subgingival zone.
6. Porosity within restorations contacting tissue.
7. Uneven or rough surfaces in restorations or prostheses contacting tissue.
8. Bridge pontics with *saddle* or *ridge lap* designs.
9. Biotraps in the root canal system resulting from incomplete obturation of the root canal system.

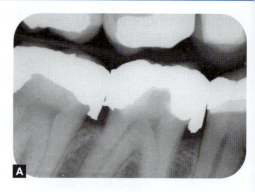

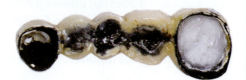

PHYSICAL FACTORS AFFECTING PULP HEALTH

MICROLEAKAGE

A great deficiency of materials used for restoring teeth is that, they do not adhere to tooth structure and preexisting restorative materials already on the tooth (except those systems based upon polyacrylic acid and certain dentin-bonding agents). Thus a microscopic space always exists between the restoration and the prepared cavity. The use of radioisotope tracers, dyes, scanning electron microscope and other techniques have clearly

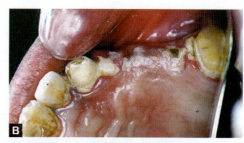

FIGURES 5.5A AND B Examples of biotraps. (A) Amalgam overhangs. (B) Saddle pontics are contraindicated because of biotraps.

shown that fluids, microorganisms and oral debris can penetrate freely along the interface between the restoration and the tooth and progress down the walls of the cavity preparation. This phenomenon is referred to as microleakage.

Microleakage can result in

1. *Recurrent or secondary caries*   The seepage of acids and microorganisms could initiate caries around the margins of the restoration *(Fig. 5.3B)*. Recurrent caries if left unchecked can lead to loss of the restoration and destruction of tooth structure.
2. *Stain or discoloration* can also develop.
3. *Sensitivity*   Sometimes because of microleakage the tooth remains sensitive even after placement of the filling. If the leakage is severe, bacterial growth occurs between the restoration and the cavity and even into the dentinal tubules. Toxic products liberated by such microorganisms produce irritation to the pulp.
4. Pulpitis from continued thermal and bacterial irritation.
5. Foul smell from trapped and decaying organic matter.
6. Inflammation of adjacent tissue caused by microorganisms or their byproducts.

THERMAL CHANGE

Tooth structure and dental restorations are continually exposed to hot and cold beverages and foods. Instantaneous temperature fluctuation during the course of an average meal may be as great as 85 °C. The temperature fluctuations can crack the restorative materials or produce undesirable dimensional changes in them because of thermal expansion and contraction.

Many restorative materials are composed of metals. Metals conduct heat and cold rapidly. Patients may often complain of sensitivity in a tooth with a metallic restoration when they are eating hot or cold foods. The problem is more in a very large restoration, where the layer of dentin remaining at the floor of the cavity may be so thin that it is not adequate to insulate the pulp against the temperature shock.

Protection from thermal changes   The dentist must place a layer of insulating cement (called base) under the restoration.

GALVANISM

Another cause for sensitivity is the *small currents* created whenever two *different* metals are present in the oral cavity. The presence of metallic restorations in the mouth may cause a phenomenon called galvanic action or galvanism. This results from a difference in potential between dissimilar fillings in opposing or adjacent teeth. These fillings in conjunction with saliva as electrolyte make up an electric cell. When two opposing fillings contact each other, the cell is short-circuited and the patient experiences pain. A similar effect may occur when a restoration is touched by the edge of a metal fork.

Studies have shown that relatively large currents can flow. The current rapidly drops if the fillings are maintained in contact, probably as a result of polarization of the cell. The magnitude of the voltage is not of primary importance, but the sensitivity of the patient to the current has a greater influence on whether he will feel pain. Some patients may feel pain at 10 μ amp and other at 110 μ amp (average: 20 to 50 μ amp). That is why some patients are bothered by galvanic action and others are not despite similar conditions in the mouth.

The galvanic current magnitude depends on the composition and surface area of the metals. Stainless steel develops a higher current density than either gold or cobalt chromium alloys when in contact with an amalgam restoration. As the size of the cathode (e.g. a gold alloy) increases relative to that of the anode (e.g. amalgam), the current density may increase. The larger cathode can enhance the corrosion of the smaller anode. Current densities associated with non γ_2-containing amalgams appear to be less than those associated with γ_2-containing amalgam.

CLASSIFICATION OF ADVERSE REACTIONS FROM DENTAL MATERIALS

A number of biological responses are possible from materials. However, they may be broadly grouped into

1. Toxic
2. Inflammatory
3. Allergic
4. Mutagenic

Fortunately, most materials are screened very early on for toxicity and mutagenicity, therefore, most of the possible responses if any to dental materials usually fall in the inflammatory or allergic category.

Adverse effects may also be classified as

1. Local
2. Systemic

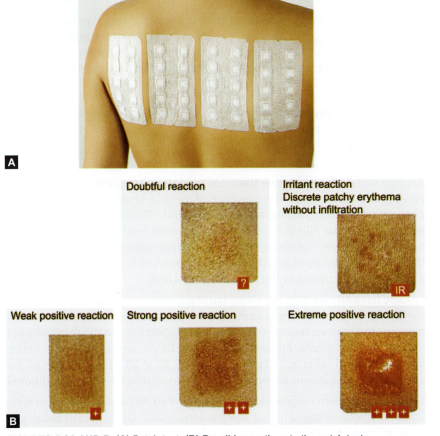

FIGURES 5.6A AND B **(A)** Patch test. **(B)** Possible reactions to the patch test.

A local effect is a result of the direct contact of the material to the regions immediately adjacent to the material. Example of a local reaction is the allergic response of the oral mucosa to the denture seen in some individuals.

A systemic reaction is caused by the absorption of the material into the body through local absorption, ingestion or inhalation.

TOXICITY EVALUATION

Toxicity tests are classified as

1. Level I tests (screening tests)
2. Level II tests (usage tests)
3. Level III tests (human trials)

LEVEL I TESTS (SCREENING TESTS)

The material is first checked for acute systemic toxicity and for its cytotoxic, irritational, allergic and carcinogenic potentials.

❍ *Acute systemic toxicity test* is conducted by administering the material orally to laboratory animals. If more than 50% of the animals survive, the material is safe.

○ *Cytotoxic screening* may be done *in vivo* or *in vitro*. *In vitro* tests are conducted on cultured cells like mouse L-929 fibroblasts and human Hela cells. There are many *in vitro* tests. *Example,* Agar overlay technique; Agar is spread over a layer of culture cells in a culture plate. The test material is then placed on it and incubated. A toxic material will show a clear zone of dead cells.

○ *Irritational properties* are checked by placing the material beneath the skin in rats or intramuscularly in rabbits. The animals are killed at different time intervals. The tissue response is then examined and compared.

○ *Allergic potential* The material is first placed inside the skin of guinea pigs. Later the material is placed on the skin surface. Erythema and swelling at the site show allergic reaction.

○ *Carcinogenic potential* (i) *In vivo* tests A material is placed beneath the skin (subcutaneously) of mice. They are then killed after 1 and 2 years and examined for tumors (ii) *In vitro* tests Include *Ames test.* Here the material is tested with the help of mutant histidine dependent bacteria.

LEVEL II (USAGE TESTS)

The material is tested in experimental animals similar to how it is used in humans, e.g. pulp reaction is studied by placing the material into class V cavities in teeth of primates (apes or monkeys). The teeth are then extracted periodically and compared with negative controls (ZOE cement) and positive controls (silicate cement).

LEVEL III (HUMAN TRIALS)

Once the material has passed screening and usage tests in animals, it is ready for trials in humans. The reactions and performance under clinical conditions are studied.

THERAPEUTIC EFFECTS OF DENTAL MATERIALS

Certain dental materials are utilized for their beneficial biological effects. For example, zinc oxide eugenol cement has a pain relieving effect on irritated pulp. Calcium hydroxide pulp capping agent promotes the formation of secondary dentin and helps repair dentinal tissue.

OSSEOINTEGRATION

The osseointegration potential of titanium has been well-documented in the literature. It is this property which allowed the successful use of materials like titanium as an implant material. The surface of titanium forms a very thin layer of oxide which promotes osseointegration. Materials that allow osseointegration have a very low degradation rate. Osseointegration with intervening connective tissue is called fibrous osseointegration and is generally considered a failure. When the bone closely approximates the implant without intervening connective tissue, it is called *osseointegration*. If the bone actually fuses with the implant, it is called *biointegration (refer chapter on Implants).*

EFFECT OF PRESSURE ON TISSUES

It was once believed that pressure from the pontic of a fixed dental prosthesis on the ridge resulted in permanent inflammation based on an article by Stein in 1966 (Pontic-residual ridge relationship: A research report, JPD 1966). With the increasing popularity of the ovate pontic it is now known that pressure results in remodelling of the tissues and does not invariably lead to permanent inflammation. Pressure from the pontic may result in short-term injury and inflammation as a result of tissue response to trauma. The tissues usually recover in 10 to 12 days. Porcelain restorations were relative uncommon prior to the 1960's. Acrylic was commonly used for masking the metal for bridges and saddle pontics were widely used. Both saddle pontics and acrylic have been implicated in ridge inflammation and thus the inflammation reported by Stein may have been related to the pontic design or material *(Figs. 5.7A and B)*.

EFFECT OF PONTIC DESIGN

Saddle or ridge lap pontics designs usually result in inflammation as they act as biotraps. Ovate pontics on the other hand present a convex interface *(Fig. 5.8A)* with the tissues with little or no biotrap. It has a biocleansing effect on the tissues. Relatively little inflammation is seen underneath a porcelain ovate pontic even when the patient has not performed subpontic flossing *(Fig. 5.8B)*.

EFFECT OF MATERIAL – PORCELAIN VERSUS RESIN

In a fixed dental prostheses, the pontic is often in continuos contact with the tissue. Among the various materials polished or glazed, porcelain is the most inert. However, the pontic design must be taken into consideration. Except for saddle design, long-term contact with porcelain shows little or no inflammation *(Fig. 5.8B)*. On the other hand long-term contact with resin pontics can result in inflammation of tissues regardless of the design *(Figs. 5.7A and B)*.

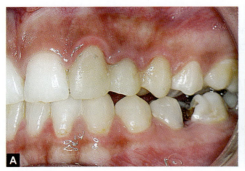 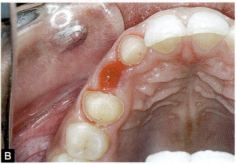

FIGURES 5.7A AND B Tissue response to 2-year old temporary resin bridge. **(A)** 2-year old temporary bridge with ovate pontic design made from resin based composite (Protemp 2). **(B)** Inflamed tissue is evident on removal of the bridge.

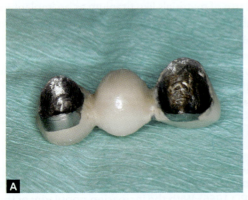 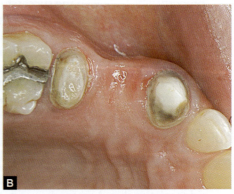

FIGURES 5.8A AND B Tissue response to 3-year old porcelain fused to metal bridge. **(A)** 3-year PFM bridge with ovate pontic requiring replacement due to ceramic chipping. **(B)** Tissues show little or no inflammation in spite of the patient not having flossed for 3 years.

INFECTION CONTROL

There is increased interest in expanding infection control measures to the dental laboratory. Concern over possible cross-contamination to dental office personnel by microorganisms, including hepatitis-B virus and human immunodeficiency virus (HIV), through dental impressions has promoted the study of the effect of disinfecting techniques on dental materials.

INFECTION ROUTES

There are many ways by which microorganisms can spread.

1. Contaminated instruments and needles.
2. Direct splashing of saliva and blood into the mouth or onto wounds.
3. Breathing of contaminated aerosol from the air-rotor handpiece.
4. Through contaminated dental materials.

Except for contamination occurring through dental materials, the other routes are beyond the scope of this book.

DISINFECTION OF DENTAL MATERIAS

Impressions

Impressions are the main source of spread of infection among the dental materials. However, disinfecting impression materials is more complex. The disinfectant must not affect its properties and accuracy. If the impression has not been disinfected, we must disinfect the cast.

Materials may be disinfected by

1. Immersion in a disinfectant.
2. Spraying with a disinfectant.
3. Incorporating the disinfectant into the material as part of its composition.

Immersion in a disinfectant is the most common method of disinfection in the dental office as well as laboratory. However, certain materials like alginates may be affected if immersed beyond the recommended period. Alginates imbibe water and swell thereby affecting its accuracy.

Contaminated restorations and prostheses

Crowns, dentures and other prostheses that have been tried in the mouth are also a possible source of contamination. After the try-in many of these are returned to the laboratory without disinfection. These contaminate the polishing lathe and the pumice powder used for polishing which in turn cross-contaminate other restorations and prostheses. Studies have shown complete dentures are massively contaminated with microorganisms and can serve as the primary source in the cycle of cross infection within dental laboratories. The polishing of dentures without previous disinfection leads to a high level of transfer of microorganisms.

Infection control measures such as the use of barriers during polishing, the disinfection of dentures before being sent to the laboratory and upon return to the dental clinic, the disposal or sterilization of the cone after each use, as well as the addition of disinfectants to pumice and unit doses of pumice should be adopted with the objective of reducing the risk of cross-infection.

PART-2

Direct Restorative Materials

Introduction to Restorations, Luting and Pulp Therapy

This chapter serves as an introduction to restorative dentistry, including cements, liners and varnish. An emphasis is also placed on the effect of these materials on the pulp.

RESTORATIONS

Tooth material is often lost as a result of caries and trauma. A restoration is a material which substitutes the missing tooth structure and restores the form and function of the tooth *(Fig. 6.1)*.

TYPES OF RESTORATIONS

Restorations may be classified in a number of different ways.

1. Temporary, intermediate and permanent
2. Direct and indirect
3. Esthetic and nonesthetic

TEMPORARY RESTORATIONS

Temporary restorations are often required before the placement of a permanent restoration. Materials used for temporary restorations are expected to last for only a short period of time, a few days or a few weeks

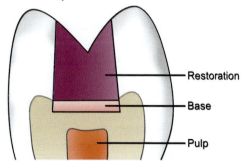

FIGURE 6.1 Restoration of a tooth.

at most. They serve as an interim restoration while the pulp heals; and/or till the permanent restoration can be fabricated and inserted. At one time gutta-percha (temporary stopping), a thermoplastic gum that is used to fill root canals was popular for this purpose. However, it did not adapt well to the cavity walls, microleakage ensued and sensitivity was a common occurrence.

Because of its excellent initial sealing ability and kind pulpal response, *zinc oxide eugenol (ZOE)* is the cement of choice for temporary restorations. This material is particularly useful when a sedative treatment is required until the pulp has healed well enough for the permanent restoration to be placed. The Type I ZOE is very popular for sedative treatment, temporary coverage and temporary cementation. Type III ZOE is used for temporary restorations.

INTERMEDIATE RESTORATIONS

Intermediate or holding type of restoration is particularly used in pedodontics. For example, in rampant caries, it is desirable to remove all the caries quickly in order to change the oral health and arrest the caries process. Once the initial 'clean up' has been done, the dentist can proceed with placement of the permanent restorations. The interval between removal of the caries and completion of final restorative work may take several months. During this time teeth are protected with a desirable intermediate restoration.

Conventional zinc-eugenol cements used as temporary restorations are deficient in toughness. They have inadequate strength and abrasion resistance to serve for a longer period. As a result polymer reinforced cement (IRM) is used. Earlier Type II zinc phosphate and Type II or Type III zinc silicophosphate cements were used. However, these materials were irritating to the pulp and required more precise cavity preparation and placement time. They are now replaced by improved ZOE formulations. The combination of surface treatment and polymer reinforcement results in good strength, improved abrasion resistance and toughness. They can last for a period of *one year or more*.

REQUIREMENTS OF A TEMPORARY FILLING MATERIAL

1. It should have adequate strength to last a few weeks, but weak enough to be dislodged easily.
2. It should be easy to insert and remove.
3. It should have adequate seal.
4. It should have antibacterial properties.
5. It should have a therapeutic effect (pain relief, healing, etc.) on the pulp.
6. It should have cariostatic properties.

PERMANENT

The term permanent is *not an absolute term*. However, it obviously serves to denote any material that is expected to last much longer than the temporary and intermediate restorations. Therefore, it is expected to have improved properties than the temporary and intermediate restorations. Examples of permanent restorative materials are direct filling gold, amalgam *(Fig. 6.1)*, composite resins, glass ionomer cement, as well as porcelain, composite and cast metal inlays and onlays.

The length of time each material lasts varies on the technical skills of the operator, the material itself and other patient related factors. A well-made amalgam restoration would probably last a lifetime or more. On the other hand the composite restoration might have to be replaced much earlier as a result of wear, fracture or discoloration.

DIRECT AND INDIRECT RESTORATIONS

Direct restorations These are materials used to build and restore the tooth structure directly in the mouth. They are usually placed in increments. They are usually soft and plastic when initially placed and harden later with time. Examples are amalgam, direct filling gold, composite (can be used both directly and indirectly) and glass ionomer.

Indirect restorations These are usually fabricated outside the mouth on models of the tooth and then cemented into place in the mouth. Examples of indirect restorations are porcelain, composite and cast metal inlays and onlays.

ESTHETIC AND NONESTHETIC

The terms esthetic and nonesthetic are again relative.

Esthetic An esthetic material is obviously something which is pleasing to an individual. At one time gold fillings and crowns were considered esthetic. Today, however, an esthetic material implies any material that is capable of reproducing the color and appearance of a *natural tooth*. Examples are resin-based composites, glass ionomer and porcelain restorations.

Nonesthetic Currently, it denotes any material that is not tooth colored. This includes amalgam, direct filling gold and metal inlays and onlays.

LUTING

Synonyms Bonding, cementing

Luting or cementation ***(Fig. 6.2)*** is the process by which crowns, restorations and other devices are fixed or attached to tooth structure using an intermediate material called cement. Cements have multiple uses. For example, glass ionomer can be used as a base, luting agent and as a restorative material. Besides attaching the restoration a luting agent must also seal the space between the restoration and the tooth structure to prevent caries and chemical and bacterial irritation of the tooth and pulp.

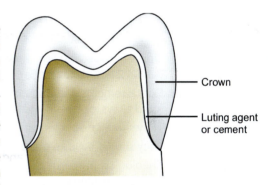

FIGURE 6.2 The luting agent attaches as well as seals the space between the restoration and tooth structure.

TYPES

1. Temporary cementation
2. Permanent cementation

TEMPORARY CEMENTATION

Temporary cementation of crowns and fixed partial dentures (FDP) are often required. Temporary crowns and FDPs are required to stay in place only until the permanent structure is ready. Therefore, it must be weak enough to be easily removed when the permanent structure is ready for cementation. In addition, this cement should have some soothing effect on the pulp of the freshly, prepared vital tooth, which would have been traumatized during the preparation. Permanent structures (e.g. crowns or FDPs) are also sometimes cemented temporarily. This allows the patient to take it for a home trial or to observe the pulpal response. Once the patient and dentist are satisfied with the results, the restoration is removed and cemented permanently. An example of such a temporary bonding cement is a zinc oxide eugenol-based cement (Temp Bond).

PERMANENT CEMENTATION

A permanent cementing material on the other hand should be strong and insoluble in oral fluids. It would also be advantageous if it had some chemical bonding to the tooth structure. In addition, it should be fluid enough to flow well to ensure the complete seating of the restoration.

Examples of permanent cementing materials are zinc phosphate cement, glass ionomer cement, resin cement, polycarboxylate cement, etc.

GENERAL REQUIREMENTS OF LUTING MATERIALS

1. They should be nontoxic and nonirritant to pulp and tissues.
2. They should be insoluble in saliva and liquids taken into the mouth.
3. Mechanical properties: These must meet the requirements for their particular applications, e.g. a cement base should develop sufficient strength rapidly to enable a filling material to be packed on it.
4. Protection of the pulp from insults.
    - Thermal insulation, a cement used under a large metallic restoration should protect the pulp from temperature changes.
    - Chemical protection, should be able to prevent penetration into the pulp of harmful chemicals from the restorative material.
    - Electrical insulation under a metallic restoration to reduce galvanic shock.
5. Optical properties: For cementation of a translucent restorations (e.g. porcelain) the cement should match the color and translucency of tooth substance.
6. Dental cements should ideally be adhesive to both tooth structure and restorative material (gold alloys, porcelain, etc.), but not to dental instruments.
7. They should be bacteriostatic in a cavity with residual caries.
8. They should have an obtundent (soothing) effect on the pulp.
9. Rheological properties: A luting cement should have sufficiently low viscosity to give a low film thickness.

PULP CAPPING

Pulp capping is the process of placing a specialized agent in contact with or in close proximity to the pulp with the intention of encouraging formation of new dentin (secondary dentin) and promote the healing of the pulp. Prior to the discovery of pulp capping agents, a pulp exposure often led to irreversible pulpitis or pulpal infection and ultimately pulp necrosis. Thanks to these pulp capping agents, it became possible to treat pulpal tissue which otherwise would have had to undergo root canal therapy. Example of a pulp capping agent is *calcium hydroxide* cement.

CRITERIA FOR PULP CAPPING

Are all exposed pulps suitable for pulp capping therapy? The answer is obviously no. The dentist has to apply certain criteria and select his cases carefully.

1. The pulp should be healthy and noninfected.

2. The area of exposure should be no more than 0.5 mm.
3. Following exposure the dentist should make all attempts to immediately isolate the tooth and prevent contamination.

TYPES OF PULP CAPPING

A. Direct pulp capping
B. Indirect pulp capping

DIRECT PULP CAPPING

Direct pulp capping is the placement of the agent directly on the exposed pulp *(Figs 6.3A and B)*. Such a situation is often encountered during

1. The excavation of deep carious lesions when the dentist accidentally exposes the pulp.
2. Traumatic fractures of the tooth.
3. Iatrogenic (caused by treatment) exposure during cavity preparation.
4. Iatrogenic exposure during crown preparation.

INDIRECT PULP CAPPING

Secondary dentin formation can be induced even when the pulp is not exposed but is near exposure. When the calcium hydroxide is placed in the region of the near exposure, it can still induce new dentin formation. This is known as *indirect pulp capping.*

Indications

1. Deep carious lesions close to the pulp.
2. During excessive crown preparation the pulp is often visible through the remaining dentin as a pinkish or reddish spot or area.
3. Similar near exposures may be seen in cases of traumatic tooth fracture.

BASES

A base is a layer of cement placed beneath a permanent restoration to encourage recovery of the injured pulp and to protect it against numerous types of insults to which it may be subjected. The type of *insults* depends upon the particular restorative material. It may be thermal or chemical or galvanic. The base serves as replacement or substitute for the protective dentin, that has been destroyed by caries or cavity preparation. Nonvital teeth do not require a base.

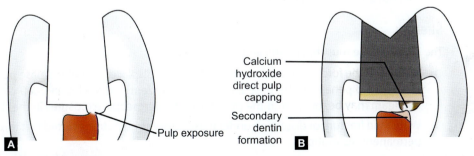

FIGURES 6.3A AND B (A) Pulp exposure. **(B)** Direct pulp capping and subsequent secondary dentin formation several weeks later

TYPES

They belong to two categories.

High strength bases

These are used to provide *thermal protection* for the pulp, as well as *mechanical support* for the restoration.

Examples of high strength bases: Zinc phosphate, Zinc polycarboxylate, glass ionomer and reinforced ZOE cements.

Some important properties of cements used as high strength bases are strength, modulus of elasticity and thermal conductivity.

Low strength bases

Low strength bases have minimum strength and low rigidity. Their main function is to act as a *barrier* to irritating chemicals and to provide *therapeutic benefit* to the pulp. Examples are: calcium hydroxide and zinc oxide eugenol.

PROPERTIES

Thermal properties

The base must provide thermal protection to the pulp. This property is important especially when the tooth is restored with *metallic restorations*.

The thermal conductivity of most cement bases is similar to tooth structure and is in the range of recognized insulators such as cork and asbestos.

For effective thermal protection the base should have minimal thickness of 0.75 mm. A thin wash of cement would not offer protection against thermal insults through metallic restorations.

Protection against chemical insults

The cement base also serves as a barrier against penetration of irritating constituents (e.g. acids, monomer, etc.) from restorative materials. Calcium hydroxide and zinc oxide eugenol are most effective for this especially in deep (close to the pulp) cavities. Polycarboxylate and glass ionomer bases are also used as chemical barriers in more moderate cavities.

Therapeutic effect

Some bases are used for their therapeutic benefit to the pulp. For example, calcium hydroxide acts as a pulp capping agent and promotes the formation of secondary dentin. Zinc oxide eugenol has an obtundent effect on the pulp.

Strength

The cement base must have sufficient strength to

○ Withstand the forces of condensation. Fracture or displacement of the base permits the amalgam to penetrate the base and contact the dentin. Likewise, in deep cavities the amalgam may be forced into the pulp through microscopic exposures in the dentin.

○ Withstand fracture or distortion under masticatory stresses transmitted to it through the permanent restoration.

Also the cement base should develop sufficient strength rapidly in order to allow early condensation of amalgam. The minimum strength requirement of a base is between 0.5 and 1.2 MPa.

CLINICAL CONSIDERATIONS

The base is selected according to

○ Design of the cavity

○ Type of permanent restorative material used

○ Proximity of the pulp to the cavity walls.

With amalgam, calcium hydroxide or zinc oxide eugenol cement is usually sufficient.

In case of direct filling gold where the condensation pressure is higher, a stronger cement is indicated as base.

With resin restorations, calcium hydroxide is the material of choice, as zinc oxide eugenol cements interfere with its polymerization. Glass ionomer cement can also be used as base.

LINERS AND VARNISH

Liners and varnishes are agents in a volatile solvent which when applied to a surface evaporates leaving behind a thin film. This film acts as a barrier which has different functions depending on the circumstance and the location where it is applied. These materials are discussed in more detail in the subsequent chapter.

Cavity Liners and Varnish

Chapter Outline

CAVITY LINERS

A cavity liner is used like a cavity varnish to provide a barrier against the passage of irritants from cements or other restorative materials and to reduce the sensitivity of freshly cut dentin. They are usually suspensions of calcium hydroxide in a volatile solvent. Upon the evaporation of the volatile solvent, the liner forms a *thin film* on the prepared tooth surface.

SUPPLIED AS

- Solutions in bottles
- Powder and liquid
- Paste in tubes

COMPOSITION

Suspension of calcium hydroxide in an organic liquid *(Fig. 7.1)* such as methyl ethyl ketone or ethyl alcohol. Acrylic polymer beads or barium sulphate calcium monofluorophosphate.

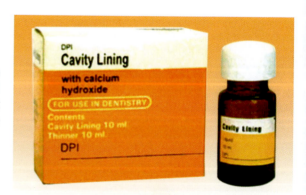

FIGURE 7.1 Calcium hydroxide suspension used for cavity lining.

PROPERTIES

Like varnishes, cavity liners neither possess mechanical strength nor provide any significant thermal insulation. The calcium hydroxide liners are soluble and *should not* be applied at the margins of restorations. Fluoride compounds are added to some cavity liners in an attempt to reduce the possibility of secondary caries around permanent restorations or to reduce sensitivity.

MANIPULATION

Cavity liners are fluid in consistency and can be easily flowed or painted over dentinal surfaces. The solvents evaporate to leave a thin film residue that protects the pulp. The paste form is applied in the cavity and then light cured.

OTHER LINERS

Some other materials have been claimed as liners. These include Type III glass ionomer and ZOE.

CAVITY VARNISH

Cavity varnish is a solution of one or more resins which when applied onto the cavity walls, evaporates leaving a thin resin film, that serves as a barrier between the restoration and the dentinal tubules.

APPLICATION

1. It reduces microleakage around the margins of newly placed amalgam restorations, thereby reducing, postoperative sensitivity.
2. It reduces passage of irritants into the dentinal tubules from the overlying restoration or base, e.g. silicate.
3. In amalgam restorations, they also prevent penetration of corrosion products into the dentinal tubules, thus, minimizing tooth discoloration.
4. Varnish may be used as a surface coating over certain restorations to protect them from dehydration or contact with oral fluids, e.g. silicate and glass ionomer restorations.
5. Varnish may be applied on the surface of metallic restoration as a temporary protection in cases of galvanic shock.
6. When electrosurgery is to be done adjacent to metallic restorations, varnish applied over the metallic restorations serves as a temporary electrical insulator.
7. Fluoride containing varnishes release fluoride.

SUPPLIED AS

Liquid in regular or-dark colored bottles *(Fig. 7.2)*.

Commercial Names   Harvard lac, Chem Varnish, Secura, Fuji Varnish (GC)

COMPOSITION

Natural gum such as copal, resin or synthetic resin dissolved in an organic solvent like alcohol, acetone, or ether. Medicinal agents such as chlorobutanol, thymol and eugenol may be added. Some varnishes also contain fluorides.

PROPERTIES

Varnishes neither possess mechanical strength nor provide thermal insulation because of the thin film thickness. The film thickness ranges from 2 to 400 μm. The solubility of dental varnishes is low; they are virtually insoluble in water.

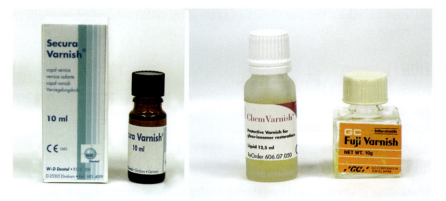

FIGURE 7.2 Some of the various commercially available varnishes.

MANIPULATION

The varnish may be applied by using a brush, wire loop or a small pledget of cotton. Several thin layers are applied. Each layer is allowed to dry before applying the next one. When the first layer dries, small pinholes develop. These voids are filled in by the succeeding varnish applications. The main objective is to attain a uniform and continuous coating.

PRECAUTIONS

1. Varnish solutions should be tightly capped immediately after use to prevent loss of solvent by evaporation.
2. It should be applied in a thin consistency. Viscous varnish does not wet the cavity walls properly. It should be thinned with an appropriate solvent.
3. Excess varnish should not be left on the margins of the restorations as it prevents proper finishing of the margins of the restorations.

CLINICAL CONSIDERATIONS

When placing a silicate restoration, the varnish should be confined to the dentin. Varnish applied on the enamel inhibits the uptake of fluoride by the enamel.

CONTRAINDICATIONS

- *Composite resins*   The solvent in the varnish may react with the resin.
- *Glass ionomer*   Varnish eliminates the potential for adhesion, if applied between glass ionomer cement (GIC) and the cavity.
- When therapeutic action is expected from the overlying cement, e.g. zinc oxide eugenol and calcium hydroxide.

FLUORIDE VARNISHES

Fluoride varnishes are used to prevent or arrest tooth decay in smooth surfaces in young children, especially when applied before age three as their teeth erupt. The taste does not appear to be offensive so is considered acceptable to young children. The technique is well accepted by parents. It hardens on contact with saliva and stays in contact with the teeth for

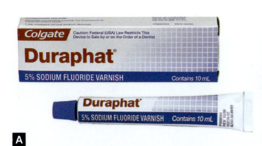
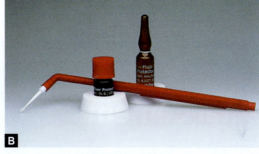

FIGURES 7.3A AND B Two commercially available fluoride varnishes. **(A)** Duraphat. **(B)** Fluor Protector.

several hours or days, but is not meant to adhere permanently. Families should be told that their child can eat and drink afterward but they should not brush the teeth until the next day, or at least 12 hours later, as it may remove some of the varnish. Most protocols suggest two applications per year, although some recommend up to four, with the first ones occurring fairly close together or in the first 1–2 weeks.

Trade names

Commonly used varnishes are Duraphat *(Figs. 7.3A and B)* (Colgate-Oral Pharmaceuticals, Inc), Duraflor (Pharmascience, Inc.), Fluor Protector (Ivoclar-Vivadent) and Cavity Shield (OMNII - Oral Pharmaceuticals).

COMPOSITION

Composition varies depending on the particular brand. It contains concentrated fluoride dissolved in an organic solvent. One varnish (Colgate Duraphat) contains 22,600 ppm (5%) sodium fluoride. Another product Fluor Protector (Ivoclar-Vivadent) contains 0.1% fluoride (Fluorsilane) in ethyl acetate (65%), isoamyl-propionate (21%) and polyisocyanate (12%).

MANIPULATION

Fluoride varnishes are painted on to the teeth using a special tiny brush. The teeth are cleaned with a toothbrush first and then dried with a gauze square; professional tooth cleaning with prophylactic paste is not indicated. Some varnishes are colored for visualization during placement *(Fig. 7.4)*.

CONTRAINDICATIONS

Varnishes should not be used in cavitated carious lesions because the caries may spread to other portions of the tooth, but can be used to remineralize white spot lesions.

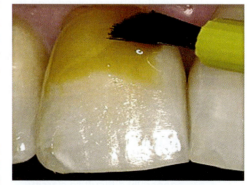

FIGURE 7.4 Application of Duraphat varnish.

8

CHAPTER

Dental Cements

Chapter Outline

Dental cements are materials of multiple uses including restorations, luting and therapeutic. They are generally materials of comparatively low strength, but have extensive use in dentistry. The first dental cement is said to have been introduced in 1785 by Sorel who created the 'zinc-oxide-chloric-cement'. Nearly a hundred years later Rostain and then Fleck developed and introduced the zinc phosphate cement. Around the same period silicates were also developed.

Cements have come a long way since then. Many of them have been improved considerably, while some like the silicate cements have been discontinued. Some like the glass ionomers and the polycarboxylate have adhesive properties and form a chemical bond to dentin and enamel. Regardless of some inferior properties, they possess so many desirable features that they are widely used in dentistry.

CLASSIFICATION

Cements have a wide variety of uses, properties and reaction mechanisms. This makes them generally difficult to classify.

ISO standards covering cements

ISO 9917-1:2007   Water-based cements–Part 1: Powder/liquid acid-based cements

ISO 9917-2:2010   Water-based cements–Part 2: Light-activated cements

ISO 3107:2011   Zinc oxide/eugenol and zinc oxide/noneugenol cements

ISO 4049:2009   Polymer-based filling, restorative and luting materials

ISO classification

Water-based cements   Zinc phosphate, glass ionomer, etc.

Oil-based cements   ZOE and noneugenol cements

Resin or polymer-based cements   Resin cements, compomer, etc.

According to setting reaction
The materials may be classified as

○   Acid-base reaction cements
○   Polymerizing cements
○   Dual cure cements
○   Tricure cements

Acid-base reaction cements   They are formulated as powder and liquid. The liquid acts as the acid and the powder as the base. On mixing the two an acid-base reaction takes placing resulting in a viscous paste, which hardens to a solid mass.

Polymerizing cements   These cements set by polymerizing reaction which may be light activated or chemically activated, e.g. resin cements.

Dual and tricure cements   Dual cure cements set by acid base and any one of the polymerization (light activated or chemically activated) mechanisms. Tricure cements utilize all three mechanisms for hardening.

Classification of cements based on application (ISO 9917-1:2007)*
a.   Luting
b.   Bases or lining
c.   Restoration

GENERAL STRUCTURE

On mixing the powder and liquid, only a part of the powder reacts with the liquid and the final set material is composed of

○   *A core* of unreacted powder, surrounded by
○   *A matrix* formed by the reaction product of the powder and the liquid.

USES OF CEMENTS

Cements have a wide variety of usage in dentistry.

Function	Cement used
Final cementation	Zinc phosphate, zinc silicophosphate, EBA cement, zinc polycarboxylate, glass ionomer, resin cement
Temporary cementation	Zinc oxide eugenol, noneugenol zinc oxide
Bases	Zinc phosphate, reinforced zinc oxide eugenol, zinc polycarboxylate, glass ionomer, zinc oxide eugenol, calcium hydroxide

(Contd...)

* Current ISO specifications no longer classify cements as Type 1, 2 or 3. The prefix 'Type' has been discontinued. Only a single type of luting cement with a maximum film thickness of 25 µm is described. Medium grain (film thickness 40 µm) from previous editions have been discontinued. Similarly, only a single class of restorative cement is described; sub-classification (a) esthetic restorative and (b) reinforced restorative cements have been discontinued.

(Contd...)

Function	Cement used
Long-term restorations	Glass ionomer, compomer, metal modified GIC
Temporary and intermediate restorations	Zinc oxide eugenol, reinforced zinc oxide eugenol, zinc polycarboxylate, glass ionomer
Pulp therapy	Calcium hydroxide
Obtundant (pain relief)	Zinc oxide eugenol
Liners	Calcium hydroxide in a suspension
Root canal sealer	Zinc oxide eugenol, zinc polycarboxylate

GENERAL PROPERTIES OF CEMENTS

Though cements are formulated to serve a variety of functions, the two most common applications of dental cements are luting and restorations. Some of the minimum requirements for water based dental cements are presented in *Table 8.1*.

NET SETTING TIME

Net setting time is the period of time, measured from the end of mixing, until the material has set (as per ISO criteria).

STRENGTH

Most cements are comparatively weak when compared to restorative materials like amalgam and composites. The strength required depends on the application. For example, a cement used as a base under amalgam should have sufficient strength to withstand condensation forces. Many dental cements as well as restorative materials continue to gain strength with time. For this reason patients are often advised to wait at least 2 hours before any food is placed in the mouth. In addition the side in which the restoration has been placed is avoided for a further 24 hours period.

MODULUS OF ELASTICITY (MOE)

This is a measure of the stiffness of the cement. Cements under ceramic crowns should have sufficient stiffness to withstand masticatory loads. A low MOE can result in flexing of the restoration resulting in fracture.

SOLUBILITY AND DISINTEGRATION

This is an important property as it can determine the long-term survivability of restorations *(Figs. 8.1, 8.2A and B)*. Solubility and disintegration of the cement at the margins can eventually lead to problems like inflammation, caries, sensitivity, etc. Most cements exhibit varying degrees of solubility. *ISO specification No. 99171:2007* uses in vitro testing with 0.1 mol/L lactic acid with pH of 2.74. However, a more reliable test would be an in vivo test as conditions in the mouth are far more complex. Solubility and disintegration can be reduced by proper manipulation, minimizing the exposure of the cement to the oral environment and protecting of the cement during setting and the initial 24 hours period.

FILM THICKNESS

Film thickness is an important property especially for luting cements. A thinner film is more advantageous for luting.

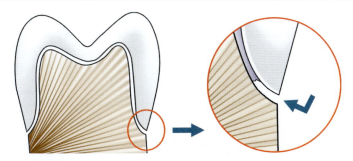

FIGURE 8.1 One cannot rely entirely on the cement for sealing an open margin. Most cements slowly dissolve and disintegrate in the oral cavity leading to microleakage and subsequent failure. A good marginal fit of the crown is therefore essential.

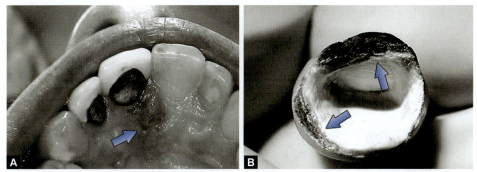

FIGURES 8.2A AND B Cement dissolution. **(A)** Area of inflammation in relation to the leaking margin (arrow). **(B)** On removing the crown, area of cement dissolution is clearly visible (arrows).

1. It improves the seating of the restoration.
2. It helps in greater flow and wetting of the tooth and restoration surface, thus improving bonding.
3. It minimizes the air spaces and structural defects present in the bulk of the cement.

Film thickness is measured in μm. ISO 9917-1:2007 specifies maximum film thickness for luting cements as 25 μm.

BIOLOGICAL PROPERTIES

Most cements are placed within the dentin and in many instances in close proximity to the pulp. Thus it is important that the cement should not be irritant or toxic to the pulp.

PH of the cement Most cements are acidic. The exceptions are zinc oxide eugenol, calcium hydroxide and resin cements. The acidity of cements is higher at the time of placement but gradually decrease with time.

Pulpal response The pulp response may be classified as mild, moderate or severe. Originally silicate cement was used as a reference to compare the pulpal response to various cements. Because of its high acidity, silicates were classed as severe irritant. High acidity can irritate and sometimes lead to irreversible pulpal damage. In some patients it can cause severe pain and sensitivity. Monomer present in resin-based cements is also a potential irritant.

Pulp protection In case of deep cavities and where the cement is classed as an irritant measures to protect the pulp are indicated.

1. Avoid thin mixes.
2. Pulp protection should be carried out in deep cavities through the use of an intervening liner or base.

BOX 8.1

Cements manufactured for various applications would have been modified slightly to suit the particular application. For example, glass ionomer manufactured for luting may be slightly different from glass ionomer used for restorations. Luting cements are usually more fine grained and have a different powder-liquid ratio. Restorative GIC has better translucency and esthetics when compared to the luting GIC which may be more opaque.

FLUORIDE RELEASE

Many cements contain fluoride which is gradually released over a period of time to impart adjacent teeth structure with caries resistance. Glass ionomer is an example of a fluoride releasing cement.

Fluoride recharging

The process by which a restorative material, specifically glass ionomer cement, absorbs fluoride from a solution with a high fluoride concentration.

SILICATE CEMENTS

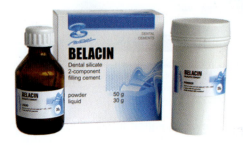

Silicate cements *(Fig. 8.3)* are said to have been introduced in *1873* by *Fletcher* as an anterior esthetic filling material. They were translucent and resembled porcelain in appearance. Though the initial esthetics was satisfactory, over a period of time silicates degraded and stained. Leakage around the margins result in dark margins. Silicates are attacked by oral fluids and in time degrade.

The average life of a silicate restoration is four years. Some may last as long as 25 years, others may require replacement in a year or even less.

FIGURE 8.3 Silicate cement.

The incidence of secondary caries is markedly less around silicate restorations. This is surprising when considering that severe leakage takes place at its margins. Also the incidence of contact caries is less when compared to amalgam restorations (contact caries is the term applied to caries occurring on the proximal surface of the tooth adjacent to the restoration). The anticariogenic property is due to presence of 15% fluoride. Fluoride release is slow and occurs throughout the life of the restoration. Silicate cements were classed as a severe irritant to the pulp because of its low pH (acidic). For many years silicate served as a standard for comparing the pulpal response to other material. In deep cavities the pulp had to be protected with varnish or calcium hydroxide.

With the development of better alternate materials like composite resin and glass ionomer cements, silicates gradually fell out of favor. By the 1980s and 1990s they were gradually phased out of the market and are rarely used. However, silicate cements are of historical interest as they were the first tooth colored filling materials. It also forms the basis for the glass ionomer system.

ZINC PHOSPHATE CEMENT

Zinc phosphate is the oldest of the luting cements and thus serves as a standard with which newer cements can be compared. The terms 'Crown and Bridge' and 'Zinc Oxyphosphate' have also been used for this cement.

APPLICATIONS

1. Luting of restorations (inlays, crowns, fixed dental prostheses, etc.)
2. High strength bases.
3. Temporary restorations.
4. Luting of orthodontic bands and brackets.

CLASSIFICATION

ISO 9917-1:2007 designates them as

a. Luting (Maximum film thickness—25 µm)
b. Bases and lining

AVAILABLE AS

○ Powder and liquid system.
○ Capsules of preproportioned powder and liquid.

Supplied in shades of yellow, gray, golden brown, pink and white.

Representative commercial products Confit, Harvard, Zinc cement (DPI), Modern Tenacin, Poscal (VOCO), De Trey Zinc (Dentsply), Hy Bond, etc. Some representative products are shown in ***Figure 8.4.***

COMPOSITION

Powder

Ingredient	Weight (%)	Function
Zinc oxide	90.2	Principal constituent
Magnesium oxide	8.2	Aids in sintering
Other oxides (like bismuth trioxide, calcium oxide, barium oxide, etc.)	0.2	Improves smoothness of mix
Silica	1.4	Filler, aids in sintering

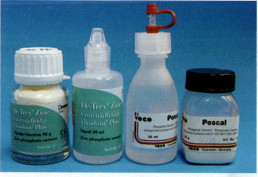
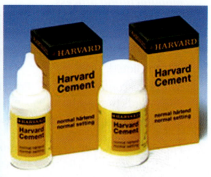

FIGURE 8.4 Three representative zinc phosphate cements.

Liquid

Ingredient	Weight (%)	Function
Phosphoric acid	38.2	Reacts with zinc oxide
Water	36.0	Controls rate of reaction
Aluminum phosphate or sometimes zinc phosphate	16.2	Buffers, to reduce rate of reaction
Aluminum	2.5	
Zinc	7.1	

MANUFACTURE

The ingredients are mixed and heated at temperatures between 1,000 °C and 1,400 °C (sintering). After sintering, the cake formed is cooled quickly. This causes the material to crack which helps in grinding of the material to a fine powder. This process is known as *fritting*.

The liquid is produced by adding aluminum and sometimes zinc or their compounds into orthophosphoric acid solution.

SETTING REACTION

When the powder is mixed with liquid, phosphoric acid attacks the surface of the particles and releases zinc ions.

The *aluminum* in the liquid is essential for cement formation. The aluminum complexes with the phosphoric acid and the zinc ions to form a *zinc aluminophosphate gel*. The reaction is *exothermic*.

STRUCTURE OF SET CEMENT

The set cement has a cored structure consisting primarily of unreacted zinc oxide particles embedded in a matrix of zinc aluminophosphate.

NET SETTING TIME

According to ISO 9917-1:2007, the net setting time can vary from 2.5 to 8 minutes for luting and 2.5 to 6 for base and lining type *(Box 8.2)*.

Control of setting time

Manufacturing process

1. *Sintering temperature* The higher the temperature, the more slowly the cement sets.
2. *Particle size* Finer particles react more quickly as a greater surface area is exposed to the liquid.
3. *Water content of liquid* Presence of excess water accelerates, whereas insufficient water retards the reaction.
4. *Buffering agents* When added slow down the reaction.

Factors under control of operator

1. *Temperature* Higher temperatures accelerate the reaction. Cooling the mixing slab is an effective way of slowing the reaction and prolonging the working time.

> **BOX 8.2**
>
> The setting time of cements in general vary widely. The setting time varies between different manufacturers. Climatic conditions too have a significant effect. Warm humid climatic conditions accelerate the setting. The portion of the material placed in the mouth sets faster than that on the table. This is because of the warm and moist conditions in the mouth.

2. *Powder-liquid ratio*   More the liquid, slower the reaction.
3. *Rate of addition of powder to liquid*   The reaction is slower if the powder is incorporated slowly.
4. *Mixing time*   The longer the mixing time (within practical limits), the slower is the rate of reaction.

PROPERTIES

COMPRESSIVE STRENGTH

The fully set zinc phosphate cement has a relatively high compressive strength ranging from 104 to 119 MPa. The set cement gains approximately 70% of its maximum strength in the first 30 minutes. The strength continues to rise with time and maximum strength is attained at the end of 24 hours *(Box 8.3)*.

The strength of zinc phosphate cement is sufficient when used as a base or luting agent. However, when it is exposed to the oral environment, e.g. temporary restorations, its brittleness and low strength causes it to fracture and disintegrate. Also, the prolonged contact with the oral fluids or water gradually reduces its strength. This may be due to the slow dissolution of the cement.

Factors affecting strength
1. *Powder-liquid ratio*   More the powder, greater the strength.
2. *Water content of the liquid*   Both loss or gain, reduces the strength.

TENSILE STRENGTH

The set cement is weaker in tension (5.5 MPa), thus making it brittle.

MODULUS OF ELASTICITY (STIFFNESS)

It is comparatively high (13.7 GPa). This makes it stiff and resistant to elastic deformation. This is beneficial when it is used to cement restorations that are subjected to high masticatory stresses.

SOLUBILITY AND DISINTEGRATION

This property is important for cements used for permanent cementation. When tested according to ISO specification, maximum solubility permitted is 0.3 *(Table 8.1)*.

However, in the mouth they show greater disintegration over a period of time. This shows that other factors are involved (like wear, abrasion, chemical attacks by products from decaying food, etc.). The solubility is greater in dilute organic acids like lactic, acetic and especially citric acids, all of which are present in the human diet. Thus it is important to minimize the exposure of the cement in the mouth by having minimum gaps at the margins of restorations.

Factors affecting solubility
1. *Powder-liquid ratio*   Thicker mixes show less solubility.
2. *Water content of liquid*   Any change in the water content is accompanied by increased solubility.

3. *Effect of moisture contamination*   Premature contact of the incompletely set cement with water results in the dissolution and leaching of the surface. Varnish application over the exposed cement margin is beneficial.

FILM THICKNESS

The smaller the particle size, less is the film thickness. The thickness is lesser than the size of the particles because, during mixing the particles are crushed and dissolved. The thickness can also be reduced by applying pressure on the casting during seating.

THERMAL PROPERTIES

Zinc phosphate cements are good thermal insulators and may be effective in reducing galvanic effects.

ADHESION PROPERTY

The primary retentive mechanism of zinc phosphate is *micromechanical*. The cemented restoration is held by mechanical interlocking of the set cement with surface roughness on the tooth and restoration.

BIOLOGICAL PROPERTIES

pH of the cement   The acidity is high at the time of insertion due to phosphoric acid. At the time of cementation, the pH is 2 (approx.). As time passes the acidity reduces. By the end of 24 hours the pH is 5.5, which is still in the acidic range (neutral value is 7).

Pulpal response   The pulp response may be classified as *moderate*.

Pulp protection   A thickness of dentin as great as 1.5 mm can be penetrated by the acid of the cement. If dentin is not protected against infiltration of this acid, pulpal injury may occur, especially during the first few hours.

1. Avoid thin mixes.
2. Pulp protection should be carried out in deep cavities through the use of an intervening liner or base
   - Zinc oxide eugenol
   - Calcium hydroxide
   - Cavity varnish
3. Some patients are extremely sensitive to the acid. Cementation of a restoration such as a crown or FDP on to vital teeth can cause severe sensitivity or pain. An anesthesia should be used in these instances.

OPTICAL PROPERTIES

The set cement is opaque.

MANIPULATION

Spatula used   Stainless steel.

Mixing time   1 min. 15 seconds.

Powder to liquid ratio 1.4 g/0.5 mL

A cool glass slab is used in order to delay the setting and allow more powder to be incorporated before the matrix formation occurs. The liquid should be dispensed just before mixing.

Procedure

The powder is added in *small increments*. Mixing is done with stainless spatula using brisk circular motion. Each increment is mixed for 15 to 20 seconds. A large area is covered during mixing in order to dissipate the exothermic heat *(Figs. 8.5A and B)*. Maximum amount of powder should be incorporated in the liquid to ensure minimum solubility and maximum strength. *Note:* An appropriate consistency is attained by addition of more powder to the liquid and not by allowing a thin mix to thicken.

Insertion

The crown should be seated immediately and held under pressure till set. Field of operation should be dry. Varnish is applied at the margins, where the cement is exposed.

ADVANTAGES AND DISADVANTAGES OF ZINC PHOSPHATE

Advantages

1. Long track record with proven reliability.
2. Good compressive strength.

Disadvantages

1. No chemical adhesion. Not indicated if the retention is poor.
2. No anticariogenic property.
3. Pulp irritation.
4. Poor esthetics; cannot be used with translucent (all ceramic) restorations like crowns and veneers.

COPPER CEMENTS

Copper cements are basically modified zinc phosphate cements. Silver salts or copper oxide are sometimes added to the powders of the zinc phosphate cements to increase their *'antibacterial'* properties. Copper cements gradually fell out of favor because of their poor biological properties. It was highly acidic and the copper was considered toxic to the cell. This may have been due to the extremely high copper content (97%) in certain cements (Ames). There has been a renewed interest in copper cements recently. New formulations have come out with lower copper content (2%). It is claimed that these new generation copper cements are safe and is especially recommended for indirect pulp capping and where there is active caries.

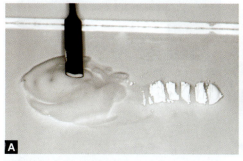 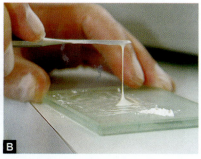

FIGURES 8.5A AND B Manipulation of zinc phosphate. **(A)** The cement is mixed over a large area to dissipate heat. **(B)** Luting consistency.

APPLICATIONS

1. Temporary fillings in children.
2. Intermediate restorations.
3. For retention of silver cap splints in oral surgery.
4. Indirect pulp capping.
5. As base beneath composite restorations.

CLASSIFICATION

Classified according to the percentage of the copper oxide that is used as a replacement for the zinc oxide.

Commercial examples Ames copper (discontinued), Doc's best red and white copper kit ***(Fig. 8.6)***.

COMPOSITION

○ Copper oxide (if cuprous oxide is used—cement is red, if cupric oxide is used, the cement is black)
○ Zinc oxide
○ Liquid used is clear phosphoric acid

PROPERTIES

1. Biological properties: They have poor biological properties. Because its pH is 5.3, it is irritant to the pulp.
2. They are bactericidal or bacteriostatic.

MANIPULATION

The chemistry of the copper cements is very similar to that of the zinc phosphate cements and they are manipulated in the same manner.

ZINC POLYCARBOXYLATE CEMENT

Canadian biochemist Smith developed the first polycarboxylate cement in 1968 by substituting the phosphoric acid of zinc phosphate cement with polyacrylic acid. Polycarboxylate became the first cement system developed with potential for adhesion to tooth structure.

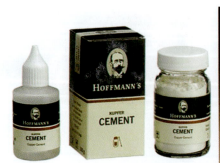
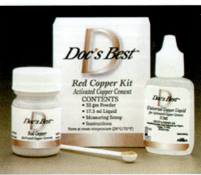

FIGURE 8.6 White and red copper cements.

APPLICATIONS

1. Primarily for luting permanent restorations.
2. As bases and liners.
3. Used in orthodontics for cementation of bands.
4. Also used as root canal fillings in endodontics.

AVAILABLE AS

- ○ Powder and liquid in bottles *(Fig. 8.7A)*
- ○ Water settable cements *(Fig. 8.7B)*
- ○ As precapsulated powder/liquid system

Commercial Examples   Poly F (Dentsply), Durelon and Durelon Maxicap (encapsulated) (3M ESPE), Carboco (Voco), Imibond P (Imicryl), Hy Bond polycarboxylate (Shofu).

Water settable cements

In these cement the polyacid is freeze dried and added to the cement powder. Water is used as the liquid. When the powder is mixed with water, the polyacrylic acid goes into the solution and the reaction proceeds as described for the conventional cements.

COMPOSITION

Powder

Ingredient	Function
Zinc oxide	Basic ingredient
Magnesium oxide	Principal modifier and also aids in sintering
Oxides of bismuth and aluminum	Small amounts
Stannous fluoride	Increases strength, modifies setting time and imparts anti-cariogenic properties

Liquid

Aqueous solution of polyacrylic acid or copolymer of acrylic acid with other unsaturated carboxylic acids, i.e. itaconic, maleic, or tricarballylic acid.

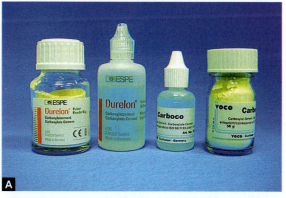
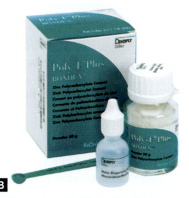

FIGURES 8.7A AND B (A) Representative zinc polycarboxylate cement products. **(B)** A water settable cement.

MANUFACTURE

The powder mixture is sintered at high temperature in order to reduce the reactivity and then ground into fine particles.

SETTING REACTION

When the powder and liquid are mixed, the surface of powder particles are attacked by the acid, releasing zinc, magnesium and tin ions. These ions bind to the polymer chain via the carboxyl groups. They also react with carboxyl groups of adjacent polyacid chains to form cross-linked salts.

Structure of set cement

The hardened cement consists of an amorphous gel matrix of zinc polyacrylate in which unreacted powder particles are dispersed.

PROPERTIES

Mechanical properties

Compressive strength ISO requires a minimum compressive strength of 50 MPa for this cement *(Table 8.1)*. Polycarboxylate cement is inferior to zinc phosphate cement in this respect.

Tensile strength 6.2 MPa. Its tensile strength is slightly higher than that of zinc phosphate cement.

The strength of the cement depends on

- Increase in P/L ratio increases strength.
- Molecular weight of polyacrylic acid also affects strength. A mix from a lower viscosity liquid is weaker.

Solubility and disintegration

It tends to absorb water and is slightly more soluble (0.6% wt) than zinc phosphate. Thus the marginal dissolution is more when used for cementing. It is more soluble in organic acids like lactic acid. Low P/L ratio results in a significantly higher solubility and disintegration in the oral cavity.

Biocompatibility

Pulpal response is classified as mild. Despite the initial acidic nature of polycarboxylate cement, the pH of the liquid is 1.0–1.7 and that of freshly mixed cement is 3.0–4.0. After 24 hours, pH of the cement is 5.0-6.0.

They are less irritant than zinc phosphate cement because:

- The liquid is rapidly neutralized by the powder. The pH of polycarboxylate cement rises more rapidly than that of zinc phosphate.
- Penetration of polyacrylic acid into the dentinal tubules is less because of its higher molecular weight and larger size. The histological reactions are similar to zinc oxide eugenol cements but more reparative dentine is observed with polycarboxylate.

Adhesion

An outstanding characteristic of zinc polycarboxylate cement is that the cement *bonds chemically* with the tooth structure. The *carboxyl group* in the polymer molecules chelates with calcium in the tooth structure.

Bond strength to enamel is 3.4–13.1 MPa and to dentine 2.07 MPa.

TABLE 8.1 Requirements for water based dental cements (ISO 9917-1:2007)

Chemical type	Application	Film thickness mm	Net setting time min		Compressive strength MPa	Acid erosion mm	Opacity $C_{0,70}$		Acid-soluble As content mg/kg	Acid soluble Pb content mg/kg
			max.	min.	min.	max.	min.	max.	max.	max.
Zinc phosphate	Luting	25	2.5	8	50	0.30			2	100
Zinc polycarboxylate	Luting	25	2.5	8	50	0.40			2	100
Glass polyalkenoate	Luting	25	1.5	8	50	0.17				100
Zinc phosphate	Base/lining		2	6	50	0.30			2	100
Zinc polycarboxylate	Base/lining		2	6	50	0.40			2	100
Glass polyalkenoate	Base/lining		1.5	6	50	0.17				100
Glass polyalkenoate	Restoration		1.5	6	100	0.17	0.35	0.90		100

Factors affecting bond

1. A clean dry tooth surface improves bonding.
2. If the inside surface of the metal crown is not clean, the cement cannot bond with the metal. So to improve the mechanical bond, the surface should be carefully abraded with a small stone or with airborne abrasives.
3. The presence of saliva reduces bond strength.
4. Unlike zinc phosphate cements, the adhesion is better to a smooth surface than to a rough surface.
5. Does not adhere to gold or porcelain.
6. Adhesion to stainless steel is excellent. Thus it is used in orthodontics.

Optical properties

They are very opaque due to large quantities of unreacted zinc oxide.

Anticariogenic properties

Some manufacturers have attempted to incorporate fluoride within the cement. However, the fluoride release is limited when compared to glass ionomer cement.

Thermal properties

They are good thermal insulators.

MANIPULATION

CONDITIONING

The tooth structure should be meticulously clean for proper bonding. To clean the surface, 10% polyacrylic acid solution followed by rinsing with water, or 1 to 3% hydrogen peroxide may be used. Then dry and isolate the tooth.

PROPORTIONING

1.5 parts of powder to 1 part of liquid by weight.

PROCEDURE

The powder and liquid are taken on a cooled glass slab. The liquid is dispensed just prior to the mixing, otherwise its viscosity increases. The powder is incorporated into the liquid in bulk (90%) with a stiff cement spatula and remaining powder is added to adjust consistency. The mix appears quite thick, but this cement will flow readily into a thin film when seated under pressure.

MIXING TIME AND SETTING TIMES

Mixing time ranges from 30 to 40 seconds. Setting time can be from 7 to 9 minutes (The setting time can be increased by cooling the glass slab. It also depends on method of manufacture of powder and liquid).

Points to note

o   The cement should be used while the surface is still *glossy*. Loss of lustre indicates that the setting reaction has progressed to an extent that proper wetting of the tooth surface by the mix is no longer possible. If the surface is not creamy and shiny and is matted and tends to form cobwebs, the mix should be discarded.

o   After insertion the excess is not removed immediately as it passes through a *rubbery stage*, it tends to get lifted from the cavity. Remove excess cement only when it has hardened and breaks off.

o   The powder may be cooled, but the liquid should not be cooled since the viscosity of the liquid increases.

Polycarboxylate cement adheres to instruments

o   Use alcohol as release agent for mixing spatula.

o   Instruments should be cleaned before the cement sets.

o   Excess cement from the spatula can be chipped off. Any remaining material is removed by boiling in sodium hydroxide solution.

ADVANTAGES AND DISADVANTAGES

Advantages

1.   Comparatively less irritating to the pulp.
2.   Chemical bond to tooth structure.

Disadvantages

Limited fluoride release when compared to GIC.

ZINC OXIDE EUGENOL CEMENT

These cements have been used extensively in dentistry since the 1890s. Depending on the use they vary widely in their properties. In general, they are cements of low strength. The are the least irritating of all dental cements and are known to have an obtundant (sedative) effect on exposed dentin.

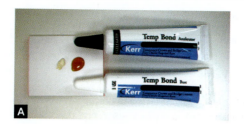

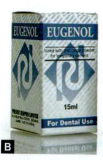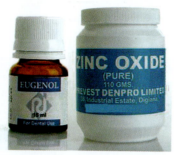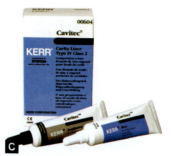

FIGURES 8.8A TO C **(A)** Type I zinc oxide eugenol for temporary cementation. **(B)** Type II zinc oxide eugenol cement for temporary restorations. **(C)** Type II zinc oxide eugenol—cavity liner (was previously Type IV).

To improve the strength many modified zinc oxide eugenol cements have been introduced, e.g. EBA—alumina modified and polymer—reinforced zinc oxide eugenol cements non-eugenol zinc oxide cements are also available. They are suitable for patients sensitive to eugenol.

CLASSIFICATION (ISO 3107:2011)*

Type I—for temporary cementation

Type II—for bases and temporary restorations

The previous version of this classification (ISO 3107:2004) * listing 4 classes, has been replaced by ISO 3107:2011, in which only 2 classes are described. (See also foot note **)

Type I cements are meant for short term luting (1 to 6 weeks—**Fig. 8.8A**). They are used to cement provisional restorations for the period it takes to make the definitive restoration. Permanent restorations are also sometimes cemented for a short period for the patient to try it. They have low strength which allows easy removal of the restoration without damage to the restoration or the tooth.

Type II cements are used for the interim period (few weeks to few months) when a tooth is undergoing treatment or until it is ready for a permanent restoration. They can also be used as bases under non-resin based permanent restorations.

AVAILABLE AS

- ○ Powder and liquid **(Fig. 8.8B)**
- ○ Two paste system **(Fig. 8.8C)**

---

* ISO 3107:2004: Type I ZOE — Temporary cementation: Class I — Setting cement, Class II — non-setting cement; Type II ZOE — Permanent cementation; Type III ZOE — Bases and temporary restorations; Type IV ZOE — Cavity liners
** A version of this classification in a popular US reference book described as ISO 3107 (Type I to Type IV with Type IV listed as intermediate filling), could not be verified in any of the original ISO sources.

Representative commercial names

	Unmodified	EBA modified	Polymer modified	Noneugenol
Type I	TempBond		TempBond clear	Nogenol, Zone Freegenol TempBond NE
Type II	DPI zinc oxide Cavitec (Kerr)	SuperEBA	IRM, Kalzinol	

COMPOSITION

Powder

Ingredient	Weight (%)	Function
Zinc oxide	69.0	Principal ingredient
White rosin	29.3	To reduce brittleness of set cement
Zinc stearate	1.0	Accelerator, plasticizer
Zinc acetate	0.7	Accelerator, improves strength
Magnesium oxide		Is added in some powders, acts with eugenol in a similar manner as zinc oxide

Liquid

Ingredient	Weight (%)	Function
Eugenol	85.0	Reacts with zinc oxide
Olive oil	15.0	Plasticizer

*Some powders may contain arsenic. ISO 3107 specifies maximum permissible arsenic content of 2 mg/kg.

SETTING REACTION

The setting reaction and microstructure are the same as that of the zinc oxide eugenol impression pastes.

In the first reaction hydrolysis of zinc oxide takes place. Water is *essential* for the reaction (dehydrated zinc oxide will not react with dehydrated eugenol).

$$ZnO + H_2O \rightarrow Zn(OH)_2$$

The reaction proceeds as a typical acid-base reaction.

$$Zn(OH)_2 + 2HE \rightarrow ZnE_2 + 2H_2O$$

Base	Acid	Salt
(Zinc hydroxide)	(Eugenol)	(Zinc eugenolate)

The chelate formed is an amorphous gel that tends to crystallize imparting strength to the set mass.

Structure of set cement

Thus, the set cement consists of particles of zinc oxide embedded in a matrix of zinc eugenolate.

Type	Setting time at 37 °C min		Compressive strength at 24/h MPa		Film thickness µm	Acid-soluble arsenic mass fraction mg/kg[a]
	min.	max.	min.	max.	max.	max.
Type I	1,5	10		35	25	2
Type II	1,5	10	5		N/A	2

TABLE 8.2 Requirements of ZOE cement as per ISO 3107:2011

GENERAL PROPERTIES OF ZINC OXIDE EUGENOL CEMENTS

Mechanical properties

Compressive strength   They are relatively weak cements. The strength depends on what it is used for, e.g. cements intended for temporary purposes like temporary restorations and cementation will have a lower strength. The compressive strength, therefore, ranges from a low of 5 to 55 MPa. Minimum requirements are presented in *Table 8.2*.

> Type I   6 to 28 MPa   (ISO—maximum of 35 MPa)
>
> Type II   45 to 55 MPa   (ISO—minimum of 5 MPa)

Particle size affects the strength. In general the smaller the particle size, the stronger the cement. The strength can also be increased by reinforcing with alumina-EBA or polymers (see EBA and polymer modified ZOE cements).

Tensile strength   Ranges from 0.32 to 5.3 MPa.

Modulus of elasticity (0.22 to 5.4 GPa)   This is an important property for those cements intended for use as bases.

Thermal properties

Thermal conductivity   3.98 [Cal. Sec-1 cm-2 (°C/cm)-1] $\times$ 10^{-4}. Their thermal insulating properties are excellent and are approximately the same as for human dentin. The thermal conductivity of zinc oxide eugenol is in the range of insulators like cork and asbestos.

Coefficient of thermal expansion $35 \times 10^{-6}/°C$.

Solubility and disintegration

The solubility of the set cement is highest among the cements (0.4 to 1.5 % wt). They disintegrate in oral fluids. This break down is due to hydrolysis of the zinc eugenolate matrix to form zinc hydroxide and eugenol. Solubility is reduced by increasing the powder/liquid (P/L) ratio.

Film thickness

This property is important for those cements (Type I) used for luting of restorations. The film thickness of zinc oxide eugenol cements (ISO maximum of 25 µm) is generally higher than other cements.

Adhesion

They do not adhere well to enamel or dentin. This is one reason why they are not often used for final cementation of crowns and other fixed dental prosthesis. The other reasons are low strength and high solubility.

Biological properties

1. pH and effect on pulp (pH is 6.6 to 8.0): They are the least irritating of all cements. Pulpal response—classified as mild.
2. Bacteriostatic and obtundent properties: They inhibit the growth of bacteria and have an anodyne or soothing effect (obtundent) on the pulp in deep cavities, reducing pain.
3. Eugenol is irritating to skin and eyes. Repeated contact may cause allergic dermatitis.

Optical properties

The set cement is opaque.

Material interactions

Eugenol interferes with the hardening/and or cause softening of resin based restorations and are therefore contraindicated as a base under these restorations.

MANIPULATION

Powder/liquid system

Powder/liquid ratio   4:1 to 6:1 by weight.

The bottles are shaken gently. Measured quantity of powder and liquid is dispensed onto a cool glass slab. The bulk of the powder is incorporated into the liquid and spatulated thoroughly in a circular motion with a stiff bladed stainless steel spatula. Zinc oxide eugenol exhibits *pseudothickening*. Although it appears to thicken early during spatulation. Further vigorous spatulation or stropping loosens the mix. Smaller increments are then added until the mix is complete.

For temporary restorations a thick *putty-like* consistency is recommended.

Oil of orange is used to clean eugenol cement from instruments.

Two paste system

Equal lengths of each paste are dispersed and mixed until a uniform color is observed.

Setting time

4–10 minutes.

ZOE cements set quicker in the mouth due to moisture and heat.

Factors affecting setting time

The complete reaction between zinc oxide and eugenol takes about 12 hours. This is too slow for clinical convenience.

1. *Manufacture* The most active zinc oxide powders are those formed from zinc salts like zinc hydroxide and zinc carbonate by heating at 3,000 °C.
2. *Particle size* Smaller zinc oxide particles set faster.
3. *Accelerators* Alcohol, glacial acetic acid and water.
4. *Heat* Cooling the glass slab, slows the reaction.
5. *Retarders* The set can be retarded with glycol and glycerine.
6. *Powder to liquid ratio* Higher the ratio, faster the set.

MODIFIED ZINC OXIDE EUGENOL CEMENTS

These were introduced to improve some of the shortcomings of the regular unmodified zinc oxide eugenol. The modified ZOE cements are

- ○ EBA-Alumina modified cements
- ○ Polymer reinforced

EBA-ALUMINA MODIFIED CEMENTS

These are modified ZOE cements *(Fig. 8.9)*. It is available as a white powder and a pinkish liquid. Its greater strength allows its use as an intermediate filling material and as a base. A part of the liquid is substituted by orthoethoxy benzoic acid. Alumina is added to the powder. These cements are increasing in popularity as a retrograde filling material because of the high cost of MTA.

USES

1. Long-term cementation.
2. Temporary and intermediate restorations.
3. Root end filling material.

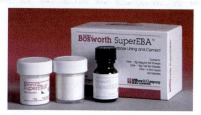

FIGURE 8.9 EBA cement.

COMPOSITION

Powder		Liquid	
Ingredient	*Weight (%)*	*Ingredient*	*Weight (%)*
Zinc oxide	60–75	EBA	
(orthoethoxy benzoic acid)	62.5		
Fused Quartz or Alumina	0–35	Eugenol	37.5
Hydrogenated Rosin	6		

PROPERTIES

Their properties are better than that of unmodified ZOE. They are more easier to handle and have improved carvability.

1. Compressive strength is higher—55 to 60 MPa (8000 psi)
2. Tensile strength—4.1 MPa (600 psi)
3. Modulus of elasticity—2.5 GPa (0.36 psi × 106)
4. Film thickness—25 µm
5. Solubility and disintegration in water—0.05% wt. Despite their low solubility, these cements disintegrated and wore more quickly clinically when compared to the polymer modified zinc oxide cements.
6. Effect on pulp—these cements are relatively mild to the pulp.
7. Adhesion—these materials adhere well to tooth structure.

MANIPULATION

A glass slab is recommended for EBA-alumina modified cements. After dispensing, the powder is incorporated into the liquid in bulk, kneaded for 30 seconds and then stropped for

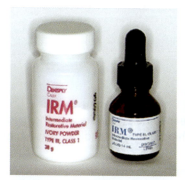
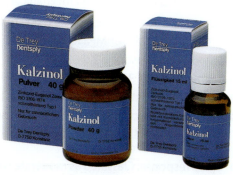

FIGURE 8.10 IRM and Kalzinol are two popular resin modified zinc oxide cements for intermediate restorations (Type II).

an additional 60 seconds with broad strokes of the spatula to obtain a creamy consistency. They have long working times.

Setting time

9.5 minutes.

POLYMER REINFORCED ZINC OXIDE EUGENOL CEMENT

The modifications take the form of resins added to the powder or the liquid. The aim is to improve the strength and reduce the solubility of the cement. Resin-modified cements are among the strongest of the zinc oxide eugenol based cements. Their high strength and low wear make them ideal intermediate restorative materials that can last as long as 1 year.

USES

1.   Luting agent
2.   As base
3.   As temporary filling material

Available as   1. Powder and liquid. 2. Capsule for mechanical mixing.

Commercial Names   IRM (Dentsply) and Kalzinol (DPI) *(Fig. 8.10).*

COMPOSITION

Powder		Liquid	
Ingredient	*Weight (%)*	*Ingredient*	*Weight (%)*
Zinc oxide	80	Eugenol	
Finely divided natural or synthetic resins	20	Acetic acid	Accelerator
		Thymol	Antimicrobial

The zinc oxide powder is surface treated. The combination of surface treatment and polymer reinforcement results in good strength, improved abrasion resistance and toughness.

SETTING REACTION

The setting reaction is similar to zinc oxide eugenol cements. Acidic resins if present, may react with zinc oxide, strengthening the matrix.

PROPERTIES

These cements have improved mechanical properties.

○   Compressive strength: 48 MPa (7000 psi)
○   Tensile strength: 4.1 MPa (600 psi)
○   Modulus of elasticity: 2.5 GPa
○   Film thickness: 32 μm
○   Solubility and disintegration: 0.03% wt
○   Material interactions: Similar to ZOE these materials interfere with the hardening/ and o▪ cause softening of composites and are therefore contraindicated as a base under resir based restorations.
○   Pulp response: Classified as moderate which is similar to unmodified ZOE.
○   Improved abrasion resistance and toughness.

MANIPULATION

The proper powder/liquid is dispensed on a dry glass slab. 50 percent of the powder is mixed into the liquid and the remainder in small portions with vigorous spatulation or stropping. The mix will appear quite stiff, however continued stropping for an additional 5 to 10 seconds improves plasticity (known as shear thinning effect).

After mixing, the plastic zinc oxide eugenol is swiped into the tooth cavity and condensed using a moist cotton pellet.

Working time These cements have a long working time.

Setting time 6 to 10 minutes. Heat and moisture in the mouth cause it to set faster than on the mixing pad.

Factors affecting setting time

1. Low powder-liquid ratio increases setting time
2. Moisture accelerates setting time.
3. Cooling the glass slab slows the setting.

OTHER ZINC OXIDE EUGENOL PRODUCTS

ENDODONTIC SEALERS

Zinc oxide eugenol is very popular as an endodontic sealer. Two traditional formulations— Rickert's formula and Grossman's formula are very popular. Along with gutta-percha, these materials are used in endodontic therapy to seal the canals. Some materials are used as therapeutic sealers and are formulated with ingredients such as iodoform, paraformaldehyde or trioxymethylene which have therapeutic value. Others contain antibiotics such as tetracyclines and steroids as anti-inflammatory agents. Some formulations can also be used for pulp capping. Endodontic sealers also contain radiopaque materials such as barium sulphate, bismuth salts or silver powder. These products are discussed in further detail in a subsequent section.

ZINC OXIDE/ZINC SULPHATE CEMENTS

These are single component temporary filling materials. Their main advantage is their ease of placement.

SUPPLIED AS

As putty in small tubes, syringes or plastic containers ***(Fig. 8.11)***.

Representative products Cavit (ESPE), Caviton (GC), Coltosol (Coltene).

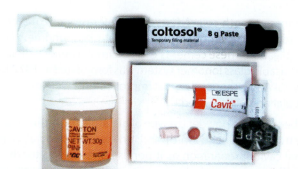

FIGURE 8.11 Various zinc oxide/ sulphate temporary restorations.

USE

Short-term restorations after caries excavation, root canal therapy, etc.

COMPOSITION

○ Zinc oxide 40–60 %
○ Zinc sulphate-1-hydrate 1–20 %
○ Calcium sulphate-hemihydrate 15–35 %
○ Ethylene bis (oxyethylene) diacetate - 15–35 %
○ Barium sulphate 0–20 %
○ Poly (vinyl acetate)
○ Diatomaceous earth

SETTING REACTION

The material sets by reacting with water which it absorbs from the mouth or from the cavity. The setting occurs slowly. It expands on setting.

PROPERTIES

It may be white or pink colored putty-consistency material. It has good initial sealing. Since it expands on setting (up to 18%), the marginal seal is further improved. The seal gradually decreases with time as it disintegrates. Unfortunately, the strength is low and its life is short. The material should be used for not more than 1 to 2 weeks. It slowly disintegrates with time and is therefore not indicated for any longer term temporary restorations. The material is radiopaque. Short-term pain may be experienced because of dehydration of the cavity.

MANIPULATION

The material is dispensed and inserted into the cavity using a cement carrier. The container should be closed immediately. It is condensed into the cavity using a plastic filling instrument (condenser). Since it sets by hydration, the cavity should not be fully dried before placing the material.

Setting time

The surface hardens in about 20 to 30 minutes. Complete hardening takes place in 2 to 3 hours.

GLASS IONOMER CEMENTS

Glass ionomer cements are adhesive tooth-colored anticariogenic restorative materials which were originally used for restorations of eroded areas. Current glass ionomers have been modified to allow a wider application. These cements evolved from a general dissatisfaction with silicate cements. The first usable glass ionomer system was formulated in **1972** by **Wilson and Kent** and was known as ASPA. Subsequently great improvements were made and today these materials are very popular and widely used.

It was named glass ionomer because, the powder is a type of glass and the setting reaction and adhesive bonding to tooth structure is due to ionic bond. Unlike other restorative materials, this cement requires minimal cavity preparation as it bonds adhesively to tooth structure. Compared to composite resin they are less technique sensitive. Glass ionomer cement is often known as a *biomimetic* material, because of its similar mechanical properties to dentine. For this reason it is one of the most popular cements in dentistry.

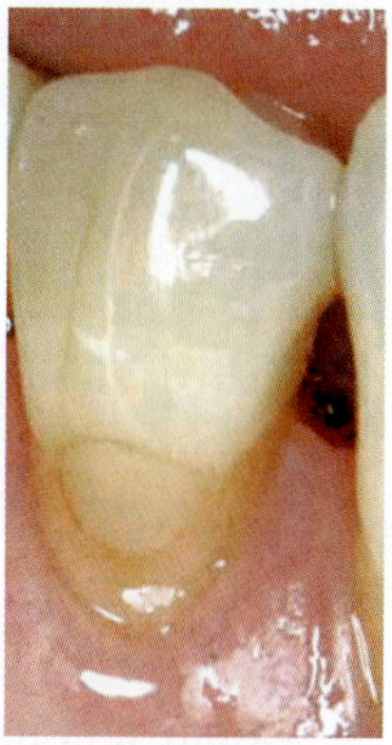

Synonyms
○ Poly (alkenoate) cement
○ GIC (glass ionomer cement)
○ ASPA (alumino silicate polyacrylic acid)

APPLICATION

1. Anterior esthetic restorative material for Class III cavities.
2. Restorative material for eroded areas and Class V restorations *(Fig. 8.12)*.
3. As a luting agent for restorations and orthodontic brackets.
4. As liners and bases.
5. For core build up.
6. To a limited extent as pit and fissure sealants.
7. Intermediate restorative material.
8. Atraumatic restorative treatment (ART) technique.

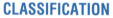

FIGURE 8.12 A four-year-old glass ionomer restoration.

Glass ionomer cements are not recommended for Class II and Class VI restorations, since they lack fracture toughness and are susceptible to wear.

CLASSIFICATION

The general ISO classification of cements apply to glass ionomer (ISO 9917-1:2007)*

a. Luting
b. Bases and liners
c. Restorations

Difference between various types

The various types of GIC cements are chemically identical. They vary primarily in the powder/liquid ratio and particle size. The GICs used for luting have a lower powder/liquid ratio and a smaller particle size when compared to the restorative variety. These features enable the luting GIC to have a thinner film and better flow.

They may also be classified as

1. Conventional GIC
2. Resin-modified GIC
3. Metal-modified GIC

Representative commercial products

Aquacem, Fuji I — Luting
Ketac bond   — Bases and liners
Chem Fil, Fuji II — Restorations
Vitra bond   — Light cure GIC

AVAILABLE AS

1. Powder/liquid in bottles *(Figs. 8.13 and 8.14)*

* see footnotes on page 85

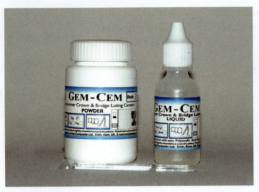 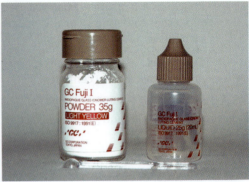

FIGURE 8.13 Representative glass ionomer luting cements (Type I).

2. Preproportioned powder/liquid in capsules
3. Light cure system
4. Powder/distilled water (water settable type)

COMPOSITION

Powder

The powder is an acid-soluble calcium fluoroaluminosilicate glass. It is similar to that of silicate, but has a higher alumina-silica ratio. This increases its reactivity with liquid.

Ingredient	Weight (%)
Silica (SiO_2)	41.9
Alumina (Al_2O_3)	28.6
Aluminum fluoride (AlF_3)	1.6
Calcium fluoride (CaF_2)	15.7
Sodium fluoride (NaF)	9.3
Aluminum phosphate ($AlPO_4$)	3.8

The fluoride component acts as a 'ceramic flux'. Lanthanum, strontium, barium or zinc oxide additions provide radiopacity.

Liquid

Originally the liquid was a 50% aqueous solution of polyacrylic acid. It was very viscous and had a tendency to gel. Modern glass ionomer liquids are in the form of copolymers.

Component	Function
Polyacrylic acid in the form of copolymer with itaconic acid, maleic acid and tricarballylic acid	*Copolymerizing* with itaconic, maleic acid, etc. tends to increase reactivity of the liquid, decrease viscosity and reduce tendency for gelation.
Tartaric acid	Improves the handling characteristics, increases working time and shortens setting time.
Water	*Water* is the most important constituent of the cement liquid, it is the medium of reaction and it hydrates the reaction products. The amount of water in the liquid is critical. Too much water results in a weak cement. Too little water impairs the reaction and subsequent hydration.

Water settable cements

The polyacrylic acid copolymer is *freeze dried* and then added to the glass ionomer powder. The liquid is water or water with tartaric acid. An example of a water settable cement is shown in *Figure 8.14.*

When the powder is mixed with water, the polyacrylic acid powder goes into solution to form liquid acid. Then the chemical reaction takes place as in the conventional powder and liquid systems. These cements are known as water settable cements and they set *faster* than those with polyacrylic acid.

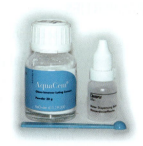

FIGURE 8.14 Water settable glass ionomer luting cement.

MANUFACTURE

The components are sintered at 1100 °C to 1500 °C. The glass is then ground to particle sizes ranging from 15 to 50 um.

SETTING REACTION

Leaching When the powder and liquid are mixed together, the acid attacks the glass particles. Thus calcium, aluminum, sodium and fluoride ions leach out into the aqueous medium.

Calcium cross-links The initial set occurs when the calcium ions cross-links (binds) the polyacrylic acid chains. This forms a solid mass.

Aluminum cross-links In the next phase, the aluminum also begins to cross-link with polyacrylic acid chains.

Sodium and fluorine ions These ions do not take part in the cross-linking. Some of the sodium ions may replace the hydrogen ions in the carboxylic groups. The rest combine with fluorine to form sodium fluoride which is uniformly distributed within the cement.

Hydration Water plays a very important role in the cement. Initially it serves as the medium. Later it slowly hydrates the matrix, adding to the strength of the cement (maturation process).

Silica gel sheath The unreacted glass (powder) particle is sheathed (covered) by a silica gel. It is formed by the leaching of the ions (Ca^{2+}, Al^{3+}, Na^+, F^-) from the outer portion of the glass particle.

Structure of set cement

The set cement *(Fig. 8.15)* consists of agglomeration of unreacted powder particles surrounded by a silica gel sheath and embedded in an matrix of hydrated calcium and aluminum cross-linked polyacrylic gel.

Sensitivity to air and moisture

Exposure of the cement to water before the hardening reaction is complete, leads to loss of cations and anions which form

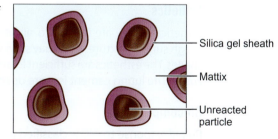

FIGURE 8.15 Representation of structure of set glass ionomer.

the matrix as they can be dissolved. Thus it is very important to protect the cement surface (by applying varnish, etc.) after it is placed in the mouth.

PROPERTIES

Some of minimum requirements for the different types of GI cements are presented in *Table 8.1*.

Mechanical properties

Compressive strength   Because of differences in the powder-liquid ratio GIC used for different applications show variations in their physical properties. Restorative GIC has a compressive strength of 150 MPa. The luting GIC has a lower compressive strength of about 85 MPa.

Tensile strength   Luting type—6.2 MPa

                          Restorative type—6.6 MPa

Hardness (49 KHN)   Less harder than silicates. The hardness is also far lower when compared to composites.

Fracture toughness   A measure of energy required to produce fracture. Type II GIC's are far inferior to composites in this respect.

Elastic modulus (7.3 GPa)   It is a measure of their stiffness. The MOE is half that of zinc phosphate cement.

Wear resistance   They are more susceptible to tooth brush abrasion and occlusal wear when compared to composites.

Solubility and disintegration

The initial solubility is high due to leaching of intermediate products. The complete setting reaction takes place in 24 hours; therefore, the cement should be protected from saliva in the mouth during this period. Glass ionomer cements are more resistant to attack by organic acids.

○   Solubility in water for Luting type—1.25% wt.

○   Solubility in water for Restorative type—0.4% wt.

Adhesion

It adheres well to enamel and dentin. Shear bond strength ranges from 3–5 MPa.

Mechanism of adhesion Glass ionomer bonds chemically to tooth structure. The exact mechanism has not been fully understood. The bonding is due to the reaction between the carboxyl groups of the polyacids and the calcium in the enamel and dentin. The bond to enamel is always higher than that to dentin, probably due to the greater inorganic content of enamel and its greater homogeneity.

Esthetics

Esthetically they are inferior to silicates and composites. They lack translucency and have a rough surface texture. They may stain with time. The restorative GICs are available in different shades. The esthetics are sufficient for restoring cervical lesions and minor defects in nonesthetic zones. The luting cement is more opaque than the restorative cement.

Biocompatibility

Pulpal response to GIC is classified as *mild*.

Type II glass ionomers are relatively biocompatible. The pulpal reaction is greater than that from zinc oxide eugenol cements but less than that produced by zinc phosphate cement. Polyacids are relatively weak acids.

The water settable cements show higher acidity. Luting type GIC is more acidic than Restorative type because of the lower powder/liquid ratio. Occasionally sensitive patients show a painful response to GIC luting cement.

Pulp protection   In deep cavities, the smear layer should not be removed as it acts as a barrier to acid penetration. Deep areas are protected by a thin layer of calcium hydroxide cement.

Anticariogenic properties

Type II glass ionomer releases fluoride in amounts comparable to silicate cements initially and continue to do so over an extended period of time.

In addition, due to its adhesive effect they have the potential for reducing infiltration of oral fluids at the cement-tooth interface, thereby preventing secondary caries.

MANIPULATION

○ Conditioning of tooth surface.

○ Proper manipulation.

○ Protection of cement during setting.

○ Finishing.

PREPARATION OF TOOTH SURFACE

The tooth should be clean for effective adhesion of cement. The smear layer present after cavity preparation tends to block off the tooth surface and so should be removed to achieve adhesive bonding.

This is achieved by

○ Rubbing with a cotton pellet and pumice slurry

○ Etching with 10% polyacrylic acid or 37% phosphoric acid.

(The objective is to remove the smear layer but still leave the collagenous plug in place. The plug acts as a barrier to the penetration of acid from the cement).

Conditioning   This is achieved with 10% polyacrylic acid or 37% phosphoric acid for about 10 to 20 seconds. Next rinse with water for 20 seconds. Very deep areas of the preparation should be protected by a dab of calcium hydroxide.

After conditioning and rinsing, the surface is dried but not desiccated. It should be kept free of saliva or blood as these will interfere with bonding. If contaminated the whole procedure is repeated.

PROPORTIONING AND MIXING

Powder/liquid ratio

Powder/liquid ratio varies according to the type of GIC and intended use.

Most manufacturers provide a plastic scoop which is useful for measuring. The manufacturers recommended ratio should be followed. Low P/L ratio reduces mechanical properties and increase the chances of cement degradation. Moisture contamination alters the acid-water balance.

Spatula used   Stiff plastic or metal spatula.

Mixing

Manual mixing   The powder bottle is tumbled gently. The powder and liquid is dispensed just prior to mixing. A nonabsorbent paper pad or a cool and dry glass slab may be used.

The powder is divided into two or more increments *(Figs. 8.16A to C)*. The first increment is incorporated rapidly into the mix with a stiff bladed spatula in about 5–10 seconds. The material should not be spread over a large area. Subsequent increments are incorporated and mixed using a swiping and folding technique. The material is collected and folded on to itself. Total mixing time should not exceed 30–40 seconds.

A good mix should have a glossy surface *(Fig. 8.17A)*. This indicates the presence of residual polyacid (which has not been used up in the setting reaction) and ensures proper bonding to the tooth. A mix with dull surface *(Fig. 8.17B)* is discarded as it indicates prolonged mixing and reduces the adhesion.

Mixing time   45 seconds.

Insertion   The mix is packed into the cavity without delay using a plastic filling instrument. If the mix loses its gloss or forms a skin it should be discarded.

Mechanical mixing   GIC supplied in capsule form containing preproportioned powder and liquid is mixed in an amalgam triturator. The capsule has a nozzle and so the mix can be injected directly into the cavity or crown *(Figs. 8.18A and B)*.

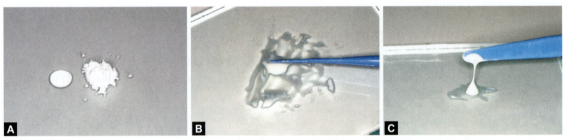

FIGURES 8.16A TO C (A) Dispensed powder and liquid. **(B)** Mixing of glass ionomer. **(C)** Mixed glass ionomer showing right consistency for luting.

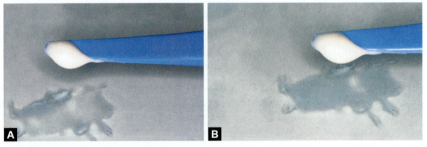

FIGURES 8.17A AND B (A) A good mix should have a *glossy surface*. This indicates the presence of residual polyacid and ensures proper bonding to the tooth. **(B)** A mix with dull surface (right) is discarded.

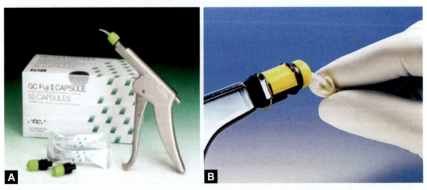

FIGURES 8.18A AND B (A) Glass ionomer in capsule form. Mixing is done in a triturator (similar to an amalgam triturator). **(B)** The cement is expressed through the nozzle with the help of a special gun.

Consistency after mixing

This varies according to the type of GIC and its intended use. For example, restorative consistency differs from luting consistency. For *luting* the material should have sufficient flow to ensure complete seating. Care should be taken not to make it too fluid as it can reduce strength. For restorations, a thicker consistency is required to provide sufficient body for manipulation and placement into the cavity. In the ART (atraumatic restorative treatment) technique the material has a very heavy or putty like consistency for improved packability.

Advantages

1. Better properties due to controlled P/L ratio.
2. Less mixing time required.
3. Convenient delivery system.

Disadvantages

1. Cement quantity limited by the manufacturer.
2. Shade selection is limited, colors cannot be blended.

Setting time

Luting type — 7 minutes

Restorative type — 4 to 5 minutes

PROTECTION AND SHAPING OF CEMENT DURING SETTING

Glass ionomer cement is sensitive to air and water during setting. It should be protected from moisture contamination as well as drying during setting and for a few days after setting. After placement into the cavity, a *preshaped matrix* **(Figs. 8.19A and B)** may be applied to

1. Protect the cement from the environment while setting.
2. Provide maximum contour so that minimal finishing is required.
3. Ensure adequate adaptation on to the walls of the cavity.

PROTECTION OF CEMENT AFTER SETTING

The matrix is removed after complete set. Immediately after removal, the cement surface is again protected from drying with

1. A special varnish supplied by manufacturer, or
2. An unfilled light cured resin bonding agent, or
3. Cocoa butter or petroleum jelly

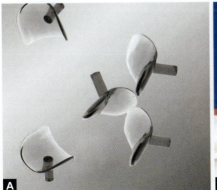
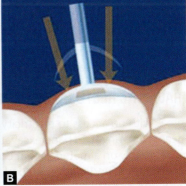

FIGURES 8.19A AND B **(A)** Commercially available cervical matrixes. **(B)** Demonstration of matrix application.

This protects the cement from drying while the dentist proceeds with the finishing. Failure to protect the cement surface from contact with air results in a chalky or crazed surface.

The causes for chalky or crazed surface are

○ Inadequate protection of freshly set cement (from air)
○ Low powder/liquid ratio
○ Improper manipulation

FINISHING

Excess material is trimmed from the margins. Hand instruments are preferred to rotary tools to avoid ditching. Further finishing if required is done after 24 hours.

Before dismissing the patient, the restoration is again coated with the protective agent to protect the trimmed areas. Failure to protect the cement from saliva for the first 24 hours can weaken the cement.

Precautions

1. If the liquid contains polyacids, it should not be placed in a refrigerator as it becomes very viscous.
2. The restorations must be protected from drying at all times, even when other dental procedures are to be carried out later.
3. The glass slab should not be below dew point, as moisture may condense on the slab and change the acid-water balance.

PACKABLE GLASS IONOMER FOR POSTERIOR RESTORATIONS

A packable GIC (Fuji VIII for anterior teeth and Fuji IX *or posterior teeth—**Figs. 8.20A and B***) with a dough like consistency is available as a cheaper alternative to compomers and composites for posterior restorations.

Indications for packable GIC

1. Pediatric and geriatric restorations.
2. Intermediate restorative material.
3. Permanent restorative material in non-stress zones.
4. As a core material.

Advantages

1. Higher wear resistance than conventional GICs.
2. Packable and pressable.
3. Fluoride release.
4. Simple to place (single step).
5. Less technique sensitive

ATRAUMATIC RESTORATIVE DENTISTRY (ART)

In areas with no access to electricity or equipment, patients may be treated using the ART concept which involves hand excavation of caries. Since hand excavation is often incomplete, one has to rely on a materials that bonds adhesively to enamel and release fluoride in order to protect teeth under adverse conditions. The material of choice in this case is packable GIC *(Figs 8.20A and B)*.

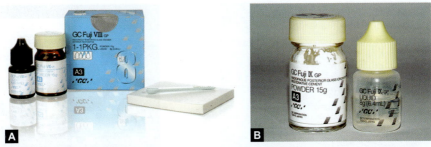

FIGURES 8.20A AND B High viscosity GIC. **(A)** Fuji VIII for anterior. **(B)** Fuji IX for posterior.

FISSURE SEALING (SPECIAL APPLICATIONS)

The traditional glass ionomer cement is somewhat viscous, which prevents penetration to the depth of the fissure. Thus the fissure orifice in general must exceed 100 um in width. Fissures or pits that are smaller are better treated with acid etching and light cured resin sealants. The use of glass ionomer in sealant therapy will increase as formulations are developed that are less viscous (e.g. light cured) and have good wear resistance.

MODIFIED GLASS IONOMERS

Over the years glass ionomer has been modified by manufacturers in order to compensate for some of their deficiencies. This has resulted in new products. The modified glass ionomers are:

1. Metal modified GIC
2. Resin modified GIC

METAL MODIFIED GLASS IONOMER CEMENT

Metal-reinforced glass ionomer cements were first introduced in 1977 to improve the strength, fracture toughness and resistance to wear and yet maintain the potential for adhesion and anticariogenic property. The addition of silver-amalgam alloy powder to conventional materials also provided radiodensity. Subsequently, silver particles were sintered onto the glass and a new product called cermet was launched. These materials are currently considered old-fashioned, as the conventional glass ionomer cements have comparable physical properties and far better esthetics.

TYPES

Two methods are employed

1. *Silver alloy admixed*   Spherical amalgam alloy powder is mixed with restorative type GIC powder (Miracle Mix—*Fig. 8.21*).
2. *Cermet*   Silver particles are *bonded* to glass particles. This is done by sintering a mixture of the two powders at a high temperature (Ketac-Silver) *(Fig. 8.22)*.

USES

1. Restoration of small Class I cavities as an alternative to amalgam or composite resins. They are particularly useful in young patients who are prone to caries.
2. For core-build up of grossly destructed teeth.

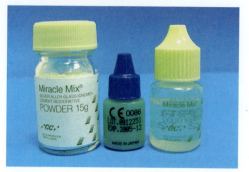

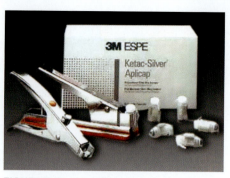

FIGURE 8.21 Miracle Mix. The bottle in the center contains the silver alloy. **FIGURE 8.22** Ketac-Silver.

PROPERTIES

Mechanical properties

1. The *strength* of either type of metal modified cement (150 MPa) is not greatly improved over that of conventional cement.
2. *Diametral tensile* strength of the cement is similar to conventional GIC.
3. The *fracture toughness* of metal modified GIC is similar to that of conventional GIC.
4. In the mouth both metal modified and conventional GIC appear to have similar wear rates.

From the above properties it is clear that there is no appreciable advantage of using metal modified GIC over conventional GIC. The clinical performance of cermet cements is considered to be inferior to other restorative materials, so much so that their use is now discouraged.

Anticariogenic property

Both metal modified ionomers have anticariogenic capability due to leaching of fluoride. However, less fluoride is released from Cermet cement than restorative GIC, since the glass particle is *metal coated*. On the other hand the admixed cement releases more fluoride than restorative GIC. Here the metal filler particles are *not bonded* to the cement matrix and thus there are *pathways* for fluid exchange. This increases leaching of fluoride.

Esthetics

These materials are gray in color because of metallic phases within them; therefore, they are unsuitable for use in anterior teeth.

RESIN-MODIFIED GLASS IONOMER

These are relatively new materials having various names like compomer, resin-ionomers, RMGI (resin-modified glass ionomer), light cured GIC, dual cure GIC, tricure GIC, reinforced GIC, hybrid ionomers, etc. These materials were developed to overcome some of the drawbacks of conventional GIC like

1. Moisture sensitivity
2. Low initial strength
3. Fixed working times.

CLASSIFICATION

Depending on which is the predominant component. These materials may be classified as (McClean *et al*).

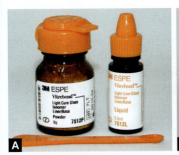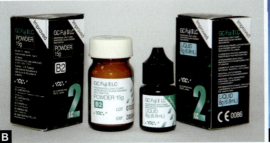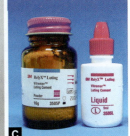

FIGURES 8.23A TO C Resin-modified glass ionomer cements. **(A)** A light cured base/liner. **(B)** GC's Fuji II LC is a radiopaque light cured restorative cement. **(C)** Resin-modified luting cement.

1. *Resin-modified glass ionomer cement* (RMGI), e.g. Fuji II LC *(Figs. 8.23A to C)*, Vitremer, Photac Fil, etc.
2. *Compomers or polyacid-modified composites (PMC),* e.g. Dyract Variglass VLC (this category will be discussed subsequently under the heading compomers).

Uses

1. Restoration of Class I, III or V cavities.
2. Bases and liners.
3. As adhesives for orthodontic brackets.
4. Cementation of crowns and FDPs.
5. Repair of damaged amalgam cores or cusps.
6. Retrograde root filling.

Note   Uses vary according to brand.

SUPPLIED AS

They are supplied as

○ Chemical cure (acid-base setting reaction of the glass ionomer portion).
○ Dual cure (combines acid-base setting reaction of the GIC portion and light curing of the resin portion).
○ Tricure (combines acid-base setting reaction, chemical and light cured polymerization of the resin portion).

All of them are usually supplied as *powder* and *liquid*. The light cured type is supplied in *dark shaded* bottles (for light protection).

COMPOSITION

Since these are combination materials, they contain components of both resin and glass ionomer. However, their proportions vary.

Powder	Liquid
Ion leachable glasses (silica, alumina)	Polyacrylic acid
Photoinitiators or chemical initiators or both	Water
Polymerizable resin	Methacrylate monomer
Hydroxyethyl methacrylate monomers	

SETTING REACTION

Setting includes both polymerization and acid-base reaction. The initial setting occurs by polymerization of the methacrylate groups giving it a high early strength. Polymerization may be light cured or chemical cured depending on the type of cement. Subsequently the acid-base reaction sets it thereby completing the setting reaction and giving the cement its final strength.

MANIPULATION

RMGI is mixed and applied after conditioning the tooth with polyacrylic acid (10–25%). The powder and liquid is mixed according to the manufacturer's instruction. Light cured RMGI is cured by exposure to blue light (which is used for curing composite).

PROPERTIES

Strength

The compressive strength is slightly lower (105 MPa) when compared to conventional GIC. The diametral tensile strength is however greater (20 MPa). They have a greater fracture toughness because of the greater resilience of the resin component.

Hardness

The hardness (40 KHN) is comparable to that of conventional GIC.

Adhesion

The bonding mechanism to tooth structure is similar to that of conventional GIC. Micromechanical retention also plays a role in the bonding process. These materials bond better to composite resins than conventional GIC. This may be because of the presence of residual unreacted monomers within the RMGI.

Microleakage

These materials have a greater amount of microleakage when compared to GIC. This may be partly due to the polymerization shrinkage and partly due to the reduced wetting of the tooth by the cement.

Anticariogenicity

These materials have a significant anticariogenic effect because of the fluoride release. Some tests indicate fluoride release may be equivalent to that of conventional GIC.

Pulpal response

The pulpal response to the cement is mild (similar to conventional GIC).

Esthetics

They are more translucent and therefore more esthetic than conventional GIC. This is due to the closeness of the refractive indices of the powder and the monomer in the liquid.

CALCIUM HYDROXIDE CEMENT

Calcium hydroxide is a relatively weak cement commonly employed as direct or indirect pulp capping agents. Due to their alkaline nature they also serve as a protective barrier against irritants from certain restorations.

A light cured calcium hydroxide base material and a calcium hydroxide root canal sealing paste is also available.

APPLICATIONS

1. For direct and indirect pulp capping.
2. As low strength bases beneath restorations for pulp protection.
3. Apexification procedure in young permanent teeth where root formation is incomplete.

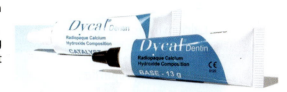

FIGURE 8.24 Dycal is a well-known brand of calcium hydroxide pulp capping agent.

AVAILABLE AS

- Two paste system containing base and catalyst pastes in soft tubes *(Fig. 8.24)*
- Light cured system
- Single paste in syringe form (Pulpdent, *Fig. 8.25*)
- Powder form (mixed with distilled water)
- Some representative commercial products
- Regular set—Dycal (Dentsply), Calcidor (Dorident), Recal (PSP), Hydrox (Bosworth)
- Light cured—Septocal LC (Septodont) and Calcimol LC (VOCO).

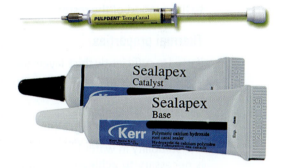

FIGURE 8.25 Calcium hydroxide root canal pastes. The syringe form (top) allows the material to be conveniently applied into the narrow root canal.

COMPOSITION

Base paste

Ingredient	Weight (%)	Liquid
l-methyl trimethylene disalicylate	40	Reacts with $Ca(OH)_2$ and ZnO
Calcium sulphate		
Titanium dioxide		Inert fillers, pigments
Calcium tungstate or barium sulphate		Provides radiopacity

Catalyst paste

Ingredient	Weight (%)	Liquid
Calcium hydroxide	50	Principal reactive ingredient
Zinc oxide	10	
Zinc stearate	0.5	Accelerator
Titanium oxide		Provides radiopacity, filler
Ethylene toluene sulfonamide	39.5	Oily compound, acts as carrier

SETTING REACTION

Calcium hydroxide reacts with the l-methyl trimethylene disalicylate ester to form a chelate viz. amorphous *calcium disalicylate*. Zinc oxide also takes part in the reaction.

Ca (OH)$_2$ + l-methyl trimethylene disalicylate → calcium disalicylate

PROPERTIES

Calcium hydroxide cements have poor mechanical properties. However, they are better than zinc oxide eugenol.

Mechanical properties

Compressive strength (10-27 MPa after 24 hours). It has a low compressive strength. The strength continues to increase with time.

Tensile strength (1.0 MPa) is low.

Modulus of elasticity (0.37 GPa/m^2). The low elastic modulus limits their use to areas not critical to the support of the restoration.

Thermal properties

If used in sufficiently thick layers they provide some thermal insulation. However, a thickness greater than 0.5 mm is not recommended. Thermal protection should be provided with a separate base.

Solubility and disintegration

The solubility in water is high (0.4–7.8%). Some solubility of the calcium hydroxide cement is necessary to achieve its therapeutic properties. Solubility is higher when exposed to phosphoric acid and ether. So care should be taken during *acid etching* and during application of *varnish* in the presence of this cement.

Biological properties

Effect on pulp: The cement is alkaline in nature. The high pH is due to the presence of free Ca(OH)$_2$ in the set cement. The pH ranges from 9.2 to 11.7.

Formation of secondary dentin: The high alkalinity and its consequent antibacterial and protein lysing effect helps in the formation of reparative dentin.

Adhesion

The material is sensitive to moisture and does not adhere in the presence of blood, water or saliva. The adhesive bond is weak.

MANIPULATION

Equal lengths of the two pastes are dispensed on a paper and mixed to a uniform color. The material is carried and applied using a calcium hydroxide carrier or applicator (a ball-ended instrument). It is applied to deep areas of the cavity or directly over mildly exposed pulp (contraindicated if there is active bleeding).

SETTING TIME

Ranges from 2.5 to 5.5 minutes.

Factors affecting setting time The reaction is greatly accelerated by moisture and accelerators. It therefore sets faster in the mouth.

LIGHT ACTIVATED CALCIUM HYDROXIDE CEMENT

Light activated calcium hydroxide cements are available. It consists of calcium hydroxide and barium sulphate dispersed in a urethane dimethacrylate resin. It also contains HEMA and polymerization activators. Some contain fluoride.

Light activated cements have a long working time and is less brittle than the conventional two paste system. They are radiopaque. They are supplied in syringe form *(Fig. 8.26)* and is expressed directly on to the tooth through a replaceable nozzle. Examples are Septocal LC (Septodont) and Calcimol LC (VOCO).

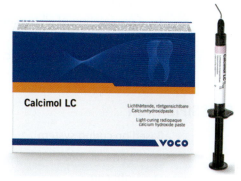

FIGURE 8.26 Light-cured calcium hydroxide.

CALCIUM HYDROXIDE ROOT CANAL SEALING PASTES

Root canal sealers containing calcium hydroxide are available *(Fig. 8.25)*. These are similar to the ones used for pulp capping but contain increased amount of *retarders* in order to extend the working time while they are being manipulated in the warm environment of the root canal. They are also radiopaque.

Commercial names Sealapex (Kerr), Pulpdent, etc.

Their advantages are

1. Effective antibacterial properties without irritation.
2. They stimulate hard tissue repair in the apical foramen.

RESIN CEMENTS

Resin cements based on methyl methacrylate have been available since 1952 for cementation of inlays, crowns and other appliances. Development of resin cements came naturally with the development of composites resins. They are essentially low viscosity flowable composites. These cements are known for their high esthetics and high bond strengths. They were widely used for the cementation of orthodontic brackets and resin-bonded restorations *(Figs 8.27 and 28)*. The development of esthetic all-ceramic restorations led to a renewed interest in an esthetic bonding system which complemented the esthetics of the restoration. The color of the underlying cement can influence the esthetics in translucent restorations. The resin cement also improves the esthetics at the margins of the restoration. According to some studies resin cements reduce fractures of all-ceramic restorations. Thus, they are popular for the cementation of all-porcelain restorations.

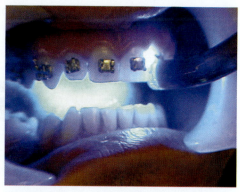

FIGURE 8.27 Bonding of orthodontic brackets.

APPLICATIONS

1. For bonding of orthodontic brackets to acid-etched enamel *(Fig. 8.27)*.
2. Cementation of porcelain veneers and inlays.
3. Cementation of all-porcelain crowns and FDPs *(Fig. 8.29B)*.
4. Cementation of etched cast restorations *(Fig. 8.28)*.

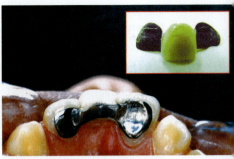

FIGURE 8.28 An etched resin-bonded cast restoration (Maryland bridge).

CLASSIFICATION

Based on curing system

○ Chemical cure

○ Light cure

○ Dual cure

Chemically activated resins can be used for all types of restorations.

Light activated resins cannot be used in all situations because of problems of light penetration. Thus their use is limited to thin ceramic restorations which allows some passage of light, composite restorations like inlays, ceramic or plastic orthodontic brackets, etc.

Dual cure resins are used when the material being bonded allows some degree of light penetration, e.g. ceramic crown, brackets, inlays, etc. The resin around the margins are cured using light to initiate setting. The portions where light cannot penetrate cure subsequently by chemical reaction.

SUPPLIED AS

They are supplied in syringes

1. Chemical cured
   – Two paste system containing base and accelerator
   – Single paste system with activator in the bonding liquid
2. Light cured: Single paste system.

Most systems also include a bonding agent and etchant.

Representative Commercial Names Panavia F, Infinity, ResiLute (Pulpdent), Transbond X (3M), Maxcem Elite (Kerr), Variolink Esthetic (Ivoclar) *(Fig. 8.29A)*, etc.

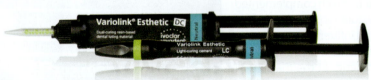
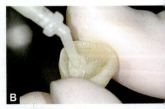

FIGURES 8.29A AND B (A) Representative resin luting cement (dual cured). **(B)** Resin cement is directly injected into the crown through the static mixing tip.

COMPOSITION

The resin cements have a composition similar to that of modern composites (refer chapter on composites). The filler content has to be lowered and diluent monomers are added to adjust the viscosity. Some contain fluoride (e.g. Panavia F).

To promote adhesion to enamel and dentin, organophosphates (MDP), HEMA and 4 META are used as bonding agent (refer chapter on resin-based composites for details).

POLYMERIZATION

1. Chemically by peroxide-amine system
2. Or by light activation
3. Or by both chemical and light activation (dual cure).

Polymerization mechanisms are similar to those of resin-based composites.

PROPERTIES

Compressive strength	:	180 MPa (26000 Psi)
Tensile strength	:	30 MPa (4000 Psi)
Film thickness	:	10–25 µm
Biological properties	:	Irritating to the pulp. Pulp protection with calcium hydroxide or GIC liner is necessary for areas close to the pulp.
Solubility	:	Insoluble in oral fluids.
Polymerization shrinkage	:	Is high
Adhesion properties	:	They do not adhere to tooth structure, which may lead to microleakage if used without etching and bonding.
Bond strength to enamel	:	7.4 MPa (1070 Psi). Bond strength to enamel is usually strong. Failure most often occurs at the metal-resin interphase.

MANIPULATION AND TECHNICAL CONSIDERATIONS

Like composites, resin cements are technique sensitive. Improper procedure can lead to poor bond strength and failure. The following processes are involved.

1. Etching the restoration
2. Etching the tooth surface
3. Bonding and curing
4. Removal of excess cement

ETCHING THE RESTORATION

Etching metal   The metal surface can be etched or roughened by blasting with 30–50 µm alumina to improve retention. Etching is usually more effective. The process is carried out in a electrolytic bath containing an acid like sulfuric acid—also known as *electrochemical etching*. The non-bonding surface is protected with wax. Silica coating can also be used to improve bonding.

Etching porcelain   Ceramic is a highly inert material and is immune to attack by most acids. However, it can be etched by using hydrofluoric acid (refer chapter on ceramics). The esthetic surfaces are protected with a coating of wax.

Orthodontic brackets In the case of orthodontic brackets, a fine mesh on the bonding side of the bracket helps to improve its retention. The cement flows into the mesh and locks to provide good mechanical retention. Coating with organosilane also improves bond strength.

ETCHING THE TOOTH SURFACE

The tooth surface is etched with phosphoric acid (similar to procedure described in restorative resins). This is followed by an application of bonding agent.

BONDING AND CURING

Chemically activated systems

Two paste systems The two components are combined by mixing on a paper pad. Mixing time is 20–30 seconds.

Single paste system with activator in bonding agent In some systems, the activator is present in the bonding agent. The bonding agent is painted on to the etched tooth surface as well as on to the restoration. Setting occurs when the cement on the restoration contacts the bonding agent on the tooth.

Dual cure system

- The two components are mixed and light cured.
- Time of exposure should never be less than 40 seconds.
- Light curing gives high initial strength.
- Light curing polymerizes the exposed cement at the margins of the restoration which is affected by air inhibition.

REMOVAL OF EXCESS CEMENT

Excess cement removal is critical. Removal of excess cement can sometimes be very difficult because of the high strength of the material. Therefore, removal of the excess cement should be attempted soon after seating before the material has fully hardened. Some manufacturers recommend a partial light cure to facilitate removal followed by completion of curing.

COMPOMER (POLYACID-MODIFIED COMPOSITE RESINS)

Shortly after the introduction of RM GICs, 'compomers' were introduced to the market. They were marketed as a new class of dental materials that would provide the combined benefit of composites (the 'comp' in their name) and glass ionomers ('omer'). These materials had the fluoride release features of GIC with the durability of composite. Based on their structure and properties, these materials belong to the class of dental composites. Often they have been erroneously referred to as 'hybrid glass ionomers', 'light-cured GICs' or 'resin-modified glass ionomers'. The proposed nomenclature for these materials is polyacid-modified composite resins, a nomenclature that is widely used in the literature.

APPLICATIONS

1. Restorative materials in pedodontics.
2. Restorative material in nonstress bearing areas.
3. Class V lesions.

4. Bases.
5. Luting (permacem) *(Fig. 8.33)*.

Their applicability as orthodontic adhesives, amalgam bonding systems and veterinary restorative materials has also been reported.

UPPLIED AS

These materials are sensitive to moisture. They are usually supplied as
- Light cured single paste in moisture proof packets (Dyract, Compoglass) *(Fig. 8.30)*
- Powder/liquid (Principle) *(Fig. 8.32)*
- Two paste static mixing system (PermaCem) *(Fig. 8.31)*.

Commercial names Restorative —Dyract (Dentsply), Compoglass (Ivoclar).

Luting   —Permacem, Principle (Dentsply), etc.

OMPOSITION

These materials have two main constituents: dimethacrylate monomer(s) with two carboxylic groups present in their structure and a filler that is similar to the ion-leachable glass present in GICs. The ratio of carboxylic groups to backbone carbon atoms is approximately 1:8. There is no water in the composition of these materials and the ion-leachable glass is partially silanized to ensure some bonding with the matrix.

Single component system   - Silicate glass, sodium fluoride, and polyacid modified monomer, photoinitiator.

Double component system   *Powder* - Glass fillers, accelerators, initiator, TiO_2

Liquid - Acrylic monomers, photoinitiator, water, carboxylic acid dimethacrylate.

ETTING REACTION

The initial set is via a free radical polymerization reaction activated by light. Subsequently water from saliva is absorbed by the cement and an acid-base reaction sets in between the carboxylic groups and areas of filler not contaminated by the silane coupling agents. It is this reaction which releases fluoride.

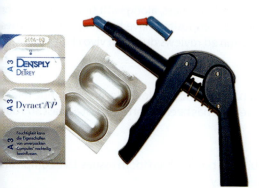

GURE 8.30 Single component compomer restorative ment (Dyract, Dentsply).

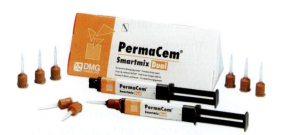

FIGURE 8.31 Two paste static mixing compomer luting cement (PermaCem by DMG).

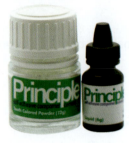

FIGURE 8.32 Powder/liquid type luting cement (Principle by Dentsply).

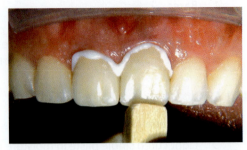

FIGURE 8.33 Luting procedure of 2 all ceramic anterior crowns. Excess cement is removed.

BONDING AND CURING

Bonding and curing mechanisms are similar to the resin luting cements.

- ○ Light cured
- ○ Chemically cured
- ○ Dual cured

Etching and bonding are similar to the resin luting cements. Some current materials are self etching and bonding (e.g. Permacem by DMG, *Fig. 8.31*). No additional etching and bonding are required in these materials.

MANIPULATION

For the single component system the tooth is etched and bonding agent applied. The material is injected into the cavity and cured by light.

For the powder/liquid system the powder and liquid is dispensed and mixed according to the manufacturer's instruction for 30 seconds.

For the static mixing system, the material comes out mixed when it is extruded through the spirals in the mixing tips.

PROPERTIES

Considering the low volume fraction filler and the incomplete silanization of the filler, it could be postulated that they are inferior to composites. Both in vitro and in vivo investigation have confirmed this expectation. Lower flexural strength, modulus of elasticity, compressive strength, flexural strength fracture toughness and hardness, along with significantly higher wear rates compared to clinically proven hybrid composites, have been reported for these materials. Their clinical performance received mixed reviews during in vivo clinical trials.

Fluoride release

Though these materials release fluoride they have significantly lower levels of fluoride release than GICs. Although low, the level of fluoride release has been reported to last at least 300 days.

Adhesion

Unlike glass ionomer they do not have the ability to bond to hard tooth tissues. Like composite acid etching and use of bond agents are necessary.

Biocompatibility

With the exception of concerns about the release of HEMA from these materials, no other biocompatibility issues have been associated with their usage.

ADVANTAGES AND DISADVANTAGES

The prime advantage of these materials are their fluoride release anticariogenic potential. The disadvantage is their lack of adhesion. Thus bonding agents are required which increase in the number of steps and time required for placement.

Constant reformulations of these types of materials may eventually make them comparable or even superior to existing composites, but as long as they do not set via an acid-base reaction and do not bond to hard-tooth tissues, they cannot and should not be classified with GICs.

9
CHAPTER

Dental Amalgam

An amalgam is defined as a special type of alloy in which mercury is one of the componen[?] Mercury is able to react with certain alloys to form a *plastic mass*, which is conveniently pack[?] into a prepared cavity in a tooth. This plastic mass hardens and is stronger than any den[?] cement or anterior filling material. Dental amalgam is *the most widely used* filling material f[?] posterior teeth.

The alloys before combining with mercury are known as dental amalgam alloys. Stric[?] speaking, however, this is a misnomer as they are not dental amalgam alloys but alloys fro[?] which dental amalgam is prepared.

In dentistry, amalgam has been successfully used for more than a century as a restorati[?] material for tooth decay. Over the years its quality has greatly improved, thanks to a low[?] amount of mercury and the addition of new components which can reduce its corrosion [?] the oral cavity.

History of Dental Amalgam

There are indications that dental amalgam was used in the first part of the T'ang Dynasty in China (618-907 CE). Prior to amalgam, dentists restored teeth using filling material such as stone chips, resin, cork, turpentine, gum, lead and gold leaf, among other metals. The renowned physician Ambroise Paré (1510–1590) used lead or cork to fill teeth.

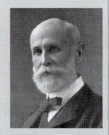

In 1603, a German named Tobias Dorn Kreilius described a process for creating an amalgam filling by dissolving copper sulfide with strong acids, adding mercury, bringing to a boil and then pouring onto the teeth. In France, D'Arcet's Mineral Cement was popular, but it had to be boiled into a liquid before being poured on patient's teeth. Louis Regnart added mercury to the mixture, lowering the temperature required significantly, and for this became known as the 'Father of Amalgam'. Amalgam was placed by Taveau of Paris as early as 1826, although he had developed it in 1816. Early amalgam had drawbacks including marginal breakdown. Some mixtures caused expansion resulting in fractured teeth.

GV Black

In the 1830s, a fusible alloy of lead, bismuth and tin, known as "Darcet's metal" was used to fill teeth. This material was heated and then poured into the tooth in the molten state, after which it quickly hardened.

Amalgam was introduced into the USA by the Crawcour brothers (from France) in 1833. However, at that point the use of dental amalgam was declared to be malpractice, and the American Society of Dental Surgeons (ASDS), the only US dental association at the time, forced all of its members to sign a pledge to abstain from using the mercury fillings. This was the beginning of what are known as the first dental amalgam war. The war ended in 1856 with the rescission of the old association. The American Dental Association was founded in its place in 1859, which has since then strongly defended dental amalgam from allegations of being too risky from the health standpoint.

Early amalgam was made by mixing mercury with the filings of silver coins. The early amalgams expanded on setting. In 1895, GV Black developed a balanced formula (67% silver, 27% tin, 5% copper, 1% zinc) for modern amalgam alloy. Black's formula overcame the expansion problems of the existing amalgam formulations.

INDICATIONS

1. As a permanent filling material for
   - Class I and class II cavities *(Fig. 9.1)*
   - Class V cavities where esthetics is not required *(Fig. 9.1)*
2. In combination with retentive pins to restore a crown.
3. For making dies.
4. In retrograde root canal fillings.
5. As a core material in abutment teeth.

CONTRAINDICATIONS

1. Amalgam should not be placed in patients with impaired kidney function.
2. Individuals with allergic hypersensitivity to mercury or components of the alloy
3. New amalgam fillings should not be placed in contact with nonamalgam restoration like gold and metal devices, such as orthodontic braces.

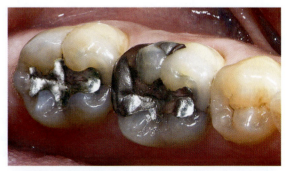

FIGURE 9.1 Amalgam restorations—Class I, class II and class V.

BOX 9.1	ISO standards covering dental amalgam and related products and equipment

ISO 24234:2015   Dentistry—Mercury and alloys for dental amalgam
ISO 7488:1991   Dental amalgamators
ISO 8282:1994   Dental equipment—Mercury and alloy mixers and dispensers
ISO 13897:2003   Dentistry -- Amalgam capsules

CLASSIFICATION OF AMALGAM ALLOYS

BASED ON COPPER CONTENT

- *Low copper alloys*   Contain less than 6% copper (conventional alloys)
- *High copper alloys*   Contain between 13–30% copper

The high copper alloys are further classified as

- Admixed or dispersion or blended alloys.
- Single composition or unicompositional alloys

BASED ON ZINC CONTENT

- *Zinc-containing alloys*   Contain more than 0.01% zinc
- *Zinc-free alloys*   Contain less than 0.01% zinc

BASED ON SHAPE OF THE ALLOY PARTICLE

- Lathe-cut alloys (irregular shape)
- Spherical alloys
- Spheroidal alloys

BASED ON NUMBER OF ALLOYED METALS

- Binary alloys, e.g. silver-tin
- Ternary alloys, e.g. silver-tin-copper
- Quaternary alloys, e.g. silver-tin-copper-indium

BASED ON SIZE OF ALLOY POWDER PARTICLE

- Microcut
- Macrocut

MANUFACTURE OF ALLOY POWDER

The various components of the amalgam alloy are combined together by melting to form ingots. The ingots have to be heat-treated in an oven for a set period of time. This process is called *annealing*. Annealing improves the homogeneity and grain structure of the alloy.

LATHE-CUT ALLOY POWDER

An annealed ingot of silver-tin alloy is placed in a lathe and fed into a cutting tool. The resulting chips obtained are often needlelike and some manufacturers reduce the chip size by ball-milling *(Fig. 9.2A)*.

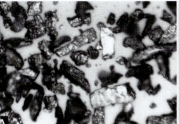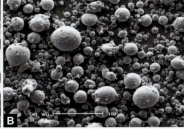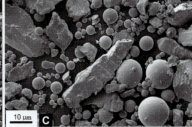

FIGURES 9.2A TO C Photomicrograph of the various alloy powders. **(A)** Lathe cut. **(B)** Spherical. **(C)** Admixed.

AGING, ACID TREATMENT AND ANNEALING OF PARTICLES

A freshly cut alloy reacts *too rapidly* with mercury. If the alloy filings are stored at room temperature for a *few months,* the reactivity gradually decreases. Such alloys are said to have been aged. The filings can be aged faster by boiling in water for 30 minutes. Aging also improves the shelf life of the product.

Some manufacturers treat the filings with *acid* to improve reactivity.

The stresses induced during the cutting and grinding process must be relieved by an *annealing* process (100 °C for several hours). Failure to anneal results in a slow release of stress over time (during storage) which can adversely affect the properties of the amalgam.

SPHERICAL ALLOY POWDER

The spherical alloy *(Fig. 9.2B)* is prepared by an *atomization* process. The liquid alloy is sprayed under high pressure of an inert gas through a fine crack into a large chamber. If the droplets solidify before hitting a surface, the spherical shape is preserved. Like the lathe-cut powders, spherical powders are aged. A comparison of two types of powders is detailed in *Table 9.1*.

SUPPLIED AS

- Bulk powder and mercury in separate containers *(Figs. 9.3A and B)*.
- Alloy and mercury in disposable capsules *(Figs. 9.4, 9.7 and 9.9)*.
- Preweighed alloy as tablet form in tubes *(Fig. 9.5)* and mercury in sachets.

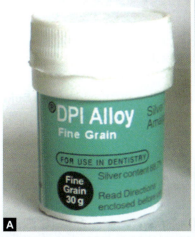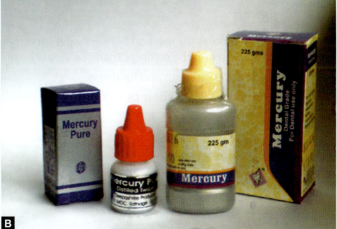

FIGURES 9.3A AND B **(A)** DPI alloy powder. **(B)** Various brands of commercially available mercury (*Courtesy:* Vijay Dental, Chennai).

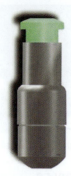

FIGURE 9.4 Alloy/mercury in preproportioned capsule form.

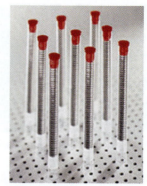

FIGURE 9.5 Alloy in tablet form.

COMPOSITION

	Low copper	High copper		Unicomposition
		Admixed		
	Lathe-cut or spherical	Lathe-cut 2/3	Spherical 1/3	Spherical
Silver	63–70%	40–70%	40–65%	40–60%
Tin	26–29%	26–30%	0–30%	22–30%
Copper	2–5%	2–30%	20–40%	13–30%
Zinc	0–2%	0–2%	0	0–40%

FUNCTION OF CONSTITUENTS

Silver

- Major element in the reaction.
- Whitens the alloy.
- Decreases the creep.
- Increases the strength.
- Increases the expansion on setting.
- Increases tarnish resistance in the resulting amalgam.

Tin

- Tin *controls the reaction* between silver and mercury. Without tin the reaction would be too fast and the setting expansion would be unacceptable.
- Reduces strength and hardness.
- Reduces the resistance to tarnish and corrosion, hence the tin content should be controlled.

Copper

- Increases hardness and strength.
- Increases setting expansion.

Zinc

- In small amounts, it does not influence the setting reaction or properties of amalgam. Zinc acts as a *scavenger* or *deoxidizer* during manufacture, thus prevents the oxidation of important elements like silver, copper or tin. Oxidation of these elements would seriously affect the properties of the alloy and amalgam. Alloys without zinc are more brittle, and amalgam formed by them are less plastic.

❏ Zinc causes *delayed expansion* if the amalgam mix is contaminated with moisture during manipulation.

Mercury

In some brands, a small amount of mercury (up to 3%) is added to the alloy. They are known as *pre-amalgamated alloys*. Pre-amalgamation produces a more rapid reaction.

Platinum

Hardens the alloy and increases resistance to corrosion.

Palladium

Hardens and whitens the alloy.

Indium

Indium when added to the mercury reduces mercury vapor and improves wetting. Indium can also added to the powder. Though it reduces early strength it increases the final strength. It reduces creep.

COMPARISON OF LATHE CUT AND SPHERICAL ALLOYS

A comparison of the two types of powders is presented in *Table 9.1.*

TABLE 9.1 Comparison of lathe cut and spherical alloys	
Spherical alloys	*Lathe-cut alloys*
Particles are spherical	Particles are irregular
Manufactured by atomization of molten alloy	Manufactured by milling an annealed ingot of alloy
More plastic (a contoured matrix is essential to establish proximal contour)	Less plastic and resists condensation pressure
Requires less mercury hence has improved properties	More mercury required hence has inferior properties

LOW COPPER ALLOYS

Historically amalgam alloys were low copper alloys. The composition recommended by GV. Black in the late 18th century remained virtually unchanged until the late 1960s when the high copper amalgams were introduced.

COMPOSITION

Constituents	Percent
Silver	63–70%
Tin	26–29%
Copper	2–5%
Zinc	0–2%

AVAILABLE AS

- ○ Lathe-cut alloys, which are further available as *coarse* or *fine grain* (fine grain type is preferred, because of the ease of carving).
- ○ Spherical alloys.
- ○ Blend of lathe-cut and spherical particles.

SETTING REACTION

When alloy powder and mercury are triturated, the silver and tin in the outer portion of the particles *dissolve* into the mercury. Simultaneously, the mercury diffuses into the alloy particles and starts reacting with the silver and tin within forming crystals of silver-mercury (Ag_2Hg_3) and tin-mercury compounds (Sn_8Hg).

Silver-tin compound (unreacted alloy powder) is known as the *gamma* (γ) *phase*. The silver-mercury compound is known as *gamma 1* (γ_1) *phase* and the tin-mercury as the *gamma 2* (γ_2) *phase* **(Table 9.2).**

A simplified reaction is outlined below

$$Ag_3Sn + Hg \rightarrow Ag_2Hg_3 + Sn_8Hg + \text{(unreacted)}\ Ag_3Sn$$
$$(\beta+\gamma)\ \ (\gamma_1)\ (\gamma_2)\ (\beta+\gamma)$$

The alloy particles do not react completely with mercury. About 27% of the original Ag_3Sn remains as *unreacted particles*, which as previously mentioned is known as the gamma (γ) phase.

The properties of the hardened amalgam depends on the proportion of the reaction phases. If more unconsumed Ag_3Sn (γ phase) is present, the stronger the amalgam. The γ_2 phase is the weakest component and is least stable to corrosion.

MICROSTRUCTURE

Set amalgam consists of unreacted particles (γ) surrounded by a matrix of the reaction products (γ_1 and γ_2) **(Fig. 9.6).**

TABLE 9.2 Amalgam reaction phases and symbols

Phases	Symbol	Chemically
Gamma	γ	Ag_3Sn
Beta	β	$AgSn$
Gamma 1	γ_1	Ag_2Hg_3
Gamma 2	γ_2	Sn_8Hg
Eta	η	Cu_6Sn_5
Epsilon	ε	Cu_3S

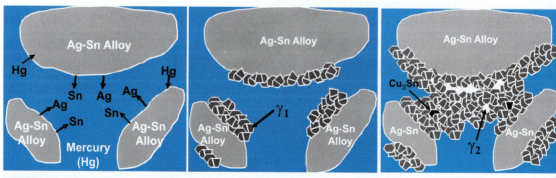

FIGURE 9.6 Schematic representation of setting reaction and microstructure of low copper amalgam.

Note   The properties of the hardened amalgam depends upon the proportion of each of the reaction phases. If more unconsumed Ag_3Sn (γ phase) is present, the stronger the amalgam. The γ_2 phase is the weakest component and is least stable to corrosion process. Also present are Cu_3Sn phase (ε or epsilon) formed from the small amounts of copper present in the composition.

HIGH COPPER ALLOYS

High copper alloys contain between 13 to 30% wt. copper. The majority of amalgam restorations placed currently are high copper. They are preferred because of their improved mechanical properties, resistance to corrosion and better marginal integrity.

TYPES

1.   Admixed alloy.
2.   Single-composition alloy.

ADMIXED ALLOY POWDER

The admixed alloy *(Figs. 9.2C and 9.7)* was introduced in 1963 and were originally made by mixing 1 part silver-copper eutectic alloy (high copper spherical particles) with 2 parts silver-tin alloy (low-copper lathe-cut particles).

(An eutectic alloy is one in which the components exhibit complete liquid solubility but limited solid solubility. The silver-copper phase exhibits a eutectic structure at the composition of silver 71.9% and copper 28.1%).

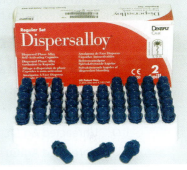

FIGURE 9.7 Admixed alloy (Dentsply).

Amalgam made from *admixed* powders is *stronger* than amalgam made from lathe-cut low-copper powder, because of three reasons

1.   A change in the nature of the filler particles. The silver-copper particles are present in greater amounts, in addition to the silver-tin particles.
2.   A greater residual filler content thereby changing the filler to matrix ratio.
3.   A reduction in the weaker γ_2 phase.

Synonyms   Dispersed phase alloy.

TYPES

Admixed alloys are of two types

1.   *Regular or conventional admixed alloy*—contains irregular and spherical alloy particles having different compositions (low copper and high copper).
2.   *Unicomposition admixed alloys*—contains irregular and spherical particles of uniform composition.

COMPOSITION

Admixed alloy powders usually contain between 30 to 55 weight percent spherical high-copper alloy powder. The total copper content ranges from 9 to 20 weight percent. A sample composition is presented below.

Constituents	Percent
Silver	69%
Tin	17%
Copper	13%
Zinc	1%

SETTING REACTION

When the components are mixed the mercury begins to dissolve the outer portion of the particles. Silver from the silver-copper eutectic alloy particles, and both silver and tin from the silver-tin alloy particles enter the mercury. The tin dissolved in the mercury reacts with the copper of the silver-copper particles and forms the Cu_6Sn_5 (η or Eta). The η crystals form around the unreacted silver-copper particle. At the same time γ_1 phase is also formed. As in the low copper alloys γ_1 surrounds everything forming the matrix. γ_2 is also formed at the same time but is later replaced by η. Thus in admixed alloy the undesirable γ_2 phase is greatly reduced.

The reaction may be simplified as follows

$$Ag_3Sn + Ag\text{-}Cu + Hg \rightarrow Ag_2Hg_3 + Cu_6Sn_5 + Ag_3Sn \text{ unreacted} + Ag\text{-}Cu \text{ unreacted}$$
$$(\beta+\gamma) \quad (eutectic) \qquad (\gamma_1) \quad (\eta) \qquad (\beta+\gamma) \qquad \qquad (eutectic)$$

Note   In this reaction, γ_2 has been eliminated and is replaced by η phase. To accomplish this, it is necessary to have a net copper content of at least 12 percent in the alloy powder.

MICROSTRUCTURE OF SET HIGH COPPER ADMIXED AMALGAM

The Cu_6Sn_5 is present as a 'halo' surrounding the Ag-Cu particles.

The final set material consists of

Core particles of

○   Unreacted Ag_3Sn, (γ phase) and
○   Unreacted Ag-Cu surrounded by a halo of Cu_6Sn_5 (η).

Embedded in a matrix made up of

○ γ_1 (Ag_2Hg_3).

Schematic representation of the setting reaction and microstructure is shown in **Figs. 9.8A to C**.

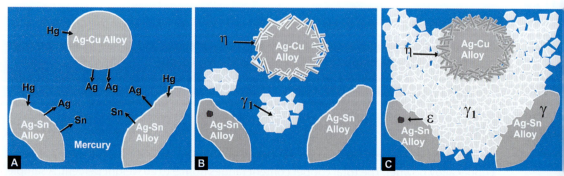

FIGURES 9.8A TO C Schematic representation of setting reaction and microstructure of admixed amalgam.

SINGLE COMPOSITION ALLOYS

High copper amalgam was developed by a Canadian metallurgist, Dr. William Youdelis in 1963. Single composition alloys are high copper amalgam alloys. Unlike admixed alloy powders, each particle of the alloy powder has the same composition. Therefore they are called single composition or 'unicompositional alloys' **(Fig. 9.9)**. The spherical alloy particles are 5 to 40 µm in size.

Synonyms   Single composition, unicompositional, non-gamma 2.

COMPOSITION

Constituents	Percent
Silver	40–60%
Tin	22–30%
Copper	13–30%
Zinc	0–4%
Indium or palladium	Small amounts

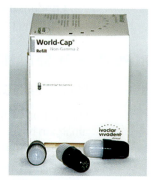

FIGURE 9.9 Single composition high copper alloy (Ivoclar).

SETTING REACTION

Though each particle has the same composition, the silver, tin and copper present exist in various phases within the particle. Thus each particle contains Ag_3Sn (γ), AgSn (β) and Cu_3Sn (ε). When triturated, silver and tin from the particle dissolve in mercury forming the γ_1 (Ag_2Hg_3) crystal matrix that binds together the partially dissolved alloy particles. At this stage very little copper dissolves. Later, a layer of η (Cu_6Sn_5) crystals are formed at the surface of alloy particles. Some η (Cu_6Sn_5) crystals also form in the matrix.

The overall simplified reaction is

$$Ag\text{-}Sn\text{-}Cu + Hg \rightarrow Cu_6Sn_5 + Ag_2Hg_3 + Ag\text{-}Sn\text{-}Cu$$
$$(\gamma + \beta + \varepsilon) \qquad (\eta) \quad (\gamma_1) \quad (\text{unreacted})$$

Note   The undesirable γ_2 does not usually form in most single composition alloys. The η (Cu_6Sn_5) crystals are much larger and rod-shaped than those in the admixed amalgam.

MICROSTRUCTURE OF SET SINGLE-COMPOSITION AMALGAM

Final set material **(Fig. 9.10)** consists of

Particles of

○ Unreacted Ag_3Sn (γ phase) and surrounded by a mesh of rod shaped η (Cu_6Sn_5).

Embedded in a matrix made up of

○ γ_1 (Ag_2Hg_3)

ADVANTAGES/DISADVANTAGES OF SPHERICAL HIGH-COPPER AMALGAM

ADVANTAGES

1. Faster set.
2. Lower residual mercury.

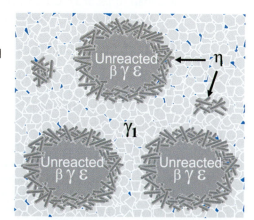

FIGURE 9.10 Schematic representation of setting reaction and microstructure of admixed amalgam.

3. Lower creep during condensation.
4. Faster finishing.
5. Higher early strength.
6. Low condensation pressure.

DISADVANTAGES

1. Less working time.
2. Condensation pressure not sufficient to displace matrix during condensation (while restoring proximal cavities). Contouring of matrix band required.

PROPERTIES OF SET AMALGAM

MICROLEAKAGE

Penetration of fluids and debris around the margins may cause secondary caries. Dental amalgam has an exceptionally fine record of clinical performance because of its tendency to minimize marginal leakage (see tarnish and corrosion).

Self sealing   The small amount of leakage under amalgam restorations is unique. If the restoration is properly inserted, leakage decreases as the restoration *ages* in the mouth. This may be due to the formation of *corrosion products* in the tooth-restoration interface. Over a period of time they *seal the interface* and reduce leakage. Thus amalgam is a *self sealing* restoration. Both low and high copper amalgams are capable of sealing against microleakage but the accumulation of corrosion products is slower with the high-copper alloys. Initial leakage can be reduced through the application of varnish on the cavity walls. Use of dentin bonding agents (bonded amalgam technique) also show promise.

DIMENSIONAL CHANGE

The earliest amalgams exhibited expansion while setting. This was because of the greater mercury/alloy ratio used. Amalgams may expand or contract, depending on its manipulation. Ideally, dimensional change should be small. Excessive contraction can lead to microleakage, sensitivity and secondary caries. Excessive expansion can produce pressure on the pulp and *postoperative sensitivity. Protrusion* of the restoration can also occur.

ISO Sp. 24234:2015 requires that amalgam should not expand more than 0.15% or contract less than –0.1% at 37 °C, during hardening. Mechanically, triturated modern amalgams, both low and high copper, prepared from low mercury/alloy ratios show a slight contraction.

Theory of dimensional change

Contraction   When the alloy and mercury are mixed contraction results initially as the particles dissolve and the γ_1 grows. The final volume of γ_1 is less than the initial volumes of silver and mercury that go into making the γ_1. Therefore, contraction will continue as long as growth of γ_1 continue.

Expansion   The γ_1 crystals as they grow, impinge against one another, and produce an outward pressure tending to oppose contraction. If there is sufficient mercury present to provide a plastic matrix, an expansion will occur when γ_1 crystals impinge on each other. After a rigid γ_1 matrix has formed, growth of γ_1 crystals cannot force the matrix to expand. Instead γ_1 crystals will grow into interstices containing mercury, consuming mercury, and producing continued reaction. Therefore, reducing mercury in the mix will favor contraction.

Thus, factors favoring contraction are

❍ Low mercury/alloy ratio
❍ Higher condensation pressure (squeezes out mercury)
❍ Smaller particles (consumes more mercury because of increased surface area)
❍ More trituration (accelerates setting)

Modern amalgams show a net contraction, whereas older amalgams always showed expansion. Two reasons for this difference are

❍ Older amalgams contained larger alloy particles and were mixed at higher mercury/alloy ratios.
❍ Hand trituration was used before. Modern amalgams are mixed with high speed amalgamators (equivalent to increase in trituration time).

EFFECT OF MOISTURE CONTAMINATION (DELAYED EXPANSION)

If a zinc-containing-low-copper or high-copper amalgam is contaminated by moisture during trituration or condensation, a large expansion can take place. It usually starts after 3-5 days and may continue for months, reaching values greater than 400 µm (4%). This is known as *delayed expansion* or *secondary expansion* *(Fig. 9.11)*. The expansion is caused by the releases of hydrogen gas from the reaction of zinc with water.

$$H_2O + Zn \rightarrow ZnO + H_2 \text{ (gas)}$$

This hydrogen gas does not combine with the amalgam, but collects within the restoration, creating extreme internal pressure and expansion of the mass. This causes protrusion of the restoration out of the cavity, increased creep, increased microleakage, pitted surfaces and corrosion. Dental pain, recurrence of caries, and fracture of the restoration are seen as a result of these poorly inserted restorations.

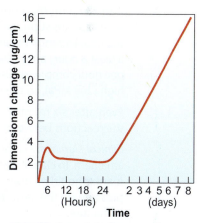

FIGURE 9.11 Delayed expansion of amalgam.

Note

Moisture contamination *after* the cavity has been filled does not cause delayed expansion. *Nonzinc alloys* do not show this type of expansion when contaminated with water. However, moisture contamination of the mix of any alloy results in inferior physical properties.

Indications for zinc free alloys

Amalgam without zinc tends to be less plastic and less workable. These alloys are used only for cases where it is difficult to control moisture, e.g. patients having excessive salivation, retrograde root canal filling, subgingival lesions, etc.

STRENGTH

Well designed amalgam restorations have sufficient compressive strength to withstand normal intraoral masticatory forces.

Compressive strength	Hour	7 Days
Low copper (lathe cut)	45 MPa	302 MPa
Low copper (spherical)	141 MPa	366 MPa
Admixed	137 MPa	431 MPa
Single composition	262 MPa	510 MPa

TENSILE STRENGTH

Amalgam cannot withstand high tensile or bending stresses and can fracture easily in improperly designed restorations *(Fig. 9.12)*. Therefore, the *cavity should be designed* so that the restoration will receive *minimal tension* or shear forces in service.

Low Copper	Admixed	Single composition
60 MPa	48 MPa	64 MPa

Factors affecting strength

Effect of rate of hardening Amalgams do not gain strength as rapidly as might be desired. After 20 minutes, compressive strength may be only 6% of the one week strength. ISO specifications stipulates a minimum of 100 MPa at one hour and 350 MPa after 24 hours. Since the initial strength of amalgam is low, patients should be cautioned not to bite too hard for a least *8 hours* after placement, the time at which at least 70% of its strength is gained. The one hour compressive strength of high-copper single-composition amalgams is exceptionally high (262 MPa), so the chances of accidental fracture is less.

Even after six months, some amalgams may still be increasing in strength, suggesting that the reactions between the matrix phases and the alloy particles may continue indefinitely.

Clinical significance The rate of hardening should be considered during the placement of amalgam. In class II restorations where a supporting matrix has been placed, removal of the matrix should be done at the appropriate time. *Early removal* can result in fracture. Excessive pressure on the restoration by the patient *prematurely* to test the occlusion can also result in fracture.

Effect of trituration Either undertrituration or overtrituration will decrease the strength for both low-copper, and high-copper amalgams.

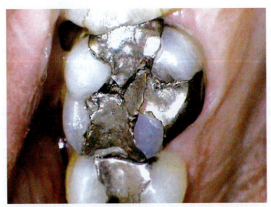

FIGURE 9.12 A fractured amalgam restoration. Amalgam is technique sensitive. If improperly placed it can result in many problems including fracture, leakage, sensitivity, periodontal problems, etc.

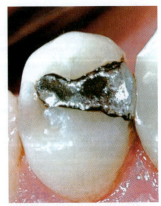

FIGURE 9.13 Amalgam with high creep rate displaying marginal breakdown.

Effect of mercury content   Sufficient mercury should be mixed with the alloy to wet each particle of the alloy. Insufficient mercury produces a *dry, granular mix **(Fig. 9.18)*** which can result in a rough and pitted restoration which is prone to *corrosion*.

Excess mercury in the mix can produce a marked reduction in strength because of the higher γ_2 content (which is the weakest phase—see setting reaction).

Effect of condensation   Higher condensation pressure results in higher compressive strength (only for lathe-cut alloys).

Reason   A good condensation technique will minimize porosity and remove excess mercury from lathe-cut amalgams. If heavy pressures are used in spherical amalgams, the condenser will punch through. However, spherical amalgams condensed with lighter pressures produce adequate strength.

Effect of porosity   Voids and porosities reduce strength.

Porosity is caused by

1.   Decreased plasticity of the mix (caused by too low Hg/ alloy ratio, under trituration and over trituration).
2.   Inadequate condensation pressure.
3.   Irregularly shaped particles of alloy powder.
4.   Insertion of too large increments.

Increased condensation pressure improves adaptation and decreases voids. Fortunately, voids are not a problem with spherical alloys.

Effect of cavity design
○   The cavity should be designed to reduce tensile stresses.
○   Amalgam has strength in bulk, therefore, the cavity should have adequate depth and width.

CREEP

It is defined as a time dependent plastic deformation. Creep of dental amalgam is a slow progressive permanent deformation of set amalgam, which occurs under constant stress (static creep) or intermittent stress (dynamic creep).

BOX 9.2	Creep test

Creep is tested by subjecting a 7 day old cylindrical specimen to a load of 36 MPa (at 37 °C) for a specified time usually between 1 and 4 hours.

Significance of creep
Creep is related to *marginal breakdown* of low-copper amalgams. The higher the creep, the greater is the degree of marginal deterioration *(Fig. 9.13)*.

According to ISO 24234:2015 creep should be below 2% See ***Box 9.2***.

Creep values
In general lathe-cut low-copper alloys show the highest creep values, often exceeding ADA limits. The lowest creep values are shown by the high copper amalgams.

Amalgam Type	Creep
Low-copper lathe cut amalgam	6%
Low-copper spherical	1.5%
High-copper admixed amalgam	0.5%
High-copper unicompositional amalgam	0.05 to 0.09%

Factors affecting creep

Microstructure   The γ_1 (Ag-Hg) phase has a big effect on low-copper amalgam creep rates. Increased creep rate is shown by larger γ_1 volume fractions. Decreased creep rate is shown by larger γ_1 grain sizes. The γ_2 phase is associated with higher creep rates.

Single composition high-copper amalgams have very low creep rates, due to absence of γ_2 phase and due to the presence of η (Cu_6Sn_5) rods, which acts as barrier to deformation of the γ_1 phase. Increased zinc content reduces creep.

Effect of manipulative variables   For increased strength and low creep values

- Mercury/alloy ratio should be minimum.
- Condensation pressure should be maximum for lathe-cut or admixed alloys.
- Careful attention should be paid to timing of trituration and condensation. Either under or over-trituration or delayed condensation tend to increase the creep rate.

RETENTION OF AMALGAM

Amalgam does not adhere to tooth structure. Retention of the amalgam filling is obtained through mechanical locking. This is achieved by proper cavity design (see cavity design in technical considerations). Additional retention if needed can be obtained by placing pins within the cavity. Amalgam can also be bonded using special bonding agents.

TARNISH AND CORROSION

Amalgam restorations often tarnish and corrode in the mouth. Black silver sulfide can form on the surface of an amalgam restoration in some patients. Both high and low-copper amalgams show corrosion. However corrosion in high-copper amalgams is limited because η phase is less susceptible.

Factors related to excess tarnish and corrosion

- High residual mercury.
- Surface texture—small scratches and exposed voids.
- Contact of dissimilar metals, e.g. gold, and amalgam.
- Patients on a high sulphur diet.
- Moisture contamination during condensation.
- Type of alloy—low copper amalgam is more susceptible to corrosion (due to higher γ_2 content) than high copper. Also η (Cu_6Sn_5) phase of high copper is less susceptible to corrosion.
- A high copper amalgam is cathodic in respect to a low-copper amalgam. Therefore, mixed high copper and low copper restorations should be avoided.

Corrosion of amalgam can be reduced by

- Smoothing and polishing the restoration.
- Correct Hg/alloy ratio and proper manipulation.
- Avoid dissimilar metals including mixing of high and low copper amalgams.

BIOLOGICAL CONSIDERATIONS

Two types of potential biological effects can occur.

1. Adverse systemic effects of the mercury component.
2. Contact reaction of the mucosa with amalgam or amalgam corrosion products. (Oral lichenoid reaction).

Mercury   Mercury is toxic to the human body and to the environment. Fortunately risk to the patient of mercury exposure from dental restorations is very low even with multiple restorations *(Boxes 9.3 and 9.5)*. However, mercury vapors pose a greater risk to the dental personnel as they as they are more easily inhaled and absorbed through the lungs. Mercury vapors may be produced during trituration and condensation of amalgam and removal of old restorations. Further information is under the section mercury toxicity at the end of the chapter.

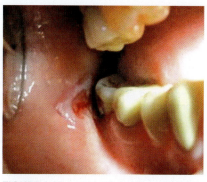

FIGURE 9.14 Lichenoid reaction on mucosa adjacent to amalgam restoration.

Contact reactions   Reactions occurring from proximity or contact with amalgam are rare. The symptoms are normally classified as delayed hypersensitivity reactions (type IV), and they were called oral lichenoid reactions (OLRs) by Finne et al. These are lesions that clinically and histologically resemble lichen planus *(Fig. 9.14)*, but have an identifiable etiology. These reactions are presumably due to allergic or toxic reactions to compounds released or generated from the restoration.

It is recommended that patch tests should be performed in patients with OLR if the lesions are in close contact with amalgam fillings. Replacement of such restorations is recommended if there is a positive patch test reaction to mercury or components of amalgam and if there are no signs of concomitant generalized lichen planus.

TECHNICAL CONSIDERATIONS

MANIPULATION OF AMALGAM

The clinical success of amalgam restorations is highly dependent on the correct cavity design and selection and manipulation of the alloy. If a restoration is defective, it is usually the fault of the operator and not the material.

CAVITY DESIGN

Providing retention   Since amalgam does not adhere to tooth structure, proper design of the cavity is very important. The amalgam cavity is designed to provide maximum mechanical locking of the amalgam *(Fig. 9.15)*. This is achieved by creating a cavity with walls that diverge towards the floor of the cavity (or converge towards the mouth of the cavity). This results in a cavity mouth that is narrower, effectively locking the amalgam within the cavity. Additional retention if needed can be obtained by placing pins within the cavity.

BOX 9.3	Current position on safety of dental amalgams

Although dental amalgam is the single largest source of mercury exposure for many individuals, current evidence does not indicate that dental amalgam is causing illness in the general population. However, there is a small percentage of the population which is hypersensitive to mercury and can suffer health effects from even a low exposure.

A total ban on amalgam is not considered justified. Neither is the removal of sound amalgam fillings in patients who have no indication of adverse health effects attributable to mercury exposure.

As recently as May 2005, the ADA endorsed amalgam as being safe for pregnant women.

As a general principle, it is advisable to reduce human exposure to heavy metals in the environment, even if there is no clinical evidence of adverse health effects, *provided* the reduction can be achieved by other materials at reasonable cost and without introducing other adverse effects.

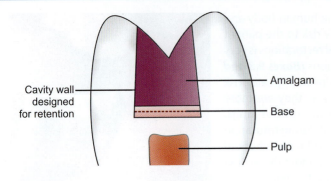

Cavity wall designed for retention

Amalgam

Base

Pulp

FIGURE 9.15 The cavity walls are designed to lock the amalgam restoration. This is achieved by creating walls that taper, effectively making the mouth of the cavity narrower than the base.

Four wall support For effective condensation, the cavity should have *four walls* and *a floor*. If one or more of the walls of the cavity is absent, a stainless steel matrix *(Figs. 9.21 and 9.22)* can compensate for the missing walls. Failure to have a four wall support can result in inadequate condensation which can weaken the amalgam. Additional retention can be obtained with amalgam pins or screws.

Preventing tensile fracture Since amalgam has poor tensile strength, the cavity should have sufficient depth and width in order to provide *sufficient bulk* to the amalgam, especially those in high stress areas.

Cavosurface angle The junction of the cavity with the external surface should be as close to a right angles as possible. Beveling is *not indicated* for amalgam as it can cause fracture of the amalgam at the margins.

SELECTION OF MATERIALS

Alloy

The alloy is selected based on clinical need.

- For restorations subjected to occlusal forces, an amalgam with high resistance to marginal fracture is desirable.
- If strength is needed quickly the best choice is spherical or high copper alloys, but they require a fast operator.
- A nonzinc alloy is selected in cases where it is difficult to control moisture.
- *Indium containing alloys* Indium performs the same functions as zinc and in addition, it decreases the γ_2 phase.

Mercury

There is only one requisite for dental mercury and that is its purity. Common contaminating elements such as arsenic, can lead to pulpal damage. A lack of purity may also adversely affect physical properties. High purity mercury is labelled as 'triple distilled'.

- Freezing point $-38.87\,°C$
- Boiling point $356.9\,°C$

ADA Sp. No. 6 for dental mercury requires that the mercury should possess no surface contamination and less than 0.02% nonvolatile residue.

DISPENSERS

Because proportioning is important, manufacturers have developed some simple dispensers for alloy and mercury *(Fig. 9.16)*. Dispensing by volume is unreliable because it is affected by particle size and the degree of packing (trapped air and voids) in the dispenser.

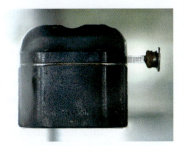

FIGURE 9.16 Mercury/alloy dispenser.

TABLETS

This is the most accurate method of dispensing. Manufacturers compress alloy powder into tablets of controlled weight which is used with measured amounts of mercury.

PREPROPORTIONED CAPSULES

Preproportioned capsules containing alloy powder and mercury in compartments separated by a membrane are available *(Figs. 9.17A and B)*. They usually contain 400, 600, 800 or in rare cases 1200 mg of alloy powder with corresponding proportion of mercury. Before use, the membrane is ruptured by compressing the capsule, and the capsule is then placed in a mechanical amalgamator.

Advantages
1. Consistent proportioning.
2. Low mercury/alloy ratio.
3. Physical handling not required thus reducing health hazard.

Disadvantages
Mercury and alloy may leak. The dentist is forced to use one alloy/mercury ratio for all situations when using disposable capsules. Also, the disposable capsules are expensive.

MERCURY: ALLOY RATIO (PROPORTIONING)

Prior to mechanical triturators, when amalgam was triturated manually excess mercury had to be used in order to achieve smooth and plastic amalgam mixes.

This excess mercury was removed from the amalgam by

1. Using a *squeeze cloth to* squeeze out the excess mercury.
2. *Increasing dryness technique*   During condensation of each increment, a mercury rich soft layer comes to the surface. This is removed by condensing excess amalgam and carving off the excess.

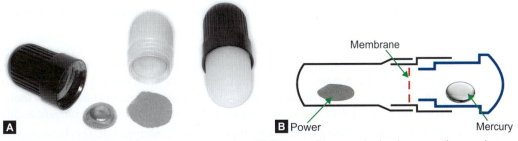

FIGURES 9.17A AND B (A) Preproportioned capsules. **(B)** Diagram of the capsule showing separating membrane.

Eames' technique

The better method of reducing mercury content is to reduce the original mercury/alloy ratio. In 1959 Dr. Wilmer Eames proposed 1:1 ratio of mercury: alloy. This is came to be known as the *minimal mercury* or *Eames' technique* (mercury/alloy 1:1). (Prior to this manufacturers usually recommended higher mercury/alloy ratios of 6.5:5,7:5 and even 8:5 to ensure adequate amalgamation.) However, it is still necessary to squeeze mercury out of the mix using the *increasing dryness technique*. Hence, with this technique, 50% or less mercury will be in the final restoration, with obvious advantages.

Mercury alloy ratios ranges from 43 to 54%. In preproportioned capsule the mercury/alloy ratio is determined by the manufacturer and is usually less than 50%.

Low mercury/alloy ratios are not easy to triturate manually. In order to benefit from a low mercury/alloy ratio a high speed mechanical triturator (amalgamator) is absolutely essential.

TRITURATION

The objective of trituration is to wet all the surfaces of the alloy particles with mercury. For proper wetting, the alloy surface should be clean. Rubbing of the particles mechanically removes the oxide film coating on alloy particles.

Trituration is achieved either by

- Manually by hand
- Mechanical mixing

Manual mixing

A glass mortar and pestle is used *(Fig. 9.18)*. The mortar has its inner surface roughened to increase the friction between amalgam and glass surface. A rough surface can be maintained by occasional grinding with carborundum paste. A pestle is a glass rod with a round end.

The three factors to obtain a well mixed amalgam mass are

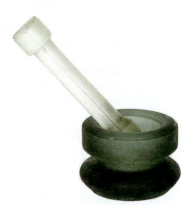

FIGURE 9.18 Glass mortar and pestle.

1. The number of rotations,
2. The speed of rotation and
3. The magnitude of pressure placed on the pestle. Typically a 25 to 45 second period is sufficient.

Mechanical trituration

Mechanical amalgamators are more commonly used to triturate amalgam alloy and mercury *(Fig. 9.19)*.

- The disposable capsule serves as a mortar. Some capsules have a cylindrical metal or plastic piece in the capsule which serves as the pestle. The capsule is inserted between the arms on top of the machines. When switched on, the arms holding the capsule oscillate at high speed thus triturating the amalgam. Most amalgamators have hoods that cover the arms holding the capsule in order to confine mercury spray and prevent accidents.
- Reusable capsules are available with friction fit or screw-type lids. This type uses alloy in tablet form and capsulated mercury. At one time not more than two pellets alloy should be mixed in a capsule.

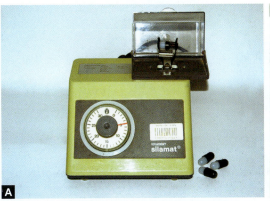
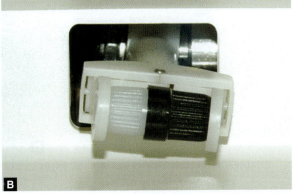

FIGURES 9.19A AND B **(A)** Mechanical amalgamator for preproportioned capsules. **(B)** Close-up of the mechanical arm that grips and vibrates the capsules (right).

With either type, the lid should fit the capsule tightly, otherwise, the mercury can spray out from the capsule, and the inhalation of fine mist of mercury droplets is a health hazard.

Amalgamators have automatic timer and speed control device. The speed ranges from 3200 to 4400 cycles per minute. High copper alloys require higher mixing speeds.

Mixing time   The mixing time can vary depending on the speed, oscillating pattern, and capsule designs. Spherical alloys usually require less amalgamation time than do lathe-cut alloys. A large mix requires slightly longer mixing time than a smaller one. Manufacturer's recommendations should be followed when determining mixing speed and time.

Advantages of mechanical trituration

1. Shorter mixing time.
2. More standardized procedure.
3. Requires less mercury when compared to hand mixing technique.

Under-triturated mix

○ It is rough and grainy and may crumble *(Fig. 9.20 A).*
○ It gives a rough surface after carving and tarnish and corrosion can occur.
○ Strength is less.
○ Mix hardens too rapidly and excess mercury will remain.

Normal mix

○ It has a shiny surface and a smooth and soft consistency *(Fig. 9.20 B).*
○ It may be warm (not hot) when removed from the capsule.
○ It has the best compressive and tensile strength.
○ The carved surface retains its lustre after polishing, hence increased resistance to tarnish and corrosion.

Over-triturated mix

○ The mix is soupy, difficult to remove from capsule and too plastic to manipulate *(Fig. 9.20 C).*
○ Working time is decreased.
○ Results in higher contraction of the amalgam.
○ Strength increases for lathe-cut alloys, whereas it is reduced in high copper alloys.
○ Creep is increased.

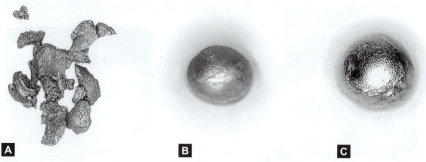

FIGURES 9.20A TO C Three possible mixes. **(A)** An under-triturated mix. **(B)** Correct mix. **(C)** An over-triturated mix.

MULLING

Mulling is actually a continuation of trituration. It is done to improve the homogeneity of the mass and get a single consistent mix. It can be accomplished in two ways

○ The mix is enveloped in a dry piece of rubber dam and vigorously rubbed between the first finger and thumb, or the thumb of one hand and palm of another hand for 2–5 seconds.

○ After trituration the pestle is removed and the mix is triturated in the pestle-free capsule for 2–3 seconds.

Mulling is not required for mechanical triturated amalgams.

CONDENSATION

The amalgam is placed in the cavity after trituration, and packed (condensed) using suitable instruments.

Aims

1. To compact the mass to increase the density of the restoration.
2. To reduce voids.
3. To remove excess mercury.
4. To adapt the amalgam to the preparation walls and margins.

Proper condensation increases the strength and decreases the creep of the amalgam. Condensation *must always* be done within the *four walls and floor*. If one or more walls of the cavity are missing, a steel *matrix* **(Figs. 9.21 and 9.22)** may be used to compensate for it. Failure

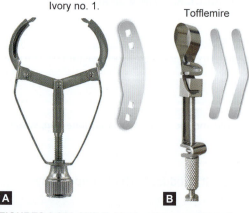

Ivory no. 1.

Tofflemire

FIGURES 9.21A AND B Matrix retainers and bands.

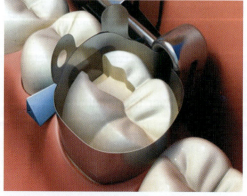

FIGURE 9.22 Tofflemire matrix. Wooden pegs help seal the embrasure area and contain the amalgam.

to use a matrix can result in a poorly condensed and weak restoration. Amalgam can also escape into the interdental space (amalgam overhang—*Fig. 9.23*) resulting in inflammation, bleeding and pain.

Condensers

Condensers are instruments with serrated tips of different shapes and sizes *(Figs. 9.24A and B)*. The shapes are oval, crescent, trapezoidal, triangular, circular or square. The condenser type is selected as per the area and shape of the cavity. Smaller the condenser, greater is the pressure exerted on the amalgam. Condensation can be done manually or mechanically. For spherical amalgams, a large condenser tip should be selected to reduce punching through and improve condensation.

Manual condensation

The mixed amalgam is held in an amalgam well *(Fig. 9.25)*. The mixed material is packed in *increments*. Each increment is carried to the prepared cavity by means of a small forceps or an *amalgam carrier (Fig. 9.26)*.

Once inserted, it should be condensed immediately with sufficient pressure (approximately 3 to 4 pounds). Condensation is started at the center, and the condenser point is stepped sequentially towards the cavity walls.

The smaller the condenser the greater the force. Serrated condensers are preferable. The shape of the condenser should conform to the area under condensation. A large circular condenser may be ineffective for cavity corners. For corners a smaller point or a triangular or rectangular condenser is more effective.

As the mix is condensed some *mercury rich material* rises to the surface. Some of this can be removed, to reduce the final mercury content and improve the mechanical properties. The remainder will assist bonding with the next increment.

Modern amalgams are fast setting and so working time is short. Therefore, condensation should be as rapid as possible. A fresh mix of amalgam should be ready if condensation takes more than 3 or 4 minutes. Long delays between mixing and condensation, results in weaker amalgam.

Spherical alloys have little 'body' and thus offer only mild resistance to the condensation. When condensing these alloys, a *larger* condenser is recommended.

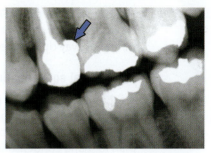

FIGURE 9.23 Amalgam overhang resulting from failure to use matrix effectively.

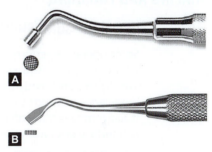

FIGURES 9.24A AND B Amalgam condensers. **(A)** Circular serrated. **(B)** Rectangular serrated.

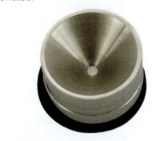

FIGURE 9.25 Amalgam well.

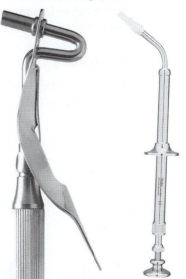

FIGURE 9.26 Two commonly used amalgam carriers.

The cavity is *overfilled (Fig. 9.27)* so that the excess *mercury rich layer* can be subsequently trimmed away during the carving process.

Mechanical condensation

Mechanical condensers *(Figs. 9.28A and B)* provide vibration or impact type of force to pack the amalgam mix. Less effort is needed than for hand condensation.

SHAPING AND FINISHING

PRECARVE BURNISHING

Some operators perform a *precarve burnishing*. This condenses and smooths the surface amalgam and reduces the voids and irregularities caused by the serrated condenser. It also removes some of the overfilled *mercury rich* surface layer from the surface.

CARVING

The restoration is carved to reproduce the tooth anatomy. Carving also removes the weaker *mercury rich* surface layer. The carving should not be started until the amalgam is hard enough to offer resistance to the carving instrument. A *scraping* or *ringing* sound should be heard when it is carved. If the carving is started too soon, the amalgam may be so plastic that it may *pull away* from the margins. Sharp carvers are used with strokes proceeding from tooth surface to amalgam surface. Various carving instruments are shown in *Fig. 9.29*.

BURNISHING

After the carving, the restoration is smoothened, by burnishing the surface and margins of the restoration. Burnishing is the plastic deformation of a surface casued by sliding contact

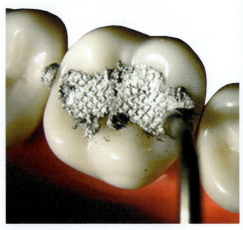
FIGURE 9.27 Amalgam condensation.

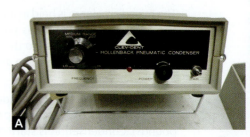

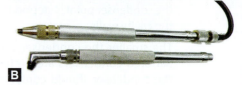
FIGURES 9.28A AND B A mechanical pneumatic condenser **(A)** with handpieces **(B)**.

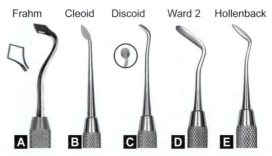

Frahm   Cleoid   Discoid   Ward 2   Hollenback

A   **B**   **C**   **D**   **E**

FIGURES 9.29A TO E Various amalgam carving instruments.

Ball   Ovate   T-Ball   Acorn

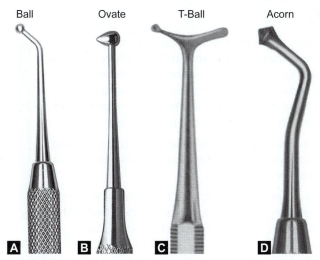

FIGURES 9.30A TO D Various types of amalgam burnishers.

with another object. Fast setting alloys gain sufficient strength by this time to resist rubbing pressure. Burnishing slow setting alloys can damage the margins of the restoration.

Burnishing is done with various types of burnishers *(Figs. 9.30A to D)* using light stroke proceeding from the amalgam surface to the tooth surface. Final smoothing can be done by rubbing the surface with a moist cotton pellet.

POLISHING

Polishing minimizes corrosion and prevents adherence of plaque. The polishing should be delayed for at least *24 hours* after condensation, or preferably longer. Wet polishing is advised, so a wet abrasive powder in a paste form is used. Dry polishing powders can raise the temperature above 60°C. If the temperature rises above 60°C, mercury is released which may cause corrosion and fracture at the margins. High copper unicompositional alloys with high early strength may be polished at the same sitting after the materials has hardened sufficiently. However, polishing should be carried out delicately using soft abrasives and gentle pressure. A completed amalgam restoration is shown in *Fig. 9.31.*

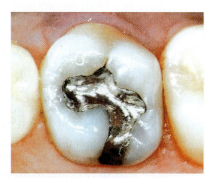

FIGURE 9.31 A completed amalgam restoration.

AMALGAM BONDING

Amalgam restorations do not reinforce the teeth. Teeth with MOD cavities are susceptible to cuspal fractures. Bonding of the amalgam with a suitable adhesive (4-META) has been shown to improve fracture resistance of the tooth (twice as much as nonbonded restorations). Amalgam bonding also reduces marginal leakage and postoperative sensitive. The bonding mechanism is similar to that of resin bonding agents. The bonding agent penetrates the dentinal tubules and forms a hybrid zone. The bond with the amalgam is micromechanical through the formation of resin tags when amalgam is condensed into the uncured bonding agent. However, amalgam to amalgam bond is not so effective and therefore repair with bonding agents is not recommended. A variety of amalgam bonding agents are available commercially *(Fig. 9.32).*

MERCURY TOXICITY

Mercury is toxic to living creatures. Free mercury should not be sprayed or exposed to the atmosphere. This hazard can arise during trituration, condensation and finishing of the restoration, and also during the removal of old restorations at high speed. Mercury *vapors* can be inhaled. Skin contact with mercury should be avoided as it can be absorbed.

Any excess mercury should not be allowed to get into the *sink*, as it reacts with some of the alloys used in plumbing. It also reacts with *gold ornaments.*

Mercury has a cumulative toxic effect. Dentists and dental assistants, are at high risk. Though it can be absorbed by the skin or by ingestion, the primary risk is from *inhalation.*

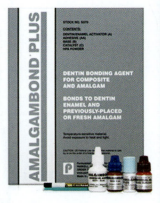

FIGURE 9.32 Amalgam bond.

Precautions

In placing and removing amalgam fillings, dentists should use techniques and equipment to minimize the exposure of the patient and the dentist to mercury vapor and to prevent amalgam waste from being flushed into municipal sewage systems

1. The clinic should be *well ventilated.*
2. Use preproportioned capsules possible to control mercury alloy ratio .
3. The alloy mercury capsules, should have a tightly fitting cap to avoid leakage.
4. Whenever possible use of protective barriers such as rubber dam isolation.
5. High volume evacuation should be used when condensing and carving amalgam.
6. While removing old fillings, a water spray, mouth mask and high volume suction should be used.
7. The use of ultrasonic amalgam condenser is not recommended as a spray of small mercury droplets is observed surrounding condenser point during condensation.
8. All excess mercury and amalgam waste should be stored in *well-sealed containers* under fixer solutions.
9. Amalgam scrap and materials contaminated with mercury or amalgam should not be subjected to heat sterilization.
10. Proper disposal systems should be followed, to *avoid environmental pollution*. Amalgam separators should be used to capture the amalgam from the spittoon and the suction devices and to prevent amalgam waste from being flushed into public sewage systems
11. Amalgam scrap should be disposed or recycled through the appropriate agencies.
12. Extracted teeth containing silver restorations should *not be* disposed in the infectious waste and incinerated. Rather they should treated as hazardous amalgam scrap and disposed accordingly.
13. Spilled mercury is cleaned as soon as possible. Avoid carpeted floors in the operatory as it is extremely difficult to clean it from carpets. Vacuum cleaners *are not* used because they disperse the mercury further through the exhaust. Mercury suppressant powders are helpful but these are temporary measures. A *mercury spill kit* **(Fig. 9.33)** is commercially available for management of mercury spills.

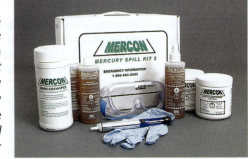

FIGURE 9.33 Mercury spill kit.

14. Skin contacted with mercury should be washed with *soap and water.*
15. Annually, a *program for handling toxic materials* is monitored for actual exposure levels.

AMALGAM DISPOSAL

Residual amalgam and empty amalgam capsules must be disposed of separately in special containers. These containers contain fixing salts or other chemical substances to bind mercury vapours. These containers must be disposed of according to legal requirements, returning them to the respective manufacturer. Local/regional instructions for waste disposal must be observed.

Amalgam separators (ISO 11143:2008)

Dentists should use dental amalgam separators to catch and hold the excess amalgam waste coming from office spittoons. The amalgam separators separate the heavier metal particles from the liquid. Removal of old fillings and placement of new amalgam restorations are sources of amalgam contamination. Without dental amalgam separators, the excess amalgam waste will be released to the sewers via drains in the dental offices.

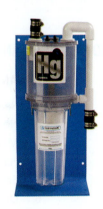

Many companies market amalgam separators *(Fig. 9.34)*. The unit acts as a collection tank allowing settling and decantation, thus separating liquids from solids. The maintenance is done on a periodic basis to decant off the liquid in your canister that will build up faster than the sediment. When full the heavy metal sediment unit is emptied into a separate container. The collected sludge is either shipped directly to a recycler or collected by an appropriate hauler who will ship it to a recycler.

FIGURE 9.34 Amalgam separator.

Extracted teeth containing amalgam fillings

Extracted teeth (not containing amalgam) are considered potentially infectious material and should be disposed into medical waste containers subject to the containerization and labelling provisions of the Occupational Safety and Health Administration (OSHA) blood-borne Pathogen Standard. However, *extracted teeth containing amalgam* should not be placed in a medical waste container that uses an incinerator for final disposal. Incinerating teeth releases mercury directly into the atmosphere. Many metal recycling companies will accept extracted teeth with amalgam. A recycler may be contacted and ask about their policies and any specific handling instructions they may have.

How does amalgam waste affect the environment?

If improperly managed by dental offices, dental amalgam waste can be released into the environment. If an amalgam separator is not used, the excess amalgam waste will be released to the sewers via drains in the dental offices *(Box 9.4)*. Not all public sewage management facilities are equipped to manage hazardous waste like amalgam. At the treatment plant, the amalgam waste settles out as a component of sewage sludge that is then disposed through various means.

1. In landfills thereby contaminating the surrounding land and water sources.
2. Through incineration, thereby contaminating the air.
3. As sludge when used as fertilizer contaminates agricultural land and water bodies and enters the food source.

ADVANTAGES AND DISADVANTAGES OF AMALGAM RESTORATIONS

ADVANTAGES

1. Reasonably easy to insert.
2. Not overly technique sensitive.
3. Maintains anatomic form well.
4. Has adequate resistance to fracture.
5. Self-sealing; minimal-to-no shrinkage and resists leakage.
6. Durable and long lasting.
7. Wears well and causes minimal wear of natural teeth.
8. More economic than other alternative posterior restorative materials like cast gold alloys and composite.

DISADVANTAGES

1. The color does not match tooth structure.
2. They are more brittle and can fracture if incorrectly placed.
3. Requires removal of some healthy tooth structure for cavity designing.
4. They are subject to corrosion and may darken as it corrodes.
5. Corrosion products may stain teeth over time
6. Galvanic action. Contact with other metals may cause occasional, minute electrical flow.
7. They eventually show marginal breakdown.
8. Temporary sensitivity to hot and cold because it is a metal.
9. They do not bond to tooth structure.
10. Environmental mercury concerns.

In the US, the Assistant Secretary for Health established in 1991, a research committee with the aim of carefully reviewing nearly 500 scientific publications on amalgam. The study, which appeared in 1995, failed to show any harmfulness for the amalgam fillings.

Following the advice of the General Surgeon and the Center for Disease Control and Prevention of the Food and Drug Administration, the US Public Health Service recently published an article in a magazine with a very high circulation. The purpose was to clarify the issue and reassure the American people, who had been alarmed by the many news reports on the amalgam risk.

In Switzerland, Chairmen from the four Dental Departments at Universities of Berne, Basel, Geneva and Zurich replied to the alleged charges of amalgam-induced damages which appeared on newspapers and nonscientific journals with a review article. Amalgam was judged as a safe and effective material for posterior tooth filling, with the only exception of allergic patients.

At two meetings of the Federation Dentaire Internationale held in 1994 in Vancouver and Budapest, amalgam was acquitted on the charge of toxicity and was judged as a valid, cheap and still irreplaceable material.

In 1995, a joint statement from the World Health Organization (through two of its agencies, the Oral Health Program and the Office for Global and Integrated Environmental Health, and from the FDA, amalgam fillings were considered to be safe and inexpensive, although their color was different from that of natural teeth. For *environmental reasons,* the document also reported, there could be in the future some limitation to the use of amalgam. Unfortunately, such restrictions were misinterpreted by the mass media, causing unjustified fears in the public opinion and a rising demand for substitution of the restorations.

Ever since the first environmentalist protests against the use of amalgam, a research center was created in Germany by the University Departments of Münster and Erlangen. After reviewing several scientific papers and following hundreds of patients, including 200 pregnant women, the center concluded that: (i) no harmful effects from amalgam had been found in both the general population and the newborns; (ii) high plasma levels of mercury had been found as a consequence of elevated fish consumption.

After careful studies, the Swedish Medical Research Council concluded that all restoration materials currently in use, including amalgam and composite resins, are safe and effective. Nevertheless the Swedish government, through the Department of Environment, recently issued a series of rules to limit the use of amalgam for filling purposes. The main argument was based on an ecological ground, as it was estimated that between 40 and 60 tons of amalgam are carried in the mouth of Swedish people. It was feared that, as a consequence of crematory habits, mercury would be massively released in the environment. In Sweden alone, nearly 300 kilograms of mercury are estimated to be dispersed in the atmosphere, and between 200 and 400 kilograms in the water mains, every year.

There is no question about the fact that the international dental community has been strongly reducing the use of amalgam for filling carious teeth; the main reason, however, has been an esthetic demand from patients rather than a toxicological need. Not unexpectedly, most colleagues from all over the world have kept using amalgam in their own or their offspring's mouth, whenever needed.

As reported in the literature, a certain number of patophobic or easily influenced patients still prefer to have restorations with materials other than amalgam, even after receiving all possible information. Their demands should be satisfied as long as this decision may have a placebo effect; however, these patients should be discouraged from having their still perfect amalgam restorations substituted by other materials. In fact removal of these restorations pose a bigger risk of releasing mercury into the environment.

As a useful reminder to the student, the best filling is *the one that has never been applied*; the most effective therapy is *prevention*.

10
CHAPTER

Direct Filling Gold

CHAPTER OUTLINE

- Applications
- Contraindications
- Composition and Purity
- Gold Foil
  - Manufacture
  - Supplied As
  - Preformed Foils
  - Platinized Foil
  - Cohesive and Noncohesive Gold
- Electrolytic Precipitate
  - Available As
  - Mat Gold

- Mat Foil
- Alloyed Electrolytic Precipitates
- Powdered Gold
  - Synonym
  - Manufacture
  - Available As
- Manipulation of Direct Filling Gold
  - Desorbing or Degassing
  - Electric Annealing
  - Flame Desorption
  - Compaction

- Hand Mallet
- Condensers
- Finishing
- Mechanical Condensers
- Properties of Compacted Gold
  - Strength
  - Hardness
  - Density
  - Effect of Voids
  - Tarnish and Corrosion
  - Biocompatibility
  - Disadvantages
  - Advantages

Prior to the discovery of amalgam, pure gold was very popular as a filling material. The use of gold foil in modern dentistry starts around 1400 in renaissance Italy. Its use is described in a medical text written in 1425 by Giovanni Arcolani (Johannas D'Arcola) a professor of the University of Bologna. Robert Woofendale is credited to have introduced it to the USA in 1766 on his arrival from England. However, its use became widespread in the USA only towards the beginning of the 19th century *(Fig. 10.1)*.

It is the most noble of metals and rarely tarnishes in the oral cavity. Gold in its pure form is very soft (25 BHN). Its malleability and lack of a surface oxide layer permit increments to be welded together. This unique

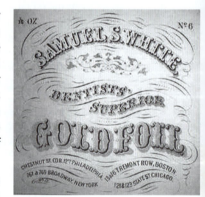

FIGURE 10.1 An example of gold foil marketed in the early 1900s.

characteristic of gold *to be welded at room temperature (cold-welded),* allows gold to be used as a direct filling material.

Although the dental profession sometimes refers to all direct filling golds (DFGs) as 'Gold Foils' the present products may be divided into three categories. All are of 99.99% or higher purity, except two (Platinized foil and Electraloy RV).

Currently, direct filling gold is not as widely used as it once was. However, it will continue to be described because it is still used and is an excellent restorative material when placed properly.

APPLICATIONS

1. Pits and small class I restorations *(Fig. 10.2)*.
2. For repair of casting margins.
3. For class II, class V and class VI restorations *(Fig. 10.3)*.
4. Repair of cement vent holes and perforations in gold crowns *(Figs. 10.4A to C)*.

CONTRAINDICATIONS

1. Teeth with very large pulp chambers.
2. Periodontally compromised teeth.
3. Handicapped patients who are unable to sit for the long dental appointments required for the procedures.
4. Root canal filled teeth because these teeth are brittle.

TYPES

Many categories of direct filling gold are available and is based on its physical form and manufacturing process.

1. *Foil (fibrous gold)*
   - Sheet
     - Cohesive
     - Noncohesive
   - Ropes
   - Cylinders
   - Laminates
   - Platinized
2. *Electrolytic precipitate (crystalline gold)*
   - Mat

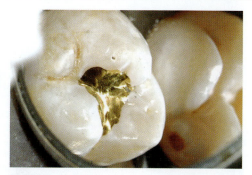

FIGRUE 10.2 Class I gold restoration. Gold restorations are esthetic, corrosion resistant and long lasting if placed properly. (*Courtesy:* Sechena).

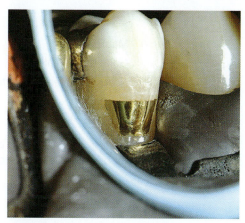

FIGURE 10.3 Class V gold restoration on a premolar. (*Courtesy:* Sechena).

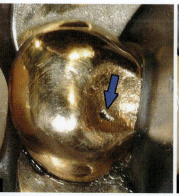
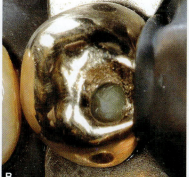
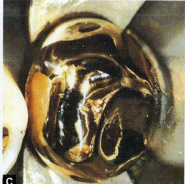

FIGURES 10.4A TO C Above illustrations demonstrate how a perforation in a cast gold crown can be repaired with DFG. (*Courtesy:* Sechena).

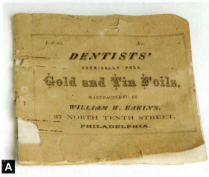

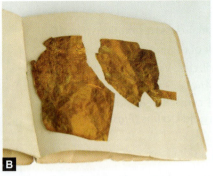

FIGURES 10.5A AND B **(A)** Gold foil booklet from the early twentieth century. **(B)** Gold foil.

- Mat foil
- Gold-calcium alloy

3. *Granulated gold (encapsulated powder)*

FIGURES 10.6A AND Gold foil cylinders (Morga Hastings).

COMPOSITION AND PURITY

Most modern gold restorations are made of gold of high purity (99.99 % or higher) exceptin for the platinized and alloyed gold.

GOLD FOIL

Gold foil is the oldest of all products described. It was manufactured for dental application as early as 1812 by Marcus Bull (USA). It is manufactured by beating gold into sheets.

MANUFACTURE

Gold is malleable. A cast ingot of 15 mm thickness is beaten to a submicroscopic thicknes of 15 or 25 µm. The product is called gold foil *(Figs. 10.5A and B)*. The crystals of the origin cast metal are deformed and elongated so that they have a fibrous structure, hence it is als known as fibrous gold.

SUPPLIED AS

1. Flat square sheets (of varying thickness) in booklet form, 12 sheets (each 10 cm × 10 cm per booklet.
   - No. 4 wt. 4 grains (0.259 gram) 0.51 µm thick.
   - No. 3 wt. 3 grains (0.194 gram) 0.38 µm thick.

   The number denotes the weight of the gold. Other sheets also available are Nos. 20, 4 60 and 90. No. 3 foil is used to manufacture electrolytic and powder gold.
2. Preformed cylinders *(Figs. 10.6A and B)* and ropes. These are made by cutting the No. gold foil sheets into strips of varying widths (3.2, 4.8, etc.) and then rolling and compressin them into pellets or cylinders. They may be 'carbonized'.
3. A number of sheets of foil may be placed one top of each other to form laminated gol foil. One type of laminated foil is the *platinized foil*, which is a sheet of pure platinum fo sandwiched between two sheets of pure gold foil.

Carbonized or corrugated gold

Rolling into a pellet or cylinder form is convenient for carrying and compacting into cavities. Many dentists cut and roll their own gold. Preformed gold foil in the form of ropes and cylinders may be available in *'carbonized' or 'corrugated' form* (made from No. 4 foil that has been *'carbonized' or 'corrugated'*). This form of gold foil is of historical interest because it was an outcome of the *great Chicago fire* in 1871. Corrugated foil is obtained by placing the gold foil in between sheets of paper and igniting it in a closed container. On igniting, the paper gets charred, but the gold foil is left unharmed except that it becomes 'corrugated'. This is because of the shriveling of the paper while oxidizing in the airtight safe. After the carbon is removed it is found that the gold exhibits *superior welding property*.

Platinized foil

This is a laminated foil in which pure platinum foil is sandwiched between two sheets of No. 4 gold foil. The sheets are beaten and joined together. Platinum is added to gold foil to increase the hardness of the restoration. This product is available only in No. 4 sheet form.

Cohesive and noncohesive gold

In practice only the sheet foil is furnished in both conditions, though all forms of direct filling gold could be supplied in cohesive and noncohesive form.

Noncohesive   The earliest gold foils were 'noncohesive' in nature. The manufacturer subjects the foil to a volatile agent such as *ammonia*, which is absorbed on the surface of the gold. Ammonia-treated foil is called noncohesive foil. This adsorption of ammonia gas onto the surface of the gold prevents the gold foil from adhering if it folds back on itself, or contacts other pieces of foil. This is also useful when pellets or cylinders are packed together in containers. It prevents premature cohesion of pellets in their container. It also protects the surface of the gold from contamination which can't be removed. This treatment enables the user of the foil to handle it with a little more ease.

Noncohesive gold can also have adsorbed agents like iron salt or an acidic gas (sulfur or phosphorous containing groups) on its surface. The volatile film is readily *removed by heating (see annealing)*, thereby restoring the cohesive character of the foil. Noncohesive gold is rarely used currently, but may be used to build-up the bulk of a direct gold restoration.

Disadvantage of noncohesive gold   Because the gold wouldn't stick to itself one could not build contour above the cavosurface. Fillings were pretty much flat from cavosurface to cavosurface.

Cohesive   Cohesive gold is also called 'sticky gold'. It was introduced in 1854 by Dr. Robert Arthur when he published his paper on sticky gold (cohesive gold), "A New Method of Using Gold Foil".

For cold-welding, gold should have a clean surface free from impurities. Gold attracts gases, e.g. oxygen to its surface and any absorbed gas film *prevents cohesion* of individual increments of gold during their compaction. The manufacturer, therefore, supplies the gold essentially free of surface contaminants. This type of gold is known as cohesive gold foil.

Representative commercial products   Jensen Gold Foil

ELECTROLYTIC PRECIPITATE

Crystalline gold powder is formed by electrolytic precipitation. The powder has a dendritic crystalline structure. The powder is formed into shapes or strips by sintering (heat fusion) at high temperatures but below their melting point. The particles coalesce or join together at this temperature.

AVAILABLE AS

Mat, mat foil and alloyed.

MAT GOLD

Mat gold is electrolytically precipitated gold sandwiched between sheets of foil and the formed into strips. The strips can be cut by the dentist into the desired size. Mat gold is use to build-up the bulk of the restoration, as it can be more easily compacted and adapted to th cavity. However, mat gold has lots of voids and results in a pitted external surface. Therefore foil gold is used to cover the mat gold and form the surface of the restoration.

MAT FOIL

It is a sandwich of electrolytic precipitated gold powder between sheets of No. 3 gold foil. Th sandwich is sintered and cut into strips of differing widths. The dentist can then cut these t the desired lengths. Sandwiching mat between foil sheets was done to try to eliminate th need to veneer the restoration with a layer of foil. This type is no longer marketed.

ALLOYED ELECTROLYTIC PRECIPITATES

A form of electrolytic gold is an alloy of gold and *calcium* (0.1% by wt.) called 'Electralc RV'. For greater ease of handling, the alloy is sandwiched between two layers of gold fo Calcium produces stronger restorations by *dispersion strengthening*, which locks in cold wor strengthening. Thus, alloying with calcium changes the crystalline structure and makes harder and stronger.

POWDERED GOLD

Synonym Granular gold

Since the 19th century, chemically precipitated gold powders have been available i agglomerated form with a liquid such as alcohol or dilute carbolic acid, which held th agglomerate together. The agglomerates usually disintegrated when compaction wa attempted, so the gold powder was mixed with a wax binder and *enclosed in a No. 3 go foil*. This form was first marketed commercially in the 1960s as 'Goldent' (Morgan Hasting Co.) *(Figs. 10.6A and B)*. In the 1980s another brand 'EZ Gold' (Ivoclar North America) wa introduced.

MANUFACTURE

A fine powder is formed by *chemical precipitation* or by *atomizing* the metal. The particle size vary (average 15 μm). The pellets are mixed with soft wax (0.01% organic wax, which is burr off prior to use) and then wrapped with gold foil (No. 3), rather than sintering the mass, lik for mat gold.

AVAILABLE AS

The powdered gold pellets have a cylindrical or irregular shape and a diameter of 1 to 2 mr The ratio of gold foil to powder varies from 1 to 3 for the smallest pellets to approximate 1 to 9 for the largest.

The foil acts as an effective container and matrix for the powdered metal, while it is condensed. Some operators believe that the use of powdered gold pellets increases cohesion during compaction and reduces the time required for placing the restoration. This is because each pellet contains 10 times more metal by volume than comparable sized pellet of gold foil.

MANIPULATION OF DIRECT FILLING GOLD

There are three processes involved

- Desorbing
- Compaction
- Finishing

DESORBING OR DEGASSING

Synonym Degassing, annealing

The direct filling golds are received by the dentist in a cohesive condition, except for the noncohesive golds. However, during storage and packaging, they absorb gases from the atmosphere. Adsorbed gases *prevent gold from fusing*. Hence, it is necessary for the dentist to *heat* the foil or pellet immediately before it is carried into the prepared cavity. This heating process which *removes surface gases* (oxygen, nitrogen, ammonia, moisture or sulfur dioxide) and ensures a clean surface is called *desorbing* or *degassing* (rather than annealing). Storage in air tight containers is advised and the operator should wear chamois finger tips to protect the gold from contamination. A totally *dry cavity* is essential throughout the compaction process in order to allow complete cohesion.

Direct filling golds may be heated by one of two methods

- In bulk on a tray by gas-flame or electricity *(Figs. 10.7A and B)*.
- Piece by piece, in a well-adjusted alcohol flame *(Fig. 10.8)*.

In practice, all but powder gold may be desorbed on a tray. Powder gold must be heated in a flame to ensure the complete burning away of the wax.

Precaution during bulk heating Excessive amounts should be avoided, since the difficulties arising from prolonged heating can arise from repeated heating as well. Care should be taken to handle pieces with stainless steel wire points or similar instruments that will not contaminate the gold.

Electric annealing

The electric 'annealer' is maintained at a temperature between 340 °C and 370 °C. The time required varies from 5 to 20 minutes depending on the temperature and the quantity of gold on the tray.

Problems associated with electric annealing are

1. Pellets may stick together, if the tray is moved.
2. Air currents may affect the uniformity of heating.
3. Difficult to anneal appropriate amounts of gold.
4. Over sintering.

BOX 10.1	Chamois finger tips

Moisture from the fingers can contaminate the gold. When the operator prepares his own pellets, ropes, etc., and the foil is handled with the fingers, it is advisable always to wear chamois finger-tips.

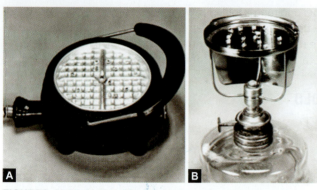

FIGURES 10.7A AND B **(A)** Electric annealer with compartments.
(B) Annealing on a mica tray over an alcohol flame.

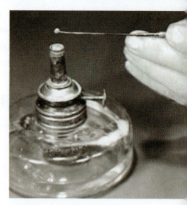

FIGURE 10.8 Flame desorption.

5. Greater exposure to contamination.
6. Size selection among the pieces of desorbed gold is limited.

To prevent their sliding and sticking together, the tray of a recent electric annealer (Neibert electric gold foil annealer) provides individual compartments for each piece of foil **(Figs. 10.7A and B)**.

Flame desorption

Each piece is picked individually by a clean sharp pointed nonoxidizing instrument (nickel chrome, stainless steel, iridioplatinum, etc.), heated directly over the open flame **(Fig. 10.8)** and placed in the prepared cavity. The fuel for the flame may be alcohol or gas. Alcohol is preferred as there is less danger of contamination. The alcohol should be pure methanol or ethanol without colorants or other additives.

Advantages of flame desorption are

1. Ability to select a piece of gold of the desired size.
2. Desorption of only those pieces used.
3. Less exposure to contamination between degassing and use.
4. Less danger of oversintering.

Under-heating does not remove impurities well and results in incomplete cohesion. Carbon deposited by the flame can cause pitting and flaking of the surface.

Overheating leads to oversintering and possibly contamination from the tray, instruments or flame. This results in incomplete cohesion, embrittlement of the portion being heated and poor compaction characteristics. Overheating can result from *too long a time* even at a proper temperature or from *too high a temperature*.

COMPACTION

The gold may be compacted by

○ Hand mallet
○ Pneumatic vibratory condensers
○ Electrically driven condensers

Hand mallet

Earlier gold was compacted entirely with a mallet. Starting points are cut in the prepared cavity. The first pieces of foil are wedged into these areas and compacted. The condenser

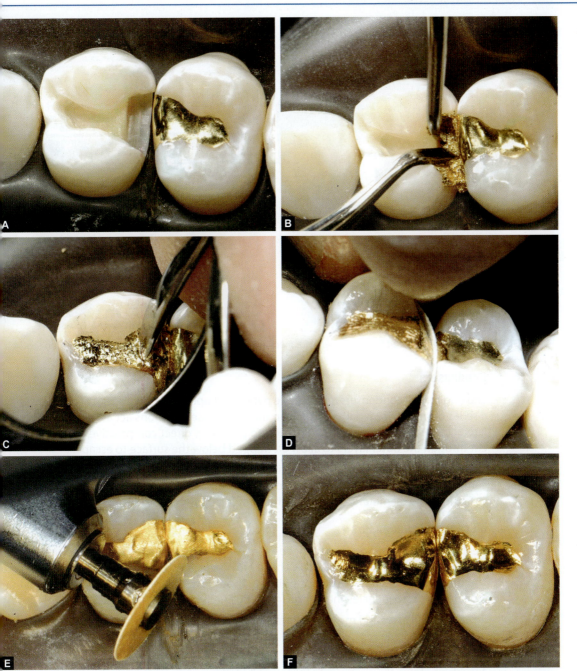

FIGURES 10.9A TO F Some of the steps in the placement of a direct filling gold restoration. **(A)** The cavity is designed for retention and resistance. **(B)** Gold is wedged into the corners of the box and condensed. **(C)** No. 4 gold foil is used on the surface of the restoration to reduce porosity. **(D)** Shaping the proximal side with an abrasive strip. **(E)** Finishing and polishing is done with a variety of burs, stones, abrasive points and disks (sof-lex). **(F)** The completed restoration. (*Courtesy:* John Sechena).

is placed against the foil and struck sharply, with a small mallet. Subsequently additional foil is wedged in the same manner, till the cavity is filled (*Figs. 10.9A to F*). Each increment of gold must be carefully 'stepped' by placing the condenser point in successive adjacent positions. This permits each piece to be compacted over its entire surface so that voids are not bridged.

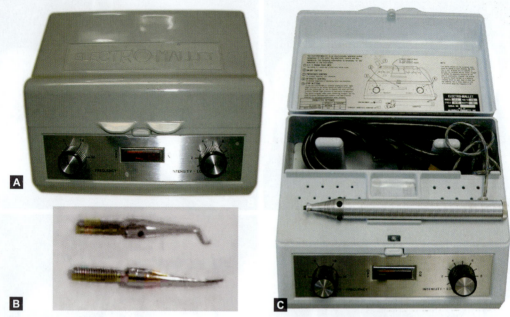

FIGURES 10.10A TO C (A and C) Electromallet for mechanical compaction of gold. **(B)** Gold condensation tips.

Condensers

The original foil condensers had a single pyramid-shaped face, but current instruments have a series of small pyramidal serrations on the face. These serrations act as swaggers, exerting lateral forces on their inclines in addition to providing direct compressive forces. They also cut through the outer layers to allow air trapped below the surface to escape.

Size of the condenser point   This is an important factor in determining the effectiveness of compaction. Small condenser points compact without using forces that might damage oral structures. The diameter of circular points should be 0.5 mm and 1 mm.

Mechanical condensers

Electromagnetic or spring-loaded (not used now a days), pneumatic (compressed air powered) and electric mallet *(Figs. 10.10A to C)* have provided a mechanical means of applying force. The mechanical devices consist of points activated by comparatively light blows that are repeated with frequencies that range from 360–3600/minute.

Advantages   Faster and more comfortable for the patient.

FINISHING

As with amalgam the cavity is slightly overfilled. The surface is probed with a explorer to test for proper compaction and to make sure all voids are eliminated. If the probe penetrates easily condensation is continued with more force. The excess is removed with a gold file or burs. The surface is burnished with a ball burnisher to strain harden the surface. Final polish (optional) is achieved with sof-lex disks *(Figs. 10.9A to F)* or other commercially available gold polishing kits.

PROPERTIES OF COMPACTED GOLD

STRENGTH

The greatest strength is in the most dense area and the weakest part is the porous area where layers or crystals are not closely compacted *(Table 10.1)*. In direct filling gold, the

TABLE 10.1 Physical properties of compacted gold

Type	Transverse	Hardness	Density
Mat gold	161-169 MPa	52-60 KHN	14.3-14.7 g/cm³
Powdered gold	155-190 MPa	55-64 KHN	14.4-14.9 g/cm³
Gold foil	265-296 MPa	69 KHN	15.8-15.9 g/cm³
Mat/gold foil	196-227 MPa	70-75 KHN	15.0-15.1 g/cm³

failure occurs from tensile stress, due to *incomplete cohesion*. Thus transverse strength is a measure of cohesion.

HARDNESS

The hardness indicates the overall quality of compacted gold. A reduction in hardness probably indicates the presence of porosity.

DENSITY

True density of pure gold is 19.3 g/cm³. However in DFGs this is not achieved, because it is not possible to eliminate voids completely during compaction. Thus density of DFGs is usually less than ideal.

The transverse strength, hardness and (apparent) density are somewhat greater when gold foil is used alone or in combination with mat gold, as compared with other forms. The difference in physical properties among the various forms of gold including the gold-calcium alloy and the method of compaction are not clinically significant. The physical properties are probably more greatly *influenced by the competence of the operator* in manipulating and placing the gold.

EFFECT OF VOIDS

The amount of voids is estimated by the apparent density of compacted gold. Voids on the restoration surface (pits) increase the susceptibility to corrosion and deposition of plaque. Voids at the restoration-tooth interface may cause gross leakage and secondary caries development (in properly compacted gold, microleakage is minimum).

TARNISH AND CORROSION

Resistance to tarnish and corrosion is good, if compacted well.

BIOCOMPATIBILITY

The pulpal response is minimal if compacted well. The technique, however, does involve a certain amount of trauma to the tooth and its supporting tissues. In smaller teeth, this is an important consideration. The mechanical condenser causes less trauma than the manual technique.

ADVANTAGES AND DISADVANTAGES

ADVANTAGES

1. Esthetic because of its gold color and high lustre.
2. Tarnish and corrosion resistant.

3.   Good mechanical properties.
4.   Good biocompatibility.

DISADVANTAGES

1.   Nonesthetic because it is not tooth colored.
2.   High CTE (coefficient of thermal conductivity).
3.   Problems of temperature sensitivity if not insulated with a base
4.   Manipulation is technically challenging.

The technical skill of the dentist is very important for the success of the direct gold restoration. A gold restoration of poor quality can be one of the most inferior of all restorations.

Resin-based Composites and Bonding Agents

Evolution of Tooth Colored Restorative Materials

Silicates

The earliest tooth colored restorative materials were the *silicate cements*. These were used extensively in the early 20th century. Though, they had a fluoride release mechanism they eroded quickly and had a problem of marginal discoloration.

Acrylic Resin Restorations

Silicates were subsequently replaced by the *tooth colored acrylic resins*. These were basically polymethyl methacrylate (PMMA) resins similar to those used in dentures. They were widely welcomed at the time because of their superior esthetics, ease of manipulation, low cost and insolubility in oral fluids.

The material was supplied as a powder and liquid (in brown bottles). With time however, many restorations began to fail, due to microleakage, staining and caries. This happened primarily because these materials shrink on setting causing them to pull away from the cavity walls. Their high thermal expansion and contraction caused further stresses at the margins. In addition, they had poor wear resistance. The monomer within was also implicated in pulpal irritation especially in deep restorations. Manufacturers tried to offset these problems by adding quartz filler particles. This greatly reduced the shrinkage by reducing the proportion of resin in the mix. It also reduced the thermal expansion. However, the quartz did not bond to the resin which resulted in staining and poor wear resistance.

Bowen's Resin

The real breakthrough came with the discovery by Ray L Bowen in 1962 of a new type of resin called bisphenol-A glycidyl methacrylate (popularly called bis-GMA or Bowen's resin). He also developed a process by which the resin was bonded to the filler particles within the composite (silane coupling). The acrylic resin restorative materials soon became obsolete and were replaced by these new composite resins (see traditional composites - ***Box 11.1***). Composite resins continued to evolve as manufacturers tried to increase the filler content as well as reduce the size of the fillers for improved esthetics and strength. Today composite resins are widely used for both posterior and anterior restorations.

COMPOSITE RESINS

Essentially, it is a resin which has been strengthened by adding silica particles called fillers. The pioneering research of Bowen together with the development of the acid etching technique and bonding agents, revolutionized restorative dentistry. It largely replaced the earlier silicate and restorative acrylics.

The composite is a system composed of a mixture of two or more macromolecules, which are essentially insoluble in each other and differ in form. The composite material's properties are superior to those of its individual components, e.g. fiberglass has a resin matrix which is reinforced by glass fibers. The resulting composite is harder and stiffer than the resin matrix material, but less brittle than glass. Examples of natural composite materials are tooth enamel and dentin. Matrix is made of collagen, with hydroxyapatite crystals acting as fillers. Though the early composites were developed for restorative purposes their uses subsequently expanded to include provisional restorations, luting, etc.

USES

1. Restoration of anterior ***(Figs. 11.1A and B)*** and posterior teeth (directly or indirectly).
2. To veneer metal crowns and fixed partial dentures (prosthodontic resins).
3. To build-up cores (post core).
4. Bonding of orthodontic brackets, etched cast restorations, ceramic crowns, posts, inlays, onlays and laminates.
5. Pit and fissure sealant.
6. Esthetic laminates.
7. Repair of chipped porcelain restorations.

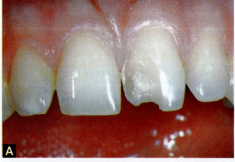 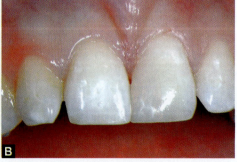

FIGURES 11.1A AND B The Illustrations show a fractured central incisor **(A)** restored quite realistically with composite resin **(B)**.

(Different composites are available for the above purposes. Each of them have their properties adjusted to suit the specific application for which it was intended. They are usually not interchangeable).

TYPES

Composite resins are difficult to classify because of the wide range of overlapping filler sizes. Therefore, a wide range of classifications exist. No single classification is deemed satisfactory.

ISO 4049:2009

Type 1   Polymer-based materials suitable for restorations involving occlusal surfaces

Type 2   All other polymer based materials and luting agents

Based on curing mechanism (ISO 4049:2009)

Type 1 and 2 are further grouped into 3 classes based on curing mechanism.

Class 1 — Self cured materials

Class 2 — Light cured materials

   Group 1 — Energy applied intraorally

   Group 2 — Energy applied extraorally

Class 3 — Dual cured materials

Based on filler particle size (Willems 1993)

Willems developed an extensive classification based on a number of parameters, such as Young's modulus, the percentage (by volume) of inorganic filler, the size of the main particles, surface roughness and compressive stress. Though the classification is not presented, terminology from Willems classification is still used today to describe some commercially available composites. With the inclusion of nanosized particles the particle sizes can be described as

- ○ Fine   Particle size > 3 μm
- ○ Ultrafine   Particle size < 3 μm
- ○ Microfine   Average particle size — 0.04 μm
- ○ Nano   Nano range (5–100 nm or 0.005–0.01 μm)

Based on filler particle size

Fillers play an important role in the composite performance. However, a universal system of classifying fillers has not been agreed upon. Differences exist on the nomenclature and the size range of the filler particles.

- ○ Macrofillers (10-100 μm)
- ○ Midifillers   (1-10 μm)
- ○ Minifillers   (0.1-1 μm)
- ○ Microfillers   (0.01-0.1 μm)
  - a. Homogenous — contains only microfillers

  b. Heterogenous — microfillers combined with prepolymerized fillers
    — splintered prepolymerized particles
    — spherical prepolymerized particles
  c. Agglomerated — microfiller sintered to form larger filler complexes
○ Nanofillers (0.005–0.01 µm)
○ Hybrid (range of sizes which usually includes micro or nanofillers with macro, midi or mini fillers

Based on viscosity

○ Conventional
○ Flowable
○ Packable

Viscosity determines the flow characteristics during placement. A flowable composite flows like liquid or a loose gel. A packable composite is firm and offers some resistance to condensation.

Based on applications and commercial availability

1. Restorative composites—direct intraoral restorations
   – Hybrid composites *(Fig. 11.2)*
     - Macrofilled hybrids
     - Midifilled hybrids
     - Minifilled hybrids
     - Nanofilled hybrids
   – Microfilled *(Fig. 11.3)*
   – Nanofilled composites *(Fig. 11.4)*
   – Flowable *(Fig. 11.5)*
   – Packable
   – Core build-up composites
2. Prosthodontic composites (for fabrication of inlays, veneers, crowns and FDPs)
3. Provisional composites (for temporary crowns, FDPs, etc.)
4. Luting composites
5. Repair composites (intraoral repair of fractured ceramic or acrylic or composite veneer)

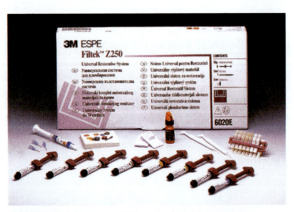

FIGURE 11.2 Representative microhybrid composite.

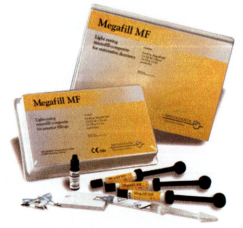

FIGURE 11.3 A microfilled composite.

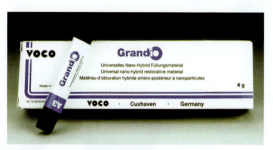

FIGURE 11.4 Universal nano-hybrid composite.

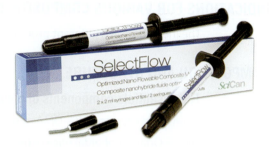

FIGURE 11.5 Flowable composites are often identified by the syringe like dispensing tips.

RESTORATIVE COMPOSITE RESINS

The first tooth colored restorative system were developed in the late 1950s and early 1960s by Bowen (also known as Bowen's resin). The early composite resins were generally macrofilled resins and were referred to as conventional composites. These were chemically activated. This was followed by U-V light activated and later visible light activated systems. The early composites had poor wear resistance and stained easily. This was attributed to the large sized (macrofillers) filler particles used. The introduction of the microfilled composites improved wear resistance and better esthetics. However, they had poor mechanical properties. The hybrid composites attempted to combine the esthetics and wear resistance of the microfilled with the mechanical properties of the macrofilled composites. The latest entry into the field - the *nanocomposites* *(Fig. 11.4)* holds the promise of high polishability with further improvement in mechanical properties.

SUPPLIED AS

Composites used for restoring teeth are usually supplied as a kit *(Fig. 11.2)* containing the following

- Composite resin (either chemical or light cured)
- Etching liquid (37% phosphoric acid)
- Bonding agent
- Shade guide.

Chemically activated composite resins are available as

Two paste (base and catalyst) system   Supplied in small jars or syringes *(Fig. 11.6)*.

Powder-liquid systems   Powder (inorganic phase plus the initiator) is supplied in jars. Liquid (BIG-GMA diluted with monomers) in bottles.

Light activated resins are available as

Single paste form in dark or light proof syringes *(Fig. 11.5)*.

Trade names   Various commercial products available are presented in *Table 11.1*.

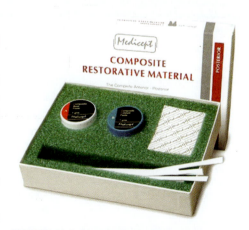

FIGURE 11.6 Chemically cured composite.

INDICATIONS FOR VARIOUS COMPOSITE RESINS

The indications for different products are presented in **Table 11.2**.

COMPOSITION AND STRUCTURE

The essentials components of a composite resin *(Fig. 11.7)*

Resin matrix/binder—Bis-GMA or urethane dimethacrylate

Filler—Quartz, colloidal silica or heavy metal glasses

Coupling agent—Organosilanes.

In addition they contain

A curing system—Chemical or light curing chemicals.

Inhibitors (0.01%)—Prevents premature polymerization, e.g. butylated hydroxytoluene (BHT).

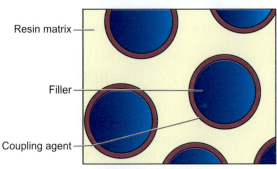

FIGURE 11.7 Essentials of a composite.

TABLE 11.1 Representative commercial products	
Type	*Commercial name*
Chemically Activated	Isopast, Alfa comp (voco), Brilliant (coltene), Medicept
Light Activated	
Hybrid (Universal)	Filtek Z250(3M), Herculite (Kerr), TPH spectrum, Venus,Charisma (Heraeus), Tetric Ceram (Ivoclar), Point-4 (Kerr)
Microfilled	Helio Progress, Durafil VS (Heraeus), A110 (3M-ESPE), Sculpt-it (Jeneric/Pentron), Amelogen Microfill (Ultra-dent), Renamel Microfill (Cosmedent).
Flowable	C- Fill Flow, Synergy D6 Flow (Coltene), Tetric flow, Venus Flow (Heraeus), Flow Plus (Medicept), etc.
Packable	Surefil (Dentsply), Heliomolar HB (Ivoclar), Solitaire 2 (Heraeus), Tetric Ceram HB, etc.
Nanocomposite	Grandio (Voco), Filtek Supreme (3 M), Venus Diamond, (Heraeus), Composite-nanohybrid (Medicept)

TABLE 11.2 Various restorative composites currently marketed and their uses	
Type	*Indications*
Hybrid or universal (microhybrids)	Anterior and posterior restorations in high stress areas requiring improved polishing (e.g. Classes I, II, III, IV)
Packable Hybrids	Class II cavities where greater packability is needed for improved contact with adjacent teeth
Flowable Hybrids	• Class V lesions subjected to flexing stresses • Mini cavities • Repair of composite • In layered composite restorations as first layer (for better adaptation)
Microfilled (homogenous and heterogeneous)	• Low stress areas • Areas requiring high polish (to reduce plaque accumulation, e.g. subgingival areas, Class V lesions, etc.)
Hybrid or universal (nanohybrids)	Anterior and posterior restorations in high stress areas requiring greater polishability, e.g. Classes I-IV and Class V cervical lesions

UV absorbers—to improve color stability

Opacifiers—(0.001 to 0.007%) e.g. titanium dioxide and aluminum

Color pigments—to match tooth color.

RESIN MATRIX

Dental composites use a blend of monomers that are aromatic or aliphatic dimethacrylates. Of these, bis-GMA (Bisphenol-A-glycidyl methacrylate), urethane dimethacrylate (UDMA) and bis-EMA (Bisphenol-A-polyethylene glycol diether dimethacrylate) are most commonly used. Triethylene glycol dimethacrylate (TEGDMA) is added to control the viscosity.

Bis-GMA was developed by RL Bowen (Bowen's resin) in the early 1960s. Its properties were superior to those of acrylic resins. However, it had a few limitations like

- ○ A high viscosity which required the use of diluent monomers
- ○ Difficulty in synthesizing a pure composition
- ○ Strong air inhibition to polymerization
- ○ High water sorption because of diluents used
- ○ Polymerization shrinkage and thermal dimensional changes still existed
- ○ Like other resins it does not adhere to tooth structure

To make it clinically acceptable, diluent monomers are added to the resin matrix to reduce the viscosity of the resin. It also allows more fillers to be incorporated.

Diluents allow extensive cross-linking between chains, thereby increasing the resistance of the matrix to solvents. The commonly used diluent monomer is TEGDMA (triethylene glycol dimethacrylate). Thus composite resins have to be blended with different monomers to optimize their properties.

Drawbacks of TEGDMA include
1. High shrinkage.
2. Contributes to reduced shelf-life by migration in to the plastic walls.
3. Being hydrophilic it makes the composite susceptible to moisture leading to thickening or softening of the paste in certain climatic conditions.

(Because of these drawbacks some manufacturers have replaced the majority of the TEGDMA with a blend of UDMA and bis-EMA).

The refractive index is an important property for anterior restorative materials. To have acceptable esthetics composite resins must match the translucency of enamel. Bis-GMA and TEGDMA have a refractive index of 1.55 and 1.46 respectively which average to around 1.5 when combined together.

FILLER PARTICLES

Fillers play a crucial role in the composite resin. Most of the important properties of the resin is determined by its filler content. Composite fillers are classified by material, shape and size. Many different classifications of fillers have been proposed. They are broadly classified into 3 groups - macrofillers, microfillers and nanofillers. A mixture of different particle sizes is referred to as a hybrid. For details of filler size and nomenclature see 'classification of composite resins.'

Functions of fillers

Addition of filler particles in to the resin significantly improves its properties.

1. Improves strength—Fillers reinforce the resin and improve mechanical properties like strength, stiffness, hardness, etc.

2. Reduces shrinkage—As less resin is present, the curing shrinkage is reduced thereby reducing marginal leakage.
3. Reduces Wear—Fillers play a crucial role in reducing the wearing of composite resins. The smaller the size and higher the concentration of fillers the better the wear resistance.
4. Surface smoothness and esthetics—Fillers affect the surface smoothness and subsequent esthetics of the composite. The smaller the particle size, the greater the polishability. Larger particle sizes in the early composites contributed to surface roughness and staining.
5. Reduces water sorption—Resins absorb water and makes it more prone to wear and staining. Filler reduce water sorption by reducing the overall resin content.
6. Reduces thermal expansion and contraction—Fillers have a lower CTE in comparison to the resin.
7. Improves clinical handling (increased viscosity makes them easier to handle clinically).
8. Imparts radiopacity—Radiopaque fillers help improve diagnostics (e.g. caries detection through roentgenograms, etc.).

Important attributes of fillers
Important attributes of fillers, that determine the properties and clinical application of composites are
○ Amount of filler added (filler loading)
○ Size of particles and its distribution
○ Shape of fillers
○ Index of refraction
○ Radiopacity
○ Hardness

Filler size The size of the fillers affect the surface smoothness and the wear resistance. The smaller the fillers the greater the surface smoothness. Microfilled composites have the best surface smoothness and lowest wear. This is because the particles are removed at the same rate as the resin matrix if they are smaller. Larger particles result in a rougher surface. The introduction of the nanoparticles hold *great promise* of improved smoothness, good wear resistance as well as improved mechanical properties.

Filler loading Filler loading refers to the amount of fillers that can be practically incorporated into the resin. The amount of filler that can be added depends on the type of filler and the purpose for which it is intended. Most hybrid composites have a filler loading ranging from 60 to 70% volume. The introduction of the newer nanofillers allow a greater filler loading of up to 79.5% vol. Microfillers thicken the resin quickly. Thus microfilled resins usually do not have the same filler loading as resins with larger particle sizes such as the hybrids.

Particle size distribution Most modern hybrid composites have particles range in size from 0.01 to 10 μm. Microfillers are usually in the range of 0.01 – 0.07 (average 0.04 μm). In order to increase the filler amount in the resin, it is necessary to add the fillers in a range of particle sizes. If a single particle size is used, a space will exist between the particles. Smaller particles can then fill-up these spaces, thus increasing the filler content ***(Figs. 11.8A to E)***.

Shape of fillers Based on shape 3 types of fillers are used—irregular, spherical and fibrous. The shape affects the filler loading and the handling characteristics of the composite.

Refractive index For esthetics, the filler should have a translucency similar to tooth structure. To achieve this, the refractive index of the filler should closely match that of the resin. Most glass and quartz fillers have a refractive index of 1.5, which match that of bis-GMA and TEGDMA.

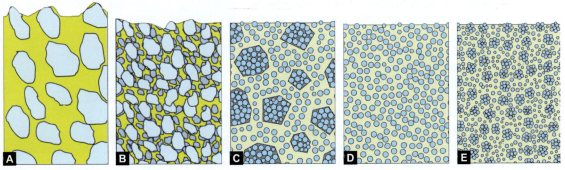

FIGURES 11.8A TO E Effect on particle size on surface smoothness. **(A)** Traditional composite. **(B)** Hybrid composite. **(C)** Microfilled heterogenous type (showing prepolymerized fillers). **(D)** Microfilled homogenous type. **(E)** Nanocomposite showing nanoparticles and nanoclusters.

Measurement of filler content—volume versus weight percentage

Filler content is designated in percent volume (vol.%) or percent weight (wt.%). Weight percent is usually higher in value than percent volume. The volume percentage may be a *more reliable indicator* of filler content than the weight percentage. This is because of differences in density between different fillers. For example, composites can have a similar volume percentage of fillers yet different weight percentages. This is because the composite containing a larger fraction of heavy metal glass fillers will have a higher weight percentage.

FILLERS TYPES

Composite resins may contain a variety of fillers

○ Ground quartz

○ Glasses or ceramic containing heavy metals

○ Boron silicates

○ Lithium aluminum silicates

○ Ytterbium trifluoride

○ Colloidal silica

Quartz fillers   They are obtained by grinding or milling quartz. They were mainly used in conventional composites. They are chemically inert and very hard. This makes the restoration more difficult to polish and can cause abrasion of the opposing teeth and restorations.

Glasses/ceramics containing heavy metals   These fillers provide radiopacity to the resin restoration. Increased radiopacity make composites detectable on radiographs which aid diagnostics. Examples are barium, zirconium, ytterbium fluoride, zinc and strontium glasses. The most commonly used is barium glass. It is not as inert as quartz. Some barium may leach out with time.

Fluoride releasing fillers   Some current composites have fluoride releasing capability. This includes fillers like *ytterbium trifluoride* and *Ba-Al-fluorosilicate glass*. In one commercial product (Tetric ceram) the YbF_3 content is as high as 17 wt.%. The Ba-Al-fluorosilicate glass content was 5 wt.%.

Colloidal silica   They have the same composition and refractive index as quartz but not as hard or abrasive. This is due to their 'amorphous' (or noncrystalline) form. They are also referred to as 'microfillers'. They are obtained by a *pyrolytic* or a precipitation process. Colloidal silica particles *(Fig. 11.9)* have a large surface area (50 to 400 m²/g), thus, even small amounts of microfillers thicken the resin. They are added in small amounts in hybrid composites (5 wt. %) to adjust the paste viscosity. The hybrid varieties have a microfiller loading of 10 to 15% weight. In *microfilled composites* it is the main filler used (20 to 59% volume). Since they cannot be added in large amounts the overall filler loading of microfilled composites is lower than conventional or hybrid varieties.

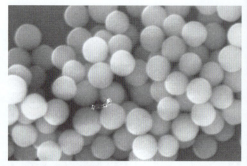

FIGURE 11.9 Electron microscopic picture of colloidal silica 0.06 μm.

METHODS TO INCREASE MICROFILLER LOADING

Manufacturers are constantly on the look out for methods to increase the filler content of the microfilled composites.

1. One method is to sinter (fuse) the colloidal silica particles, thereby reducing surface area. These are known as agglomerated silica.
2. Addition of *prepolymerized fillers*   This is the more common method. Also known as 'organic fillers'. They are prepared by adding 60 to 70 wt.% of silane coated colloidal silica to the monomer, which is held at a slightly higher temperature to reduce its viscosity. It is then heat cured and ground.

The composite is obtained by adding these prepolymerized fillers along with more silane coated microfillers into unpolymerized resin matrix *(Fig. 11.13)*.

Silica nanoparticles   These are currently the smallest filler particles used in dental composites. Nanoparticles are *defined as* particles between *1 and 100 nanometers* in size. In nanotechnology, a particle is defined as a small object that behaves as a whole unit with respect to its transport and properties.

Adoption of nanoparticle technology have ushered in the next generation of composite resins. Incorporation of silica nanoparticles into the composite resins have improved many of the properties of composite resins, particularly wear resistance and polishability. Nanoparticles in composites can be used in 2 forms.

○ Nanoparticle—a single nanoparticle (size ranges from 5-25 nm)
○ Nanoclusters—a group of nanoparticles (forms larger sized particles).

Manufacture of fillers

Filler particles can be generated: (1) by crushing, grinding, and sieving large blocks of ceramic, (2) by condensation of SiO_2 from the vapor phase as small droplets of microfiller, or (3) by precipitation of filler particles from solution (sol-gel). The smallest fillers can only be manufactured in a practical way from the vapor phase or by sol-gel processes.

COUPLING AGENTS

Coupling agents bond the filler particles to the resin matrix. The earliest composites did not use coupling agents. This resulted in microscopic defects between the filler and surrounding resin. Microleakage of fluids into these defects led to surface staining and failure. Typically the manufacturer treats the surface of the filler with a coupling agent to bond the filler to the resin matrix.

Functions of coupling agents

1. They improve the properties of the resin through transfer of stresses from the more plastic resin matrix to the stiffer filler particles.
2. They prevent water from penetrating the filler-resin interface.
3. They bond the fillers to the resin matrix thereby reducing the wear.

The most commonly used coupling agents are *organosilanes* (i.e. 3-methacryloxypropyl-trimethoxysilane).

$$CH_2\!\!=\!\!C\!-\!\overset{\displaystyle O}{\overset{\displaystyle \|}{C}}\!-\!O\!-\!CH_2CH_2CH_2\!-\!Si\!-\!OCH_3$$
with CH_3 below the C and OCH_3 above and OCH_3 below the Si

The agent is a molecule with a methacrylate groups on one end and methoxy groups (OCH_3) on the other end. In the presence of adsorbed water the methoxy groups hydrolyze to form silanol groups (-Si-OH) which then form ionic bonds with the silanol groups of the filler forming a siloxane bond (-Si-O-Si-). The other end has a methacrylate group which forms a covalent bond with the resin when it is polymerized. This completes the coupling process. *Zirconates* and *titanates* can also be used as coupling agents.

POLYMERIZATION (SETTING) MECHANISMS

They polymerize by the addition mechanism that is initiated by *free radicals* as described in resins. The free radicals can be generated by chemical activation or external energy (heat, light or microwave).

Based on the mode of activation of polymerization, there are three main types

A. Chemically activated resins
B. Light-activated resins
C. Combination of the above (dual cure).

CHEMICALLY ACTIVATED COMPOSITE RESINS

This is a two-paste system

○ Base paste contains—benzoyl peroxide initiator
○ Catalyst paste—tertiary amine activator (i.e. N, N-dimethyl-p-toluidine).

Setting

When the two pastes are spatulated, the amine reacts with the benzoyl peroxide to form the *free radicals* which starts the polymerization.

Disadvantages

1. No control of curing time.
2. No control of curing shrinkage.
3. Hand mixing increases possibility of voids.

LIGHT ACTIVATED COMPOSITE RESINS

Under normal light they do not interact. However, when exposed to light of the correct wavelength the photoinitiator (camphorquinone) is activated and reacts with the amine to form *free radicals* which then start the polymerization.

UV light activated systems

The earliest systems used ultraviolet (UV) light for curing. Light activation put control of the working time in the hand of the dentist.

Limitations of UV light curing were
1. Limited penetration of the light into the resin. Thus, it was difficult to polymerize thick sections.
2. Lack of penetration through tooth structure.

Visible-light activated resins

These have totally replaced UV light systems. They are also more widely used than the chemically activated resins.

These are single paste systems containing

○ Photoinitiator: Camphorquinone 0.2 wt.%

○ Amine accelerator: Dimethylaminoethyl-methacrylate (DMAEMA 0.15 wt.%).

Camphorquinone has light absorption range between 400 and 500 nm. This is in the *blue region* of the visible light spectrum. In some cases inhibitors are added to enhance its stability to room light or dental operatory light.

DUAL CURE RESINS

A combination of chemical and light curing is used to overcome some of the drawbacks of light curing. Dual cure resins are supplied as two pastes. When mixed together a slow setting reaction is initiated. These resins are used for cementing crowns or bulk restorations where there is limited or no light penetration. After the initial light cure, the remainder of the resin cures over a period of time by the chemical process.

CURING LAMPS

A number of curing lights are manufactured. Most use visible light in the blue spectrum (between 400 and 500 nm). In some units the light source is remote and is transmitted to the site of restoration through a light guide which is a long, flexible fiber-optic cord. There are also hand held light curing devices which transmit the light through short light guides *(Fig. 11.10)*.

Important features of curing lamps
1. *Spectral range* Light emitted by curing lamps should fall in the photoabsorbtion spectral range of camphorquinone. This is in the violet-blue region of the spectrum and is between 400-500 nm. Some curing lamps produce light within this spectrum whereas others produce more broad spectrum light which then needs to be filtered to emit only the light in the blue range.

2. *Light intensity* Light intensity should be high for a shorter curing time and greater depth of cure. Light intensity of lamps vary from 300 to 1200 milliwatts/cm². For maximum curing a radiant energy of 16 J/cm² is needed for a 2 mm thick section of composite.

Types of lamps

Currently many forms of curing lights are available. These include

QTH (Quartz-tungsten-halogen) These were the earliest visible light lamps. The light source is a *tungsten-halogen-quartz bulb (Fig. 11.11)*. The white light generated passes through a filter that removes all wavelengths except those in the blue range. Heat is also generated

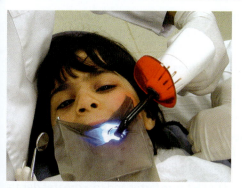

FIGURE 11.10 A dental curing light in the visible blue range (QTH).

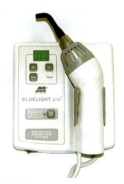

FIGURE 11.11 A wired curing light device (QTH).

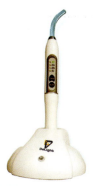

FIGURE 11.12 A wireless LED lamp.

thus requiring a cooling fan. The intensity of light gradually reduces with time (aging) and so calibration is required at intervals.

LED (Light emitting diodes) LED *(Fig. 11.12)* is increasingly popular as a light source in all spheres including dentistry ever since the discovery of the blue diode in the 1990s. It is similar in power to QTH lamps (700 mW/cm²). Research has shown that the curing depth and degree of conversion is significantly better with LEDs than with QTH. It emits light only in the blue part of the spectrum. Thus, it does not require filters. Its advantages also include low power consumption (can even be operated by batteries), no heat generation (eliminating cooling fan), and low noise (due to the absence of cooling fan).

PAC (Plasma arc curing) These lamps generate an intense white light by ionizing xenon gas to produce a plasma. Filters are required to remove heat and the unwanted wavelengths. Their high power allows faster cures as well as greater depth of cures.

Argon laser These produce light of the greatest intensity. They emit light of a single wavelength around 490 nm and therefore do not require filters. They do not produce little heat because of the limited infrared. However, these lamps are more expensive. They have a narrow light tip (spot size) requiring clinicians to increase number of overlaps in case of a larger restoration.

The high intensity lights like the PAC and the laser provide a faster cure (as short as 5 seconds for a 2 mm section). Besides being expensive the accelerated curing can introduce substantial stresses. Further studies are needed.

EYE PROTECTION

Staring into the curing lights for prolonged periods can cause retinal damage. It is best to look away while the curing is in progress. Various kinds of eye protection are available and should be used when working with composites.

DEGREE OF POLYMERIZATION AND DEPTH OF CURE

The total amount of resin polymerized depends on several factors.

❍ *Transmission of light through the material* This is controlled by absorption and scattering of light by the filler particles, as well as any tooth structure interposed between the light source and the resin. For this reason, microfilled composites with smaller and more numerous particles will not cure to as great a depth as conventional composites.

❍ *Shade of resin Darker shades* require longer exposure time.

- ❍ *Amount of photoinitiator and inhibitor present*   For polymerization to take place at any depth, a particular amount of photons must be available. This is directly related to the intensity of light and time of exposure.
- ❍ *Curing time*   Manufacturers recommend curing times for each material and shade. This depends on the output of the particular curing device. Thus, 80 to 240 seconds is required with a low intensity light whereas to achieve the same result, a high intensity light requires only a 20 to 60 second exposure.
- ❍ *Intensity of light*   Light intensity is measured in milliwatts/cm^2. The time required for curing a 2 mm depth of resin by a QTH lamp is 40 seconds. The same thickness can be cured in 20 seconds if the light intensity is increased to 800 mW/cm^2.
- ❍ *Type of light*   High intensity lights like PAC and LASER cure faster and to a greater depth than the QTH and LED generated lights.
- ❍ *Thickness of resin*   Thickness greater than 2–3 mm are difficult to cure because of the lack of light penetration.
- ❍ *Distance from light* Optimum distance is 1 mm with the light positioned 90 degrees from the surface of the resin.

BOX 11.1 | Traditional composite

Traditional composites are also referred to as 'conventional' or 'macrofilled composite' (because of the large size of the filler particles). Traditional composites are rarely used currently and have been largely replaced by other hybrids. However, their discussion will continue largely for comparison to the newer composites.

Composition
Ground quartz was most commonly used as filler. There is a wide distribution of particle sizes. Although average size is 8 to 12 μm, particles as large as 50 μm may also be present.
Filler loading: 70-80 wt.% or 60-70 vol.%.

Composition
Ground quartz was most commonly used as filler. There is a wide distribution of particle sizes. Although average size is 8 to 12 μm, particles as large as 50 μm may also be present.
Filler loading: 70-80 wt.% or 60-70 vol.%.

Properties
The conventional composites have significantly improved properties when compared to the unfilled restorative resins which preceded them. The improvement is the result of the improved resin, the filler loading and the strong bond between the filler and the resin matrix.

Compressive Strength   It is four to five times greater than that of unfilled resins (250 to 300 MPa).

Tensile Strength   It is double that of unfilled acrylic resins (50 to 65 MPa).

Elastic Modulus   It is four to six times greater than the unfilled resins (8 to 15 GPa).

Hardness   It is considerably greater (55 KHN) than that of unfilled resins.

Water Sorption   It is less than that of unfilled resins (0.5 to 0.7 mg/cm^2).

Coefficient of Thermal Expansion   The high filler-to-resin ratio reduced the CTE (25 to 35 × 10^{-6}/°C) significantly.

Esthetics   Polishing of the conventional composite results in a rough surface. This is due to the selective wear of the softer resin matrix leaving the hard filler particles elevated. This resulted in a tendency to stain over a period of time.

Radiopacity   Radiopacity is measured by a ***photo densitometer***. Radiopacity allows proper assessment of the restoration as well as future diagnosis of caries. The heavy metal fillers contribute to the radiopacity of composites. Aluminum is used as a standard reference for radiopacity. A 2 mm thickness of dentin and enamel is equivalent to 2.5 and 4 mm of aluminum respectively. Traditional composites have a radiopacity of 2-3 mm of aluminum equivalent.

Adhesion   Composites do not adhere to tooth structure and require special bonding techniques to provide adhesion to the tooth structure.

Disadvantages

Although the conventional composites were superior to unfilled resins, they had certain disadvantages
- High surface roughness
- Polishing was difficult
- Poor resistance to occlusal wear
- Tendency to discolor—the rough surface tends to stain.

Because of these disadvantages as well as the introduction of improved composites this type was gradually phased out. It is probably no longer marketed.

MICROFILLED COMPOSITE

The microfilled composites *(Fig. 11.3)* were introduced soon after the traditional composites. They were developed to overcome the problems of surface roughness of traditional composites. The resin achieved the smoothness of unfilled acrylic direct filling resins and yet had the advantage of having fillers. Unfortunately, they could not achieve high levels of filler loading and therefore had somewhat inferior mechanical properties when compared to the traditional composites. For this reason, these composites are primarily used for esthetic restorations in stress free areas and in areas close to the gingiva where a smooth finish is required for reduced plaque accumulation.

Synonyms Also referred to as microfine composites.

COMPOSITION

The smoother surface is due to the incorporation of microfillers. *Colloidal silica* is used as the microfiller and is the only type of filler present in this type. The problem with colloidal silica was that it had a large surface area that could not be adequately wetted by the matrix resin. Thus, addition of even small amounts of microfillers resulted in *thickening* of the resin matrix. Thus, it was not possible to achieve the same filler loading as conventional composites.

Manufacturers tried to overcome this problem by

1. Using prepolymerized or organic fillers (see section on fillers). These composites were referred to as 'heterogenous'.
2. Using silica in cluster or agglomerate form. These were referred to as 'homogenous' microfilled composites.

Filler size The colloidal silica is 200-300 times smaller than the quartz fillers of conventional composite. Size ranges from 0.04 to 0.4 μm.

Filler content With the inclusion of prepolymerized (organic) fillers, the filler content is 70 wt.% or 60 vol.%. However, the actual inorganic filler content is only 50 wt.%.

CLINICAL CONSIDERATIONS

With the exception of compressive strength their mechanical properties are inferior to the other types of composites. This is because of their higher resin content (50 vol.%). Their biggest advantage is their esthetics. The microfilled composite is the resin of choice for esthetic restoration of anterior teeth, especially in non-stress bearing situations. For most applications, the decreased physical properties do not create problems. However, in stress bearing situations like Class IV and Class II restorations they have a greater potential for fracture. Sometimes, chipping occurs at the margins.

HYBRID COMPOSITE RESINS

The hybrid type forms the majority of the composites used in dentistry currently *(Fig. 11.2)*. These were developed to obtain better surface smoothness than that of the conventional large particle composites, yet maintain the properties of the latter. Hybrid composites have a surface smoothness and esthetics competitive with microfilled composites for anterior restorations. The hybrids are generally considered as multipurpose composites suitable for both anterior and posterior use.

Filler volume

The total filler content is 75–80 wt.% or 60–65 vol.%. The overall filler loading is not as high as small particle composites because of the higher microfiller content.

Filler type

Two kinds of filler particles are employed

1. *Heavy metal glasses*   Average particle size is 0.4 to 1 µm. 75% of the ground particles are smaller than 1.0 µm.

2. *Colloidal silica*   Size—0.04 µm. It is present in higher concentrations (*10 to 20 wt.%*) and therefore, contributes significantly to its properties.

The hybrids are generally considered as multipurpose composites suitable for both anterior and posterior use. They are widely used for anterior restorations, including class IV because of its smooth surface and good strength.

The hybrids are also widely employed for stress bearing restorations.

NANO AND NANOHYBRID COMPOSITE RESINS

Continued interest in the reduction of the size of fillers has led to the adaptation of nanotechnology to the field of composite resins. A new type of composite resin based on nanosized filler particles has been recently introduced. Nanocomposites *(Fig. 11.6)* are similar to the microfilled, comprising of uniformly sized nanofillers. Nanohybrids like the conventional hybrids, come in a range of filler sizes including nanofillers. Unfortunately conflicting reports exist on the efficacy of these relatively new materials. Initial reports indicate that these materials have the mechanical properties of the hybrid composites with the esthetics and polishability of the microfilled composites. Thus they can be used for both anterior and posterior restorations. Nanohybrids are generally stronger than the nanocomposites. However, nanocomposites have improved polishability. Continued development along these lines might eventually lead to the phasing out of conventional hybrid and microfilled composites. However, further research is required to establish the efficacy of the nano and the nanohybrid composites.

Filler volume and type

The predominant fillers are zirconium/silica or nanosilica particles measuring approximately 5 to 25 nm and nanoaggregates of approximately 75 nm. The aggregates are treated with silane so that they bind to the resin. The aggregates and nanoparticles filler distribution gives a high load, up to 79.5%.

PROPERTIES OF COMPOSITE RESINS

Composite resins were developed after amalgam and therefore it is a useful material with which to compare restorative composite resins. The mechanical properties of these materials have steadily improved over the years. Hovever, when compared to amalgam these materials are highly technique sensitive and therefore optimal properties can be achieved only if proper techniques of manipulation and insertion are followed. The common factor affecting most physical and mechanical properties of the composite is the filler content.

FLEXURAL STRENGTH

| Hybrid | 80–160 | MPa | | Nanohybrids | 180 | MPa |
| Microfilled | 60–120 | MPa | | Amalgam | 90–130 | MPa |

COMPRESSIVE STRENGTH

| Hybrid | 240–290 | MPa | | Nanohybrids | 460 | MPa |
| Microfilled | 240–300 | MPa | | Amalgam | 510 | MPa |

TENSILE STRENGTH

| Hybrid | 30–55 | MPa | | Nanohybrids | 81 | MPa |
| Microfilled | 25–40 | MPa | | Amalgam | 64 | MPa |

MODULUS OF ELASTICITY

Hybrid	8.8–13	GPa		Amalgam	62	GPa
Microfilled	4–6.9	GPa		Enamel	83	GPa
Nano	18	GPa		Dentin	19	GPa

HARDNESS

Hardness determines the degree of deformation of a material and it is generally accepted as an important property and a valuable parameter for comparison with tooth structure. To assure an optimized clinical performance of restorations, it is of paramount importance to employ materials with hardness at least similar to that of the dentinal substrate, not only superficially, but also in depth, since an accentuated decrease in hardness would adversely affect their mechanical properties and marginal integrity.

❍ Enamel   343 KHN
❍ Dentin   70 KHN

Composites generally show lower hardness than enamel. The hardness varies between different products and depends on the amount and type of filler used.

❍ Hybrid   60–117 KHN
❍ Microfilled   22–80 KHN
❍ Amalgam   110 KHN

Factors affecting hardness

Time period   Composites show an increase in surface hardness with time due to continued polymerization. The best results are seen 7 days after polymerization. For those unable to wait for a subsequent appointment a 15 minute delay is recommended before start of polishing procedures.

Polishing   Polishing has been shown to increase the surface hardness of composites. Polishing removes the surface organic layer and exposes the harder fillers below. However, polishing is best delayed at least 24 hours after polymerization.

POLYMERIZATION SHRINKAGE

Polymerization in composite resins is accompanied by a shrinkage which varies between different composites depending on the resin to filler ratio. Thus, the polymerization shrinkage ranges from 0.6–1.4% (in composites with higher filler content) to 2–3% (in composites with lower filler content like microfilled composites). This creates tensile stresses as high as 130 kg/cm² which severely strains the bond and can lead to marginal leakage. Sometimes, it may also cause the enamel at the restoration margin to crack or fracture.

The total polymerization shrinkage between light activated and chemically activated resins do not differ. However, the pattern of shrinkage is different (see differences). The polymerization shrinkage is highest in case of the microfilled composites because of the higher resin content.

Clinical techniques to reduce polymerization shrinkage include

1. *Ramped curing*   Polymerizing the composite resin in layers or ramps **(Fig. 11.13)**.

2. *Soft start*   In this technique polymerization is initiated slowly. The device automatically begins with a low intensity light, gradually increasing and ending with high intensity light. This gives time for stress relaxation.

3. *Delayed curing*   The restoration is partially cured with a low intensity light. The operator continues working on the restoration and then follows it with a final high intensity exposure.

4. Fabricating and curing the restoration extraorally on a cast (indirect technique) and then cementing on to the tooth, thereby completing the polymerization before cementing.

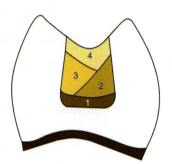

FIGURE 11.13 Ramped curing.

AIR OR OXYGEN INHIBITION

Polymerization is inhibited by air or oxygen. To avoid this the surface of the restoration should be protected by a transparent matrix strip or celluloid crown former. If the composite is unprotected during polymerization the surface of the composite remains tacky. This is known as the *air or oxygen inhibited layer (OIL)*.

THERMAL PROPERTIES

Thermal expansion coefficient (TEC)

Thermal expansion and contraction is cyclic in nature in the mouth and this can place additional strain on the tooth-resin bond. Over time this can lead to material fatigue, bond failure and percolation of fluids into the gap. Ideally the TEC of a restorative material should be close to that of tooth structure.

- Dentin $8.3 \times 10^{-6}/°C$
- Enamel $11.4 \times 10^{-6}/°C$

The TEC of composite resins is again related to the proportion of resin. Thus composites with higher resin content like microfilled will show a greater TEC.

- Hybrid $25–38 \times 10^{-6}/°C$
- Microfilled $55–68 \times 10^{-6}/°C$

Thermal conductivity

The thermal conductivity influences the rate at which heat or cold is transmitted through the restoration. Ideally restorative materials should have low thermal conductivity to reduce transfer of excessive thermal stimuli to the pulp.

- Hybrid $25–30 \times 10^{-4}$ cal/sec/cm^2 (°C/cm)
- Microfilled $12–15 \times 10^{-4}$ cal/sec/cm^2 (°C/cm)

WATER SORPTION

Water sorption is related to the resin content. The water sorption of hybrid composites are comparatively lower than that of the microfilled resins. ISO 4049 requirements limit the water sorption to a maximum of 40 µg/mm^2.

- Hybrid   5–17 µg/mm^2
- Microfilled 26–30 µg/mm^2

DIMENSIONAL STABILITY

A slow expansion (hygroscopic expansion) is associated with water sorption. The expansion which starts 15 minutes after polymerization reaches equilibrium in about 7 days. Microfilled resins show more expansion than hybrid varieties.

RETENTION

Composite resins do not adhere chemically to tooth structure. Micromechanical retention together with bonding agents have to be used to enhance adhesion to tooth structure.

ESTHETICS

Composites are highly esthetic direct restorative materials. Composites are supplied in a variety of shades. Special composite stains and other effects are also available to create lifelike restorations.

Ideally, with wear the silica filler should be removed along with the resin in which it is embedded. This is possible by using smaller filler sizes. In nanofilled and microfilled composites, the higher resin content and presence of microfillers is responsible for the increased surface smoothness. The inorganic filler particles are smaller than the abrasive particles used for finishing the restoration. Composites with larger fillers have a reduced surface smoothness which results in staining over a period of time. Age related effects also include stress cracks, a partial debonding of the filler-resin bond. This results in a loss of opacity/and or loss of shade match over time.

BIOCOMPATIBILITY OF COMPOSITE RESINS

The resin components are cytotoxic *in vitro*. Composites release some resin components for weeks after insertion. The level of release depends on the type of composite and efficiency of the cure.

Thus composites resins have biocompatibility issues from three aspects.

- Inherent chemical toxicity of the material on the pulp.
- Pulpal involvement due to microleakage.
- Allergic potential on contact with the oral mucosa.
- Allergic potential for personnel handling the material.
- Chronic inflammatory response in the periodontium when compared to amalgam in animal studies (monkeys).
- More cytotoxic than amalgam in vitro studies.
- Resin composite components have been shown to cause immunosuppression or immunostimulation and to inhibit DNA and RNA synthesis.
- Concerns over estrogenicity of Bisphenol A and its dimethacrylate.

In spite of the controversies properly polymerized composites appear to be relatively biocompatible as long as there is sufficient thickness of dentin. In cases where the pulp is exposed some form of pulp capping overlayed with a glass ionomer liner is recommended.

When used in proximity to gingival tissues, proper care should be taken to ensure correct technique of placement to prevent inflammatory responses associated with overhangs and microleakage. Issues concerning estrogenicity have not been proven to be of sufficient concern under intraoral conditions.

Pulp protection

Glass ionomer liners are applied as pulp protection in deep cavities. *Zinc oxide-eugenol is contraindicated* as it interferes with polymerization. Bacterial contamination should be avoided by using rubber dam isolation.

WEAR RATES AND LIFE EXPECTANCY OF COMPOSITES

Composites are ideal as an anterior restorative material where wear rates are low. For posterior teeth amalgam has long been the standard direct filling material. Due to the increasing demand for esthetics, concern about mercury toxicity and aggressive marketing, there is an increasing interest in the use of composites for class I and II restorations. The older generation composites showed high attrition rates. Newer formulations have shown improvements in wear resistance.

All types of composites have been used for posterior restorations. Current guidelines require posterior composites to show less than 50 µm wear over 18 months. For posterior use, the cavity preparation should be conservative, and the manipulation technique meticulous.

PROBLEMS IN THE USE OF COMPOSITES FOR POSTERIOR RESTORATIONS

1. In Class V restorations, when the gingival margin is located in cementum or dentin, the material shrinks away from the margin leading to a gap.
2. The placement technique is more time consuming and demanding.
3. Composites wear faster than amalgam. However, the newer materials like hybrids and nanocomposites have less wear (20 µm per year), which approaches that of amalgam (10 µm). In terms of years the average life expectancy of the composite resin is around 8 years, which is near to that of amalgam (10 years).

The major indications of composites for posterior use are
1. When esthetics is the prime consideration.
2. When a patient is allergic to mercury.

ADHESION

Composites do not adhere to tooth structure or any dental related surface. Acid etch technique and bonding agents have to be used to ensure adhesion.

Adhesion to instruments   Composite adhere to the sculpting and packing instruments which interfere with adaptation to the cavity walls, increase porosity and reduce operator comfort. Some clinicians use alcohol or the bonding agent as a release agent. However, both these techniques should be avoided as these materials are solvents that can weaken the resin.

RADIOPACITY

Radiopacity is a useful feature for any restorative material. Posterior restorations must demonstrate adequate radiopacity to permit detection of secondary caries, excess or inadequate quantities of material, air bubbles and other imperfections. ISO norm states that the minimum radiopacity of a restorative material should be equal or greater than that of the 2 mm-thick aluminum step wedge. Composites containing heavy metal glass fillers are radiopaque (2–3 mm/Al).

Enamel	4	mm/Al	Hybrid	2–5	mm/Al
Dentin	2.5	mm/Al	Microfilled	2–3	mm/Al
Amalgam	10	mm/Al			

MANIPULATION AND PLACEMENT OF COMPOSITE RESINS

Steps in the manipulation of composite resin are illustrated in *Fig. 11.14*

Placement of rubber dam Composite resins are highly technique sensitive and contamination from saliva, gingival fluid or blood is best avoided with rubber dam isolation *(Figs. 11.15A to C)*.

Cavity preparation   The cavity is prepared and margins bevelled.

Cleaning   The tooth is cleaned with a mild abrasive.

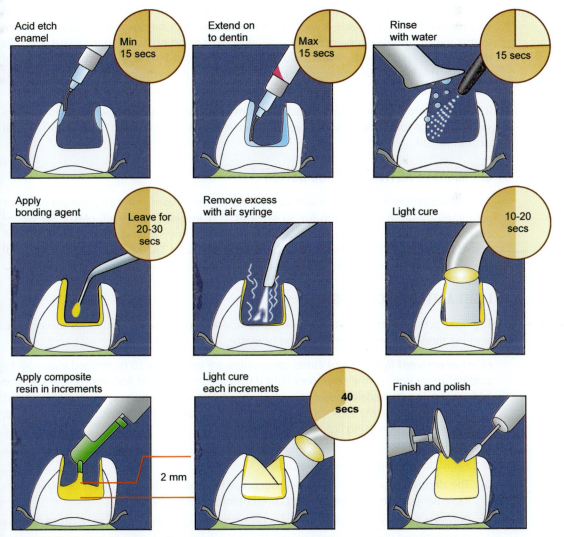

FIGURE 11.14 Technique for placing a light-cured composite restoration.

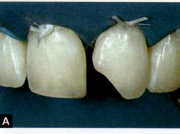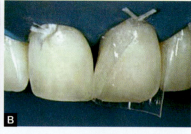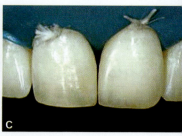

FIGURES 11.15A TO C **(A)** Rubber dam isolation is critical. **(B)** Preformed celluloid crown formers or matrix strips are used to shape and protect the restoration from air inhibition. **(C)** The completed restoration.

Etching The enamel at the cavity margins is acid etched. The acid is rinsed off and the area is dried thoroughly.

Bonding agent An enamel or dentin bond agent is applied and polymerized. (Discussed in detail subsequently). The cavity is now ready for the composite.

TECHNIQUES OF INSERTION

Resins are manipulated with plastic or plastic coated instruments. Metal instruments should be avoided as it may abrade and discolor the composite. Composites are tacky and stick to metal instruments. Some operators use alcohol or bonding liquid as a release agent to reduce tackiness. However, this should be avoided as it can interfere with the properties of the resin. This is especially true of the bonding agent as it can dissolve the resin matrix and cause dilution.

It is inserted into the cavity using a plastic instrument or a special syringe. Some manufacturers supply it in the form of a capsule which can be injected directly into the cavity with a special extruding gun.

CHEMICALLY ACTIVATED COMPOSITES

The correct proportions of base and catalyst pastes are dispensed onto a mixing pad and combined by rapid spatulation for 30 seconds. It is inserted while still plastic for better adaptation to cavity walls. Air inclusions can be avoided by swiping the material into one side of the cavity and filling the cavity from bottom outward. The cavity is slightly overfilled. A *matrix strip* is used to apply pressure and to avoid inhibition by air.

LIGHT ACTIVATED COMPOSITES

The light activated composites are single component pastes and require no mixing. The working time is under the control of the operator.

Effect of ambient light Light cured composites are vulnerable to prolonged exposure to ambient room light or the operatory light if they are left exposed and unprotected on the mixing pad. The composite begins slow polymerization as soon as it is exposed to ambient light and within 60 to 90 seconds it may lose its ability to flow. Therefore, some precautions to be observed when using light activated materials.

❍ The paste is dispensed just before use

❍ Avoid dispensing excessive quantities

❍ The depth of cure is limited, so in deep cavities the restorations must be built up in increments, each increment being cured before inserting the next

❍ Between cures any excess material is protected by covering with a light proof dark or orange tinted cover

The material hardens rapidly, on exposure to the curing light. To ensure maximal polymerization a high intensity light unit should be used. The light tip should be held as close as possible to the restoration. The exposure time should be no less than 40 to 60 seconds. The resin should be no greater than 2.0 to 2.5 mm thick. Darker shades require longer exposure times, as do resins that are cured through enamel. Microfilled resins also require a longer exposure.

Retinal damage   The high intensity light can cause retinal damage if one looks at it directly. Avoiding looking at the light directly and use of protective eye glasses is recommended. Even greater care should be exercised when using laser as even a short exposure can cause damage.

Control of polymerization shrinkage   As mentioned earlier composites exhibit polymerization shrinkage and build-up of stresses. This can be controlled by

1. *Incremental curing* The restoration is built-up in increments each increment being cured before inserting the next.
2. *Soft-start technique* The curing is started with low intensity and finished with high intensity. This extends the time for stress relaxation. Some commercially available lamps have this feature built in. Ramped curing is a variation of this technique.
3. *Delayed curing* In delayed curing the restoration is partially cured at low intensity. The operator then completes the shaping and contouring and follows it with a second exposure for the final cure.

FINISHING AND POLISHING

Finishing is best done after 24 hours during which time the polymerization is complete. However, if a subsequent appointment is not desired finishing procedures can be started 15 minutes after curing. The initial contouring can be done with a knife or diamond stone. The final finishing is done with rubber impregnated abrasives or rubber cup with polishing pastes or aluminium oxide disks. The best finish is obtained when the composite is allowed to set against a *matrix or mylar strip*.

Special glazes and coatings are available. These are basically lightly filled resins. They are applied with a brush on the surface of the restoration and cured.

BONDING

One of the initial problems when resin restoratives were introduced was microleakage which resulted from the shrinkage of the resin while curing. The problem was overcome to a great extent by the introduction of the '*acid etch technique*' by Buonocore in 1955. The acid etch technique used a combination of acid to etch the tooth and a bonding agent to improve the retention of the composite resin to the tooth (***Box 11.2***).

BOX 11.2	Essentials of current bonding systems
Etchant	The etchant is an acid which selectively dissolves the tooth structure to provide retention for the restoration. They are also known as conditioners. The most popular etchant is 37% phosphoric acid.
Primer	Primers are hydrophilic monomers usually carried in a solvent. Because of their hydrophilic nature they are able to penetrate the moist tooth structure especially the dentin and its collagen mesh thus improving the bond. Thus they serve as a bridge connecting the tooth structure to the adhesive. The solvent used are acetone, ethanol or water. Some are used without solvents.
Adhesive	Adhesives are generally hydrophobic monomers. Being hydrophobic they do not wet the tooth leading to air entrapment, air inhibition and thereby poor bonding. Thus they have to be used in combination with primers to form an effective bond to tooth structure. The adhesive bonds the resin to the primer which in turn penetrates and binds to the tooth structure thus completing the bonding sequence.

ACID ETCH TECHNIQUE

The acid etch technique was initially developed to improve retention to enamel. Initial bond agents did not appear to bond to the dentin.

At the time it was widely believed that

○ Dentin could not be etched as well as enamel

○ Acid etching of dentin would cause injury to the pulp

One reason for the low bond strength to dentin was because of the hydrophobic nature of the early adhesive resins. In 1979 Fusyama demonstrated that dentin could be etched without causing any significant harm to the pulp. This together with the development of hydrophilic bonding agents significantly improved the bond strength to dentin.

The acid etch technique together with the application of current bonding agents is one of the most effective ways of improving the bond and marginal seal between resin and tooth structure.

ETCHANT/CONDITIONER

The etchants are acidic in nature. They may be grouped as

○ Mineral (e.g. phosphoric, nitric acid, etc

○ Organic (e.g. maleic, citric, ethylene-diamine-tetracetic (EDTA), etc.)

○ Polymeric (e.g. polyacrylic acid).

The most frequently used etchant is **37% phosphoric acid**. The acid in concentrations greater than 50% results in the formation of *monocalcium phosphate monohydrate* that reduces further dissolution. It may be supplied as clear or colored gel or liquid. Brushes are used to apply or the acid is supplied in a syringe for direct application on to the enamel **(Fig. 11.16)**.

Another acid used is **10% maleic acid**.

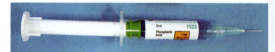

FIGURE 11.16 37% phosphoric acid in a syringe.

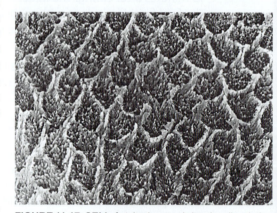

FIGURE 11.17 SEM of etched enamel showing dissolution of rod centers (*Courtesy:* Mario Fernando).

MODE OF ACTION ON ENAMEL

1. It creates microporosities by discrete etching of the enamel, i.e., by selective dissolution of enamel rod centers **(Fig. 11.17)**, or peripheries, or both.

2. Etching increases the surface area.

3. Etched enamel has a high surface energy, allowing the resin to wet the tooth surface better and penetrate into the microporosities. When polymerized, it forms resin 'tags' which forms a mechanical bond to the enamel **(Fig. 11.18)**.

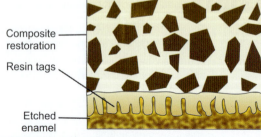

Composite restoration

Resin tags

Etched enamel

FIGURE 11.18 Diagrammatic representation showing mechanism of composite adhesion to etched enamel.

MODE OF ACTION ON DENTIN

1. Removes smear layer and partially opens the dentinal tubules *(Fig. 11.19)*.
2. Provides modest etching of the intertubular dentin.

PROCEDURE

The tooth is cleaned and polished with *pumice* before etching. The phosphoric acid is then applied onto the enamel and then on to the dentin (also known as *total-etch technique*). Originally the length of application was set at 60 seconds but now it has been shown that *15 seconds* is sufficient. The etching time also depends on the history of the tooth, e.g. a tooth with high fluoride content and primary teeth requires longer etching time (to produce a similar etch pattern and bond strength 10% maleic acid needed at least 60 seconds of etching time).

The acid along with dissolved minerals should be *rinsed off* with a stream of water for 15 seconds and the enamel dried using compressed air. After drying the enamel should have a *white, frosted* appearance *(Fig. 11.20)*.

This surface must be kept *clean and dry* until the resin is placed. Even momentary contact of saliva, or blood can prevent effective resin tag formation and severely reduce the bond strength.

Avoiding desiccation of dentin

Desiccation (excessive drying) of the dentin should be avoided. Desiccation can result in the collapse of the *collagen mesh (Fig. 11.21A)* or network which forms a dense film that is difficult to penetrate by the bond agent. The collagen mesh is crucial in the formation of the *hybrid layer (Fig. 11.21B)*. The monomers impregnate and became entangled with the collagen fibrils of surface demineralized dentin, creating a hybrid layer after their polymerization. The hybrid layer together with the resin tags forms the prime mechanism for the adhesion of the composite restoration in dentin.

After drying the tooth the dentin may be lightly remoistened with cotton and then blotted dry.

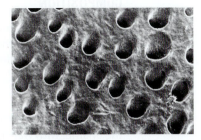

FIGURE 11.19 SEM of etched dentin showing the open dentinal tubules (*Courtesy:* Mario Fernando).

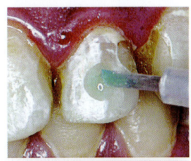

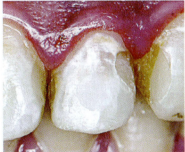

FIGURE 11.20 Frosted appearance after a 15 second etch with 37% phosphoric acid.

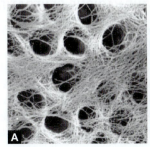
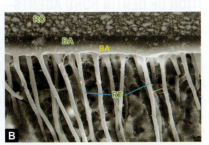

FIGURES 11.21A AND B **(A)** SEM of etched non-desiccated dentin showing collagen mesh (x 5000). **(B)** SEM of resin-dentin interphase. RC - Resin composite, BA - Bond agent, HL - Hybrid layer, RT - Resin tags. (x 2000).

ENAMEL BOND AGENTS

These were the earliest bond agents. The more viscous composite did not bond well to the etched enamel. The enamel bond agent helped improve the bond by flowing into all the microporosities of the etched enamel and creating a mechanical retention.

COMPOSITION

They are unfilled resins similar to that of the resin matrix of composite resin, diluted by other monomers to lower the viscosity. These materials have been replaced by agents that bond to both enamel and dentin.

BOND STRENGTH

Bond strengths to etched enamel range from 16 MPa (230 Psi) to 22 MPa (3200 Psi). Drying the enamel with warm air or using an ethanol rinse can increase the bond strength.

ENAMEL/DENTIN BOND SYSTEMS

The term dentin bond agent is no longer relevant as current bond agents bond to both enamel and dentin. The usage of the term is relevant only to discuss their evolution. Due to acid etching, microleakage or loss of retention is no longer a hazard at the resin-enamel interface. The problem lies at the resin-dentin/cementum interface. Thus agents that could bond to dentin were needed. Developing agents that will adhere to dentin was more difficult because

- It is heterogenous.
- The high water content interferes with bonding. Its tubular nature provides a variable area.
- Presence of a *smear layer* on the cut dentin surface (The smear layer is the layer of debris which adheres tightly to the dentin and fills the tubules after cavity cutting).

Ideally, the bond agent should be hydrophilic to displace the water and thereby wet the surface, permitting it to penetrate the porosities in dentin as well as react with the organic/inorganic components.

Restorative resins are hydrophobic, therefore, bonding agents should contain both hydrophilic and hydrophobic parts. The hydrophilic part bonds with either calcium in the hydroxyapatite crystals or with collagen. The hydrophobic part bonds with the restorative resin.

SUPPLIED AS

Dentin bond systems are supplied in one or more bottles containing conditioners (etchant)/primers/ and adhesive depending on the generation (see box below and also evolution of dentin bond agents - the various generations).

EVOLUTION OF DENTIN BOND AGENTS—THE VARIOUS GENERATIONS

For ease of description the evolution of bonding agents for composite resins are described under various generations (see also *Table 11.3*).

First generation (1950 to 1970) Mineral acids were used to etch enamel. *Dentin etching was not recommended* as it was believed it would harm the pulp. They used glycerophosphoric acid dimethacrylate to provide a bifunctional molecule. The hydrophilic phosphate part reacted with calcium ions of the hydroxyapatite. The hydrophobic methacrylate groups bonded to the acrylic restorative resin. These were generally self cured. The main disadvantage was their

TABLE 11.3 Various generations of bond agents

Generation	Enamel etchant	Dentin conditioner/primer	Adhesive
1st generation	37% phosphoric acid	(not recommended)	GPDM
2nd generation	37% phosphoric acid	(not recommended)	Phenyl-P BisGMA/TEGDMA MPPA
3rd generation	37% phosphoric acid	Citric acid (10%)/CaCl (20%) Oxalic acid/aluminium nitrate EDTA	NPG-GMA/BPDM BisGMA/TEGDMA HEMA/BPDM 4 META/MMA HEMA/GPDM
4th generation	37% phosphoric HEMA/ BPDM	(total etch technique)	NPG-GMA/BPDM BisGMA/TEGDMA HEMA/BPDM 4 META/MMA HEMA/GPDM
5th generation	37% phosphoric	(total etch technique)	PENTA, Methacrylated phosphonates
6th generation			Methacrylated phosphates in water (acidic primer-adhesive)
7th generation			Methacrylated phosphates in water (acidic primer-adhesive)

Abbreviations

BisGMA	– Bisphenol-A-glycidyl methacrylate		MMA	– Methyl methacrylate
BPDM	– Biphenyl dimethacrylate		MPPA	– 2-methacryloxyphenyl phosphoric acid
EDTA	– Ethylenediaminetetraacetic acid		TEGDMA	– Triethylene glycol dimethacrylate
GPDM	– Gylcerophosphoric acid dimethacrylate		PENTA	– Dipentaerythritol pentacrylate phosphoric acid
GA	– Glutaraldehyde		ester	
HEMA	– 2-Hydroxyethyl methacrylate		NPG-GMA	– N-Phenyl glycine glycidylmethacrylate
4-META	– 4-Methyloxyethyl trimellitic acid		NTG-GMA	– N-Tolyl glycine glycidylmethacrylate

low bond strength (2 to 6 MPa) because of their high polymerization shrinkage and the high CTE. Leakage was a concern at the dentin-resin interphase.

Second generation (1970s)   Developed as adhesive agents for composite resins which had by then replaced acrylic restorations. One system used NPG-GMA. It was proposed that the NPG portion bonded to the calcium of the tooth by chelation. Other products included phenyl-P, 2-methacryloxy phenyl phosphoric acid. Bond strengths achieved were three times more than the earlier generations.

Disadvantage   Bond strengths were still low. The adhesion was short term and the bond eventually hydrolysed, e.g. Prisma, Universal Bond, Clearfil, Scotch Bond.

Third generation (1980s)   The third generation bond agents made a serious attempt to deal with the smear layer which is formed when dentin is cut. It was believed that the smear layer prevented proper bonding to the underlying dentin. Yet its complete removal by aggressive etching was contraindicated because it was believed that it protected the pulp by preventing direct contact with the monomer. The third generation bond agents had bond strengths comparable to that of resin to etched enamel. Thus bond strengths improved to 12 to 15 MPa. However, their use is more complex and requires two to three application steps.

- ❍ Etching of enamel using 37% phosphoric acid
- ❍ Conditioning of dentin using mild acids
- ❍ Application of separate primer
- ❍ Application of polymerizable monomer
- ❍ Placement of the resin.

Examples are Tenure, Scotch bond 2, Prisma, Universal bond, Mirage bond, etc.

Fourth generation (early 1990s)   The fourth generation systems were possible because of some important ideological breakthroughs - like the *total etch* technique and the development of the *hybrid zone*. Research showed that acid etching of dentin did not significantly harm the pulp as long as bacterial contamination and microleakage was avoided. Thus, the *total-etch technique* was introduced.

The hybrid layer (Fig. 11.21 B)   In 1982, Nakabayashi and Fusayama reported the formation of a hybrid layer. The hybrid layer is defined as "the structure formed in dental hard tissues (enamel, dentin, cementum) by demineralization of the surface and subsurface, followed by infiltration of monomers into the *collagen mesh (Fig. 11.21)* and subsequent polymerization. However, dealing with the collagen mesh was not easy. It is delicate and can be destroyed by desiccation. *Kanca* (1991) introduced the idea of wet bonding again breaking with the traditional belief that thorough drying was necessary to improve bonding.

Examples are All Bond 2, Scotch bond multipurpose *(Fig. 11.22)*, Optibond, etc.

The All Bond consists of 2 primers (NPG-GMA and Biphenyl dimethacrylate (BPDM) and an unfilled resin adhesive (40% BIS-GMA, 30% UDMA, 30% HEMA). This system bonds composite not only to dentin but to most dental related surfaces like enamel, casting alloys, amalgam, porcelain and composite. Bond strengths were high but as with the earlier system, multiple application steps were required.

Fifth generation (mid 1990s)   Because of the clinical complexity and multiple steps of the fourth generation dentists began asking for more simple adhesives. The fifth generation combined the primer and adhesive in to one bottle (self priming adhesive). Examples of the fifth generation self-priming adhesives are Single Bond (3M) *(Fig. 11.23)*, One Step (BISCO) Prime and Bond (Dentsply).

The advantages claimed are

1.   Reduced application steps.
2.   Less technique sensitive as it can bond to moist dentin.
3.   Less volatile liquid.
4.   Pleasant odor.
5.   Higher bond strength.

Sixth generation (mid to late 1990s)   A separate etchant is not required. These are 2 bottle systems. Two varieties are seen—Type I and Type 2.

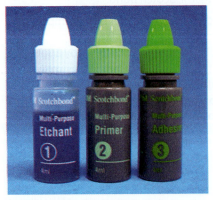

FIGURE 11.22 4th generation bonding system consisting of the conditioner (etchant), primer and the adhesive.

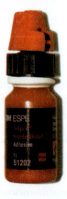

FIGURE 11.23 A 5th generation self priming adhesive (3M single Bond 2).

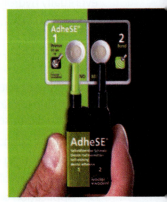

FIGURE 11.24 A 6th generation Type I - self etching primer (AdheSe - Ivoclar).

Type I   2 bottle 2 step system. Etchant and primer are combined in one bottle (called self etching primer). Other bottle contains adhesive. Examples are Clearfil SE bond (Curare), Adhese (Ivoclar -*Fig. 11.24*), Optibond solo plus(Kerr), Nano bond (Pentron) etc.

Type II   2 bottle 1 step system. Liquid A contains the primer. Liquid B contains a phosphoric acid modified resin (self etching adhesive). Both liquids are mixed just before application. For example, Xeno III (Dentsply - *Fig. 11.25*), Adper prompt L-pop (3 M), Tenure unibond (Dent Mat) etc.

Seventh generation (early 2000)   Attempts to combine all three (etchant, primer and adhesive) into a single product. Thus, seventh generation adhesives may be characterized as - '*no mix self etching adhesives*'.

Examples include iBond (Heraeus Kulzer - *Fig. 11.26*), G bond (GC), Xeno IV (Dentsply) (glass ionomer based), Clearfil S3 (Curare). Unfortunately, insufficient research exists of the efficacy of the newer systems. Composition *(Table 11.4)* and procedure *(Box 11.3)* for one such product is presented.

INDICATIONS FOR USE OF BOND AGENTS

1. For bonding composite to tooth structure.
2. Bonding composite to porcelain and various metals like amalgam, base metal and noble metal alloys.
3. Desensitization of exposed dentin or root surfaces.
4. Bonding of porcelain veneers.

Contraindication   Bonding should not be done immediately after bleaching a tooth. It is advisable to wait at least a week following the procedure.

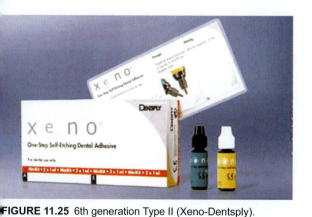

FIGURE 11.25 6th generation Type II (Xeno-Dentsply).

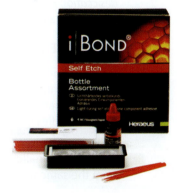

FIGURE 11.26 7th generation iBond (Heraeus kulzer).

BOX 11.3	Procedure for iBond

1. Isolate the tooth from saliva contamination during the adhesive procedure.
2. Clean the preparation, removing all debris with water. Remove excess water.
3. Saturate the microbrush with iBondTM liquid from either the bottle or single dose vial.
4. Apply 3 consecutive coats of iBondTM to both the enamel and dentin followed by gentle rubbing for 30 seconds.
5. Use gentle air pressure or vacuum to remove the acetone and water solvent.
6. Cure for 20 seconds with a dental curing light of at least 500 mW/C2.
7. Place composite.

TABLE 11.4 Composition of a 7th generation bonding agent (iBond)

Component	Function
UDMA	Matrix component Wetting of the surface Promotion of infiltration Bonding to collagen via hydrogen bonding Bonding to Ca^{2+} ions of the apatite via chelation complexes
4-Meta (pH = 2.2)	Matrix component Film-forming properties Cross-linking
Acetone	Solvent for monomers Facilitates solvent evaporation
Water	Solvent for monomers Hydrolysis of 4-Meta to 4-Meta (= acid) Provides water for etching process
Camphorquinone	Photoinitiator
Glutaraldehyde	Disinfectant/Desensitizer agent Cross-linking of collagen fibrils
Stabilizers	

BONDING MECHANISMS

Though chemical bonding schemes have been proposed, there is little evidence supporting it. The bonding is more probably micromechanical, due to the penetration of the polymerizable monomer into the finely textured primed dentin. A fine collagen mesh exists on the surface of the dentin which current bond agents are able to infiltrate because of their hydrophilic components. One more precaution is that the dentin should not be dried excessively as *desiccation* can cause the collapse of the fine collagen meshwork **(See Fig. 11.19)** thereby reducing the bond strength.

BOND STRENGTH OF DENTIN BOND AGENTS

Current dentin bond agents generate bond strengths comparable to that of resin to etched enamel. Bond strength is difficult to measure because of the wide variations in the dentin itself, test methods, and other factors. Bond strength reduces with increased depth of dentin. Various studies have shown values ranging from 15 to 35 MPa.

An increasing number of studies are using the microtensile test methodology. The size of the specimen is smaller (1 mm² in cross section). Thus, a number of specimens can be prepared from the same tooth thereby increasing the uniformity of the study.

DYE PENETRATION TESTS

These are important tests related to the performance of the bonding system. A test for microleakage is indicative of the success or failure of a bond. These tests are done using tracers and staining to determine the depth of penetration.

REPAIR OF COMPOSITES

Composite resins may be repaired by adding new material over the old. This is useful in correcting defects or altering contours of an existing restoration. The procedure differs depending on whether the restoration is fresh or old.

- Freshly polymerized restoration still has an inhibited layer of resin on the surface. More than 50% of unreacted methacrylate groups are available to copolymerize with the newly added material.
- In older composites, the presence of fewer methacrylate groups and the greater cross-linking reduces the ability of fresh monomer to penetrate into the matrix.

Method

Remove contaminated material from the surface and roughen it. Place fresh composite after applying bonding agent.

SANDWICH TECHNIQUE

Composite does not bond adequately to dentin, therefore during polymerization, a gap may result if the cavity margin is situated in dentin. The bond to dentin can be improved by placing a glass ionomer liner between the composite restoration and dentin. The glass ionomer bonds to the dentin through chemical adhesion whereas the resin bonds mechanically to porosities and crazing present on the surface of the glass ionomer liner. The glass ionomer can also be etched with the help of phosphoric acid to improve retention. In addition it also provides an anticariogenic effect due to its fluoride release. When used in this context it is often referred to as 'sandwich technique'.

Indications

1. Lesions where one or more margins are in dentin, e.g. cervical lesions.
2. Class II composite restorations.

Procedure

Dentin is conditioned and a thin layer of GIC cement is placed. The cement must be exposed at the margins in order to achieve fluoride release. Phosphoric acid is used to etch the enamel portion. Some operators also *etch the GIC surface* with the same phosphoric acid for 15 to 20 seconds to increase surface roughness (light cured GIC is not etched). The surface is then washed for 25 to 30 seconds. After adequate drying, a bond agent is applied to the cement surface and to the etched enamel. The composite resin is then inserted in the usual manner.

SPECIALIZED COMPOSITE RESINS

FLOWABLE COMPOSITES

As suggested by the name these are hybrid composites modified to have an increased flow *(Fig. 11.27)*. The increased flow is achieved by a reduction in the filler content (30–55 vol % or 40–60 wt.%). When placed in the cavity the material flows readily and intimately adapts to the cavity wall. The reduced filler content affects some of the properties.

Thus these materials

- Are more prone to wear
- Have half the stiffness (more flexible) of regular hybrids (4–8 GPa)
- Greater polymerization shrinkage (3–5 vol%)

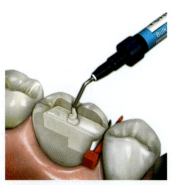

FIGURE 11.27 Flowable resin.

These materials are intended for specialized usage

1. As a preventive material (fissure sealant and small class I cavity).
2. Cervical lesions and Class V restorations.
3. As a base or liner.
4. Areas of reduced access.

PACKABLE COMPOSITES

These are composites that have very high viscosity and low surface tackiness. They have a high filler loading (66–70% vol) with porous or irregularly shaped particles. They are not condensable like classic amalgam, rather they can be compressed and forced to flow using flat faced instruments, hence the term packable *(Fig. 11.28)*. They are considered as posterior composites. The distinguishing characteristics of all packable compositions are less stickiness or stiffer viscosity than conventional composites, which allow them to be placed in a manner that somewhat

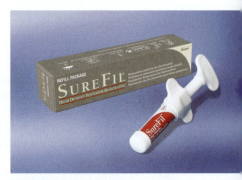

FIGURE 11.28 Example of packable composite–Sure Fil by Dentsply.

resembles amalgam placement. They have a higher wear resistance. Claims also include a greater depth of cure and low polymerization shrinkage. Iin general, mechanical propertie of packable composites are not substantially better than those of most conventional universa composites.

Commercial examples   Solitaire (Heraeus), ALERT (Jeneric), and SureFil (Dentsply).

Indications

They are indicated for use in Classes I and II cavities. In class II cavities where improved contact with adjacent teeth are desired.

PROSTHODONTIC VENEER COMPOSITES (LABORATORY COMPOSITES)

Resin may be used as a veneer (a tooth colored layer used to hide the underlying metal for crowns and fixed partial dentures. They are also known as *composites for dental indirec restorations*. The earliest recorded use was in the Hollywood film industry where they were used to temporarily mask the teeth of actors. The early materials were heat cured poly (methy methacrylate) improved by fillers and cross-linking agents. Current veneer materials are hybrid, micro or nanofiller reinforced resins such as bis-GMA, urethane dimethacrylate o 4,8-di(methacryloxy methylene) tricyclo-(5.2.1.02,6) -decane *(Fig. 11.29A to C)*. Some are fiber reinforced. The newer resins have superior physical properties and are polymerized b light or heat and pressure.

The resins are mechanically bonded to the metal using wire loops or retention beads *(Fig 11.29B)*. Recent improvements, include micromechanical retention created by acid etching the base alloy and the use of chemical bonding systems such as 4-META, phosphorylated methacrylate, epoxy resin, or silicon dioxide that is flame sprayed to the metal surface followed by the application of a silane coupling agent (silicoating).

Commercial examples   SR Adoro (Ivoclar), GC Gradia (GC), Targis Vectris, etc.

Available as   A kit containing various materials which include—incisal, dentin and othe specialized resins, masking resins *(Fig. 11.29B)*.

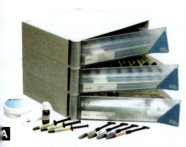 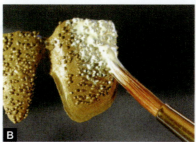 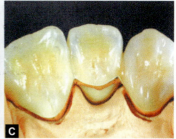

FIGURES 11.29A TO C **(A)** Prosthodontic resin kit (SR Adoro (Ivoclar Vivadent). **(B)** Opaquer resin is applied to mask the metal. Multiple tiny nodules provide retention for the resin. **(C)** The completed restoration.

Indications

1. Inlays, onlays, veneers and anterior crowns (metal free).
2. As veneer over metal supported crowns and FDPs.
3. Long term temporaries (alone or in combination with Kavo C-temp blanks).

The advantages of resin when compared to porcelain

1. Ease of fabrication.
2. Easily repairable intraorally.
3. Less wear of opposing teeth or restorations.

Disadvantages

1. Microleakage of oral fluids and staining under the veneers due to thermal cycling and water sorption.
2. Surface staining and intrinsic discoloration.
3. Susceptibility to toothbrush wear.
4. Cannot be used in crowns serving as abutments for removable partial dentures. The clasp arm will abrade the resin.
5. Not as durable as other prosthodontic materials like ceramics and PFM.

RESIN INLAY SYSTEMS

These were introduced in an attempt to overcome some of the limitations of traditional posterior composite resin restoration. The resin inlay is completely polymerized outside the mouth by light, heat, pressure or combination and then luted to the tooth using a resin cement. They may be fabricated using the direct method or indirect method.

Direct inlay system (fabricated in the mouth)

Hybrid or microfilled resins are used. A separating medium (agar solution or glycerine) is applied to the prepared tooth. The restoration is then formed, light-cured, and removed from the tooth. The rough inlay is subjected to additional polymerization by light (6 minutes) or heat (100 °C for 7 minutes). After this the prepared tooth is etched and the inlay luted to place with a dual-cure resin cement and then polished.

Indirect inlay system (fabricated on a die)

The inlay is fabricated with prosthodontic resin (described earlier) in the laboratory on a die made from an impression of the prepared tooth. Conventional light and heat or heat and pressure may also be used for polymerization.

Advantages of inlays
1. Improved physical properties and wear resistance due to the higher degree of polymerization attained.
2. Induced stresses and potential for microleakage is reduced as polymerization shrinkage occurs outside the mouth.
3. Being resins they do not abrade opposing teeth and are repairable in the mouth.

PREFORMED COMPOSITE RESIN LAMINATES

Composite resins are used as preformed laminate veneers to mask tooth discoloration or malformation. These shells are adjusted by grinding and are bonded to teeth using acid-etch technique and resin cement.

CORE BUILD-UP COMPOSITE RESINS

Modified highly filled resins are used as core materials in combination with prefabricated posts during the restorations of broken down teeth. They are highly colored opaque materials. They are usually chemically cured or dual cured with a longer working time and shorter setting time. Some concerns exist regarding the strength of composite cores when compared to cast post and cores. Failures are often seen when these materials form the bulk of the support for crowns and FDPs. The lower stiffness

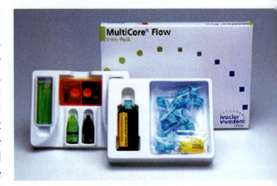

FIGURE 11.30 Core composite resin.

(greater flexibility) can result in slightly more frequent debonding of crowns and other restoration. Therefore, when using composite cores *shared* support from remaining tooth structure is indicated. *MultiCore (Ivoclar Vivadent)* **(Fig. 11.30)** is an example of a core build-up composite. The product also contains fluoride.

RESIN CEMENTS

Lower viscosity filled resins (e.g. Panavia Ex, Infinity) are used for the cementation of laminates crowns and orthodontic brackets. Etching and bonding is done before cementing (described in detail in chapter on cements).

PROVISIONAL COMPOSITES

A temporary restoration is necessary to protect the teeth after preparation and in the interim period while the definitive restoration is being constructed. Composite resins are available for making provisional inlays, onlays, crowns and FDPs. E.g. Protemp (ESPE) **(Fig. 11.31)**, Structur (VOCO), Integrity (Dentsply), etc.

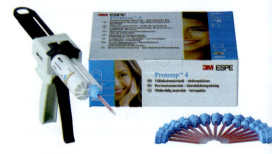

FIGURE 11.31 Composite for provisional crowns and fixed partial dentures.

Advantages
1. Can be made directly in the mouth because of its low exothermic heat 18 to 28 °C.

2. It is easily ground and shaped using regular high speed diamond burs without melting and clogging the burs (unlike the conventional acrylic provisional resins).
3. Improved mechanical properties including low wear rates when compared to acrylic provisionals.
4. Good radiopacity.

Available as

Syringe form It comes as base and catalyst. Currently, two shades are available. It is supplied in a syringe form and is dispensed by rotating the plunger until a clicking sound is heard, this represents one unit. The catalyst is a two component system and only a small amount is required. As the plunger is rotated the two components are dispensed simultaneously. The base and catalyst are mixed with a spatula and used. Setting occurs in approximately two to three minutes.

Cartridge form The material is also available in the cartridge form for use with a *static mixing* device. It consists of a caulking gun which forces the materials through special static mixing tips. The material comes out mixed and ready to use when expressed through these tips. After curing in the mouth the hardening can be accelerated by placing in hot water.

Precautions

1. As with all materials expressed from cartridges, the material that comes initially should be discarded as it may not be in the correct proportions.
2. Oxygen inhibited layer This reaction is strongly inhibited by oxygen diffusing from the atmosphere into the curing resins is responsible for the formation of a soft, sticky, superficial layer on the surface of the prepared tooth. This layer can affect inhibit the setting of polyvinyl siloaxane impression materials In some techniques where a putty impression is used as a template, this layer can prevent the bonding

COMPOSITE RESIN BLANKS FOR CAD-CAM SYSTEMS

Composite resin blanks are available for the fabrication of long term (up to 1 year) provisional restorations including crowns and fixed partial dentures. They are fabricated by a CAD/CAM process (see chapter on ceramics for further details of the process). One such product is the *Everest C-Temp* (Kavo) **(Fig. 11.32)**. The whole restoration may be fabricated as one piece or it may be fabricated as a framework which is subsequently veneered with conventional prosthodontic resins. These resins are characterized by high flexural strength.

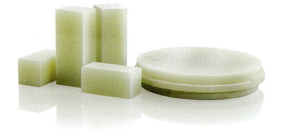

FIGURE 11.32 Composite resin CAD/CAM blanks.

PORCELAIN REPAIR COMPOSITE RESINS

Composite resins are occasionally used to repair fractured or chipped ceramic restorations. The kit consists of an silane based bonding agent, a metal masking agent (opaquer). Conventional composite is then used to carry out the final repair. The material and procedure is discussed in further detail (refer chapter on porcelain).

PIT AND FISSURE SEALANTS

Deep pits and fissures on posterior teeth are susceptible to decay as they provide shelter for organisms. They are often too narrow making it difficult to clean. Various materials have been used to seal these areas, especially in the child patient. The *objective* is for the resin to penetrate into the pits and fissures, thereby, sealing these areas against oral flora and debris *(Figs. 11.33A and B)*.

Indications

Sealants are most effective in children with high risk of caries. Both deciduous molars and young permanent molars with deep pits and fissures are common candidates. Commonly surfaces that are free of caries should be selected. However, a recent study where the sealant was placed intentionally in pits and fissures having caries showed that the lesion did not progress.

Types

1. Based on filler content 2 types are available—Filled and Unfilled.
2. Based on curing mechanism—they may be light cured or chemical cured.
3. Color—The sealants are available as transparent, tooth colored, opaque, tinted or white materials. The color contrast helps to determine the efficacy of the application. Recent products include photosensitive color reversible sealants. These sealants are normally colorless but change to a pink or green when exposed to a curing light. The color change which lasts about 5–10 minutes is useful for diagnosis during periodic recalls.

Composition

The most commonly and successfully used sealant is bis-GMA *(Figs. 11.33B and C)*. It may be cured chemically (amine-peroxide system) or by light. The bis-GMA resin is mixed with a diluent to obtain a low viscosity sealant that flows readily. In filled sealants small amounts of filler (up to 40%) are added to improve its stiffness and wear resistance. Other resins systems include polyurethanes and cyanoacrylates.

Properties

Important properties of sealants are flow, wear resistance, fluoride release and long term retention.

Sealants must have low viscosity so that they will flow readily into the depths of the pits and fissures *(Fig. 11.33A)* and wet the tooth. Wettability is also important for proper adaptation and penetration. Acid etching improves the wettability.

Proper retention of the sealant is important for caries prevention. Acid etching with bonding agents is necessary for the retention of the sealant.

The sealant must have sufficient mechanical properties like strength, stiffness and wear resistance for effective function and durability. Sealants with fillers usually have better mechanical properties than unfilled resins.

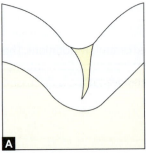
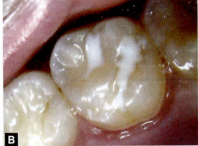
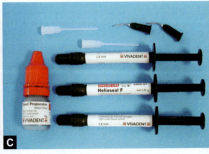

A **B** **C**

FIGURES 11.33A TO C Pit and fissure sealants. **(A)** Diagrammatic representation of a sealant in a fissure. **(B)** A pit and fissure sealant on a deciduous molar. **(C)** A typical pit and fissure sealant kit.

Current products have been formulated for fluoride release during service. Initial fluoride release is high especially during the first 24 hours but gradually tapers to low levels which may not be effective for long term protection.

Air inhibition during polymerization is also a problem in sealants. The tacky air inhibited layer is removed using a pumice paste on a cotton pellet or rotary cup or brush. The operator must ensure that sufficient thickness of sealant is applied to compensate for this loss.

The unpolymerized surface layer was once a health concern because of the presence of BPA (bisphenol A) which is chemical similar to estrogen. However, this has since been discredited and is no longer a major concern.

Efficacy of sealant therapy

Early clinical studies showed a retention rate of 42% and a caries reduction rate of 35% over 5 years. Improvements in materials and technique over the years have dramatically improved the success rates. Current studies indicate a success rate of over 90% in caries reduction.

Periodic recall

Evidence has shown that sealant therapy cannot be taken for granted. The sealant should be re-examined every six months. If the sealant is missing it should be reapplied. Improper case selection and application of sealant may actually enhance caries.

COMPOSITE RESIN DENTURE TEETH

Over the years various types of materials have been used for denture teeth. Traditionally conventional acrylic (Biotone), cross-linked acrylics (SR-Postaris, Genios-P, etc.) and porcelain denture teeth are used.

Since their introduction composite resins too have been tried as denture teeth. Some examples are nano-filled (Veracia) and micro-filled composites (SR-Orthosit, Endura, Duradent, Surpass). In one study, the composites and cross-linked acrylic resins did not show significant difference in wear resistance properties. However, both were significantly better than conventional resin acrylic teeth.

ADVANTAGES AND DISADVANTAGES OF RESTORATIVE COMPOSITE RESINS

ADVANTAGES

1. Highly esthetic tooth colored restorations possible.
2. Multiple curing systems allow choice of working time.
3. Relatively ease of placement.
4. Moderately strong and durable.
5. Does not corrode when compared to amalgam.
6. Easy to repair.

DISADVANTAGES

1. Highly technique sensitive.
2. High shrinkage.
3. Does not bond to tooth structure; requires dentin bonding techniques.
4. Sticks to instruments.
5. Not condensable like amalgam.

6. Possibility of microleakage and recurrent caries if improperly placed.
7. Some materials exhibit slumping.
8. Not as wear resistant as other metallic restorative materials.
9. Shorter life span when compared to other more durable restorative materials like ceramics, DFGs, amalgam and cast metal restorations.
10. Higher allergic, inflammatory response, cytotoxic and other biologically adverse effects when compared to amalgam.
11. Potential for color instability and staining over time.

PART-3

Endodontic Materials

Endodontic Medicaments and Irrigants

Jacob Kurien

CHAPTER OUTLINE

- Root Canal Irrigants
  - Sodium Hypochlorite
  - Chlorhexidine
  - Hydrogen Peroxide
  - MTAD
  - EDTA
  - RC-Prep
- Intracanal Medicaments
- Phenol and Related Compounds
  - Phenolic Compounds
  - Eugenol
  - Parachlorophenol (PCP)

- Formocresol
- Cresatin
- Camphorated Monochlorophenol (CMCP)
- Glutaraldehyde
- Formaldehyde based (N2)
- Antibiotics
  - PBSC and PBSN (Polyantibiotic Pastes)
  - Sulfonamides
  - Grossman's Paste
  - Corticosteroids - Antibiotics

- Combinations
- Halogens
- Aminoacridine
- Quaternary Ammonium Compounds
  - Chloramine
  - Iodine
  - Calcium Hydroxide
  - Chlorhexidine (CHX) Gluconate

Endodontics is the specialty of dentistry that manages the prevention, diagnosis, and treatment of the dental pulp and the periradicular tissues that surround the root of the tooth.

The main objectives of root canal therapy are

1. Removal of the pathological pulp.
2. Cleaning and shaping of the root canal system.
3. Three dimensional obturation to prevent reinfection *(Fig. 12.1)*.

Irrigation is an essential part of root canal debridement because it allows for cleaning beyond what might be achieved by root canal instrumentation alone. Disinfection of the root canal system is one of the primary aims of root canal treatment. This can be achieved through the use of various antimicrobial agents in the

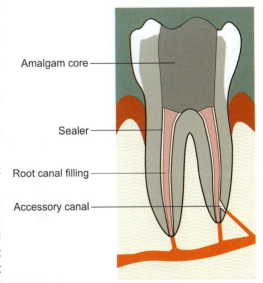

FIGURE 12.1 A root canal treated tooth.

form of irrigants (only used for relatively short periods of time) and medicaments (days or several weeks). The main objective of root canal obturation is to achieve a three dimensional well filled root canal with fluid tight seal *(Fig. 12.1)*. It serves to prevent percolation and microleakage of periapical exudate into the root canal space and create a favorable environment for the healing process.

Materials used in endodontics

The materials used in Endodontics may be grouped as follows.

1. Root canal irrigants
2. Root canal medicaments
3. Obturating materials
4. Endodontic sealers

ROOT CANAL IRRIGANTS

Several irrigants and irrigant delivery systems are available, all of which behave differently and have relative advantages and disadvantages. Root canal irrigants must not only be effective for dissolution of the organic portions of the dental pulp, but also effectively eliminate bacterial contamination and remove the smear layer (the organic and inorganic layer) that is created on the walls of the root canal during instrumentation.

Desirable properties

1. Irrigants should have a broad antimicrobial spectrum and high efficacy against anaerobic and facultative microorganisms organized in biofilms.
2. Dissolve necrotic pulp tissue remnants.
3. Inactivate endotoxin.
4. Should be nontoxic, noncarcinogenic and nonantigenic.
5. Should be able to disinfect and penetrate dentin and its tubules.
6. Prevent the formation of a smear layer during instrumentation or dissolve the latter once it has formed.
7. Should not have adverse effect on dentin.
8. Should not discolor dentin.
9. Not irritate or damage vital periapical tissue (caustic or cytotoxic effects).
10. Should not weaken tooth structure.
11. Should not affect the sealing ability of filling materials.

Function of irrigants

Irrigants are used to clean the root canal and are used along with the shaping instruments. The functions of irrigants include

1. Rinsing and flushing (helps remove debris).
2. Lubricant function to reduce instrument friction during preparation.
3. Dissolve inorganic tissue (dentin).
4. Dissolve organic matter (dentin collagen, pulp tissue, biofilm).
5. Penetrate to the peripheries of the root canal system.
6. Kill bacteria and yeasts (antimicrobial).

Classification

Chemically inactive irrigants
1. Water
2. Saline
3. Local anesthetic solution

Chemically active irrigants
1. Tissue dissolving agents [e.g. Sodium hypochlorite (NaOCl)]
2. Oxidizing agents [e.g. Hydrogen peroxide (H_2O_2), Sodium hypochlorite]
3. Antibacterial agents (e.g. Chlorhexidine, NaOCl, MTAD, Iodine)
4. Chelating agents (e.g. EDTA)

CHEMICALLY ACTIVE IRRIGANTS

SODIUM HYPOCHLORITE

Sodium hypochlorite is used widely as a household bleach and disinfectant. In dentistry, sodium hypochlorite (NaOCl) is a popular as an irrigating solution for Endodontic use.

Available as

Solutions in various concentrations between 0.5% and 6% in bottles *(Fig. 12.2).*

Chemical reaction

NaOCl ionizes in water into Na^+ and the hypochlorite ion, OCl^-. The OCl^- ion in turn combines with water to form Hypochlorous acid (HOCl).

$$NaOCl + H_2O \rightarrow Na^+ + Cl^- + 2\,HO$$

In commercial NaOCl solutions, the following species are in equilibrium

$$H^+ + OCl^- \leftrightarrow HOCl$$
$$HOCl + Cl^- + H^+ \leftrightarrow Cl_2 + H_2O$$

Hypochlorous acid is responsible for the antibacterial activity; the OCl ion is less effective than the undissolved HOCl. Hypochlorous acid disrupts several vital functions of the microbial cell resulting in cell death. At acidic and neutral pH, chlorine exists predominantly as HOCl, whereas at high pH of 9 and above, OCl predominates.

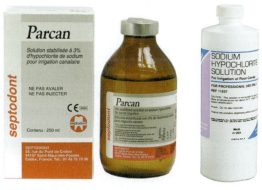

FIGURE 12.2 Representative commercially available sodium hypochlorite solutions.

It is a potent antimicrobial agent, killing most bacteria instantly on direct contact. It also effectively dissolves pulpal remnants and collagen, the main organic components of dentin. Hypochlorite is the only root canal irrigant of those in general use that dissolves necrotic and vital organic tissue. Although hypochlorite alone does not remove the smear layer, it affects the organic part of the smear layer, making its complete removal possible by subsequent irrigation with EDTA or citric acid (CA). It is used as an unbuffered solution at pH 11 in the various concentrations mentioned earlier, or buffered with bicarbonate buffer (pH 9.0), usually as a 0.5% (Dakin solution) or 1% solution.

Sodium hypochlorite is the most important irrigating solution and the only one capable of dissolving organic tissue, including biofilm and the organic part of the smear layer. It should be used throughout the instrumentation phase.

Biological considerations

Extrusion of NaOCl into periapical tissues can cause severe injury to the patient *(Fig. 12.3).* To minimize NaOCl accidents, the irrigating needle should be placed short of the working length, fit loosely in the canal and the solution must be injected using a gentle flow rate. Constantly moving the needle up and down during irrigation prevents wedging of the needle in the canal and provides better irrigation. The use of irrigation tips with side venting reduces the possibility of forcing solutions into the periapical tissues. Treatment of NaOCl accidents is palliative and consists of observation of the patient as well as prescribing antibiotics and analgesics.

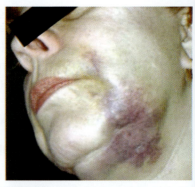

FIGURE 12.3 Sodium hypochlorite injury caused by irrigant leaking into the periapical areas.

Storage

Sodium hypochlorite is generally not utilized in its most active form in a clinical setting. For proper antimicrobial activity, it must be prepared freshly just before its use. It should be stored at room temperature and not exposed to oxygen for extended periods of time. Exposure of the solution to oxygen and light can inactivate it significantly.

Disadvantages

1. Unpleasant taste
2. Relative toxicity
3. Inability to remove smear layer (inorganic)

CHLORHEXIDINE

Chlorhexidine *(Fig. 12.4)* has a broad-spectrum antimicrobial action and relatively little toxicity. Chlorhexidine (CHX) however, lacks the tissue-dissolving ability. It penetrates the cell wall and attacks the bacterial cytoplasmic or inner membrane or the yeast plasma membrane. It may be used in concentrations between 0.2% and 2%. Its activity is pH dependent and is greatly reduced in the presence of organic matter.

HYDROGEN PEROXIDE

It is a clear, colorless liquid *(Fig. 12.5)* used in a variety of concentrations. 1%–30% H_2O_2 is active against viruses, bacteria, and yeasts.

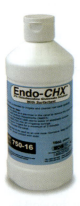
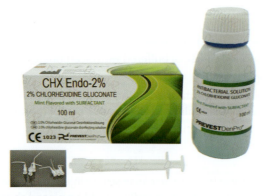
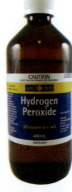

FIGURE 12.4 Chlorhexidine irrigant.

FIGURE 12.5 Hydrogen peroxide irrigant.

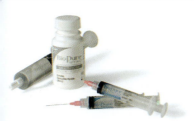

FIGURE 12.6 MTAD stands for mixture of tetracycline isomer, acid and detergent.

Functions and actions

It produces hydroxyl free radicals (OH), which attack several cell components such as proteins and DNA. In endodontics, H_2O_2 has long been used because of its antimicrobial and cleansing properties. It has been particularly popular in cleaning the pulp chamber from blood and tissue remnants, but it has also been used in canal irrigation.

MTAD

The acronym MTAD *(Fig. 12.6)* stands for mixture of tetracycline isomer, acid and detergent (doxycycline, citric acid, and the detergent Tween-80). It has sustained antibacterial activity. It has a low pH of 2.15. MTAD solubilized dentine well (70%) and pulp tissue to a lesser extent (50%). It is an alternative to EDTA.

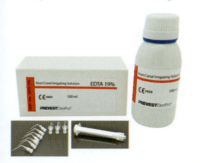

FIGURE 12.7 EDTA irrigant for root canal.

EDTA (ETHYLENEDIAMINETETRAACETIC ACID)

EDTA *(Fig. 12.7)* (17%, disodium salt, pH 7) has little if any antibacterial activity. It effectively removes smear layer by chelating the inorganic component of the dentine. It aids in the mechanical canal shaping.

RC-PREP

RC-Prep *(Fig. 12.8)* is composed of EDTA and urea peroxide in a base of Carbowax. It is not water soluble. Interaction of the urea peroxide in RC-Prep with sodium hypochlorite, produces a bubbling action thought to loosen and float out dentinal debris.

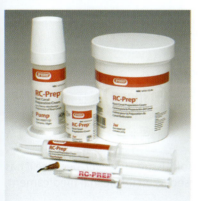

FIGURE 12.8 RC-Prep is composed of EDTA.

INTRACANAL MEDICAMENTS

If root canal treatment cannot be finished in a single visit, root canals are dressed with medicaments. A medicament is an antimicrobial agent that is placed inside the root canal between treatment appointments in an attempt to destroy remaining microorganisms and prevent reinfection.

Functions of intracanal medicaments

Primary functions
1. Antimicrobial activity
2. Antisepsis
3. Disinfection

Secondary functions
1. Hard-tissue formation
2. Pain control
3. Exudation control
4. Resorption control

Desirable properties
1. Antibacterial
2. Penetrate dentinal tubules

3. Control exudation or bleeding
4. Biocompatible
5. Eliminate pain
6. Induce calcific barrier
7. Have no effect on temporary restoration
8. Should be radiopaque
9. Should not stain tooth

Types of intracanal medicaments

1. Phenol and related volatile compounds
2. PBSC paste
3. Sulfonamide and sulfathiazole
4. Corticosteroid-antibiotic combination
5. Calcium hydroxide
6. N2
7. Halogens
8. Quaternary ammonium compounds

PHENOL AND RELATED COMPOUNDS

1. Phenol
2. Eugenol
3. CMCP
4. Cresatin
5. Formocresol
6. Glutaraldehyde
7. Cresol
8. Beechwood
9. Creosote
10. Thymol

PHENOLIC COMPOUNDS

Phenol is a protoplasm poison and produces necrosis of soft tissue. However, because it has a strong inflammatory potential, at present it is rarely used as an intracanal medicament.

EUGENOL

Eugenol is the chemical essence of the oil of clove. It is both antiseptic and an anodyne. It is a constituent of most root canal sealers and used as a temporary sealing material. It inhibits intradental nerve impulses.

PARACHLOROPHENOL (PCP)

It is a substitution product of phenol. The aqueous solution of PCP penetrates deeper into the dentinal tubules, than camphorated chlorophenol. A 1% solution of PCP is capable of killing many of the microorganisms in the root canal. It may, however, produce mild inflammation.

FORMOCRESOL

This is a combination of formalin and cresol in the ratio of 1:2 or 1:1. Formalin is a strong disinfectant that combines with albumin to form an insoluble, nondecomposable substance and fixes the tissues. It is used as a dressing for pulpotomy to fix the retained pulp tissue. Formocresol *(Fig. 12.9)* is a nonspecific bacterial medicament most effective against aerobic and anaerobic organisms found in root canals. Formocresol is also mutagenic and carcinogenic.

It is placed on a cotton pellet, squeeze dried and then placed in the pulp chamber of the tooth in treatment. The vapors will penetrate the entire canal preparation.

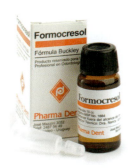

FIGURE 12.9 Formocresol.

CRESATIN

Cresatin (*Fig. 12.10*) or metacresylacetate has both antiseptic and obtundent properties. But the antimicrobial effect is less than that of formocresol and camphorated parachlorophenol. It is less irritating to the tissue.

CAMPHORATED MONOCHLOROPHENOL (CMCP)

Camphorated monochlorophenol (*Fig. 12.11*) consists of 2 parts of parachlorophenol and 3 parts of gum camphor (p-chlorophenol 35%, camphor 65%).

Camphor serves as a vehicle and diluent and reduces the irritating effect of pure PCP. It also prolongs the antimicrobial effect. It is used in the form of vapour forming intracanal medicaments. The vapours can pass through the apical foramen.

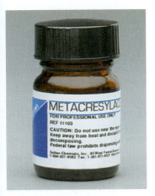

FIGURE 12.10 Cresatin.

GLUTARALDEHYDE

Glutaraldehyde is a colorless oil slightly soluble in water. It is a strong disinfectant and fixative. The antimicrobial action of glutaraldehyde is bacteriostatic in nature. The recommended concentration is 2%.

FORMALDEHYDE BASED (N2)

N2 (*Fig. 12.12*) was introduced by Sargenti. It is a compound containing paraformaldehyde as the primary ingredient. It also contains Phenylmercuric borate, eugenol, and additional ingredients like lead, corticosteroid and antibiotics. It is claimed to be both intracanal medicament and sealer. The antibacterial effect of N2 is short-lived.

ANTIBIOTICS

POLYANTIBIOTIC PASTES - PBSC AND PBSN

Polyantibiotic pastes were first introduced in 1951 by Grossman who was considered as the father of Endodontics. Grossman's paste was also known as PBSC which stood for penicillin, bacitracin, streptomycin and caprylate sodium suspended in silicone oil. Subsequently the antifungal agent caprylate sodium was replaced by Nystatin, i.e. PBSN.

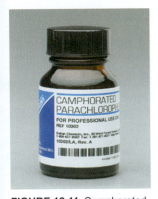

FIGURE 12.11 Camphorated monochlorophenol.

Composition

Ingredient	Proportions	Function
Penicillin G	1,000,000 units	Effective against gram positive organisms
Bacitracin	10000 units	For penicillin resistant organism
Streptomycin	1.0 g	Effective against gram negative organisms
Caprylate sodium	1.0 g	Antifungal
Silicone fluid	3 mL	Vehicle
Nystatin	10000 units	Antifungal

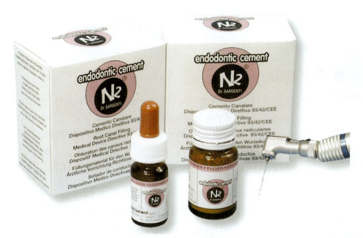

FIGURE 12.12 N2 contains paraformaldehyde as the main agent.

They are available in a paste form that may be injected into root canals impregnated on paper points.

Drawbacks and concerns

Polyantibiotic paste showed therapeutic potential, but owing to the drawbacks including ineffectiveness against anaerobic species and allergic reactions, the Food and Drug Administration (FDA) prohibited PBSC for endodontic use in 1975. Fears of development of resistant organisms was another concern. Antibiotics for use in root canal therapy should be carefully justified in order to avoid development of bacterial resistance.

SULFONAMIDES

Sulfonilanide and sulfanizole are used as medicaments by mixing with sterile distilled water or by placing a moistened paper point into a fluffed jar containing the powder. This medication is suggested for use as intracanal medicament in acute periapical abscess.

Disadvantage Yellowish tooth discoloration has been reported after use.

CORTICOSTEROIDS - ANTIBIOTICS COMBINATIONS

These medicaments are highly effective in the treatment of over instrumentation. They must be placed in the inflamed tissue by a paper point or reamer to be effective. They are more effective in vital pulps than the necrotic pulp tissue. The steroid constituent reduces the periapical inflammation and gives instant relief of pain. The antibiotic constituents are present so that overgrowth of microorganisms will be prevented. An example of this category is the Ledermix paste developed by Schroeder and Triadan in 1960 which contains an antibiotic demeclocycline—HCl (3.2%) and a corticosteroid, triamcinolone acetonide (1%), in a polyethylene glycol base. Another example is the Odontopaste released in February 2008 (zinc oxide-based root canal paste with 5% clindamycin hydrochloride and 1% triamcinolone acetonide).

HALOGENS

Sodium hypochlorite is also used as an intracanal medicament (ICM). Chlorine is the active ingredient in NaOCl. Sodium hypochlorite reacts rapidly with organic matter, and hence the longevity of its antimicrobial effect is questionable.

Disadvantage Toxic to the periapical tissues.

AMINOACRIDINE

It is a mild antiseptic. It works by inhibiting bacterial protein synthesis.

QUATERNARY AMMONIUM COMPOUNDS

CHLORAMINE

It is a chlorine compound (NH_2Cl) used in concentration of 5%. It has good antimicrobial qualities. It remains stable for a long period of time.

IODINE

Iodine is highly reactive combines with proteins and forms salts which probably destroys micro- organisms. Iodine-potassium iodide has a relatively high antibacterial effect and relatively low toxicity.

Disadvantage

1. It may cause staining of the tooth.
2. Allergic reaction.

CALCIUM HYDROXIDE

Calcium hydroxide was introduced by Herman in 1920. It is one of the commonly used ICMs (Intracanal medicaments). It is a broad spectrum antimicrobial agent. Its antiseptic action probably relates to its high pH and its leaching action on necrotic pulp tissue. It is best used in 'weeping canals', where there is a constant clear or reddish exudate associated with large periapical lesion. In such cases calcium hydroxide is an excellent medicament to be used.

CHLORHEXIDINE (CHX) GLUCONATE

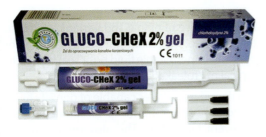

FIGURE 12.13 Chlorhexidine gel.

Chlorhexidine (CHX) (2% gel) *(Fig. 12.13)* is also shown to be an excellent intra canal medicament. It is broad spectrum antimicrobial agent. It can be used alone in gel form or mixed with Ca(OH)2. CHX gel provides antimicrobial activity for up to 21 days after contamination. When it is used in combination with Ca(OH)2, the antimicrobial activity of this mixture is greater than the combination of Ca(OH)2 and saline.

13
CHAPTER

Endodontic Sealers and Obturating Materials

Jacob Kurien

Following the cleaning, debriding and enlarging of the root canals, the canals spaces are sealed or obturated *(Fig. 13.1)* to prevent reinfection and colonization by bacteria.

Why obturate canals?

Microorganisms and their byproducts are the major cause of pulpal and periapical disease. However, it is difficult to consistently and totally disinfect root canal systems. Therefore, the goal of three-dimensional obturation is to provide an impermeable fluid tight seal within the entire root canal system, to prevent oral and apical microleakage.

Successful obturation requires the use of materials and techniques capable of densely filling the entire root canal system and providing a fluid tight seal from the apical segment of the canal to the cavosurface margin in order to prevent reinfection. This also implies that an adequate coronal filling or restoration be placed to prevent oral bacterial microleakage. It has been shown that endodontic treatment success is dependent both on the quality of the obturation and the final restoration. The quality of the endodontic obturation is evaluated using radiographic images upon completion.

The objectives of modern nonsurgical endodontic treatment are

1. To provide a clean and bacteria free.
2. To provide an apical seal. This prevents the ingress of fluids that will provide nutrients for canal bacteria and also prevents irritants leaving the canal and entering the periapical tissues.
3. To provide a 'coronal' seal. This prevents recontamination due to the ingress of oral microorganisms from the coronal end.

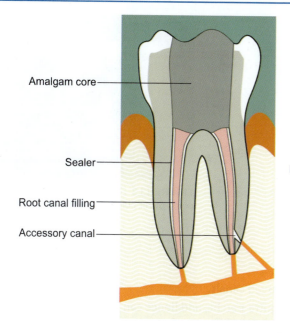

Amalgam core

Sealer

Root canal filling

Accessory canal

FIGURE 13.1 A root canal treated tooth.

ROOT CANAL OBTURATING MATERIALS

Historically a wide variety of materials and techniques have been used in an attempt to produce an impervious seal of the tooth root apex ranging from orange wood through to precious metals and dental cements. During the Civil War, a material called "Hill's stopping" *(Box 13.2)* (which contained gutta-percha, quick lime, quartz and feldspar) was used.

Related ISO Standards
ISO 6877:2006 Dentistry — Root-canal obturation points
ISO 6876:2012 Dentistry — Root canal sealing materials

The most widely used root-canal sealing technique is a combination of root obturating points and canal sealer cements.

A root canal filling material should prevent infection/reinfection of treated root canals. Together with an acceptable level of biocompatibility (inert material) this will provide the basis for promoting healing of the periodontal tissues and for maintaining a healthy periapical environment.

CLASSIFICATION OF ROOT CANAL OBTURATING MATERIALS

Root canal obturating materials may be classified as

1. Solid core, e.g. Silver
2. Plastic/Semi solid core, e.g. Gutta-percha, Resilon
3. Paste type, e.g. iRoot SP

SILVER POINTS

Silver points or cones *(Fig. 13.2)* were introduced by Jasper in 1941. Silver cones were the most widely used solid-core metallic filling material between 1940 to 1960 because of their bactericidal effect *(Fig. 13.3)*. Points of gold, iridioplatinum, and tantalum were also available. These have been largely replaced by gutta-percha and are rarely used currently. They are largely of historical interest.

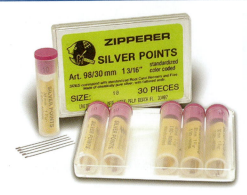

FIGURE 13.2 Silver points.

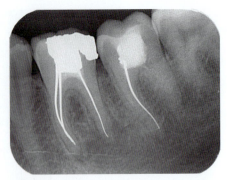

FIGURE 13.3 Root canal obturated with silver point. Silver points are rarely used currently.

Advantages

1. They had a bactericidal effect.
2. Can be used in narrow and curved canals.
3. Silver has more rigidity than gutta-percha, and hence can be pushed into tightly fitting canals and around curves where it is difficult to force gutta-percha.

Disadvantages

1. Silver points/cones have a circular cross section unlike the canals which may be oval hence a poor lateral seal.
2. Could show high levels of corrosion especially due to the dissolution of the sealers.
3. Corrosion products are cytotoxic.
4. Retrievability may be difficult in cases where retreatment is desired.
5. Preparation of canal for post and core reconstruction difficult.

The disadvantages of silver points far outweigh their advantages and their use has been largely discontinued. However, they present an important evolutionary stage in the development of root canal filling materials.

GUTTA-PERCHA

Gutta-percha is a polymeric resin-like material obtained from the coagulation of latex produced by Palaquium gutta tree (commonly known as the Isonandra gutta tree). Gutta-percha is a name derived from the Malay words 'getah' meaning gum and pertja' (name of the tree in Malay). Long before Gutta-percha was introduced into the western world, it was used in crude form by the natives of Malaysian archipelago for making knife handles, walking sticks and other purposes *(Box 13.1)*.

Manufacture of gutta-percha (Obach's technique)

The obtained pulp is mixed with water and heated to 75 °C to release the Gutta-percha threads and then cooled to 45 °C. The flocculated Gutta-percha called "yellow Gutta" contains 60% poly isoprene and 40% contaminants (resin, protein, dirt and water). Yellow Gutta is mixed with cold industrial gasoline at below 0 °C temperature. This treatment not only flocculates the Gutta-percha but also dissolves resins and denatures any residual proteins. After removal of cold gasoline, deresinated Gutta threads are dissolved in warm water at 75 °C and dirt particulate is allowed to precipitate. Residual greenish yellow solution is bleached with activated clay filtered to remove any particulate and then steam distilled to remove the gasoline. "Fina

Box 13.1   History of gutta-percha

Gutta-percha trees are native to South East Asia and Australia. Their sap is similar to rubber. It's actually a natural polymer-like rubber. Though very similar to it, unlike rubber, Gutta-percha is biologically inert - it doesn't react with biological materials - and that was the key to its usefulness. It was discovered by Western explorers in the middle of the 17th century, though local Malay people already knew about it and used it. The first Westerner to discover this material was John Tradescant, who brought this material after his travels from far-east in 1656, he named this material as "Mazer wood". But the honour of introduction of this material goes to Dr. William Montogmerie, who was a medical officer in Indian service. He was the first to appreciate the potential of this material in medicine and for which he was awarded the gold medal by the Royal Society of Arts, London in 1841. As soon as it was introduced, it found use as an insulating medium in the laying of underground seawater cables. The first Gutta-percha patent was taken by Alexander, Cabriol and Duclos for a laminate consisting of three layers called "Gutta-percha fabric". In 1845 Hancock and Bewley formed the Gutta-percha company in United Kingdom. There were even jewels and ornaments made of it as they were considered to be precious materials at that time.

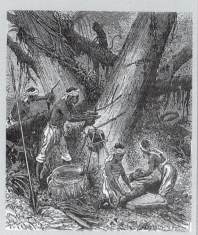

Gutta-percha and the Telecom Revolution

Back in the 19th century, the telegraph was revolutionising the way people communicated. The solution was to lay down undersea telegraph cables. However, to carry electricity an undersea cable needs to be protected and no one had succeeded in doing that. Rubber had been tried as an insulating layer for the cables but marine animals and plants just attacked it, and once the cable was open to the sea it became useless for sending signals. Gutta-percha on the other hand is a great insulator but it doesn't degrade in sea-water. As it was the only known material that worked, soon all marine cable used Gutta-percha and as a result the British businessmen who controlled its supply became very rich.

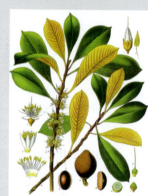

Dimpled Balls

Early golf balls were filled with feathers. In 1848 Robert Adams Paterson came up with the idea of making them out of Gutta-percha since it was much easier to make than the laborious process of sewing balls of feathers. It was quickly realised, that after they had been used a few times they would fly further. It turned out this was due to the dimples that were made in the balls each time they were hit. The dimples improved the aerodynamics of the ball. That's why modern golf balls are intentionally covered in dimples. The era of Gutta-percha golf balls lasted from 1845-1903, till the introduction of natural rubber.

Medical use of Gutta-percha

In medicine, they were used as splints for holding fractured joints and manufacture of handles of forceps, catheters, etc. It was earlier used to control hemorrhage in extracted socket wounds. They were also used for skin diseases by the dermatologists, particularly against Small pox, Erysipelas, Psoriasis and Eczema.

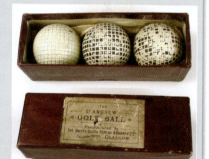

Antique gutta-percha golf balls

Gutta-percha in India

In India the species of this genus is very scanty. The species found are Palaquium obavatum, Palaquium polyanthum, Palaquium ellipticum and Palaquium gutta trees in Assam and Western ghats. Palaquium gutta was recently introduced and planted in Botanical gardens, Bangalore.

Gutta-percha in Dentistry

Gutta-percha made its appearance in dentistry in the mid-1800s, when it was first used for filling cavities *(Box 13.2)*. In 1887, S.S. White Manufacturing Co. began producing "points" of rolled gutta-percha for stuffing root canals. The material was valued for its plasticity when heated, which permits it to be 'stuffed into the odd nooks and crannies'. And that's how its still done today, with a material derived from the sap of a tropical tree. The annual market for gutta-percha in the US is estimated to be $30 million to $40 million, and most of it comes from Brazil. Even though it is the closest thing to an ideal root-canal filling material, it is hard to work with, and sometimes it still leaks. Developing a better material is what's on the horizon. Indeed, the big dental-supply firm Dentsply International, based in York, Pa., is working on a synthetic replacement for gutta-percha that it hopes to introduce in the near future. The final retirement of a historical material with a magnificent name seems too sad to contemplate.

So gutta-percha revolutionised global communications, changed the game of golf and even helped people with rotting teeth. Not bad for a tree.

ultra pure" gutta-percha has a gasoline scent, before it is modified with fillers into its final commercial product formulation.

Chemical structure of gutta-percha

Gutta-percha is 1,4-trans-polyisoprene isomer (natural gutta-percha) CH_2 groups are on opposite sides of the double bond for each successive monomer.

Since its molecular structure is close to that of natural rubber, which is a cis-isomer of polyisoprene, it has a number of similarities but a difference in form makes it to behave more like crystalline polymers. Thus it not exhibit the classic elastic properties of rubber

Forms of gutta-percha

Gutta-percha exists in three forms

α – (or alpha form)—runny, tacky and sticky

β – (or beta form)—solid, compactible and ductile

γ – (or gamma form)—amorphous and unstable form

The β form is used with mechanical condensation techniques.

The α form is used with the thermomechanical and injectable techniques.

Box 13.2   Evolution into dentistry

Gutta-percha was first introduced to dentistry as a temporary filling material by Edwin Truman.

1847 - Hill Developed "Hill's-stopping" a restorative material, a mixture of bleached Gutta-percha and carbonate of lime and quartz.

1867 - Bowman was the first to use Gutta-percha for root canal filling.

1883 - Perry used pointed gold wire wrapped with soft Gutta-percha, rolled and packed it into the canal.

1887 - S.S White Company was the first to start the commercial manufacture of Gutta-percha points.

1893 - Rollins used Gutta-percha with pure oxide of mercury into root canal filling.

1914 - Callahan introduced softening and dissolution of Gutta-percha with the use of rosins in obturation.

1959 – Ingle and Levine were the first persons to propose standardization of root canal instruments and filling materials and at their behest, standardized Gutta-percha was introduced to the profession in 1959 after the 2nd International Conference of Endodontics at Philadelphia.

1976 - A group was formed for the approval of specifications of root canal instruments and filling materials which subsequently evolved into the present day International Standards Organization (ISO).

Supplied as

1. Solid core Gutta-percha points
   - Standardized points *(Figs. 13.4A and B)*
   - Nonstandardized points
2. Thermomechanical compactible Gutta-percha points
3. Thermoplasticized Gutta-percha
   - Solid core system
   - Injectable form *(Figs. 13.7 to 13.9)*
4. Medicated Gutta-percha
   - Iodoform containing
   - Calcium hydroxide containing
   - Chlorhexidine containing
   - Tetracycline containing

Gutta-percha used for the above techniques are supplied in point or pellet form.

○ Tapered points of varying sizes. The sizes range from 15 to 80 *(Fig. 13.4B)*. The various sizes are usually color coded for easy identification.

○ Pellet form is used for the injectable technique *(Fig. 13.7)*

Composition of commercial gutta-percha

Ingredient	Wt %	Function
Gutta-percha	8–22%	Matrix
Zinc oxide	59–76%	Filler
Waxes or resins	1–4%	Plasticity
Metal sulphates	1–18%	Radiopacity (barium or strontium)

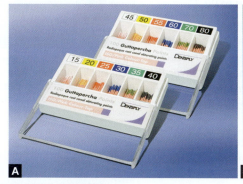
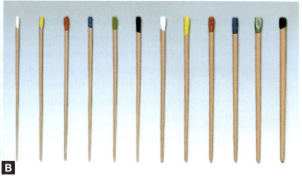

FIGURES 13.4A AND B Commercially available Gutta-percha points of varying sizes. They are color coded for differentiation.

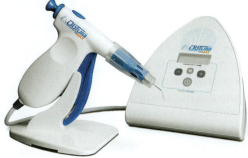
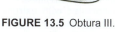

FIGURE 13.5 Obtura III.

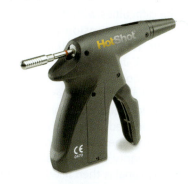

FIGURE 13.6 Hot Shot is a wireless battery operated.

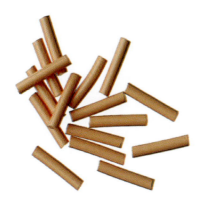

FIGURE 13.7 Gutta-percha pellets for use in the thermoplastic technique.

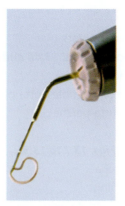

FIGURE 13.8 Extrusion of gutta-percha.

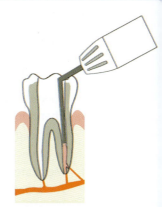

FIGURE 13.9 Backfill technique.

THERMOPLASTICIZED GUTTA-PERCHA

Gutta-percha may also be delivered to the canal in fluid form through a syringe *(Fig. 13.8)*. The gutta-percha is melted in the chamber of the device and injected into the canal starting apically and proceeding coronally. This is known as "backfilling" *(Fig. 13.9)*.

There are many such devices available in the market. The Obtura III *(Fig. 13.5)*, Calamus, Elements, HotShot *(Fig. 13.6)*, and Ultrafil 3D are examples of such devices. The Obtura III system heats the gutta-percha to 160 °C, whereas the Ultrafil 3D system employs a low-temperature gutta-percha that is heated to 90 °C.

The Obtura III system (Obtura Spartan) consists of a hand-held "gun" that contains a chamber surrounded by a heating element into which pellets of gutta-percha are loaded. Silver needles (varying gauges of 20, 23, and 25) are attached to deliver the thermoplasticized material to the canal. The control unit allows the operator to adjust the temperature and thus the viscosity of the gutta-percha.

Thermoplastic techniques are often indicated in cases with irregularities in the canal or internal resorption *(Fig. 13.10)*

Drawbacks

The difficulties with this system include lack of length control. Both overextension *(Fig. 13.11)* and underextension can occur. To overcome this drawback, a hybrid technique may be used, in which the clinician begins filling the canal by the lateral compaction technique. When the master cone and several accessory cones have been placed so that the mass is firmly lodged in the apical portion of the canal, a hot plugger is introduced, searing the points off approximately 4 to 5 mm from the apex. Light vertical compaction is applied to restore the integrity of the apical plug of gutta-percha. The remainder of the canal is then filled with thermoplasticized gutta-percha injected as previously described.

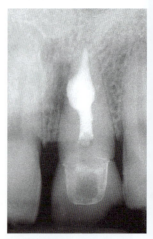

FIGURE 13.10 Thermoplastic techniques are often used in cases with significant canal irregularities like internal resorption.

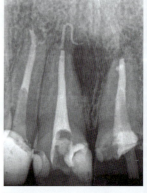

FIGURE 13.11 Thermoplastic backfilling techniques are often associated with extrusion of gutta-percha beyond the apex.

Properties

At raised temperatures, gutta-percha behaves like other plastic materials (thermoplastic), softening above 65 °C, melting at 100 °C, and in the a-form beyond 160 °C without decomposing while remaining soft and fluid.

Removal of gutta-percha

Occasionally gutta-percha requires to be removed for retreatment or placement of a post for reconstruction of the tooth.

This can be achieved with the aid of

1. Rotary instruments like NiTi (Protaper retreatment series)
2. Gutta-percha solvents like Chloroform or xylol
3. Thermosoftening.

ADVANTAGES AND DISADVANTAGES OF GUTTA-PERCHA

Advantages

1. It is compactible and adapts excellently to the irregularities and contour of the canal by the lateral and vertical condensation method.
2. It can be softened and made plastic by heat or by organic solvents (eucalyptol, chloroform, xylol, turpentine).
3. It is inert.
4. It is dimensional stable; when unaltered by organic solvents, it will not shrink.
5. It is tissue tolerant (nonallergenic).
6. It will not discolor the tooth structure.
7. It is radiopaque.
8. It can be easily removed from the canal when retreatment is indicated.

Disadvantages

1. It lacks rigidity. The smallest, standardized gutta-percha cones are relatively more difficult to use unless canals are enlarged above size no. 25.
2. It lacks adhesive quality. Gutta-percha does not adhere to the canal walls; consequently, a sealer is required. The necessary use of a cementing agent introduces the risk of tissue-irritating sealers.
3. Gutta-percha does not bond to any sealers.
4. It can be easily displaced by pressure.
5. Gutta-percha is almost wholly dependent on a coronal seal to prevent the apical migration of bacteria if it is challenged by coronal leakage.

RESILON-EPIPHANY ROOT CANAL OBTURATING SYSTEM

This system is an alternative to gutta-percha. It consists of resin obturating points sealed with dual cure, hydrophilic resin sealer.

The system consists of three parts (Figs. 13.12 and 13.13)

A. *Resilon* – A thermoplastic synthetic polymer-based (polyester) root canal filling material, as the major component.
B. *Epiphany sealer* – A resin-based composite that forms a bond to the dentin wall and the core material. It sets with a chemical reactions and halogen curing light.
C. *Primer* - Which prepares the canal wall for contact with Resilon and the sealer.

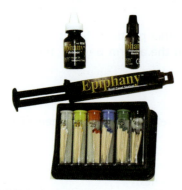

FIGURE 13.12 Epiphany root canal filling system consists of polyester points for insertion into the canal, a sealer and primer.

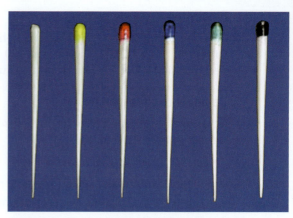

FIGURE 13.13 Resilon points for obturation.

Primer The primer is a self-etching system that is cured by the sealer. The primer penetrates all the dentinal tubules. The bonding procedure is preceded by irrigating with a 17% solution of EDTA. This last process is necessary for removing oxide radicals from the NaOCl and peroxides irrigants. Failure to do so can interfere with the curing of the dentin bonding agent.

Sealer The sealer bonds to the primer thereby eliminating potential for microleakage. The sealer used in this system is a dual cure bis-GMA, ethoxylated bis-GMA, UDMA, hydrophilic difunctional methacrylate. Fillers like calcium hydroxide, barium sulphate and barium glass are present 7% by weight. It contains the catalyst that initiates curing of self-etching primer in the dentinal tubules.

Obturator

The Resilon obturator is a thermoplastic polyester and contains the following components: (1) Bioactive glass, (2) barium sulfate and (3) bismuth oxychloride. The bioglass is a unique component that forms calcium/phosphate when in contact with body fluid. It does not dissolve in fluid but instead it releases ions to stimulate the formulation of osseous tissue. As already mentioned, its radiopacity is better than gutta-percha, condenses laterally and vertically like gutta-percha and softens at around 70 to 85 °C. The Resilon obturator bonds to the surface of the sealer which in turn bonds to the primer that has hybridized with the tubular surfaces.

Thinning Resin In addition to the above, many systems include a thinning resin, which may be added to thin the sealer to the desired viscosity.

PASTE-TYPE OBTURATING MATERIALS

Various paste-type products have been tried as the sole obturating materials because they have sufficient volume stability to maintain a seal. These include zinc oxide-eugenol based pastes, epoxy resins (AH-26), AH-Plus, Ketac-Endo, polyvinyl resins (Diaket), calcium hydroxide, etc. Many of these are dual use, i.e. they may be used as sole obturating material or as sealer (when combined with gutta-percha).

Disadvantages

1. Removal of a hard set cement can be a challenge if retreatment is required.
2. Risk of microleakage when used as the sole obturating material.

Because of these inherent problems, use of a hard setting non-thermoplastic, non-soluble cement type filling material as the sole obturating material is not routinely recommended.

ROOT CANAL SEALERS

The sealer plays an important role in the obturation of root canal. Gutta-percha cannot entirely obliterate the spaces within the root canal because of its physical limitations. The sealer fills all the spaces, the gutta-percha is unable to fill. Factors like the shape of the canal, defects within the canal, internal resorption, iatrogenic damage, accessory canals, etc., make intimate sealing of the root canal system a challenging task. A total hermetic seal of the root canal system is necessary to prevent the ingress of bacteria and reinfection of the canal. The sealer also acts as a binding agent, to the dentin and to the core material, which usually is gutta-percha.

Ideal requirements of a root canal sealer

1. It should be tacky when mixed.
2. It should adhere well to the gutta-percha and the canal wall when set.
3. It should make a hermetic seal.
4. It should be radiopaque so that it can be visualized in the radiograph.
5. The particles should be very fine so that they can mix easily with the liquid.
6. It should not shrink upon setting.
7. It should not stain tooth structure.
8. It should be bacteriostatic.
9. It should set slowly to provide suitable working time.
10. It should be insoluble in tissue fluids.
11. It should be tissue tolerant, that is, nonirritating or toxic to periradicular tissue.
12. It should be soluble in a solvent if it is necessary to remove the root canal filling.
13. It should not provoke an immune response in periradicular tissue.
14. It should be neither mutagenic nor carcinogenic.

Classification

Endodontic sealers can be broadly classified based on the principal components that react and set to form the binding matrix *(Table 13.1)*

TABLE 13.1 Showing classification of different root canal sealers

	Type	Sub-type	Commercial examples
A.	Zinc oxide-Eugenol based	Silver-containing (Rickert's formula based)	Pulp Canal Sealer (SybronEndo)
		Grossman's formula based (Silver free)	Wach's paste, Tubliseal (SybronEndo), Roths, Intrafill (SS White), Roth Root 801 (Roth)
		Therapeutic - Formaldehyde - Iodofor - Steroid	N2/RC2B, Endomethasone, SPAD, Riebler's paste Zical (Prevest Denpro) Endomethasone N (Septodont), Endofill (Dentsply)
B.	Resin based	BisGMA UDMA based	Real Seal SE (SybronEndo), Acroseal (Septodont), Epiphany (Pentron), EndoREZ (Ultradent), Diaket (3M)
		Epoxy resin based	Sealer 26 (Dentsply), AH Plus & AH-26 (Dentsply),
C.	Calcium hydroxide based		CRS (Hygienic), Sealapex (SybronEndo), Life Apexit (Ivoclar) Vitapex
D.	Silicone based		GuttaFlow (Coltene), RoekoSeal (Coltene)
E.	Glass ionomer based		Ketac-Endo (ESPE)
F.	MTA based		MTA Fillapex (Angelus), Endo CPM Sealer (EGEO), MTA Obtura (Angelus), ProRoot Endo Sealer (Dentsply)

ZINC OXIDE-EUGENOL-BASED SEALERS

Commercial names Tubli-Seal (SybronEndo), Pulp canal sealer (SybronEndo), Roth's cement, Proco-sol

RICKERT'S FORMULA BASED (SILVER CONTAINING)

The earliest sealers were made by dissolving gutta-percha in solvents like chloroform and was termed '*chloropercha*'. These sealers had problems resulting from shrinkage. Rickert's formula was developed in 1931 as an alternative to the chloropercha technique.

Composition

Powder	%	Liquid	%
Zinc oxide	41.2	Oil of clove	78
Precipitated silver	30	Canada balsam	22
White resin	16		
Thymol iodide	12.8		

The silver was added for its radiopacity and germicidal qualities. It has excellent lubricating and adhesive qualities, and sets in about half an hour. However the silver content caused discoloration of tooth structure. Pulp canal sealer **(Fig. 13.14)** is based on Rickert's formula.

GROSSMAN'S AND ROTH'S FORMULA BASED (SILVER FREE ZOE SEALERS)

This includes most current ZOE sealers. In 1958, Grossman introduced a nonstaining ZOE cement as a substitute for Rickert's formula. This formulation is considered standard by which other cements are measured because it reasonably meets most of Grossman's requirements for sealers. Many current sealers are still based on Grossman's formula **(Fig. 13.16)**.

Composition

Powder	wt %	Liquid
Zinc oxide, reagent	42	Eugenol
Staybelite resin	27	
Bismuth subcarbonate	15	
Barium sulphate	15	
Sodium borate, anhydrous	1	

Roth's sealer **(Fig. 13.15)** was similar to Grossman's except for the addition of Bismuth subnitrate instead of Bismuth subcarbonate.

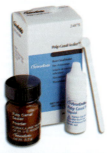

FIGURE 13.14 Rickert's sealer is sold under the trade name Pulp canal sealer.

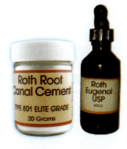

FIGURE 13.15 Roth's root canal sealer. It is a silver ZOE formulation.

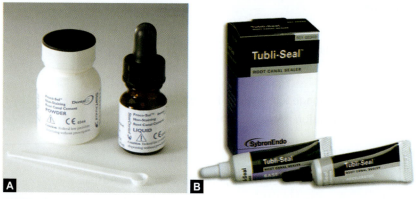

FIGURES 13.16A AND B Two other representative zinc-oxide eugenol based sealers.
(A) Proco-sol. **(B)** Tubli-seal.

THERAPEUTIC SEALERS

The first formaldehyde containing sealer was introduced by Sargenti in 1954 (also called Sargenti's Paste). These sealers constantly release antimicrobial formalin. Formalin is highly cytotoxic.

Therapeutic sealers contain antibiotics, bactericidal and anti-inflammatory agents. Bactericidal agents include formaldehyde and iodoform. Antiinflammatory agents include hydrocortisone, prednisolone, etc.

Commercial names

Formaldehyde containing - N2/RC2B **(Fig. 13.17A),** SPAD, Riebler's paste (drug combination consisting of zinc oxide, barium sulfate, formalin and resorcinol), etc.

Corticosteroid containing - Endomethasone **(Fig. 13.17B),** Endofill, etc.

Composition

Powder		Liquid
Zinc oxide	Bismuth subcarbonate	Eugenol
Barium sulphate	Hydrocortisone	Geraniol
Prednisolone	Paraformaldehyde	
Titanium dioxide	Phenyl mercuric borate	
Lead tetraoxide		

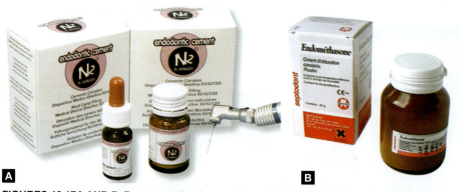

FIGURES 13.17A AND B Representative therapeutic sealers. **(A)** N2. **(B)** Endomethazone.

Advantages

1. Good antibacterial effect.
2. Good anti-inflammatory effect.

Disadvantages

1. Irreversible damage to the nerve tissue.
2. Causes coagulation necrosis of the tissues.

EPOXY RESIN-BASED SEALERS

Commercial names   Diaket, AH-26, AH Plus (Dentsply), Adseal.

DIAKET

Diaket *(Fig. 13.18 A)* was introduced by Schmidt in 1951. During setting, a resin-reinforced chelate is formed between zinc oxide and diketone. It has a high resistance to absorption.

Advantages

1. Good adhesion.
2. Sets quickly in the root canal.
3. Low solubility and good volume stability.
4. Superior tensile strength.

Disadvantages

1. It is highly toxic.
2. It is nonresorbable and forms fibrous encapsulation if extruded into the periapical tissues.

AH-26

AH-26 *(Fig. 13.18B)* was introduced by Schroeder 1957. It is an epoxy resin based sealer. It is a powder-liquid system.

Composition

Powder	Wt%	Liquid
Silver powder	10%	Bisphenol diglycidyl ether
Bismuth oxide	60%	
Hexamethylene tetramine	25%	
Titanium oxide	5%	

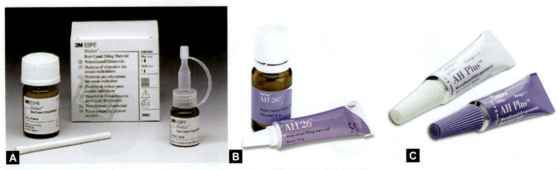

FIGURES 13.18A TO C Resin-based sealers. **(A)** Diaket. **(B)** AH-26. **(C)** AH Plus.

Manipulation and setting

AH 26 powder and resin are mixed to produce a root canal filling material. As it sets traces of formaldehyde are temporarily released, which initially makes it antibacterial. It is not sensitive to moisture and will even set under water.

However, it will not set in the presence of *hydrogen peroxide*. It sets slowly, in 24 to 36 hours. It has strong adhesive properties.

Disadvantages

1. Slight contraction while setting.
2. Delayed setting.
3. Staining.

AH- PLUS

AH Plus *(Fig. 13.18C)* is an epoxy-amine resin based two paste root canal sealer. Epoxy paste contains radiopaque fillers.

Composition

Epoxide paste contains bisphenol-A and F as epoxy resin, calcium tungstate, zirconium oxide, silica and iron oxide pigments and

Amine paste contains dibenzylediamine, aminoadmantace, tricyclodecane-diamine, calcium tungstate zirconium oxide, silica and silicone oil.

Advantages over AH-26

1. Less toxic.
2. New amines added to maintain the natural color of the tooth.
3. Half the film thickness.
4. Better flow.
5. Four-hour working time.
6. Eight-hour setting time allows for corrections of fillings.
7. Increased radiopacity.

EPIPHANY ROOT CANAL SEALER

Epiphany as described earlier is a dual cure, hydrophilic resin obturating material/sealer system.

CALCIUM HYDROXIDE BASED SEALERS

Dentists have been using calcium-based chemicals in clinical practice for over a century. Calcium hydroxide was introduced to endodontics by Herman in 1920 for its pulp-repairing ability. In endodontics, it is mainly used for pulp-capping procedures, as an intracanal medicament, in some apexification techniques, and as a component of several root canal sealers.

The two most important reasons for using calcium hydroxide as a root-filling material are stimulation of the periapical tissues in order to maintain health or promote healing and secondly for its antimicrobial effects. The exact mechanisms are unknown, but the following mechanisms of actions have been proposed.

1. Calcium hydroxide is antibacterial depending on the availability of free hydroxyl ions. It has a very high pH (hydroxyl group) that encourages repair and active calcification.

There is an initial degenerative response in the immediate vicinity followed rapidly by a mineralization and ossification response.

2. The alkaline pH of calcium hydroxide neutralizes lactic acid from osteoclasts and prevents dissolution of mineralized components of teeth. This pH also activates alkaline phosphatase that plays an important role in hard tissue formation.

3. Calcium hydroxide denatures proteins found in the root canal.

4. Calcium hydroxide activates the calcium-dependent adenosine triphosphatase reaction associated with hard tissue formation.

5. Calcium hydroxide diffuses through dentinal tubules and may communicate with the periodontal ligament space to arrest external root resorption and accelerate healing.

Setting of calcium hydroxide-based sealers in root canals

The setting time of calcium hydroxide-based sealers the root canal is dependent upon the availability of moisture. The setting reaction can progress very quickly even in canals which have been inadequately dried. The amount of moisture required for the setting reaction reaches the root canal by means of the dentinal tubules. The material begins to set at the apex, as dentin is thinnest in this region and the apical foramen admits additional moisture.

CRCS (CALCIOBIOTIC ROOT CANAL SEALER)

CRCS *(Fig. 13.19A)* is essentially a ZOE/eucalyptol sealer to which calcium hydroxide has been added for its called osteogenic effect.

CRCS takes 3 days to set fully in either dry or humid environments. It also shows very little water sorption. This means it is quite stable, which improves its sealant qualities, but brings into question its ability to stimulate cementum and/or bone formation. If the calcium hydroxide is not released from the cement, it cannot exert an osteogenic effect, and thus its intended role is negated

SEALAPEX

Sealapex *(Fig. 13.19B)* is a zinc oxide based calcium hydroxide sealer containing polymeric resin. It is available as a two paste system.

Advantages

1. Biocompatible
2. Extruded material resorbs in 4 months
3. Good therapeutic effect.

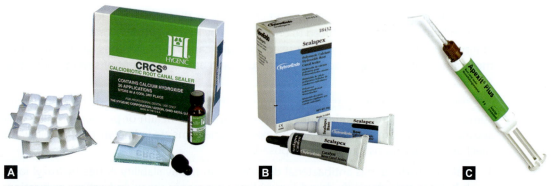

FIGURES 13.19A TO C Representative calcium hydroxide-based sealers. **(A)** CRCS. **(B)** Sealapex. **(C)** Apexit plus.

Disadvantages
1. Long setting time.
2. Absorbs water while setting and expands.
3. Poor cohesive strength.

APEXIT PLUS

Apexit Plus *(Fig. 13.19C)* is a radiopaque, non-shrinking root canal sealer paste that is based on calcium hydroxide. It is available as a two paste system. It is used for the permanent obturation of root canals and it is suitable for use in conjunction with all obturation techniques involving gutta-percha.

Working and setting characteristics
1. Long working time (over 3 hours at room temperature)
2. Setting Time - 3–5 hours in normal canals. Up to 10 hours in extremely dry canals.

Advantages
1. Excellent tissue tolerance.
2. Durable sealing of the root canal due to the slight setting expansion.
3. Its easy flowing composition allows the material to adapt well even to morphologically complicated canals.
4. Convenient application (static mix syringe and intracanal tip).
5. Better seal than that provided by Sealapex.

GLASS IONOMER-BASED SEALERS

Commercial name   Ketac-Endo *(Fig. 13.20)*

Advantages
1. Biocompatible.
2. Chemical bonding with the root dentine, hence strengthens the root.
3. Less solubility.
4. Dimensionally stable.
5. Less technique sensitive.

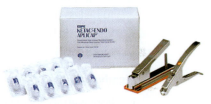

FIGURE 13.20 Glass ionomer-based sealers.

Disadvantages
1. Extruded sealer is highly resistant to resorption (delayed resorption).
2. Retrievability is difficult.

SILICON-BASED SEALERS

The silicon-based sealers are based on the polydimethyl siloxane system.

Commercial names RoekoSeal (Coltene) and Guttaflow (Langenau) *(Figs. 13.21A and B).*

Composition

RoekoSeal - Polydimethylsiloxane, silicone oil, zirconium oxide.

Gutta flow - Polydimethylsiloxane, silicone oil, zirconium oxide, gutta-percha.

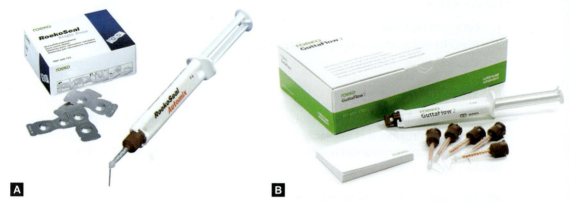

FIGURES 13.21A AND B Silicon-based sealers. **(A)** Roekoseal. **(B)** GuttaFlow.

Properties

1. Excellent flow properties and good spreadability.
2. Contains nanosilver which prevent further spread of bacteria.
3. Good adaptability and tight seal of the root canal.
4. Flowable cold filling system.
5. Solubility is virtually zero.
6. Excellent radiopacity.
7. The included nanosilver can also have a preserving effect in the canal. The chemical type and concentration of the silver does not cause corrosion or color changes in the GuttaFlow.
8. A Gutta-percha containing silicone sealer expands slightly and thus leakage was reported to be less than the AH-26 over a period of 12 months.
9. Very good biocompatibility with lower cytotoxicity than the AH Plus.
10. More easily removed from the canals than a resin-based sealer.

Disadvantages

1. Poor wettability of GuttaFlow
2. GuttaFlow does not adhere chemically to the canal wall.
3. Due to its viscosity, it is more likely to be extruded into the periapical tissue when placed under pressure.

MINERAL TRIOXIDE AGGREGATE (MTA)

The first reported use of Portland cement in dental literature dates to 1878, when Dr. Witte in Germany published a case report on using Portland cement to fill root canals. At the time the material itself was relatively new as Portland cement was invented in 1824. Mineral trioxide aggregate (MTA) was first described in modern dental scientific literature in 1995. It was developed at Loma Linda University, California, USA, by Torabinejad and Dean White who subsequently obtained two US patents for this Portland cement-based endodontic material, which became known as mineral trioxide aggregate (MTA). Since then, over 20 patents have been issued in the USA and the EU for materials that include Portland cement for dentistry.

The term *mineral trioxide aggregate* (MTA) was coined from the *three oxides* present in Portland cement namely, calcia, silica and alumina (CaO, SiO_2 and Al_2O_3). Furthermore, the powder particles of cement are in aggregate form.

Indications

Mineral trioxide aggregate materials are indicated for various restorative, endodontic, and regenerative dental procedures.

1. Vital pulp therapy (pulp capping and pulpotomy)
2. Apexification
3. Perforation repair (lateral and furcation) *(Figs. 13.22A and B)*
4. Root-end filling
5. Internal bleaching
6. Resorption repair
7. As sealer and as obturating material (partial or complete).

Commercial names

The first commercially available product was a *gray* mineral trioxide aggregate, marketed as ProRoot® MTA (Dentsply) *(Fig. 13.23A)*. Subsequently for esthetic reasons a *tooth-colored or white* formulation of MTA was introduced (Dentsply) in 2002.

Currently Many MTA sealer formulations are available. These include Endo CPM Sealer (EGEO SRL, Argentina), MTA Obtura (Angelus, Brazil), MTA Fillapex (Angelus) *(Fig. 13.23B)*, *Endocem MTA (Maruchi, Korea)* and ProRoot Endo Sealer (Dentsply Maillefer, Switzerland).

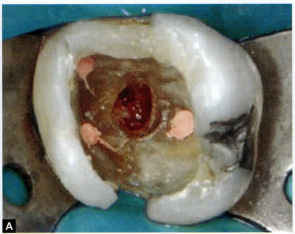
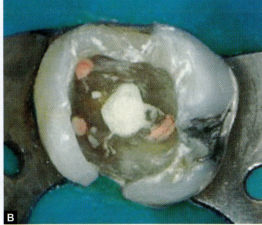

FIGURES 13.22A AND B **(A)** Perforation in the floor of maxillary molar. **(B)** Perforation repaired with MTA.

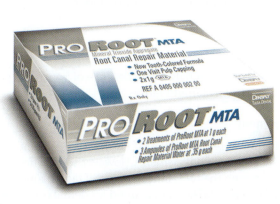
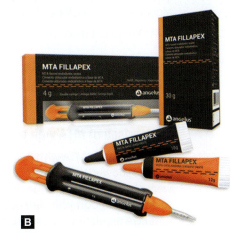

FIGURES 13.23A AND B MTA based sealers. **(A)** ProRoot MTA. **(B)** MTA Fillapex.

Supplied as

1. Powder and liquid form (e.g. ProRoot MTA)
2. Two paste - base and catalyst in tubes (MTA Fillapex)
3. Two paste - in plunger tubes as static mixing system (MTA Fillapex).

Composition

A wide variation in composition exists between the different products.

ProRoot MTA is calcium silicate-based endodontic sealer. The major components of the powder of are tricalcium silicate and dicalcium silicate, with inclusion of calcium sulfate (gypsum) as setting retardant, bismuth oxide as radiopacifier, and a small amount of tricalcium aluminate. Tricalcium aluminate is necessary for the initial hydration reaction of the cement.

Powder *

Ingredient	Formula	Wt%	Function
Tricalcium silicate	$(CaO)_3.SiO_2$	45–75	
Dicalcium silicate	$(CaO)_2.SiO_2$	7–32	
Tricalcium aluminate	$(CaO)_2.Al_2O_3$	0–13	Initial hydration
Bismuth or tantalum oxide	Bi_2O_3 or Ta_2O_5	20–35	Radiopacity
Calcium sulphate dihydrate (gypsum)	$CaSO_4.2H_2O$	2–10	Retarder
Tetracalcium aluminoferrite	$(CaO)_4.Al_2O_3.Fe_2O_3$	0–18	Impart gray color in MTA. Absent in white MTA.

* Adapted from Phillips Science of Dental Material. Ed. 12.

Liquid

The liquid component consists of viscous aqueous solution of a water soluble polymer to improve the workability.

MTA Fillapex **(Fig. 13.23B)** is a mineral trioxide aggregate-based, salicylate resin root canal sealer. It is designed to provide a high flow rate and a low film thickness for easy penetration of lateral and accessory canals. It contains 13% MTA and salicylate resin for their antimicrobial and biocompatibility properties. The working time is 23 minutes with a complete set time is approximately 2 hours. MTA Fillapex is a two-paste system and is provided in a 4 g static mixing syringe and 30 g tubes.

CPM sealer The composition of CPM sealer after mixing is reported to be 50% MTA (SiO_2, K_2O, Al_2O_3, SO_3, CaO, and Bi_2O_3), 7% SiO_2, 10% $CaCO_3$, 10% Bi_2O_3, 10% $BaSO_4$, 1% propylene glycol alginate, 1% propylene glycol, 1% sodium citrate, and 10% calcium chloride.

MTA Obtura is a mixture of white MTA with a proprietary viscous liquid.

Difference between white and gray MTA

The difference between the gray and the white materials is the presence of iron in the gray material, which makes up the phase tetracalcium alumino-ferrite.

Comparison of MTA with portland cement

The similarity of MTA with Portland cement was reported in 2000. Further studies comparing the two showed the cements to have similar constituent elements. However, some differences were also noted. The prime difference between the two is the addition of radiopaque fillers to enable radiographic differentiation. Secondly, MTA manufactured for dental use have to pass FDA regulations to enable it to be used in humans, thus components considered harmful have to be eliminated or minimized. A comparison of the two are presented in **Table 13.2.**

TABLE 13.2 Comparison of MTA and Portland cement

	MTA	Portland cement
Radiopaque fillers	Present	Absent
Tricalcium aluminate	Present	Absent
Tricalcium silicate	Lower levels	Higher level
Calcium sulphate hemihydrate	Absent	Present
Particle size	Fine	Coarser
Heavy metal content	Minimal or absent	Present

Biological properties

When placed in the canal, it releases calcium activity and causes cell attachment and proliferation, increases the pH, modulates cytokines like interleukin (IL4, IL6, IL8, IL10), and hence causes proliferation, migration, and differentiation of hard tissue producing hydroxyapatite which aids in the formation of physical bond between sealer and MTA.

The polymer did not seem to affect the biocompatibility of the materials and the hydration characteristics were similar to those reported for MTA. Sealers based on MTA have been reported to be biocompatible, stimulate mineralization, and encourage apatite-like crystalline deposits along the apical- and middle-thirds of canal walls. These materials exhibited higher push-out strengths after storage in simulated body fluid and had similar sealing properties to epoxy resin-based sealer when evaluated using the fluid filtration system. Fluoride-doped MTA demonstrated stable sealing up to 6 months, and was significantly better than conventional MTA sealers and comparable to AH Plus. The study supports the suitability of MTA sealers in association with warm GP for root filling.

Manipulation

P/L Ratio   The powder liquid ratio of MTA can vary according to its intended use. For use as a sealer a creamy consistency is preferred. For use in perforation repair a putty consistency may be preferred. P/L therefore ranges from 4 to 1 to 2 to 1.

Open a pouch of ProRoot MTA root repair material and dispense the powder onto a mixing pad. Liquid from the ampoule squeeze out onto the mixing pad next to the powder. Gradually incorporate the liquid into the cement with a plastic spatula.

Mixing time   Mix the material with the liquid for about one minute to ensure all the powder particles are hydrated.

If needed (one extra ampoule is provided, sterile water can also be used), one or two drops of liquid can be added to make the material into a thick, creamy consistency.

Working time   The ProRoot MTA root repair material will set over a period of four hours, but the working time is about five minutes. If more working time is needed, cover the mixed material with a moist gauze pad to prevent evaporation.

Setting time

Traditionally these materials generally have long setting times. Newer products currently being marketed have shorter setting times. Examples include Endocem MTA and Biodentine.

	ProRoot MTA	**Endocem MTA**	**Biodentine**
Initial setting time	165 minutes	2 minutes	
Final setting time	4 to 6 hours	4 minutes	9–12 minutes

It has also been stated that the faster setting time is achieved by increasing particle size, adding calcium chloride to the liquid component, and decreasing the liquid content.

Chemistry and setting reaction

MTA sets through a hydration reaction when mixed with water.

MTA + water → calcium hydroxide + calcium silicate hydrate

When MTA is mixed with water a highly alkaline (pH 12) cement matrix comprising of calcium hydroxide and calcium silicate hydrate is formed. A setting expansion of 0.1% is seen which contributes to its sealing ability.

An acidic environment does not interfere with the setting of the MTA.

Properties

1. *Compressive strength* It has been shown that once it is set, it has a compressive strength equal to IRM and Super EBA but less than amalgam. Compressive strength of MTA within 24 hours of mixing was about 40.0 MPa and increases to 67.3 MPa after 21 days. In comparison gray MTA exhibited greater compressive strength than white MTA.
2. *Setting Expansion* Set MTA exhibits a low setting expansion of less than 0.1%.
3. *Radiopacity* MTA is less radio opaque than IRM, amalgam or gutta-percha and has similar radiodensity as Zinc Oxide Eugenol. The mean radiopacity of MTA is 7.17 mm of equivalent thickness of aluminium, which is sufficient to make it easy to visualize radiographically.
4. *Solubility* Although the set MTA shows no signs of solubility, the solubility might increase if more water is used during mixing. The set MTA when exposed to water releases calcium hydroxide is responsible for its *cementogenic property.*
5. *Marginal adaptation and sealing ability* This property is most vital for any restorative material especially when used for root end filling, repair of perforations, pulp capping or pulpotomy procedures. Bates et al found MTA superior to the other traditional root-end filling materials. MTA expands during setting which may be the reason for its excellent sealing ability. According to Torabinejad et al MTA seals very superiorly and no gaps were found in any of the experimental specimen. However, amalgam, Super EBA and IRM exhibited gaps ranging from 3.8 to 14.9 microns. MTA has also proved itself to be superior in the bacterial leakage test by not allowing the entry of bacteria at the interface. MTA thickness of about 4 mm is sufficient to provide a good seal.
6. *Antibacterial and antifungal property* Torabinejad et al reported that MTA shows no antimicrobial activity against any of the anaerobes but have some effect on five (*S. mitis, S. mutans, S. salivarius,* Lactobacillus and *S. epidermidis*) of the nine facultative bacteria. Since most of the flora in the root canal are strict anaerobic bacteria with few facultative anaerobes, MTA may not be beneficial as a direct antibacterial in endodontic practice. However, it can be proclaimed as an antibacterial agent only by virtue of providing a good seal and preventing micro leakage.
7. *Reaction with other dental materials* MTA does not react or interfere with any other restorative material. Glass Ionomer cements or composite resins, used as permanent filling material do not affect the setting of MTA when placed over it. Residual calcium hydroxide may interfere with the adaptation of MTA to dentin thereby reducing its sealing ability either by acting as a mechanical obstacle or by chemically reacting with MTA. This may be important when calcium hydroxide is placed in the cavity in between the appointments prior to the placement of MTA.
8. *Biocompatibility* Kettering and Torabinejad studied MTA in detail and found that it is not mutagenic and is much less cytotoxic compared to Super EBA and IRM. This supports the superiority of MTA over formocresol as a pulpotomy medicament. Genotoxicity tests of

cells after treatment of peripheral lymphocytes with MTA showed no DNA damage. On direct contact they produce minimal or no inflammatory reaction in soft tissues and in fact are capable of inducing tissue regeneration.

9. *Tissue regeneration* MTA is capable of activation of cementoblasts and production of cementum. It consistently allows for the overgrowth of cementum and also facilitates regeneration of the periodontal ligament. MTA allows bone healing and eliminates clinical symptoms in many cases. In animal studies, MTA produced cementum growth which was very unique compared to other root-end filling materials. Arens and Torabinejad reported osseous repair of furcation perforations treated with MTA. MTA showed good interaction with bone-forming cells. Investigations by Koh et al revealed that MTA offers a biologically active substrate for bone cells and stimulates interleukin production. MTA is also said to stimulate cytokine production in human osteoblasts.

10. *Mineralization* MTA, just like calcium hydroxide, induces dentin bridge formation and is believed to be due to its sealing property, biocompatibility, alkalinity and other associated properties. Tricalcium oxide in MTA reacts with tissue fluids to form calcium hydroxide, resulting in hard-tissue formation in a manner similar to that of calcium hydroxide cement. In comparison the dentin bridge formed with MTA is faster, thicker with good structural integrity and more complete than with calcium hydroxide. MTA also proves to be better at stimulating reparative dentin formation and maintaining the integrity of the pulp.

Storage

Powder form MTA pouches must be kept tightly closed and stored in a dry area to avoid degradation by moisture.

ProRoot MTA root repair material must be placed intraorally immediately after mixing with liquid, to prevent dehydration during setting. Excess water will retard curing process. Excess moisture in cotton pellets should be held to a minimum. The area should not be irrigated after placement of the material.

Placement technique

Using a rubber dam, debride the root canal system using intracanal instruments, and irrigate with NaOCl. Dry the canal with paper points and isolate the perforation.

Obturate all the canal space, apical to the perforation.

The material is prepared according to the manufacturers instruction. Using the carrier, dispense the material into the perforation site. Condense the material into the perforation site using a small plugger, cotton pellets or paper points. Confirm placement material with a radiograph. If an adequate barrier has not been created, rinse the root repair material out of the canal and repeat the procedure.

Following satisfactory obturation. Take a moist cotton pellet (remove excess moisture) and place in the canal. Seal the access preparation with a temporary restoration for a minimum of four hours. After four hours, or at a subsequent appointment, use a rubber dam and examine the MTA. This cement should be hard. If not, rinse and repeat the application. When the material is hardened, obturate the remaining canal space. The ProRoot MTA root repair material remains as a permanent part of the root canal filling.

ENDODONTIC SOLVENTS

Endodontic treatment may not always be successful and failures may be seen on occasion. If retreatment is indicated, the old endodontic filling materials have to be removed to gain access to the canals. The various removal methods available are solvents, heat and mechanical instrumentation. Silver points are removed by grasping and pulling with a pair of pliers. Gutta-percha and resin-based obturating material removal is usually achieved by a combination of mechanical removal and chemical dissolution. However one must remember that the solvent must act on both the *obturating material and sealer* for effective cleansing of the canal of old material. Thus an endodontic solvent may be more effective for a particular material and not all. Materials often encountered in the canals include gutta-percha, resin-based sealers silicone, zinc oxide eugenol and glass ionomer. Most solvents are cytotoxic and potentially carcinogenic and therefore has to be used with proper precautions.

Commonly used solvents for gutta-percha and sealers are

1. Xylol or xylene
2. Orange oil
3. Chloroform
4. Halothane
5. Rectified turpentine
6. Eucalyptol

Commercial names

1. For resin-based sealers: Endosolv R (septodont)
2. For zinc oxide based sealers: Endosolv E (septodont), DMS IV (Dentsply).

XYLOL OR XYLENE

Xylene is a colorless, sweet smelling but flammable liquid. Xylene is a petrochemical product and a widely used industrial solvent. Chemically it is an aromatic hydrocarbon mixture consisting of a benzene ring with two methyl groups [dimethylbenzene or $C_6H_4(CH_3)_2$]. Xylene exists in three isomeric forms—ortho, meta and para.

It is one of the most effective solvents for gutta-percha and resin-based sealers like resilon.

CHLOROFORM

Chloroform (trichloromethane - $CHCl_3$) is a colorless, sweet-smelling, dense liquid and is considered hazardous *(Fig. 13.24)*.

It is an effective solvent for gutta-percha and resin based sealers like AH Plus.

It is not effective for GIC based sealers like Ketac Endo. It has low solubility for CaOH based sealers (Apexit).

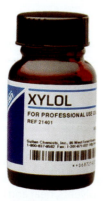 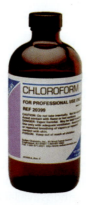 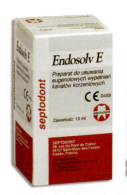 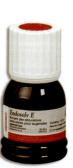

FIGURE 13.24 Endodontic solvents.

HALOTHANE

Halothane (2-bromo-2-chloro-1,1,1-trifluoroethane) is an inhalational general anesthetic. It is packaged in dark-colored bottles and contains 0.01% thymol as a stabilizing agent.

It is an effective solvents for gutta-percha and resin-based sealers like AH Plus.

It is not effective for GIC based sealers like Ketac Endo and ZOE sealers. It has low solubility for CaOH based sealers (Apexit).

RECTIFIED TURPENTINE

Spirit of turpentine (*syn:* oil of turpentine, wood turpentine) is a fluid obtained by the distillation of resin obtained from many trees other than the pines. It is an industrial solvent and paint thinner. Rectified turpentine is obtained by treating turpentine oil with sodium hydroxide, and redistilling. Medically it is used externally as a counterirritant.

It is an effective solvents for gutta-percha especially if warmed to 70 °C.

ORANGE OIL OR D-LIMONENE

Orange oil is an essential oil extracted from the rind of an orange. It is composed of mostly (greater than 90%) d-limonene. D-limonene can be extracted from the oil by distillation. It was originally introduced as a general solvent and cleansing agent for the dental office.

It is an effective solvent for zinc oxide eugenol sealers and an alternative solvent for thermoplastic gutta-percha.

It has no effect on resin-based sealers like resilon.

EUCALYPTOL

Eucalyptol ($C_{10}H_{18}O$) is a distillation product of eucalyptus oil. It is natural organic compound that is a colorless liquid with a fresh camphor-like smell and a spicy, cooling taste.

Compared to the others it is a comparatively less effective solvent for gutta-percha. Its effect increases on heating.

PART-4

Impression Materials

Rigid Impression Materials—Impression Compound and ZOE Paste

A dental impression is a negative record of the tissues of the mouth. It is used to reproduce the form of the teeth and surrounding tissues.

The negative reproduction of the tissues given by the impression material is filled up with dental stone or other model materials to get a positive cast. The positive reproduction of a single tooth is described as a 'die', and when several teeth or a whole arch is reproduced, it is called a 'cast' or 'model'.

The application of dental impression compound has also decreased with the increased use of rubber impression materials, which can also be electroformed to produce metal dies. However, impression compound is useful for checking cavity preparations for undercuts and for making impressions of full crown.

ADVANTAGES OF USING A CAST OR MODEL

1. Models provide a three-dimensional view of the oral structures, thus aiding in diagnosis and treatment planning.
2. Many restorations or appliances are best constructed on casts. It may be inconvenient to both dentist and patient if these have to be made directly in the patient's mouth.
3. Models can be used to educate the patient.
4. They serve as treatment records.
5. By using casts, technical work can be passed on to technicians, saving valuable clinical time.

DESIRABLE PROPERTIES OF AN IMPRESSION MATERIAL

1. Should be nontoxic and nonirritant to dentist and patient.
2. Acceptable to the patient.
   a. Have a pleasant taste, odor, consistency and color.
   b. Should set quickly once placed in the mouth.
3. Should be accurate.
   a. Accurate surface detail.
   b. Elastic properties with freedom from permanent deformation after strain.
   c. Dimensionally stable.
4. Have adequate shelf life for storage and distribution.
5. Be economical.
6. Handling properties.
   a. Sufficient working time.
   b. Set quickly in mouth (saves chairside time).
   c. Be easy to use with the minimum equipment.
   d. Satisfactory consistency and texture.
7. Have adequate strength so that it will not break or tear while removing from the mouth
8. Should be compatible with the die and cast materials.
9. Should be able to be electroplated.

CLASSIFICATION OF IMPRESSION MATERIALS

There are several ways of classifying impression materials.

1. According to mode of setting and elasticity.
2. According to tissue displacement during impression procedure.
3. According to their uses in dentistry.

According to mode of setting and elasticity

The terms thermoset, thermoplastic, rigid and elastic are used to describe these material *(Table 14.1)*.

According to tissue displacement

Depending on whether tissues are displaced while making impressions a material may be

1. Mucostatic
2. Mucocompressive (Mucodisplacive)

TABLE 14.1 Classification of impression materials according to mode of setting and elasticity

Mode of setting	Rigid	Elastic
Set by chemical reaction (irreversible or thermoset)	Impression plaster Zinc oxide eugenol	Alginate hydrocolloid Nonaqueous elastomers -e.g. polysulfide, silicone
Set by temperature change (reversible/ thermoplastic)	Compound, Waxes	Agar hydrocolloid

Mucostatic materials produce minimal displacement of the tissue during impression, e.g. plaster, zinc oxide eugenol, low viscosity alginates, low viscosity elastomeric materials, etc.

Mucocompressive materials are more viscous and displace the tissues while recording them, e.g. compound, high viscosity alginates, high viscosity elastomers, etc.

According to their uses in dentistry

Impression materials used for complete denture prosthesis   Impression plaster, impression compound and impression paste set to a hard rigid mass, and hence cannot be removed from undercuts without the impression being fractured or distorted. Therefore these materials are best suited for *edentulous* mouth.

Impression materials used for dentulous mouths   On the other hand alginates and rubber base impressions are sufficiently elastic to be withdrawn from undercut areas. Such elastic impression materials are suitable for impressions for fabrication of removable and fixed partial denture prostheses, where the impressions of the ridge and teeth are required.

RIGID IMPRESSION MATERIALS

As mentioned earlier the rigid impression materials are

1. Impression plaster
2. Impression compound
3. Zinc oxide eugenol impression paste
4. Impression waxes

(Impression plaster is described in the chapter on Gypsum Products).

IMPRESSION COMPOUND

Impression compound is one of the oldest of the dental impression materials. It can be described as a rigid, reversible impression material which sets by physical change. On applying heat, it softens and on cooling it hardens. It is mainly used for making impressions of edentulous ridges. A more viscous variety of compound called tray compound is used to form a tray in which a second more fluid material is placed to make a more detailed impression compound.

Synonyms   Modeling compound or modeling plastic.

CLASSIFICATION

Type I - Impression compound

Type II - Tray compound

Type II Tray compound is used to prepare a tray for making an impression. A second material is then carried in it in order to make an impression of oral tissues. Since reproduction of the fine details is not essential, it is generally stiffer and has less flow than regular impression compound. The use of dental tray compound decreased with the increased substitution of acrylic tray materials.

SUPPLIED AS

Supplied as sheets, sticks, cakes and cones in a variety of colors *(Fig. 14.1)*.

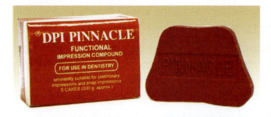
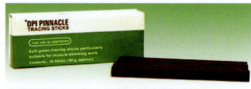
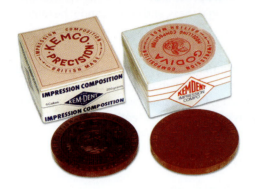
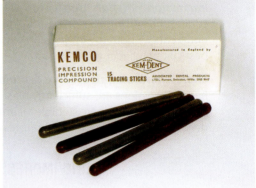

FIGURE 14.1 Impression compound cakes and sticks.

APPLICATIONS

1. For making a preliminary impression in an edentulous mouth (mouth without teeth).
2. For impressions of full crown preparations where gingival tissues must be displaced.
3. Peripheral tracing or border molding.

$\left.\right\}$ Type I

4. To check undercuts in inlay preparation.
5. To make a special tray.

$\left.\right\}$ Type II

Single tooth impression

In conservative dentistry, an impression is made of a single tooth in which a cavity is prepared. The compound is softened and carried in a copper band. The filled band is pressed over the tooth and the compound flows into the prepared cavity. It is referred to as a *tube impression*. Tube impressions were also used to make electroformed dies.

Complete denture impressions

In complete denture fabrication, it is common to make two sets of impressions—the *preliminary* and the *final impression*. The preliminary impression is made in a stock tray. A study cast made from this is used to construct a custom tray or special tray. The custom tray is used to make the final impression. The technique of making a preliminary and final impression greatly improves the accuracy of the complete denture.

REQUIREMENTS OF IMPRESSION COMPOUND

An ideal impression material should

1. Harden at or little above mouth temperature.
2. Be plastic at a temperature not injurious or harmful to oral tissues.

3.   Not contain irritating or toxic ingredients.
4.   Harden uniformly when cooled without distortion.
5.   Have a consistency when softened which will allow it to reproduce fine details.
6.   Be cohesive but not adhesive.
7.   Not undergo permanent deformation or fracture while withdrawing the impression from the mouth.
8.   Be dimensionally stable after removal from the mouth and during storage.
9.   Exhibit a smooth glossy surface after flaming.
10. Withstand trimming with sharp knife without flaking or chipping after hardening.
11. Should not boil and lose volatile components on flaming.
12. Should remain stable without losing soluble plasticizers when immersed in water for long periods.

COMPOSITION

In general impression compound is a mixture of waxes, thermoplastic resins, organic acids, fillers and coloring agents.

Ingredient	Parts
Resin	30
Copal resin	30
Carnauba wax	10
Stearic acid	5
Talc	25
Coloring agent (e.g. rouge)	

Plasticizers   Compounds, such as shellac, stearic acid and gutta-percha are added to improve plasticity and workability. These substances are referred to as *plasticizers*. Synthetic resins are being used in increasing amounts. Waxes and resin give the material its characteristic thermoplastic properties.

Fillers   These are small particles of inert materials which strengthen or improve the physical properties of many materials. Fillers are chemically different from the principal ingredient. In such a case the filler particles are sometimes referred to as the core and the surrounding ingredients as the matrix. For example, the waxes and resins in impression compound impart high flow and low strength. Consequently, a filler such as talc is added to reduce the plasticity and increase strength of the matrix material. Other fillers used are diatomaceous earth, soap stone and French chalk.

PROPERTIES OF IMPRESSION COMPOUND

FUSION TEMPERATURE

When impression compound is heated in a hot water bath the material *starts to soften* at approximately 39 °C. However at this stage, it is still not plastic or soft enough for making an impression. This temperature at which the material looses its hardness or brittleness on heating or forms a rigid mass upon cooling is referred to as *fusion temperature.* Impression compound exhibits a fusion temperature range rather than a fixed point.

On continued heating above 43.5 °C, the material continues to soften and flow to a plastic mass that can be manipulated. Thus all impressions with compound should be made above this temperature. Below this temperature an accurate impression cannot be expected.

THERMAL PROPERTIES

Thermal conductivity

Impression compound has very low thermal conductivity, i.e. they are poor conductors of heat.

Significance

1. During softening of the material, the outside will soften first and the inside last. So to ensure uniform softening the material should be kept immersed for a sufficient period in a water bath. Kneading of the material ensures further uniform softening.
2. The low thermal conductivity affects the cooling rate. The layer adjacent to the oral tissues cools faster than the inside. Removal of the impression at this stage can cause serious distortion. Thus it is important to wait for the compound to cool thoroughly before removing it from the mouth.

Coefficient of thermal expansion (CTE)

The CTE of compound is comparatively high due to the presence of resins and waxes. The linear contraction from mouth temperature to room temperature is 0.3%.

Errors from thermal distortion can be reduced

1. By obtaining an impression and then passing the impression over a flame until the surface is softened and then obtaining a second impression. During the second impression, the shrinkage is relatively lower, since only the surface layer has been softened.
2. Another way of reducing the thermal contraction is by spraying cold water on the metal tray just before it is inserted in the mouth. Thus the material adjacent to the tray will be hardened, while the surface layer is still soft. In both techniques, the impression is likely to be stressed considerably and so the stone cast should be constructed at the earliest.

FLOW

Good flow is desirable during impression making. The softened material should flow into all the details of the tissue contour. Once the compound hardens, it should have minimum flow, otherwise it will get distorted.

Dimensional stability

Since the release of strains is unavoidable, the safest way to prevent distortion is to *pour the cast immediately* or at least within the hour. Another cause of warpage is removal of the impression too early from the mouth before complete hardening.

Detail reproduction

Surface detail reproduction is comparatively less because of its high viscosity and low flow. Because of the viscosity, pressure has to be used during impression, which compresses or distorts the tissues. Thus the tissues are recorded in a distorted state.

MANIPULATION

STICKS

Small amounts of compound (stick compound) can be softened over a flame *(Fig. 14.2)*. When a direct flame is used, the compound should not be allowed to boil or ignite, otherwise, the plasticizers are volatilized.

CAKES

Larger amounts of compound are softened in warm water in a thermostatically controlled water bath *(Fig. 14.3)* usually in the range of 65 to 75 °C. After the compound is removed from the water bath, it is usually kneaded with the fingers in order to obtain uniform plasticity throughout the mass.

LOADING THE TRAY

A slightly oversized tray is selected. The softened material is loaded onto the tray and quickly seated on to the tissues to be recorded *(Figs. 14.4 to 14.6)*. Any delay can cause the impression to harden prematurely. If the compound is too hot, it may be tempered by briefly immersing in slightly cooler water. The lips are manipulated to mold the borders of the impression while it is still soft.

Precautions

1. Prolonged immersion in a water bath causes the compound to become brittle and grainy because some of the ingredients may be leached out.
2. Overheating in water makes the compound sticky and difficult to handle.
3. Avoid incorporating water while kneading.

REMOVAL OF IMPRESSION FROM THE MOUTH

The impression is removed from the mouth only after it has completely cooled and hardened.

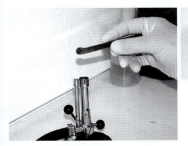
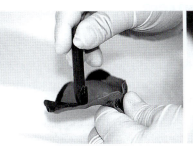
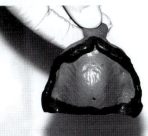

FIGURE 14.2 Manipulation of stick compound for border molding of a custom tray.

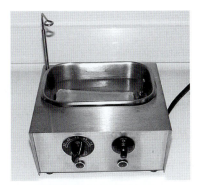

FIGURE 14.3 A thermostatically controlled water bath. This water bath maintains a steady softening temperature and is ideal for softening impression compound.

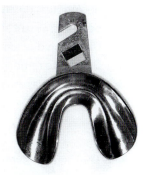

FIGURE 14.4 A slightly oversized stock metal tray.

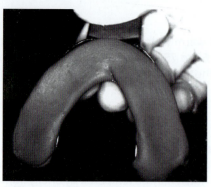

FIGURE 14.5 Placing the material in the tray is known as loading the tray.

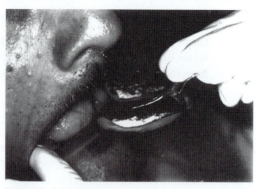

FIGURE 14.6 Positioning the loaded tray over the ridges for the impression.

DISINFECTION

The recommended disinfectant is 2% glutaraldehyde.

POURING THE CAST AND CAST SEPARATION

The cast should be poured without delay. The cast is separated from the impression by immersing it in warm water until it is soft enough. Excessively hot water is avoided as it can make the material sticky and difficult to remove from the cast.

ADVANTAGES AND DISADVANTAGES

ADVANTAGES

1. The material can be reused a number of times (for the same patient only) in case of errors.
2. Inaccurate portions can be remade without having to remake the entire impression.
3. Accuracy can be improved by flaming the surface.
4. The material has sufficient body to support itself especially in the peripheral portions. It does not collapse completely if unsupported by the tray.

DISADVANTAGES

1. Records less detail because of its high viscosity.
2. Compresses soft tissues during impression.
3. Distortion due to its poor dimensional stability.
4. Difficult to remove if there are severe undercuts.
5. There is always the possibility of overextension especially in the peripheries.

ZINC OXIDE EUGENOL IMPRESSION PASTE

Zinc oxide and eugenol based products are widely used in dentistry.

1. Cementing and insulating medium.
2. Temporary filling material.
3. Root canal filling material.

4. Surgical pack in periodontal surgical procedures.
5. Bite registration paste.
6. Temporary relining material for dentures.
7. Impressions for edentulous patients *(Fig. 14.7)*.

In dentistry, zinc oxide eugenol is popular as an impression material for making impressions of edentulous arches for the construction of complete dentures. It is classified as a rigid, irreversible impression material. It cannot be used for recording impressions of dentate arches and in areas of severe undercuts.

CLASSIFICATION

ADA specification No. 16.

○ Type I or Hard
○ Type II or Soft

AVAILABLE AS

In paste form in two tubes *(Fig. 14.8)*

○ Base paste (white in color)
○ Accelerator or reactor or catalyst paste (red in color)

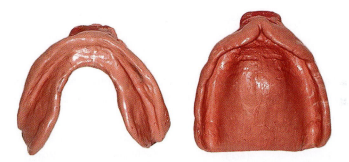

FIGURE 14.7 Impressions of the upper (right) and lower (left) edentulous arches made with zinc oxide eugenol impression paste in custom trays.

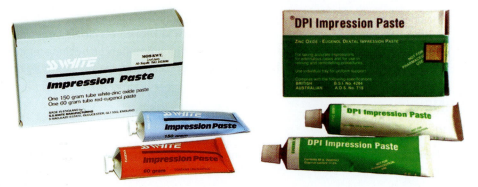

FIGURE 14.8 DPI (India) and SS white (USA) are examples of two commercially available zinc oxide eugenol impression pastes *(Courtesy:* KDC, Kannur).

COMPOSITION

Base Paste		Accelerator paste	
Ingredient	*Wt. %*	*Ingredient*	*Wt. %*
Zinc oxide	87%	Oil of cloves or eugenol	12%
Vegetable or mineral oil	13%	Gum or polymerized rosin	50%
		Filler (Silica type)	20%
		Lanolin	3%
		Resinous balsam	0%
		Calcium chloride and color	5%

Zinc oxide should be finely divided and should contain slight amount of water.

Fixed vegetable or *mineral oil* acts as plasticizer and also aids in masking the action of eugenol as an irritant.

Oil of cloves contains 70–85% eugenol. It is sometimes used in preference to eugenol because it reduces burning sensation.

Gum or polymerized rosin speeds the reaction and improves homogeneity.

Canada and Peru balsam improves flow and mixing properties.

Calcium chloride acts as an accelerator of setting reaction.

Other accelerators are   1. Zinc acetate

2. Primary alcohols

3. Glacial acetic acid

SETTING REACTION

The setting reaction is a typical acid-base reaction to form a chelate. This reaction is also known as *chelation* and the product is called *zinc eugenolate*.

1. ZnO + H_2O $\longrightarrow$ $Zn(OH)_2$

2. $Zn(OH)_2$ + $2HE$ $\longrightarrow$ ZnE_2 + $2H_2O$

   (Base)   (Acid)   (Salt)   +   (Water)

                    (Eugenol)   (Zinc eugenolate)

MICROSTRUCTURE

The chelate (zinc eugenolate) forms a matrix surrounding a core of zinc oxide particles. The chelate is thought to form as an amorphous gel that tends to crystallize giving strength to the set mass. Formation of crystalline zinc eugenolate is greatly enhanced by zinc acetate dehydrate (accelerator) which is more soluble than $Zn(OH)_2$ and can supply zinc ions more rapidly.

SETTING TIME

Working time

There should be sufficient time for mixing, loading onto the tray and seating the impression into the mouth.

Setting time

Once the material is in place, it should set fast.

Why should an impression material set quickly in the mouth?

Any material which takes a long time to set in the mouth.

- ○ Would obviously be uncomfortable to the patient.
- ○ Movement is bound to occur, resulting in stresses and errors in the impression.
- ○ Result in a wastage of time for the dentist. In a busy practice, this is unacceptable.

Initial setting time is the period from the beginning of the mixing until the material ceases to pull away or string out when its surface is touched with a metal rod of specified dimensions. The impressions should be seated in the mouth before the initial set.

The final set occurs when a needle of specified dimension fails to penetrate the surface of the specimen more than 0.2 mm under a load of 50 gm.

	Initial setting time	Final setting time
Type I	3–6 minutes	10 minutes
Type II	3–6 minutes	15 minutes

Factors controlling setting time

1. *Particle size of zinc oxide powder* If the particle size is small and if it is acid coated, the setting time is less.
2. By *varying the lengths* of the two pastes (not recommended).
3. Setting time can be decreased by adding *zinc acetate* or a drop of water or *acetic acid* (acetic acid is a more effective than water. It increases speed of formation of the zinc hydroxide).
4. Longer the *mixing time,* shorter is the setting time.
5. High atmospheric *temperature* and *humidity* accelerate setting.
6. Setting can be delayed by *cooling* the mixing slab, spatula or adding small amounts of *retarder* or *oils* or *waxes.*

PROPERTIES

Consistency and flow

These are clinically important properties. A paste of thick consistency can compress the tissues. A thin free flowing material copies the tissues without distorting them.

According to ADA specification No. 16, the spread is

- ○ Type I pastes — 30 to 50 mm
- ○ Type II pastes — 20 to 45 mm

Clinically, these materials have a very good flow. Poor quality impression pastes, thicken unduly and have a poor flow.

Detail reproduction

It registers surface details quite accurately due to the good flow.

Rigidity and strength

The impression should resist distortion and fracture when removed from the mouth after setting. The compressive strength of hardened ZOE is approximately 7 MPa two hours after mixing.

Dimensional stability

The dimensional stability is quite satisfactory. A negligible shrinkage (less than 0.1%) may occur during hardening.

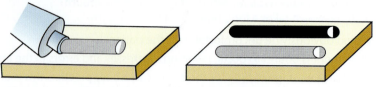

FIGURE 14.9 Proper dispensing is an important aspect of the manipulation of materials supplied in tubes. For zinc oxide eugenol both the ropes should be of equal length and width in order to ensure correct proportioning. One way of obtaining this is by ensuring the extruded paste has a uniform width and length.

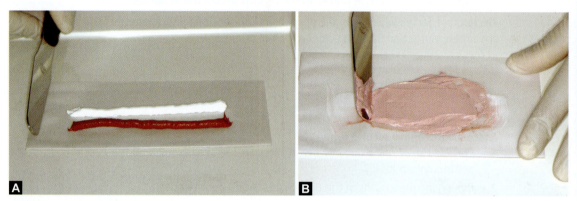

FIGURES 14.10A AND B Manipulation of zinc oxide eugenol paste. **(A)** Equal lengths of base and reactor pastes are dispensed. **(B)** Mixing is done with a stainless steel spatula using circular motions until a streak free mix is obtained (Manufacturers usually provide such materials in contrasting colors to aid in visually ascertaining completion of mix).

Biological considerations

Some patients experience a burning sensation in the mouth due to eugenol. It can also cause tissue irritation. Non-eugenol pastes can be substituted.

MANIPULATION

The mixing is done on an oil-impervious paper or glass slab. Two ropes of paste of *same length and width*, one from each tube are squeezed onto the mixing slab *(Fig. 14.9)*. A flexible stainless steel spatula is used. The two ropes are collected with the spatula and mixed until a uniform color is observed *(Figs. 14.10A and B)*.

Mixing time   1 minute.

Mechanical mixing   A rotary mixing device can also be used *(Fig. 14.11)*. Special circular mixing pads are attached to the circular table of the device. After dispensing the material, the machine is switched on. As the table rotates, the operator first collects the material using the sides of the spatula. He then spreads the material by flattening the spatula. The process of collecting and flattening is repeated alternately until a uniform mix is obtained. Mechanical mixing gives a faster, uniform mix with less voids and bubbles.

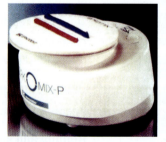

FIGURE 14.11 Mechanical mixer.

IMPRESSION TRAY

Custom impression tray made of stable resin is recommended for zinc oxide eugenol. The material adheres to the tray so no special adhesive is required. A primary compound impression can also be used as a tray. The material is loaded into the tray by swiping on to the sides of the tray and then spread in a smooth uniform motion. Loading and spreading through a patting motion can trap air.

DISINFECTION

The impression is rinsed and placed in disinfectant solution. Rinsing removes saliva and other contaminants. The recommended disinfectant solution is 2% glutaraldehyde solution. Glutaraldehyde is an organic compound with the formula $CH_2(CH_2CHO)_2$. A pungent colorless oily liquid, glutaraldehyde is used to sterilize medical and dental equipment.

POURING THE IMPRESSION

As with most impression materials the pouring of the cast should not be delayed for too long. After setting, the impression is removed off the cast after softening it through immersion in hot water.

ADVANTAGES AND DISADVANTAGES

ADVANTAGES

It has sufficient body so as to make-up for any minor under extensions in the tray itself during impression making.

1. It has enough working time to complete border molding.
2. It can be checked in the mouth repeatedly without deforming.
3. It registers accurate surface details.
4. It is dimensionally stable.
5. Does not require separating media since it does not stick to the cast material.
6. Minor defects can be corrected locally without discarding a good impression.

DISADVANTAGES

1. It requires a special tray for impression making.
2. It is sticky in nature and adheres to tissues.
3. Eugenol can cause burning sensation and tissue irritation.
4. It cannot be used for making impression of teeth and undercut areas as it is inelastic in nature.

OTHER ZINC OXIDE PASTES

SURGICAL PASTES (PERIODONTAL PACKS)

After certain periodontal surgeries (e.g. gingivectomy, i.e. surgical removal of diseased gingival tissues) where sutures cannot be placed, a zinc oxide-based surgical paste **(Figs. 14.12A and B)** may be placed over the wound to aid in the retention of the medicament, to protect the wound and to promote healing (also known as periodontal pack). Earlier pastes were eugenol based and have been around since 1923 (Ward's Wondrpak). Current surgical pastes avoid eugenol because of the potential of tissue irritation. These are called noneugenol pastes.

NONEUGENOL IMPRESSION AND SURGICAL PASTES

The chief disadvantage of zinc oxide eugenol paste is the burning sensation caused by eugenol. Some patients find the taste of eugenol disagreeable and in cases where the surgical pack

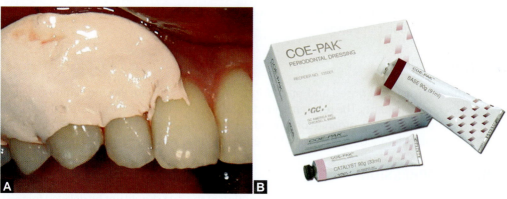

FIGURES 14.12A AND B **(A)** Periodontal dressing. **(B)** Coe-Pak is a popular brand of periodontal dressing material.

is worn for several weeks chronic gastric disturbance may result. Hence, noneugenol pastes were developed.

Noneugenol pastes consist of a base and reactor paste. The base paste contains ZnO, gum and lorothidol (fungicide). The reactor pastes contains coconut fatty acids, rosin (thickening), chlorothymol (bacteriostatic), etc. Antibiotics like tetracycline may be incorporated at the time of mixing.

Setting reaction

Zinc oxide is reacted with a carboxylic acid.

$$ZnO \ + \ 2RCOOH \ \longrightarrow \ (RCOO)_2 \, Zn \ + \ H_2O$$

The reaction is not greatly affected by temperature or humidity.

Compared to impression pastes the surgical pastes are less brittle and weaker after hardening. The setting time is longer (around 15 minutes). They are available as a 2 paste system. The paste is mixed and formed into a rope that is packed over the gingival wounds (using wet fingers) and into the interproximal spaces to provide retention. The final product after setting should be sufficiently strong so that it is not readily displaced during mastication. Light cured periodontal dressing materials and single component pastes (that set by heat and moisture in the mouth are also available). An automixing cartridge version of Coe-Pak is also available *(Fig. 14.13)*.

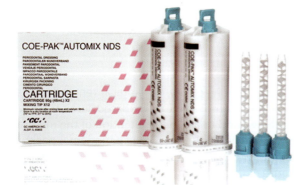

FIGURE 14.13 Cartridge dispensed static mixing version of Coe-Pak is also available.

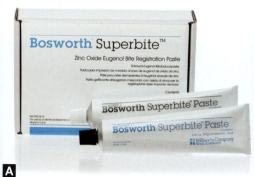
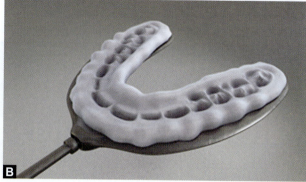

FIGURES 14.14A AND B **(A)** Bite registration paste. **(B)** Bite registration paste used for making a facebow transfer.

BITE REGISTRATION PASTES

These are materials used for recording the occlusal relationship between two occluding surfaces, e.g. teeth, occlusion rims, etc. ZOE pastes *(Figs. 14.14A and B)* used for this purpose have slightly different properties

○ Shorter setting time to prevent distortion.

○ More plasticizers to prevent it from sticking to the teeth or occlusion rims.

Other bite registration materials include wax and silicones. ZOE registrations are more rigid than registrations made in wax or silicones. They are more stable, and offer less resistance to the closing of the jaw than wax. Resistance free closure is often indicated in complete dentures where denture base movement or tissue displacement occurring from closure is not desired.

Elastic Impression Materials—Agar and Alginate

The rigid impression materials described previously are best suited for recording edentulous areas. Teeth or severe undercuts if present, would make the removal of such impressions difficult. The impression could distort or fracture on removal.

The ideal impression material for accurately reproducing tooth form and relationship would be an elastic substance which can be withdrawn from the undercut area and return to its original form without any distortion.

By definition, an elastic impression material is one that can transform from a semisolid, nonelastic state to a highly elastic solid state.

TYPES OF ELASTIC IMPRESSION MATERIALS

Two systems are used

1. Hydrocolloids
2. Elastomeric materials

HYDROCOLLOIDS

SOLUTION AND SUSPENSION

In a *solution* (e.g. sugar in water) one substance, usually a solid is dispersed in another, usually a liquid and the two phases are microscopically indistinguishable. Thus, a solution exists as a single phase because there is no separation between the solute and the solvent.

A *suspension* on the other hand, consists of larger particles that can be seen under a microscope or even by the naked eye, dispersed in a medium. Similarly, liquid distributed in liquids are *emulsions*. Suspensions and emulsions are two phase systems.

COLLOIDS

They are often classed as the fourth state of matter known as colloidal state. A colloid is a two-phase system. The 'colloidal solution' or 'colloidal sol' is somewhere between the smaller molecules of a solution and the larger particles of a suspension.

The two phases of the colloidal sol are

○   Dispersed phase or dispersed particle (the suspended particle).
○   Dispersion phase or medium (the substance in which it is suspended).

Types of colloids

Colloidal sols may be

○   Liquid or solid in air (Aerosol)
○   Gas, liquid or solid in liquid (Lyosol)
○   Gas, liquid or solid in solid.

HYDROCOLLOIDS

They consist of gelatin particles suspended in water (Lyosol). Since water is the dispersion medium it is known as hydrocolloid. The particles are larger than those in solutions and size ranges from 1 to 200 nanometers (1 nm = 10^{-9} m). There is no clear demarcation between solutions, colloids, and suspensions (emulsions).

GELS, SOLS, GELATION

Colloids with a liquid as the dispersion medium can exist in two different forms known as 'sol' and 'gel'. A *sol* has the appearance and many characteristics of a viscous liquid. A *gel* is a jelly like elastic semisolid and is produced from a sol by a process called *gelation* by the formation of fibrils or chains or micelles of the dispersed phase which become interlocked. Gelation is thus the conversion of a sol to gel. The dispersion medium is held in the interstices between the fibrils by capillary attraction or adhesion.

Gelation may be brought about in one of the two ways

1.   Lowering the temperature, e.g. agar.
2.   By a chemical reaction, e.g. alginate.

Gel strength

The gel strength depends on

1.   Density of the fibrillar structure Greater the concentration, greater will be the number of micelles and hence greater the brush heap density.

2. Filler particles trapped in the fibrillar network. Their size, shape and density determine their effectiveness. Fillers also increases the viscosity of the sol.

3. In reversible hydrocolloids, the lower the temperature, the greater is the strength, as gelation is more complete.

4. Types of hydrocolloids.

Based on the mode of gelation, they are classified as

○ *Reversible hydrocolloids* They are called reversible because their physical state can be reversed. This makes them reusable.

○ *Irreversible hydrocolloids* Once these set, it is usually permanent, and so are known as irreversible.

REVERSIBLE HYDROCOLLOIDS—AGAR

In 1925, *Alphous* Poller of Vienna was granted a British patent for a totally different type of impression material. It is said that Poller's objective was to develop a material that could be sterilized and applied without pressure to the exposed surface of the dura mater for perfectly recording its convulsion and the bony margins of the skull. Later Poller's *Negacol* was modified and introduced to the dental profession as *Dentacol* in 1928.

Agar hydrocolloid was the first successful elastic impression material to be used in dentistry. It is an organic hydrophilic colloid (polysaccharide) extracted from a type of *seaweed (Gelidium, Gracilaria, etc. **Box 15.1 and Fig. 15.1**). China and South America are major sources of farmed seaweed.

Agar is a sulfuric ester of a linear polymer of galactose. Although it is an excellent impression material and yields accurate impressions, presently it has been largely replaced by alginate hydrocolloid and rubber impression materials.

CLASSIFICATION BASED ON VISCOSITY (ISO 21563:2013)

Type 1 — Heavy bodied (for use as tray material)
Type 2 — Medium bodied (for use as tray or syringe material)
Type 3 — Light bodied (for syringe use only)
Type 3A — Light bodied for agar-alginate combination technique

USES

1. Widely used at present for cast duplication (e.g. during the fabrication of cast metal removable partial dentures, etc.).

BOX 15.1 AGAR AGAR

Agar has been used for centuries in Asia where it is called 'kanten' by the Japanese and 'dongfen' by the Chinese. It was brought to Malaysia by Chinese immigrants where it came to be known as agar.

Throughout history into modern times, agar has been chiefly used as an ingredient in desserts throughout Asia and also as a solid substrate to contain culture media for microbiological work. Agar (agar-agar) can be used as a laxative, an appetite suppressant, a vegetarian substitute for gelatin, a thickener for soups, in fruit preserves, ice cream, and other desserts, as a clarifying agent in brewing, and for sizing paper and fabrics

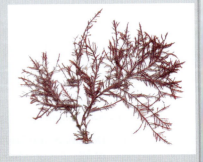

FIGURE 15.1 Gelidium seaweed.

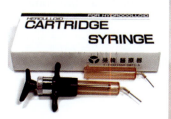
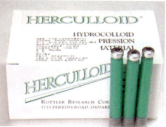

FIGURE 15.2 Agar impression syringe and syringe material.

2. For full mouth impressions without deep undercuts.
3. It was used extensively for FPD impressions prior to elastomers.
4. As a tissue conditioner.

SUPPLIED AS

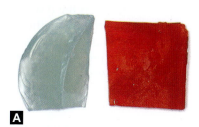

○ Gel in collapsible tubes (for impressions).

○ As cartridges or gel sticks (syringe material, *Fig. 15.2*).

○ In bulk containers (for duplication, *Figs. 15.3A and B*).

Commercial names   Syringe materials include—herculloid, cartriloids (Van R), etc. Duplicating materials include Wirogel (Bego), Dubliform (Dentaurum).

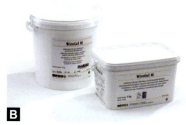

FIGURES 15.3A AND B **(A)** Agar duplication gel samples. **(B)** Bulk packing.

COMPOSITION

Ingredient	Wt. %
Agar	13–17%
Borates	0.2–0.5%
Potassium sulphate	1–2%
Wax, hard	0.5–1%
Thixotropic materials	0.3–0.5%
Alkylbenzoates	0.1 %
Coloring and flavoring agents	Traces
Water	Balance (around 84%)

FUNCTIONS OF THE INGREDIENTS

Agar   Basic constituent 13–17% for tray material 6–8% for syringe material.

Borates   Improves the strength of the gel (it also retards the setting of plaster or stone cast when poured into the finished impression—a disadvantage).

Potassium sulfate   It counters retarding effect of borates, thereby ensures proper setting of the cast or die.

Hard wax   It acts as a filler. Fillers affect the strength, viscosity and rigidity of the gel. Other fillers are zinc oxide, diatomaceous earth, silica, rubber, etc.

Thixotropic materials It acts as plasticizer. Examples are glycerine, and thymol. Thymol acts as bactericide also.

Alkylbenzoates It acts as preservative.

Coloring and flavoring For patient comfort and acceptance.

Water It acts as the dispersion medium.

GELATION OR SETTING OF AGAR

Agar changes from the sol to the gel state (and vice versa) by a physical process. As the agar sol cools the dispersed phase groups to form fibrils called *micelles*. The fibrils branch and intermesh together to form a brush-heap structure. The fibrils form weak covalent bonds with each other which break easily at higher temperatures resulting in gel turning to sol. The process of converting gel to sol is known as liquefaction which occurs at a temperature between 70 and 100 °C. On cooling agar reverses to the gel state and the process is called gelation. Gelation occurs at or near mouth temperature which is necessary to avoid injury to oral tissues.

The gelling property of agar-agar is due to the three equatorial hydrogen atoms on the 3,6-anhydro-L-galactose residues, which constrain the molecule to form a helix. The interaction of the helixes causes the formation of the gel.

MANIPULATION

The equipment and material required for an agar impression are

- Hydrocolloid conditioner *(Fig. 15.4F)*
- Water cooled rim lock trays *(Figs. 15.4E and 15.5)*
- Impression syringes *(Figs. 15.3 and 15.4C)*
- Connecting water hose *(Fig. 15.4D)*
- Agar tray material in tubes *(Fig. 15.4B)*
- Agar syringe material *(Figs. 15.2 and 15.4A)*

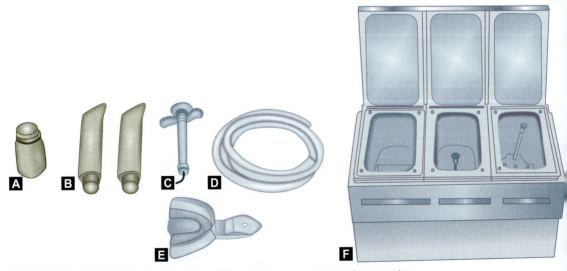

FIGURES 15.4A TO F Typical equipment and material for an agar impression procedure.

Hydrocolloid conditioner

	46 °C for about two minutes with the material loaded in the tray. This reduces the temperature so that it is tolerated by the sensitive oral tissues. It also makes the material viscous.
Boiling section or Liquefaction section	Ten minutes in boiling water (100 °C). The sol should be homogeneous and free of lumps. Every time the material is liquefied, three minutes should be added. After every use the agar brush heap structure gets more difficult to break.
Storage section	65–68 °C temperature is ideal. It can be stored in the sol condition.
Tempering section	46 °C for about two minutes with the material loaded in the tray. This reduces the temperature so that it is tolerated by the sensitive oral tissues. It also makes the material viscous.

IMPRESSION TRAYS

Rim lock trays with water circulating devices are used. The rim lock is a beading on the inside edge of the tray border which helps to retain the material (as agar does not adhere to the tray). It also has an *inlet* and *outlet* for connecting the water tubes *(Fig. 15.5)*. The tray should allow a space of 3 mm occlusally and laterally and extend distally to cover all teeth.

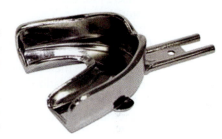

FIGURE 15.5 A water cooled tray.

MAKING THE IMPRESSION

The tray containing the tempered material is removed from the bath. The outer surface of the agar sol is scraped off, then the water hoses are connected, and the tray is positioned in the mouth by the dentist. Water is circulated at 18–21 °C through the tray until gelation occurs. *Rapid cooling* (e.g. ice cold water) is not recommended as it can induce distortion. To guide the tray into position, three *stops* of compound are prepared on non-involved teeth. A *post dam* is constructed with compound to prevent distal flow of the impression material. In a deep palate case, compound is placed on the palatal aspect of the tray in order to provide a uniform thickness of the hydrocolloid. The mandibular tray is prepared by placing compound on the distal aspect to limit the impression material. Black tray compound is used as it is not affected in the tempering bath.

WORKING AND SETTING TIME

The working time ranges between 7 minutes and 15 minutes and the setting time is about 5 minutes. Both can be controlled by regulating the flow of water through the cooling tubes. Since the cooling tubes are on the periphery, the material sets from the periphery towards the teeth surfaces.

REMOVAL OF IMPRESSION

When the agar has gelled, the peripheral seal is broken, and the impression is removed from the mouth rapidly. The impression is rinsed thoroughly with water and the excess water is removed by shaking the impression.

STORAGE OF AGAR IMPRESSION

Storage of agar impression is to be avoided at all costs. The cast should be poured immediately. Storage in air results in dehydration, and storage in water results in swelling of the impression.

Storage in 100% relative humidity results in shrinkage as a result of continued formation of the agar network agglomeration. If storage is unavoidable, it should be limited to one hour in 100% relative humidity.

SEPARATION FROM CAST

When the gypsum product has set, the agar impression must be removed promptly since the impression will dehydrate, become stiff and difficult to remove. Weaker portions of the model may fracture. In addition, prolonged contact will result in a rougher surface on the model.

PROPERTIES OF AGAR HYDROCOLLOIDS

The ISO 21563 (2013) sets the standard for properties required of agar–hydrocolloid impression materials.

Gelation, liquefaction and hysteresis

Most materials melt as well as resolidify at the same temperature. However, in agar, this does not coincide. Gelation (solidification) occurs at 37 °C approximately, whereas liquefaction (melting) occurs at a higher temperature, i.e. 60–70 °C higher than the gelation temperature. This temperature lag between liquefaction and gelation is known as *hysteresis*.

Syneresis and imbibition (dimensional stability)

Since hydrocolloids use water as the dispersion medium, they are prone for dimensional change due to either loss or gain of water. If left in a dry atmosphere, water is lost by syneresis and evaporation, and if it is immersed in water, it absorbs water by a process known as *imbibition*.

The exuding of fluid from the gel is known as *syneresis*. Some of the more soluble constituents are also lost. During syneresis small droplets of exudate are formed on the surface of the hydrocolloid and the process occurs irrespective of the humidity of the surrounding atmosphere.

Agar exhibits the properties of syneresis and imbibition. *However, when immersed in water, they do not imbibe more than original content which was lost by evaporation (unlike alginates).*

Importance   Syneresis and imbibition can result in dimensional changes and therefore inaccurate casts. To avoid this hydrocolloid impressions should be poured immediately.

Flexibility

ISO 21532:2013 requires flexibility ranging between 4% and 15%, when a stress of 12.2 N is applied. A few set materials, however, have a flexibility of 20%. On an average a flexibility of 11% is desirable.

Elasticity and elastic recovery

They are highly elastic, and elastic recovery occurs to the extent of 98.8% (ISO 21532:2013 - min. 96.5 %).

Gel strength including tear and compressive strengths

The gel can withstand great stresses particularly shear stress, without flow, provided the stress is applied rapidly. Thus, the impression should be removed as rapidly as possible in order to avoid distortion.

Agar has a tear strength of 0.8–0.9 kN/m and compressive strength of 0.5–0.9 g/cm². (ISO 21532:2013, minimum tear strength for Type 1 and 2 is 0.75 N/mm; for Type 3 is 0.50 N/mm.) The above values are for tray materials. The syringe materials have poorer mechanical properties

Factors affecting strength
1. The composition—agar concentration, borate and filler content, etc.
2. The temperature—the lower the temperature the greater the strength.

Flow

The material is sufficiently fluid to record the fine details if correctly manipulated.

Reproduction of detail

A reproduction of a groove of 25 µm (micrometers) is achievable with agar.

Accuracy and dimensional change

Some contraction takes place during gelation. If the material is retained well in the tray, the material contracts towards the tray resulting in larger dies. Agar impressions are highly accurate at the time of removal from the mouth, but shrink when stored in air or 100% relative humidity and expand when stored in water. The least dimensional change occurs when the impressions are stored in 100% humidity (for not more than one hour). However, *prompt pouring* of plaster or stone models is recommended.

LAMINATE TECHNIQUE (AGAR–ALGINATE COMBINATION TECHNIQUE)

After injecting the syringe agar on to the area to be recorded, an impression tray containing a mix of chilled alginate that will bond with the agar is positioned over it. The alginate gels by a chemical reaction, whereas the agar gels through contact with the cool alginate **(Fig. 15.6),** rather than the water circulating through the tray.

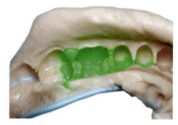

FIGURE 15.6 Agar–alginate combination or laminate technique.

Advantages
1. The syringe agar gives better details than alginate.
2. Less air bubbles.
3. Water cooled trays are not required and therefore more convenient.
4. It sets faster than the regular agar technique.

WET FIELD TECHNIQUE

In this technique the areas to be recorded are actually flooded with warm water. Then the syringe material is introduced quickly, liberally, and in bulk to cover the occlusal and/or incisal areas only. While the syringe material is still liquid, the tray material is seated. The hydraulic pressure of the viscous tray materials forces the fluid syringe hydrocolloid down into the areas to be recorded. This motion displaces the syringe materials as well as blood and debris throughout the sulcus.

CAST DUPLICATION

With the introduction of alginate, agar slowly lost its appeal as an impression material. However, it is still popular as a duplicating material primarily because
○ When liquefied it flows readily (like a fluid) over the cast to be duplicated. This makes it an ideal mould material.
○ Large quantities can be prepared relatively easily.
○ It is economical, because it can be reused.

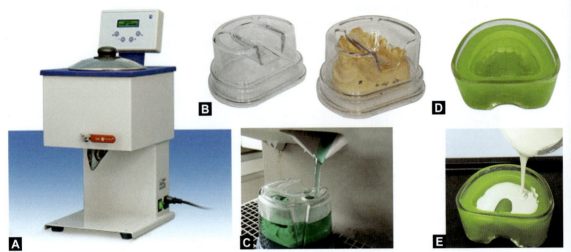

FIGURES 15.7A AND E **(A)** The agar hydrocolloid duplicating machine liquefies the agar using heat. Rotating blades in the machine further break up the agar. **(B)** Duplicating flask (left) with cast inside (right). **(C)** Liquefied agar is poured into the duplicating flask virtually surrounding the cast. **(D)** The completed mould. **(E)** Investment material is poured into the agar mould to create a duplicate in refractory material.

In the construction of cast removable partial dentures (RPD) the relieved and blocked master cast is duplicated in investment material. This is known as a refractory cast. The master cast to be duplicated is placed in a duplicating flask or mould former *(Fig. 15.7C)*. The agar is broken into small chunks and loaded into the liquefying machine *(Fig. 15.7A)* where it is liquefied and stored. The liquid agar is poured into a mould former *(Figs. 15.7B and C)* to create a mould *(Fig. 15.7 D)*. Later, investment is poured into this to create a *refractory cast (Fig. 15.7E)* which is used in the fabrication of the cast partial denture framework.

IMPRESSION DISINFECTION

Since the impression has to be sent to the laboratory, the need to disinfect it is very important. Most manufacturers recommend a specific disinfectant. The agent may be iodophor, bleach or glutaraldehyde. Apparently little distortion occurs if the recommended immersion time is followed and if impression is poured promptly.

ADVANTAGES AND DISADVANTAGES OF AGAR HYDROCOLLOID

Advantages

1. Accurate dies can be prepared, if the material is properly handled.
2. Good elastic properties help reproduce most undercut areas.
3. It has good recovery from distortion.
4. Hydrophilic, moist mouth not a problem. It also gives a good model surface.
5. It is palatable and well tolerated by the patient.
6. It is economical when compared to synthetic elastic materials.
7. It can be reused when used as a duplicating material (reuse is not recommended when used as impression material).
8. Low cost because it can be reused.

Disadvantages

1. Does not flow well when compared to newly available materials.
2. It cannot be electroplated.
3. During insertion or gelation the patient may experience thermal discomfort.
4. Tears relatively easily. Greater gingival retraction is required for providing adequate thickness of the material.
5. Only one model can be poured.
6. Has to be poured immediately. Cannot be stored for too long.
7. Requires special and expensive equipment.
8. A soft surface of the gypsum cast results unless a plaster hardener is used.
9. Although it can be reused, it is impossible to sterilize this material. Also with repeated use there may be contamination of the materials and a deterioration in its properties.

IRREVERSIBLE HYDROCOLLOID—ALGINATE

The word alginate comes from 'alginic acid' (anhydro-β-d-mannuronic acid) which is a mucous extract yielded by species of brown seaweed (*Phaeophyceae*). Alginic acid is a naturally occurring hydrophilic colloidal polysaccharide.

Alginate was developed as a substitute for agar when it became scarce due to World War II (Japan was a prime source of agar). Currently alginate is more popular than agar for dental impressions, because it is simpler to use. Alginate is perhaps the most widely used impression material in the world.

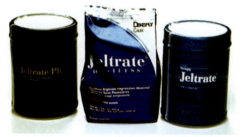

FIGURE 15.8 Representative commercially available bulk packed alginate.

TYPES

Type I — Fast setting.

Type II — Normal setting

SUPPLIED AS

A powder that is packed

- ○ Commonly in bulk packing (tins, bins or sachets) **(Fig. 15.8)**.
- ○ In preweighed packets for individual impression **(Fig. 15.9)**.
- ○ A plastic scoop is supplied for dispensing the bulk powder and a plastic cylinder is supplied for measuring the water.

Modified alginates

- ○ In the form of a *sol,* containing the water. A reactor of plaster of Paris is supplied separately.

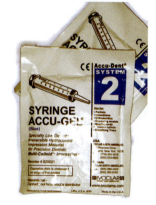

FIGURE 15.9 Preweighed sachet for individual impressions are also available. The one displayed in the illustration is a special low viscosity alginate for use with syringe. (*Courtesy:* The dental center, Chennai).

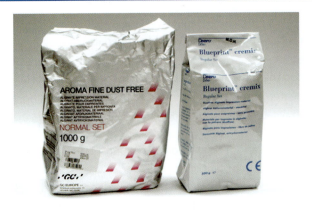
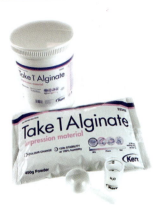

FIGURE 15.10 Other commercially available alginates including dust free (extreme left) and chromatic alginate (extreme right).

- ○ *As a two paste system* One contains the alginate sol, while the second contains the calcium reactor. These materials are said to contain silicone and have superior resistance to tearing when compared to unmodified alginates. They may be supplied in both tray and syringe viscosity.
- ○ One product is supplied in low density for use with syringe *(Fig. 15.9)*
- ○ *Dust free alginates* Concern over the inhalation of alginate dust have prompted manufacturers to introduce 'dust free alginates' *(Fig. 15.10)*.
- ○ *Chromatic alginates*   Alginates which change color on setting *(Fig. 15.10)*.
  Commercial Names   Zelgan (DPI), Jeltrate (Dentsply), Hydrogum (Zhermack), etc.

APPLICATIONS

1. It is used for impression making
   - When there are undercuts.
   - In mouths with excessive flow of saliva.
   - For partial dentures with clasps.
2. For making preliminary impressions for complete dentures.
3. For impressions to make study models and working casts.
4. For duplicating models.

COMPOSITION

Ingredients	% wt.	Function
Sodium or potassium or triethanolamine alginate	15%	Dissolves in water and reacts with calcium ions
Calcium sulfate (reactor)	16%	Reacts with potassium alginate and forms insoluble calcium alginate
Zinc oxide	4%	Acts as a filler
Potassium titanium fluoride	3%	Gypsum hardener
Diatomaceous earth	60%	Acts as a filler
Sodium phosphate (retarder)	2%	Reacts preferentially with calcium sulfate
Coloring and flavoring agent	Traces	e.g. wintergreen, peppermint, anice, orange, etc.

SETTING REACTION

When alginate powder is mixed with water a sol is formed which later sets to a gel by a chemical reaction.

The final gel, i.e. insoluble *calcium alginate* is produced when soluble *sodium alginate* reacts with *calcium sulfate* (reactor). However, this reaction proceeds too fast. There is not enough working time. So the reaction is delayed by addition of a retarder (trisodium phosphate) by the manufacturer.

Calcium sulfate prefers to react with the retarder first. Only after the supply of the retarder is over does calcium sulfate react with sodium alginate. This delays the reaction and ensures adequate working time for the dentist.

In other words, two main reactions occur during setting

Reaction 1 $2Na_3PO_4 + 3CaSO_4 \longrightarrow Ca_3(PO_4)_2 + 3Na_2SO_4$

Reaction 2 $Sodium\ alginate + CaSO_4 + H_2O \longrightarrow Ca\ alginate + Na_2SO_4$

   (Powder)   (Gel)

Initially the sodium phosphate reacts with the calcium sulfate to provide adequate working time. Next after the sodium phosphate is used up, the remaining calcium sulfate reacts with sodium alginate to form insoluble calcium alginate which forms a gel with water.

Gel structure

The final gel consists of a brush heap of calcium alginate fibril network enclosing unreacted sodium alginate sol, excess water, filler particles and reaction byproducts. It is a cross-linked structure (i.e. each fiber is tied to each other at certain points). Calcium is responsible for cross-linking.

PROPERTIES OF ALGINATE HYDROCOLLOID

TASTE AND ODOR

Alginate has a pleasant taste and smell. Over the years, manufacturers have added a variety of colors, odors and tastes to make it as pleasant as possible to the patient. Flavors include strawberry, orange, mint, vanilla, etc.

FLEXIBILITY

It is about 14% at a stress of 12.2 N. However, some of the hard set materials have lower values (5–8%). Lower W/P ratio (thick mixes) results in lower flexibility (ISO 21563:2013—minimum requirement ranges from 5 to 20%).

ELASTICITY AND ELASTIC RECOVERY

Alginate hydrocolloids are highly elastic (but less when compared to agar) and about 98.2% elastic recovery occurs. Thus, permanent deformation is more for alginate (about 1.8%). Permanent deformation is less if the set impression is removed from the mouth quickly.

REPRODUCTION OF TISSUE DETAIL

Detail reproduction is also lower when compared to agar hydrocolloid. ISO 21563:2013 requires the material to reproduce a line that is 20 µm in width. A number of products exceed this minimum value.

STRENGTH

Compressive strengths

○ Ranges from 0.5 to 0.9 MPa.

Tear strength

This is an important property for alginates. Values range from 0.4 to 0.7 kN/m

Factors affecting strength are

○ *Water/powder ratio* Too much or too little water reduces gel strength.

○ *Mixing time* Over and under mixing both reduce strength.

○ *Time of removal of impression* Strength increases if the time of removal is delayed for few minutes after setting.

SYNERESIS AND IMBIBITION

Like agar–agar alginate also exhibits the properties of synerisis and imbibition. When placed in contact with water alginates absorb water and swell *(Figs. 15.11A and B)*. Continued immersion in water results in the total disintegration of the alginate.

DIMENSIONAL STABILITY

Set alginates have *poor* dimensional stability due to evaporation, syneresis and imbibition. Therefore, the cast should be poured *immediately*. If storage is unavoidable, keeping in a humid atmosphere of 100% relative humidity (humidor) results in the least dimensional change. Alginates can also be stored in sealed plastic bags. Modern alginates, both regular and extended pour varieties have shown to have good clinically acceptable dimensional stability for periods ranging form 1 to 5 days according to some studies *(Box 15.2)*.

BIOLOGICAL PROPERTIES

No known chemical or allergic reaction have been identified for alginate. Silica particles present in the dust which rises from the can after fluffing alginate powder, are a possible health hazard. Avoid breathing the dust. Some manufacturers supply *'dust free'* alginates. Dustless alginates contain glycol. It acts by coating the powder.

ADHESION

Alginate does not adhere well to the tray. Good adhesion is important for the accuracy of the impression. Retention to the tray is achieved by mechanical locking features in the tray or by applying an adhesive.

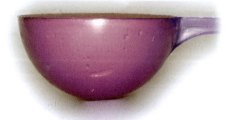
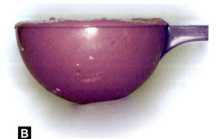

A   **B**

FIGURES 15.11A AND B Demonstration of imbibition. **(A)** Alginate shortly after setting. **(B)** The dimensional change is evident after a 48-hour storage in water.

SHELF LIFE AND STORAGE

Alginate material deteriorates rapidly at elevated temperatures and humid environment.

○ The material should be stored in a cool, dry environment (not above 37 °C).

○ The lid of bulk package can, must be replaced after every use, so as to minimize moisture contamination.

○ Stock only for one year.

MANIPULATION

○ Fluff or aerate the powder by inverting the can several times. This ensures uniform distribution of the filler before mixing. The top of the can should be taken off carefully to prevent the very fine silica particles from being inhaled.

○ Mixing equipment includes
  – A clean flexible plastic bowl and
  – A clean wide bladed, reasonably stiff metal spatula.

Note It is better to use separate bowls for plaster and alginate as plaster contamination can accelerate setting.

The proper W/P ratio as specified by the manufacturer should be used (usually one measure water with two level scoops of powder. The water measure and scoop are supplied by the manufacturer). The water is taken first. The powder is sprinkled in to the water in the rubber mixing bowl and the lid of the metal can is replaced immediately. The mixing is started with a stirring motion to wet the powder with water. Once the powder has been moistened, *rapid* spatulation by *swiping* or *stropping* against the side of the bowl is done *(Fig. 15.12A)*. A vigorous figure-eight motion can also be used.

This helps

1. Remove most of the air bubbles.

2. Wipe dissolved algin from the surface of the yet undissolved algin thereby promoting complete dissolution.

Mechanical devices (Fig. 15.13) are available for spatulating alginate.

Their main advantages are

1. Speed

2. Convenience

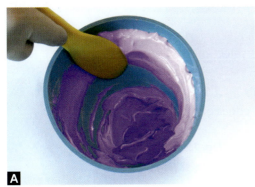 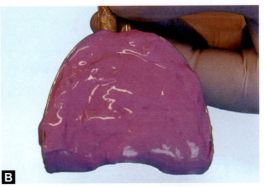

FIGURES 15.12A AND B (A) Alginate is mixed by stropping or swiping the material against the sides of the bowl. **(B)** The loaded tray.

3. Elimination of the human variable.

A proper mix is smooth and creamy with minimum voids and does not drip off the spatula when it is raised from the bowl.

MIXING TIME

For fast set alginate—45 seconds.

For normal set alginate—60 seconds.

Over mixing results in

○ Reduction in final strength as the gel fibrils are destroyed.

○ Reduction in working time.

Under mixing results in

○ Inadequate wetting, lack of homogeneity and reduced strength.

○ The mix being grainy and poor recording of detail.

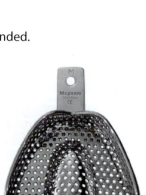

FIGURE 15.13 Alginate mixing device.

WORKING TIME

Fast set alginate—1¼ minutes.

Normal set alginate—2 minutes.

GELATION TIME (SETTING TIME)

Type I (fast set)—1.5–2.0 minutes

Type II (normal)—3–4.5 minutes

Control of gelation time

Ideal gelation time is 3–4 minutes (at 20 °C room temperature).

○ Gelation time is best controlled by adding retarders (which is in manufacturer's hands).

○ The dentist can best control the setting time by altering the *temperature* of the water for mixing alginate material.

   – Colder the water, the longer is the gelation time.

   – Warmer the water, the shorter is the gelation time.

   – Even the mixing bowl and spatula can be cooled.

Note Control of setting by changing W/P ratio is not recommended.

TRAY SELECTION

Since alginate has poor adhesion, tray selection is very important. Alginate can be retained by

○ Mechanical locking features in the tray

   – A rim lock (a beading round the edges of the tray) *(Fig. 15.14)*

   – Perforations (holes or slits) in the tray *(Fig. 15.14)*

○ Applying adhesive (available as liquid or sprays) *(Fig. 15.15)*

○ A combination of the above.

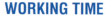

FIGURE 15.14 Tray with rim lock and perforations is recommended for alginate.

The tray should cover the entire impression area and provide a space of at least 3 mm on all sides.

LOADING THE TRAY

The mixed alginate is *pressed and swiped* **(Fig. 15.16)** into the perforated rim lock tray so that the material is forced out through the holes in the tray, thereby locking itself mechanically into the tray **(Fig. 15.17)**. A loaded tray is shown in **Fig. 15.12B**.

The surface of the alginate in the tray may be smoothened out using a moist finger. However, this is not mandatory.

A small amount of material may be taken on the index finger and applied on the occlusal surfaces of the teeth and on the rugae area. This help to reduce voids and improve accuracy.

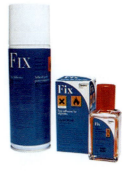

FIGURE 15.15 Tray adhesive improves the retention to the tray.

SEATING THE TRAY

Since the material sets from tissues towards periphery any movement during gelation may result in distortion. So once the tray is seated, it must be held in place firmly without any movement.

TIME OF REMOVAL AND TEST FOR SET

The alginate impression should be left in the mouth for at least 2–3 minutes after initial gelation. The strength and elasticity of the alginate gel continues to increase for several minutes after initial gelation.

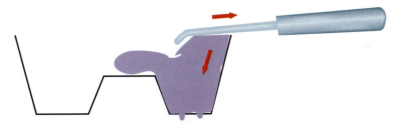

FIGURE 15.16 Alginate is loaded using the sides of the tray to force the material in to the tray and through the perforations.

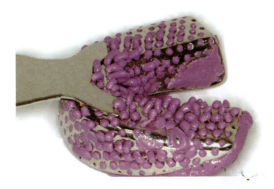

FIGURE 15.17 Alginate extruding through the holes helps in retention of the material to the tray.

Test for Set

The material loses its tackiness when set. It should rebound fully when prodded with a blunt instrument.

Color indicators   Although chromatic alginates indicate a color change after setting, it is still best to test for set by prodding the material at the periphery with a blunt instrument.

REMOVAL OF THE IMPRESSION

An alginate impression when set, develops a very effective peripheral seal. This seal should be freed by running the finger round the periphery. In addition to holding the tray handles, additional displacing force may be applied with a finger on the buccal flange of the set material and tray. A completed impression is shown in *Fig. 15.18*.

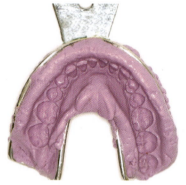

FIGURE 15.18 The completed impression.

The impression must be removed as quickly as possible. The brush-heap structure of a gel responds more favourably to a sudden force. A gentle, long, continued pull will frequently cause the alginate to tear or separate away from the tray *(Fig. 15.19)*. It also causes higher permanent deformation.

After removal from the mouth, the impression should be

○ Washed with cold water to remove saliva.

○ Disinfected by immersion in a suitable disinfectant.

○ Covered with a damp napkin to prevent drying.

○ Cast should be poured as soon as possible, preferably within 15 minutes after making the impression.

IMPRESSION DISINFECTION

Disinfection of impression is a concern because of viral diseases such as hepatitis B, AIDS and herpes simplex. The viruses can contaminate the gypsum models and present a risk to dental laboratory and operating personnel.

Recommended disinfectants include phenol, iodophor, bleach or glutaraldehyde. Irreversible hydrocolloids may be disinfected by immersion in, or spraying. Current protocol recommended

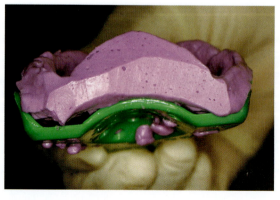

FIGURE 15.19 Separation from tray is a serious error resulting in distortion. The impression should be repeated.

BOX 15.2	Extended pour alginates

Traditionally alginates were considered to be dimensional unstable. For decades, dental professionals were taught that casts should be generated from alginate impressions immediately or within 60 minutes after the impression is removed from the patient's mouth. Studies have challenged these assumptions for currently available alginates (J Am Dent Assoc 2010;141;32-39). Many alginates today are marketed with manufacturers claiming good dimensional stability for up to 5 days (Hydrogum 5). These are known as *extended pour alginates*. Dimensional stability over a longer period is desirable for transportation of alginate impressions to distant labs. Studies have shown that both conventional and extended pour alginates meet the requirements for dimensionally stability and accuracy for periods ranging from 2 to 5 days under recommended storage conditions.

by the Center for Disease Control and Prevention is to spray the impression with disinfectant. The impression is then wrapped in disinfectant soaked paper towel. Immersion disinfection if used should not exceed 10 minutes to reduce dimensional change.

STORAGE OF ALGINATE IMPRESSION

Alginate impressions must be poured as soon as possible. If it becomes necessary to store the impression, the following methods may be used

- Wrap the impression lightly with a moist paper towel and cover with a rubber bowl or
- Keep the impression in a sealed plastic bag.

Note   Even under these conditions storage should not be done for more than one hour *(Box 15.2)*. Care should be taken not to use a *soaking we*t paper towel or gauze as it can cause imbibition of water.

CONSTRUCTION OF CAST

The early alginates required immersion in a gypsum hardening solution, such as potassium sulfate, zinc sulfate, manganese sulfate, and potash alum (most effective is 2% potassium sulfate solution). However, the formulas of presently available alginates have been adjusted so that no hardening solution is required.

Alginate is a hydrophilic material and wets easily reducing the entrapment of air. After rinsing *(Fig. 15.20)* the excess water is shaken off. The impression is held against a vibrator to reduce the trapping off air. Freshly mixed stone is placed at one end of the impression. The impression is rotated to facilitate the flow of the stone around the arch. The stone displaces water and wets the surface of the impression as it flows. It is then allowed to flow out through the other side and discarded *(Figs. 15.21A to C)*.

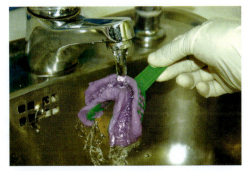

FIGURE 15.20 Rinsing removes traces of saliva, bacteria and other contaminants.

This helps to

- Reduce the trapping of air bubbles.
- Removes the water rich surface layer which can result in a weaker cast surface.
- The impression is filled with the remaining stone and placed aside to set. The stone cast should not be separated for at least 30 minutes. For alginate, best results are obtained

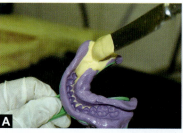 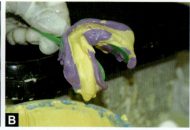 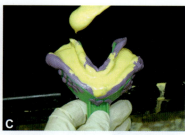

FIGURES 15.21A TO C Pouring an alginate impression. **(A)** The first portion of stone is placed in one corner of the impression. **(B)** With the help of a vibrator, the stone is flowed along the surface of the impression and round to the other side and allowed to drip off. This improves the wetting of the impression and reduces air entrapment. **(C)** The rest of the stone is poured to complete the cast.

if the cast is removed in one hour. The cast should not be left in the impression for too long a period either because it can result in a rough and chalky surface.

○ Alginate, dries and stiffens. Removal can break the teeth and other thin portions of the cast.

ADVANTAGES AND DISADVANTAGES OF ALGINATE

ADVANTAGES

1. It is easy to mix and manipulate.
2. Minimum requirement of equipment.
3. Flexibility of the set impression.
4. Accuracy if properly handled.
5. Low cost.
6. Comfortable to the patient.
7. It is hygienic, as fresh material must be used for each impression.
8. It gives a good surface detail even in presence of saliva.

DISADVANTAGES

1. Cannot be electroplated so metal dies are not possible.
2. It cannot be corrected.
3. Distortion may occur without it being obvious if the material is not held steady while it is setting.
4. Poor dimensional stability—it cannot be stored for long time.
5. Poor tear strength.
6. Because of these drawbacks and the availability of better materials, it is not recommended where a higher degree of accuracy is required, e.g. cast RPD, crowns and FDPs, etc. **(Box 15.3).**

BOX 15.3	Improper use of alginates

Because of their low cost alginates are often used to make final impressions during the fabrication of high precision restorations like RPDs, crowns and FPDs. Although they are reasonably accurate, they have a few properties which make them inferior to elastomeric materials. These include lower dimensional stability, poor tear strength, lower detail reproduction, etc. Some clinics process their impressions in distant laboratories which then involves a period of delay before it can be cast in stone. Alginate impressions are inaccurate if pouring is delayed. For these reason alginates are not recommended where high levels of accuracy is required, especially where it has to be withdrawn over severe undercuts (as in dentate subjects) and where very thin areas which can tear easily are present (gingival margins).

Elastomeric Impression Materials

The first elastomeric materials to be introduced to dentistry were the natural rubbers introduced as denture base materials in the 1850s. These were called vulcanite as they were converted into rubber from their natural latex by a process called vulcanization.

The first elastomeric or rubber-based 'impression material' to be introduced was polysulfide which was introduced in 1950. Interestingly, they were originally developed as an industrial sealant for gaps between concrete structures. This was followed by condensation silicone in 1955, polyether in 1965 and the addition silicones in 1975.

Introduction of the elastomers were a considerable technological advance in the quality of dental services. Elastomers are soft and rubber-like and far more stronger and stable than the hydrocolloids. They are known as *synthetic rubbers*. The ADA Sp. No. 19 referred to them as *nonaqueous elastomeric dental impression materials*. The term nonaqueous was used to differentiate them from agar and alginate (considered aqueous or water containing materials). Currently ISO 4823 simply refers to them as 'elastomeric impression materials'. These materials are the most accurate and dimensionally stable impression materials available in dentistry.

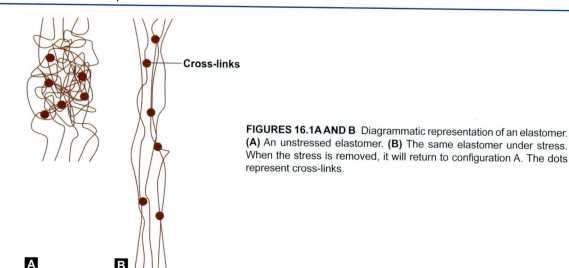

FIGURES 16.1A AND B Diagrammatic representation of an elastomer. **(A)** An unstressed elastomer. **(B)** The same elastomer under stress. When the stress is removed, it will return to configuration A. The dots represent cross-links.

Synonyms Initially they were called *rubber-base or rubber* impression materials. Currently, they referred to simply as elastomeric impression materials.

CHEMISTRY AND STRUCTURE OF ELASTOMERIC POLYMERS

The term '*elastomer*' is derived from the words elastic polymers. Thus elastomers are essentially polymers with elastic or rubber-like properties. Other polymers used in dentistry are the denture and composite resins. Gutta-percha is also a polymer (cis-polyisoprene) which is closely related to natural latex (trans-polyisoprene). Natural latex is currently used in dentistry to manufacture examination gloves and rubber dams. Gutta-percha is used as an endodontic obturation material.

Elastomeric materials contain large molecules with weak interaction between them. They are tied together at certain points to form a three-dimensional network. On stretching, the chains uncoil, and on removal of the stress they snap back to their relaxed entangled state *(Figs. 16.1A and B)*.

Elastomers are amorphous polymers existing above their glass transition temperature, so that considerable segmental motion is possible. As a result of this extreme flexibility, elastomers can reversibly extend from 5% to 700%, depending on the specific material. Without the cross-linkages or with short, uneasily reconfigured chains, the applied stress would result in a permanent deformation.

POLYMERIZATION

Polymers are long chains of large high-molecular weight macromolecules. They are formed by a chemical reaction where a large number of smaller units or monomers join to form polymer macromolecules, a process called polymerization.

Elastomers are liquid polymers which can be converted to solid rubber at room temperature. By mixing with a suitable catalyst, they undergo polymerization and/or crosslinking (by condensation or addition) reaction to produce a firm elastic solid.

Types of polymerization reactions

In elastomers 3 types of polymerization reactions are seen.

1. Addition polymerization
2. Condensation polymerization
3. Ring opening polymerization

Glass transition temperature in elastomers

The glass–liquid transition (or glass transition for short) is the reversible transition in amorphous materials (or in amorphous regions within semicrystalline materials) from a hard and relatively brittle state into a molten or rubber-like state.

TYPES

According to their chemistry

Chemically, there are four kinds of elastomers.

1. Polysulfide
2. Condensation polymerizing silicones
3. Addition polymerizing silicones
4. Polyether

Classification based on viscosity (ISO 4823:2015)

Each type may be further divided into four viscosity classes *(Fig. 16.2)* based on consistencies determined immediately after completion of mixing.

Type 0—Putty consistency (very heavy)

Type 1—Heavy-bodied consistency (tray consistency)

Type 2—Medium-bodied consistency (regular bodied)

Type 3—Light-bodied (syringe consistency)

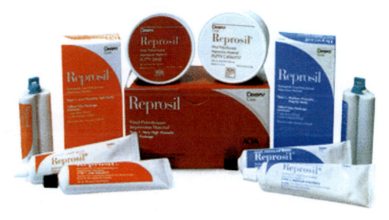

FIGURE 16.2 Elastomers are available in different viscosities and forms.

According to wettability or contact angle

Impression materials are also classified as

1. Hydrophilic, if their contact angle is from 80 to 105°.
2. Hydrophobic, if their contact angle is from 40 to 70°.

USES OF ELASTOMERIC IMPRESSION MATERIALS

1. In fixed partial dentures for impressions of prepared teeth.
2. Impressions of dentulous mouths for removable partial dentures.
3. Impressions of edentulous mouths for complete dentures.
4. Polyether is used for border molding of edentulous custom trays.
5. For bite registration.
6. Silicone duplicating material is used for making refractory casts during cast partial denture construction.

SUPPLIED AS

Regardless of type all elastomeric impression materials are supplied as *two component* (base and catalyst) systems.

○ Collapsible tubes
○ Cartridges—light and regular body material are also supplied in cartridges to be used with static mixing tips and dispensers
○ Putty consistency is supplied in jars

The various forms of elastomers are shown in **Figure 16.2**.

GENERAL PROPERTIES OF ELASTOMERIC MATERIALS

1. Excellent reproduction of surface details. The low viscosity is capable of producing very fine details (**Table 16.1** for minimum requirements as specified by ISO 4323:2015).
2. They are generally *hydrophobic* (except polyether which is hydrophilic), so the oral tissues in the area of impression should be absolutely dry for better flow of the impression material. Because of their hydrophobic (water hating) nature, care must be taken while pouring stone in the impression. The poor wetting and high contact angle can result in air entrapment. Commercial surfactants sprays are available which improve wetting.
3. Elastic properties of elastomers is good with near complete elastic recovery. Repeated pouring of impression is possible (though not recommended when high accuracy is critical).

TABLE 16.1 Property requirements (ISO 4823:2015)*

Type	Consistency (Test disc diameter) mm		Detail reproduction (Line width reproduced)ᵃ	Linear dimensional change %	Compatibility with gypsum (line width reprodcued)ᵃ	Elastic recovery %	Strain-in-compression %	
	min	max	µm	max	µm	min	min	max
0	–	35	75	1.5	75	96.5	0.8	20
1	–	35	50	1.5	50	96.5	0.8	20
2	31	41	20	1.5	50	96.5	2.0	20
3	35	–	20	1.5	50	96.5	2.0	20

* Adapted from ISO 4823:2015

4. Coefficient of thermal expansion of elastomers is high. Thermal contraction occurs when impression is transferred from mouth to room temperature.
5. In general dimensional changes and inaccuracies occur due to
   - Curing shrinkage.
   - Loss of by-products of reaction, e.g. condensation silicones lose alcohol and shrink. Polysulfides (hydroperoxide type) lose volatile accelerators causing contraction.
   - Polyether being hydrophilic absorbs water and loses soluble plasticizers causing change in dimension (e.g. when immersed in disinfectant).
   - Thermal contraction when transferred from mouth to room temperature.
   - Removing impression before complete setting can cause serious distortion.
   - Incomplete recovery after deformation during removal.
   - *Amount of filler* When filler content is increased, the polymer content is reduced and shrinkage is less. Thus, less shrinkage is seen in putty, and higher shrinkage is observed in light bodied.
   - Uniform thickness of material gives more accurate impression as the shrinkage is uniform.
   - Good adhesion of impression to the tray (using adhesives) minimizes dimensional changes as the shrinkage is directed towards the tray. In the absence of adhesion between the tray and impression, the shrinkage is directed centrally and the model prepared will be smaller in size.
   - *Time of pouring* Impression should be poured after elastic recovery but before dimensional changes set in.
6. The tear strength of these materials are excellent, thus making it more resistant to tearing even when the impression is in thin sections.
7. *Electroplating*   Elastomers can be copper and/or silver plated.
8. *Radiopacity*   Radiopacity of impression materials is important for radiographic identification of excess material which may be accidentally swallowed, aspirated or left in gingival tissues. Presently, only the polysulfide materials exhibit significant radiopacity due to their lead dioxide content.
9. *Retention to tray*   Elastomeric materials do not adhere well to the impression tray. They may be retained by
   - Mechanically by using perforated trays (only in case of putty).
   - *Tray adhesives*   These are tacky liquids that are applied with a brush. Each elastomer type has a specific adhesive which is not interchangeable.
10. The shelf life is about two years. The silicones have a slightly lower shelf life. Storage under cool conditions increases shelf life.
11. *Color*   They come in a variety of colors (**Box 16.1**).

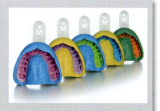

BOX 16.1   Color

Color is an important feature of elastomeric impression materials. Elastomeric impression materials come in a variety of colors. This helps to differentiate between the various consistencies while making impressions. The base and catalyst are in contrasting colors to visually determine completion of mixing.

POLYSULFIDES

This was the first elastomeric impression material to be introduced (1950). It is also known as *Mercaptan or Thiokol*. Interestingly, they were first developed as an industrial sealant for gaps between sectional concrete structures.

SUPPLIED AS

They are supplied as a two-paste system in collapsible tubes. The base paste is white colored. The accelerator may be brown or gray.

Available in three viscosities

- Light bodied
- Medium bodied
- Heavy bodied

Commercial names

Permlastic (Kerr) **(Fig. 16.3)**

Coe-flex   Lead dioxide system

Omni flex   Copper hydroxide system

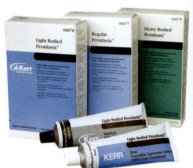

COMPOSITION

Base paste

Ingredient	Wt. percent
Liquid polysulfide polymer	80–85%
Inert fillers (Titanium dioxide, zinc sulfate, copper carbonate or silica)	16–18%

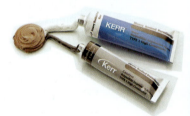

FIGURE 16.3 A representative polysulfide impression material.

Reactor paste

Ingredient	Wt. percent
Lead dioxide	60–68%
Dibutyl phthalate	30–35%
Sulfur	3%
Other substances like magnesium, stearate (retarder) and deodorants	2%

Tray adhesive   The adhesive cement should be compatible with the polysulfide impression material. Butyl rubber or styrene/acrylonitrile dissolved in a volatile solvent, such as chloroform or a ketone is used with polysulfide.

CHEMISTRY AND SETTING REACTIONS

When the base and accelerator pastes are mixed, it undergoes a chemical reaction, whereby the liquid polymer sets to form a solid, but highly elastic and flexible rubber like material.

The lead dioxide reacts with the polysulfide polymer causing

○ Chain lengthening by oxidation of terminal—SH groups
○ Cross-linking by oxidation of the pendant—SH groups

The reaction is exothermic with a 3–4 °C rise in temperature. It is accelerated by heat and moisture.

$$HS - R - SH \xrightarrow{\quad PbO_2 + S \quad} HS - R - S - S - R - SH + H_2O$$

or

Mercaptan + Lead dioxide $\longrightarrow$ Polysulfide + Water

As an alternative to lead dioxide, an organic hydroperoxide can be used (e.g. t-butyl hydroperoxide). However, these compounds are volatile and so are dimensionally unstable. The other cross-linking system successfully used are certain complex inorganic hydroxides (e.g. copper).

PROPERTIES

1. Unpleasant odor and color. It stains linen and is messy to work with.
2. These materials are extremely viscous and sticky. Mixing is difficult. However, they exhibit *pseudoplasticity*, i.e. if sufficient speed and force is used for spatulation, the material will seem easier to handle. The mixing time is 45 seconds.
3. It has a long setting time of 12.5 minutes (at 37 °C). In colder climates setting can take as longer. This adds to the patient's discomfort. Heat and moisture accelerate the setting time (sets faster in the mouth).
4. Excellent reproduction of surface detail.
5. *Dimensional stability*   The curing shrinkage is high (0.45%) and continues even after setting. It has the highest permanent deformation (3–5%) among the elastomers. Elastic recovery improves with time and so pouring of the model should be delayed by half an hour. Further delay is avoided to minimize *curing shrinkage*. Loss of the by-product (water) also causes shrinkage.
6. It has high tear strength (4000 g/cm) *(Box 16.2)*.
7. It has good flexibility (7%) and low hardness. A 2 mm spacing in the tray is sufficient for making an impression.
8. It is hydrophobic so the mouth should be dried thoroughly before making an impression. Care should also be taken while pouring the stone to avoid air pockets.
9. It can be electroplated. More with silver than copper.
10. The shelf life is good (2 years).

SILICONE RUBBER IMPRESSION MATERIALS

These materials were developed to overcome some of the disadvantages of polysulfide materials, such as their objectionable odor, the staining of linen and clothing by the lead dioxide,

BOX 16.2	Tear strength

In fixed prosthodontics the impression material is often extruded into the sulcus of the prepared tooth. When the impression is removed, the material in the sulcus being very thin, can tear away and remain in the sulcus. Therefore, a high tear strength is advantageous.

the amount of effort required to mix the base with the accelerator, the rather long setting times, the moderately high shrinkage on setting, and the fairly high permanent deformation.

TYPES

Two types of silicone impression materials are available based on the type of polymerization reaction occurring during its setting.

1. Condensation silicones
2. Addition silicones

Both silicones are available in a variety of colors, such as pastel pinks, purples, blues, greens, oranges, etc. Different viscosities may be identified by their color.

CONDENSATION SILICONE

This was the earlier of the two silicone impression materials. It is also referred to as *conventional silicones*.

SUPPLIED AS

Paste   Supplied as two pastes in unequal sized collapsible tubes. The base paste comes in a *larger tube* while the catalyst paste is supplied in a much *smaller tube* (**Fig. 16.4B**).

Putty   The putty is supplied in a single large plastic jar (**Fig. 16.4A**). The catalyst may be in paste form or sometimes it may be supplied as a *liquid*.

They come in a variety of colors. The base and accelerator are typically in contrasting colors (which aids mixing).

Available in three viscosities

❍   Light bodied
❍   Medium bodied
❍   Putty

Commercial names   Sil 21, Coltex, Dent-a-scon, etc.

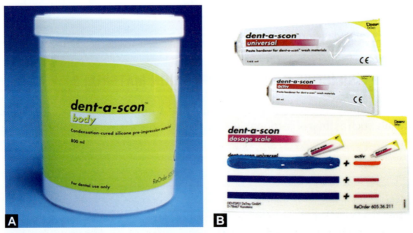

FIGURES 16.4A AND B Condensation silicone. **(A)** Putty. **(B)** Regular body base and catalyst. Notice the smaller size of the catalyst paste. Note also quantity of activator dispensed is less.

COMPOSITION

Base

Ingredient	Wt. percent
Polydimethyl siloxane (hydroxy—terminated)	80–85%
Colloidal silica or microsized metal oxide filler	35–75% (depending on viscosity)
Color pigments	16–18%

Reactor paste/accelerator

Ingredient	Action
Orthoethyl silicate	crosslinking agent
Stannous octoate	catalyst

CHEMISTRY AND SETTING REACTION

It is a condensation reaction. Polymerization occurs as a result of crosslinking between the orthoethyl silicate and the terminal hydroxy group of the dimethyl siloxane, to form a three-dimensional network. Stannous octoate acts as the catalyst. The reaction is exothermic (1 °C rise).

$$OH - \underset{\underset{CH_3}{|}}{\overset{\overset{CH_3}{|}}{Si}} - OH + C_2H_5O - \underset{\underset{OC_2H_5}{|}}{\overset{\overset{OC_2H_5}{|}}{Si}} - OC_2H_5 \xrightarrow[\text{octoate}]{\text{Stannous}} \text{Silicone rubber} + CH_3CH_2OH$$

or

$$\underset{\text{siloxane}}{\text{Dimethyl}} + \underset{\text{silicate}}{\text{Orthoethyl}} \xrightarrow[\text{octoate}]{\text{Stannous}} \underset{\text{rubber}}{\text{Silicone}} + \underset{\text{alcohol}}{\text{Ethyl}}$$

The ethyl alcohol formed as a by-product evaporates gradually from the set rubber leading to shrinkage.

Tray adhesive   The adhesive for silicones contain poly (dimethyl siloxane) or a similar reactive silicone, and ethyl silicate. Hydrated silica forms from the ethyl silicate to create a physical bond with the tray, and poly (dimethyl siloxane) bonds with the rubber.

PROPERTIES

1. Pleasant color and odor. Although nontoxic, direct skin contact should be avoided to prevent any allergic reactions.
2. Setting time is 6–9 minutes. Mixing time is 45 seconds.
3. Excellent reproduction of surface details.
4. Dimensional stability is comparatively less because of the high curing shrinkage (0.4–0.6%), and shrinkage due to evaporation of the *ethyl alcohol* by-products. To avoid this the cast should be poured immediately. The permanent deformation is also high (1–3%).
5. Tear strength *(Box 16.2)* (3000) g/cm is lower than the polysulfides.
6. It is stiffer and harder than polysulfide. The hardness increases with time. The spacing in the tray is increased to 3 mm to compensate for the stiffness.
7. It is hydrophobic. The field should be *well-dried* before making an impression. Care should also be taken while pouring the cast to avoid air entrapment.

8. Can be plated with silver/copper. Silver-plating is preferred.
9. Shelf life is slightly less than polysulfides due to the unstable nature of the orthoethy silicates.

ADDITION SILICONES (POLYVINYL SILOXANE)

These materials were introduced subsequent to the introduction of the condensation silicones These new materials had better properties when compared to the condensation silicones It is also known as *polyvinyl siloxane*. Currently, the addition silicones are very popular and is perhaps the most widely used elastomeric impression material worldwide.

SUPPLIED AS

1. *Tubes*   The base and catalyst pastes come in *equal* sized tubes (unlike condensation silicones). The different viscosities usually come in different colors like orange, blue, green, etc
2. *Cartridge form with static mixing tips*   For use with a dispensing gun.
3. *Putty jars*   Two equal sized plastic jars—containing the base and catalyst.
4. A larger electric driven autodispenser and mixing device is also available (Pentamix— ESPE). This machine stores larger quantities. At the press of the button, it dispenses and mixes the material.

Available in four viscosities (Fig. 16.2)

○ Light bodied
○ Medium bodied
○ Heavy bodied
○ Putty

Representative Commercial Products   Reprosil (Dentsply—**Fig. 16.1**), Provil, President (Coltene), etc.

COMPOSITION

Base paste	Reactor paste
Poly (methyl hydrogen siloxane)	Divinyl polysiloxane
Other siloxane prepolymers	Other siloxane prepolymers
Fillers (amorphous silica or fluorocarbons)	Platinum salt - catalyst (chloroplatinic acid)
Palladium - hydrogen absorber	Fillers
Retarders	
Coloring agents	

CHEMISTRY AND SETTING REACTION

It is an addition reaction. In this case, the base polymer is terminated with vinyl groups and is crosslinked with silane (hydride groups). The reaction is activated by the platinum salt.

$$\underset{\overset{|}{CH_3}}{\overset{\overset{|}{CH_3}}{Si}} - H + CH_2 = CH - \underset{\overset{|}{CH_3}}{\overset{\overset{|}{CH_3}}{Si}} \xrightarrow[\text{Salt}]{Pt} \underset{\overset{|}{CH_3}}{\overset{\overset{|}{CH_3}}{Si}} - CH_2 - CH_2 - \underset{\overset{|}{CH_3}}{\overset{\overset{|}{CH_3}}{Si}}$$

or

$$\text{Vinyl silozane} + \text{Silane siloxane} \xrightarrow[\text{Salt}]{\text{Pt}} \text{Silicone rubber}$$

There are no by-products as long as, there is balance between the vinyl siloxane and the silane siloxane. If unbalanced, *hydrogen gas* is produced causing air bubbles in the stone models. To avoid this, *palladium* is added to absorb the hydrogen.

PROPERTIES

1. Pleasant odor and color.
2. This may also cause allergic reaction so direct skin contact should be avoided.
3. Excellent reproduction of surface details. Polyvinyl siloxanes are currently considered to reproduce the greatest detail of all the impression materials. The international standard for dental elastomeric impression materials states that a type 3 (light bodied) impression material must reproduce a line 20 μm in width. With the exception of the very high viscosity putty materials, all polyvinyl siloxanes (light, medium and heavy body) achieve this. Very low viscosity materials can reproduce lines 1–2 μm wide.
4. Setting time ranges from 5 to 9 minutes. Mixing time is 45 seconds. Working time may be extended by chilling the tubes. Gains of up to 90 seconds have been reported when the materials are chilled to 2 °C.
5. It has the best dimensional stability among the elastomers. It has a low curing shrinkage (0.17%) and the lowest permanent deformation (0.05–0.3%).
6. Early materials had the problem of hydrogen gas formation. If hydrogen gas is liberated pouring of stone is delayed by 1–2 hours to prevent formation of air bubbles in the stone cast. Current materials do not have this problem because of the addition of palladium.
7. It has good tear strength (3000 g/cm).
8. It is extremely hydrophobic, so similar care should be taken while making the impression and pouring the wet stone. Some manufacturers add a surfactant (detergent) to make it more hydrophilic.
9. It can be electroplated with silver or copper. However, hydrophilic silicones are more difficult to electroplate because of the surfactant added.
10. It has low flexibility and is harder than polysulfides. Extra spacing (3 mm) should be provided in the impression tray. Care should also be taken while removing the stone cast from the impression to avoid any breakage.
11. Shelf life ranges from 1 to 2 years.

POLYETHER RUBBER IMPRESSION MATERIAL

Polyether was introduced in Germany in the late 1960s. It has good mechanical properties and dimensional stability. Its disadvantage was that the working time was short and the material was very stiff. It is also expensive.

AVAILABLE AS

Available as base and accelerator in collapsible tubes, cartridges for static mixing and dynamic mechanical mixing devices. The accelerator tube is usually smaller **(Fig. 16.5)**. Originally, it was supplied in a single viscosity. A third tube containing a *thinner* was provided.

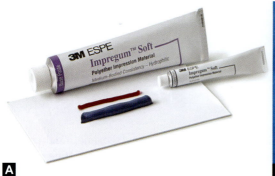
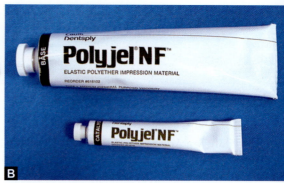

FIGURES 16.5A AND B Representative polyether impression pastes. Notice the smaller size of the reactor tubes.

Currently, it is available in three viscosities.

○ Light bodied

○ Medium bodied

○ Heavy bodied

Commercial examples   Impregum (3M ESPE), Ramitec, Polyjel (Dentsply), Permadyne (ESPE)

COMPOSITION

Base

Ingredient	Wt. Percent/Function
Polyether polymer	80–85%
Colloidal silica	Filler
Glycolether or phthalate	Plasticizer

Reactor/accelerator paste

Ingredient	Function
Aromatic sulfonate ester	Crosslinking agent
Colloidal silica	Filler
Phthalate or glycolether	Plasticizer

CHEMISTRY AND SETTING REACTION

It is cured by the reaction between aziridine rings which are at the end of branched polyether molecule. The main chain is a copolymer of ethylene oxide and tetrahydrofuran. Crosslinking is brought about by the aromatic sulfonate ester via the imine end groups. The reaction is exothermic (4 to 5 °C).

$$CH_3 - \underset{\underset{CH_2-CH_2}{\overset{|}{N}}}{\overset{\overset{H}{|}}{C}} - CH_2 - \overset{\overset{O}{\|}}{C} - O - R - O - \overset{\overset{O}{\|}}{C} - CH_2 - \underset{\underset{CH_2-CH_2}{\overset{|}{N}}}{\overset{\overset{H}{|}}{C}} - CH + ester \longrightarrow \text{Crosslinked rubber}$$

or

Polyether + Sulfonic ester $\longrightarrow$ Crosslinked rubber

PROPERTIES

1. Pleasant odor and taste.
2. The sulfonic ester can cause skin reactions. Thorough mixing is recommended before making an impression and direct skin contact should be avoided.
3. Setting time is around 6–8 minutes. Mixing should be done quickly that is 30 seconds. Heat decreases the setting time.
4. Dimensional stability is very good. Curing shrinkage is low (0.24%). The permanent deformation is also low (0.8–1.6%). However, polyethers absorb water and can change dimension. Therefore, prolonged storage in water or in humid climates is not recommended.
5. It is extremely stiff (flexibility 3%). It is harder than polysulfides and increases with time. Removing it from undercuts can be difficult, so additional spacing (4 mm) is recommended. Care should also be taken while removing the cast from the impression to avoid any breakage.
6. Tear strength is good (3000 g/cm).
7. It is hydrophilic, so moisture in the impression field is not so critical. It has the best compatibility with stone among the elastomers.
8. It can be electroplated with silver or copper.
9. The shelf life is excellent — more than 2 years.
10. It has excellent detail reproduction (20 microns).
11. Many medicaments, such as aluminum sulfate and ferric sulfate, used on gingival retraction cords have been accused of causing inhibition of set of polyvinyl siloxane materials. However, studies have not found not any inhibitory effect.
12. *Material interactions* Composite based provisional crown materials like Protemp 4 have been observed to have an inhibitory effect on the setting of polyvinyl siloxane materials. When a provisional crown is made directly in the mouth using a putty impression as a template, an oily residue called the oxygen inhibited layer (OIL) remains on the tooth and in the impression after separation of the provisional crown. Failure to adequately remove the OIL can result in impaired setting.

MANIPULATION OF ELASTOMERIC IMPRESSION MATERIALS

There are many methods of mixing and using elastomeric impression materials depending on whether it is supplied in tube, cartridge or putty form.

The 5 main mixing techniques are

1. Hand or manual spatulation
2. Manual kneading
3. Rotary table assisted mixing
4. Static or extrusion mixing
5. Dynamic mechanical mixing

HAND MIXING - PASTES IN TUBES

Hand or manual spatulation and is primarily used elastomers supplied in tubes.

Polysulfides and addition silicones

Equal lengths of base and accelerator pastes are extruded on to the mixing pad alongside each other without touching. The accelerator paste is then incorporated into the base paste. Mixing is done using a tapered stiff bladed metal or plastic spatula. Just before loading the tray the material should be spread in a thin layer to release the trapped air bubbles. A streak free mix is obtained in 45 seconds.

Condensation silicone

Unlike addition silicone, the quantity of catalyst paste needed is very little. The manufacturer usually marks the length required on the mixing pad. The two pastes therefore are of *unequal* length and diameter *(Fig. 16.4B)*.

For polyether

The required amount of thinner (when supplied) may be added to the base and accelerator depending on the viscosity needed. Again, like condensation silicone, the quantity of accelerator needed is very little. The ratio is usually displayed on the mixing pad. The mixing should be done quickly. The mixing time is 30 seconds.

KNEADING - PUTTY

Kneading is primarily employed for very heavy or putty consistency elastomers. In case of addition silicones, equal scoops of base and accelerator are dispensed. With condensation silicones, the required number of scoops of base and recommended amount of liquid or paste accelerator is taken. In either case mixing is done by kneading between the fingers. Mixing is continued until a streak free mix is obtained.

ROTARY TABLE-ASSISTED MIXING

The technique is similar to that described for zinc oxide impression pastes. The pastes are dispensed on to a rotating table *(Fig. 16.7)*. The spatula is used to scoop and flatten the pastes alternately and continuously as the table rotates until a uniform mix is obtained.

STATIC OR EXTRUSION MIXING

Static mixing also known as 'extrusion mixing' (ISO 4823:2015), has grown in popularity over the years, primarily because of its high accuracy and convenience. Extrusion mixing is a method by which two or more material components are extruded simultaneously from their separate primary containers through a special mixing tip from which the material components emerge as a homogeneous mixture *(Figs. 16.6A to D)*.

Advantages of static mixing

1. Shorter mixing time.
2. More uniform proportioning and mixing.

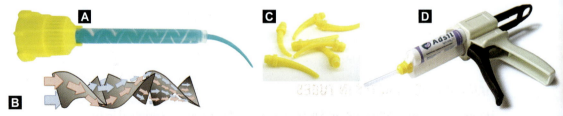

FIGURE 16.6 (A) Static mixing tip showing internal helical mixers. The used tip show set material inside the tip. (B) Internal helix demonstrating flow division. (C) Accessory tips for direct delivery to impression site. (D) Static mixing device.

3. Less voids.
4. Mix can be delivered directly to the tray or impression site.

The system consists of a gun with a dual plunger *(Fig. 16.6D)*. The cartridges are loaded onto this device. A static mixing tip is then attached to the cartridge. The tip contains helical mixing blades on the inside *(Fig. 16.6B)*. Forcing of the base and accelerator through the tip results in its mixing.

Precautions

1. The *initial portion* should be discarded as material from the right and left tubes may not have extruded evenly. This can affect its setting characteristics.
2. The material should be ejected in a continuous stream, avoiding lifting or skipping across segments. This reduces the chances of air entrapment and voids.

DYNAMIC MECHANICAL MIXING

Another device is an electrically operated dynamic mechanical mixer (ESPE Pentamix— *Figs. 16.8A and B*). The base and catalyst are supplied in large plastic bags which are loaded in to the machine. On pressing a button, the material is mixed and extruded through the tip, directly into the impression tray.

IMPRESSION TECHNIQUES

Impressions may be made in custom or stock trays. Elastomers do not adhere well to the tray. An adhesive *(Fig. 16.9A)* should be applied to the tray and allowed to dry before making impressions. The adhesive cements provided with the various elastomers are not interchangeable. A slightly roughened tray surface will increase the adhesion. For putty impressions, a perforated stock tray is used. The perforations help retain the putty in the tray *(Fig. 16.9B)*.

In case of elastomers, the bulk of the impression should be made with a heavier consistency (to reduce shrinkage). Light bodied should only be used in a thin layer as a wash impression.

CLASSIFICATION OF ELASTOMERIC IMPRESSION TECHNIQUES

Based on the viscosity used

1. Single viscosity technique
2. Dual viscosity techniques
   a. Dual viscosity technique using light body-heavy bodied
   b. Putty-wash technique

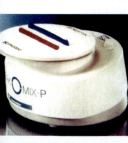

FIGURE 16.7 Rotary mixing device.

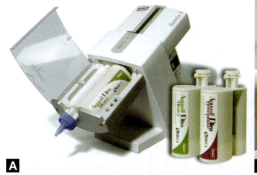

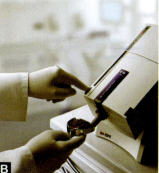

FIGURES 16.8A AND B Two representative dynamic mechanical mixing devices.

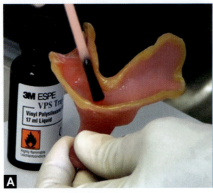 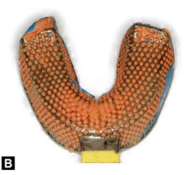

FIGURES 16.9A AND B Retention of elastomers. **(A)** Tray adhesive. **(B)** Mechanical retention through perforations in tray.

Based on the number of stages used

1. *One stage technique*—Both viscosities are dispensed and allowed to set simultaneously
2. *Two stage technique*—This is usually employed with putty. In this technique a preliminary impression is made first with the ultra-heavy or putty viscosity. This is relined later by the lighter viscosity called as wash impression.

ONE-STAGE SINGLE VISCOSITY (MONOPHASE) TECHNIQUE

Tray used   Resin custom tray with 2–4 mm spacing.

Viscosity   Medium only.

Method   The paste is mixed and part of it is loaded on to the tray and part into a syringe. The syringe material is then injected on to the prepared area of impression. The tray with material is seated over it. The material is allowed to set.

This technique utilizes the principle of shear thinning. The same material when ejected under pressure through the syringe tip it exhibits *pseudoplasticity* and behaves like a material with lower viscosity. Shear thinning allows as single material to be used as both syringe and tray material.

ONE-STAGE DUAL VISCOSITY (DUAL-PHASE) TECHNIQUE

Tray used Resin custom tray with 2–4 mm spacing.

Viscosity used   (a) Heavy bodied and (b) light bodied.

Method   The two viscosities are mixed simultaneously on separate pads. The heavy body is loaded into the tray while the light bodied is loaded into the syringe. The syringe material is injected over the preparation. The tray containing the heavy body if then seated over it. Both materials set together to produce a single impression.

TWO-STAGE PUTTY RELINE (TWO-STAGE PUTTY-WASH TECHNIQUE)

Tray used   Perforated stock tray.

Viscosity used   (a) Putty and (b) Light body.

Method (Fig. 16.10 A to J)   First a preliminary impression is made with putty in the stock tray. Before seating the tray in the mouth, a thin plastic sheet is placed over the putty (it acts as a spacer). After setting it is removed and kept aside. Mixed light bodied is loaded into a syringe and injected over the preparation. Static mixing tips fitted with special direct delivery tips can also be used for this purpose. Light viscosity material is also loaded into the putty impression. The preliminary impression is then seated over the injected material and held till it sets.

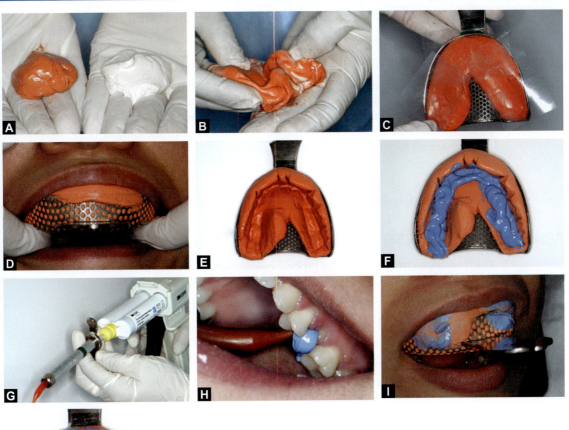

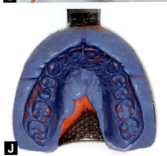

FIGURES 16.10A TO J Two-stage Putty-wash technique. **(A)** Equal quantities of base and catalyst is dispensed. **(B)** Mixing by kneading until uniform color is achieved. **(C)** A plastic sheet spacer is placed to provide space for the final impression material. **(D)** Making the preliminary impression. **(E)** The completed preliminary impression. **(F)** The final impression material dispensed in to the preliminary impression. **(G)** Simultaneously some material is loaded in to the syringe. **(H)** The syringe material is injected around the prepared tooth/teeth. **(I)** The loaded tray is seated in the mouth. **(J)** The completed impression.

Advantages

1. No special tray required.
2. Simple and quick as custom tray is not required.
3. Accurate.

Precautions

Some clinicians use the preliminary impression as a template to construct a provisional restoration (temporary crown). The same preliminary impression is then relined with the final wash material to make the final impression. If a composite based provisional restorative material [e.g. Protemp 4 (ESPE), Structur (VOCO)] has been used to construct the provisionals, a shiny oily layer called the *air or oxygen inhibited layer* (OIL) from this material forms a coating over the putty in this region. The OIL can affect both setting as well as bonding of the wash material. This can result in delayed setting, distortion or separation of the wash impression from the preliminary impression. This can be eliminated by rigorously wiping off the OIL or physically removing of a layer of putty with a trimmer.

ONE-STAGE PUTTY RELINE (ONE-STAGE PUTTY-WASH TECHNIQUE)

Tray used   Perforated stock tray.

Viscosity used   (a) Putty and (b) Light body.

Method   Unlike the previous technique, the putty and light body are dispensed and mixed simultaneously. The putty is loaded into a perforated stock tray whereas the light body is injected on to the prepared tooth. The tray is then taken to the mouth and pressed into position. The heavier putty forces the lighter material into the details. Both material set simultaneously to produce an accurate impression.

Advantage

No special tray required. The technique is simple and quick.

REMOVAL OF THE IMPRESSION

The material is checked for set by prodding with blunt instrument. When set, it should be firm and return completely to its original contour.

The impression is dislodged from the mouth as quickly as possible for the following reasons

- ○   Elastic recovery is better
- ○   Tear resistance is higher.

However, rapid removal may be difficult as well as uncomfortable to the patient. Removal is facilitated by breaking the air-seal. This can be done by teasing the borders of the tray parallel to the path of insertion until the air leaks into the tray. Compressed air through an air syringe may also be used. In addition to the holding the tray handle, a finger on the buccal portion of the tray may be used to apply additional pressure to dislodge the tray.

INFECTION CONTROL

Rubber impression materials are disinfected by immersing in disinfectant solutions. 10 minutes in 2% glutaraldehyde or 3 minutes in chlorine dioxide solutions have been found to be satisfactory. Because of its tendency to absorb water, a spray of chlorine dioxide is preferred in case of polyether. Other disinfectants used are phenol and iodophor.

IMPRESSION ERRORS

Errors in impressions do occur and can result in inaccurate casts and prostheses. Most of the errors occur due to poor technique and a failure to understand the properties of the material.

Some of the impression errors that can occur are

1.   Air entrapment
2.   Fluid entrapment
3.   Seating trails
4.   Contamination from provisional crowns
5.   Contamination from latex gloves
6.   Rough or uneven surface
7.   Distortion

AIR ENTRAPMENT

Voids in the impression mostly result from a trapping of air.

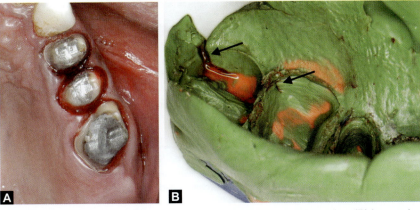

FIGURES 16.11A AND B (A) Gingival bleeding following teeth preparation. **(B)** Impression errors (fluid trails and loss of detail) caused by active bleeding and inadequate fluid control.

Voids occur from a variety of causes.

1. Air entrapment due to faulty loading of the tray. Care should be taken when loading the tray. Material should be loaded in a continuous motion from one end of the tray to the other pushing the material ahead as it is ejected from the static mixing device. The tip should be in close proximity to the surface of the tray. Lifting the tip away from the tray and moving it from place to place in a discontinuous motion can result in air entrapment.

2. Air entrapment from faulty placement of material around the prepared tooth. When placing the material on the prepared tooth using a syringe or a static mixing tip, the material should be extruded in close proximity to the sulcus and prepared tooth in a continuous motion around the prepared tooth starting from the sulcus and finish line through to the occlusal surface. Discontinuous and erratic motion with lifting of the tip from place to place can result in air entrapment.

FLUID ENTRAPMENT AND FLUID TRAILS

Elastomers with the exception of polyether are generally being hydrophobic require the impression field to be reasonably clean and dry.

Fluid entrapment and fluid trails can occur due to

○ Failure to adequately remove water or control saliva in impression field .

○ Failure to control bleeding and exudate. Continuos bleeding from injured or inflamed soft tissues near the prepared tooth can result in loss of detail and fluid trails as the blood continues to flow *(Figs. 16.11A and B)*.

SEATING VOIDS OR TRAILS

Seating voids or trails are usually seen when using a 'single stage putty-wash technique'. The putty tends to displace the light bodied resulting in voids or 'seating trails' *(Figs. 16.12A and B)*. Seating trails usually correspond to prominent cusps. The void caused by the penetration of the cusp fails to get filled by the wash material because of the displacement. This can cause inaccuracies in the impression especially if it is related to the prepared tooth. Seating trails correspond to the direction of seating.

For this reason the single stage putty reline technique is not advocated for procedures requiring a high degree of accuracy. The two-stage technique is superior in this regard.

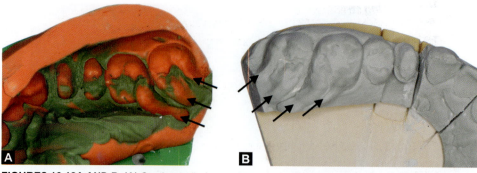

FIGURES 16.12A AND B **(A)** Seating trails (arrows) corresponding to the palatal cusps of the maxillary molars result in a significant loss of detail in the impression and the corresponding area of the cast **(B)**.

EFFECT OF PROVISIONAL CROWN MATERIALS (MATERIAL INTERACTION)

A knowledge of material interaction are important to avoid impression errors. According to one study direct contact of polyvinyl siloxane impression materials to some brands of resin based provisional interim fixed prosthodontic materials resulted in polymerization inhibition (delayed setting). The brands tested included Trim Plus, Unifast, Integrity, Systemp C&B, Tuff-Temp, Protemp IV. Among the elastomers polyether was least affected.

Composite based provisional crown materials like Protemp 4 are used to make direct intraoral provisional (temporary crowns). The material is usually placed on to the tooth in a clear vacuum-formed template (suck-down). Some clinicians use a preoperative putty impression as a template. When a provisional crown is made directly in the mouth using a putty impression as a template. An oily coating of resin also known as the *oxygen inhibited layer* (OIL) remains on the teeth as well as the impression surfaces after separation of the provisional crown. If the operator continues with the final impression by relining the putty impression in which the provisional crown was made without adequate cleansing of the OIL can result in 2 problems.

1. Impaired setting in the area resulting in an inaccurate impression.
2. Failure of the wash impression material to bond to the underlying putty resulting in physically separation from the putty **(Figs. 16.13A and B)**.

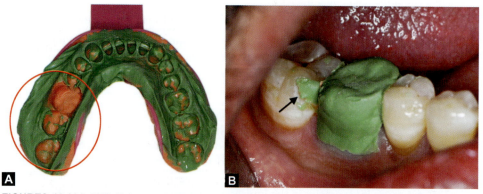

FIGURES 16.13A AND B Impression error caused by oxygen inhibited layer (OIL) contamination of the putty as well as the prepared tooth. In this instance the putty impression had been used earlier as a template to make the provisional crown using Protemp 4. The material has totally separated from the impression **(A)** and remained on the prepared tooth **(B)**. Areas of inhibited setting can be seen on the adjacent second molar (arrow).

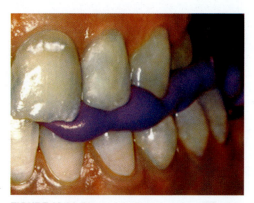

FIGURE 16.14 Bite registration procedure using bite registration silicone.

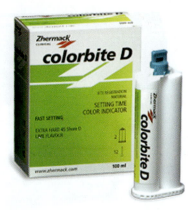

FIGURE 16.15 Bite registration silicone.

To ensure accuracy of the impression some precautions which may be observed are

❍ Thorough physical removal of the OIL from the tooth surface by rubbing with gauze.

❍ According to one study 3% H_2O_2 was found to be effective in cleaning the OIL from the tooth.

❍ Avoid reusing the putty impression template in which provisional was made.

❍ If the putty template is reused, ensure thorough removal of the OIL by vigorous rubbing with gauze or scraping with putty knife or bur.

❍ Holding the impression for a slight longer period to ensure complete set.

SPECIALIZED MATERIALS

BITE REGISTRATION SILICONES

Registering the three-dimensional relationship between two articulating surfaces is known as bite registration *(Fig. 16.14)*. Many materials are used for this purpose in dentistry. The earliest materials were wax and plaster. A specialized addition type of silicone is increasingly popular as a bite registration material. Unlike the regular impression silicone these materials show greater stiffness and greater hardness (32–45 Shore D), when set. A faster setting time is also important to reduce errors caused by movement and to reduce discomfort to the patient. Setting time ranges from as low as 20 seconds to a minute depending on the type. Other important properties required of these materials is that they should not slump or drip when initially placed. A scannable version has also been introduced for use in CAD CAM (Virtual CADbite Registration, Ivoclar). Most are supplied in cartridge form for use with a caulking gun. Some are supplied in collapsible tubes. One product (Colorbite D, Zhermack—*Fig. 16.15*) has thermochromic indicators to help the clinician ascertain setting in the mouth.

FIT CHECKING SILICONES

Another specialized addition type silicone is used for detecting errors in the internal surface of crowns and fixed partial dentures. They are available as a two-paste system *(Fig. 16.16A)*. Small but equal lengths of the two pastes are mixed and applied to the internal surface of the crown. The crown is seated on the tooth and the material allowed to set. Areas of premature contact are revealed as bare areas or areas where the internal surface of the crown is showing through *(Fig. 16.16B)*. These areas are marked and reduced. The material can also be used to assess the fit of complete and partial dentures.

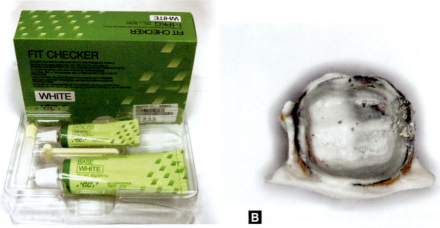

FIGURES 16.16A AND B (A) Addition silicone for locating high spots, interferences, fulcrum points and pressure spots on the fitting surfaces of restorations and prostheses (fit checking). **(B)** Crown with fit checker. The high spots show as areas of metal exposure.

DUPLICATING SILICONES

Duplicating silicones are primarily used in the fabrication process of cast removable partial dentures for constructing duplicate of the master cast in a refractory material (refractory cast) *(Fig. 16.17B)*. The duplicating silicones were introduced as an alternative to agar duplicating material.

The material is supplied as base and catalyst in the fluid consistency *(Fig. 16.17A)*. They are usually supplied in bulk containers ranging from 250 g to 10 kg.

They are mixed in a ratio of 1:1. The working time ranges from 2 to 5 minutes. The setting time of these materials are comparatively longer ranging from 10 to 30 minutes. Shore hardness of these materials range from 17 to 26. Like conventional silicones they exhibit a low shrinkage usually in the range of −0.03 to 0.05%. Because of their high dimensional stability and elastic recovery they may be used to create multiple casts.

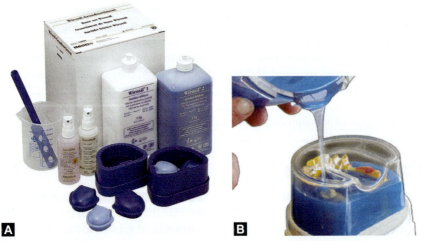

FIGURES 16.17A AND B (A) Duplicating silicone (base and catalyst) including flasks. **(B)** Duplicating silicone being poured into the mould former.

Part-5

Dental Laboratory— Materials and Processes

Model, Cast and Die Materials

Chapter Outline

Casts and models are an important part of dental services. Plaster and stone are the usual materials used to prepare casts and models. However, it must be remembered that other materials can also be used for this purpose.

MODELS

Models are used primarily for observation, diagnosis and patient education, e.g. orthodontic study models *(Fig. 17.1)*, diagnostic casts, etc.

CASTS

A working model or master cast is the positive replica on which restorations or appliances are fabricated, e.g. complete denture, removable partial denture *(Fig. 17.2)*, orthodontic appliances. Casts should be made with a high level of accuracy. They should be handled with great care, taking care not to scratch or damage its surface.

DIES

A positive replica of a prepared tooth or teeth in a suitable hard substance on which inlays, crowns and other restorations are made *(Fig. 17.3)*. Similar care should be taken in ensuring its accuracy as well as handling.

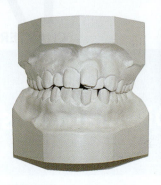

FIGURE 17.1 A study model.

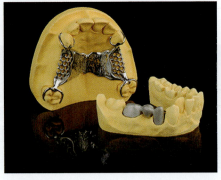

FIGURE 17.2 Casts are used to fabricate dental restorations.

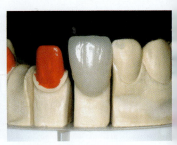

FIGURE 17.3 Dies are used to fabricate dental restorations.

TYPES OF DIE MATERIALS

Gypsum
- ○ Type IV dental stone
- ○ Type V dental stone, high strength, high expansion
- ○ Type V dental stone + lighosulfonates (this wetting agent reduces the water requirement of a stone and thus enables the production of a hard, stronger and more dense set gypsum)

Metal and metal-coated dies
- ○ Electroformed
- ○ Sprayed metals
- ○ Amalgam

Polymers
- ○ Metal or inorganic filled resins
- ○ Polyurethane
- ○ Epoxy

Cements Silicophosphate or polyacrylic acid bonded cement. These are no longer commonly used currently.

Refractory materials This includes investments and divestments. Investment casts are used to make patterns for RPD frames. Divestment dies are used in direct baking of porcelain crowns or preparation of wax patterns.

IDEAL REQUIREMENTS OF DIE MATERIALS

An ideal die material should

1. Be dimensionally accurate.
2. Have good abrasion resistance, strength and toughness to allow burnishing of foil and resist breakage.
3. Have a smooth surface.
4. Be able to reproduce all fine details in the impression.
5. Be compatible with all impression materials.
6. Have a color contrast with wax, porcelain and alloys.

7. Be easy to manipulate and quick to fabricate.
8. Be noninjurious to health by touch or inhalation.
9. Be economical.

ALTERNATE DIE MATERIALS

Polymers	They shrink during polymerization and so tend to produce an undersized die.
Cements	All cements shrink slightly and exhibit brittleness and have a tendency to crack due to dehydration.
Metal-sprayed	The bismuth-tin alloy is rather soft; care is needed to prevent abrasion of the die.

IMPROVED DENTAL STONE OR DIE STONE

The most commonly used die materials are still alpha hemihydrate type IV and type V gypsum products. Type IV gypsum products have cuboidal-shaped particles and the reduced surface area produce the required properties of strength, hardness and minimal setting expansion.

The most recent gypsum product, having an even higher compressive strength than the type IV is the high strength, high expansion type V stone. The setting expansion has been increased from 0.01 to 0.3%. This higher setting expansion is required in the stone used for the die to aid in compensation for the base metal alloy solidification shrinkage.

ADVANTAGES

1. Good strength.
2. Minimal shrinkage.
3. Easy manipulation.
4. Good working time.
5. Sets quickly.
6. Compatible with impression materials.
7. Has smooth, hard surface.
8. Can be easily trimmed.
9. Has good color contrast.
10. Is economical.

DISADVANTAGES

1. Brittle.
2. Not as abrasion resistant as the epoxy and electroformed dies. Edges and occlusal surface may be rubbed off.

ELECTROFORMED/ELECTROPLATED CASTS AND DIES

Electrodeposition of copper or silver on the impression gives a hard metallic surface to the cast. Electroformed dies are not used currently; however, they will be described for historical reasons.

ADVANTAGES

1. Dimensional accuracy.
2. Hard and abrasion resistant.
3. Imparts a smooth surface to the wax pattern in contact.
4. Not very expensive.
5. Better marginal definition.
6. Does not absorb oil or water.
7. Prevents cuspal wear due to repeated contact with opposing cast.

DISADVANTAGES

1. Difficult to trim.
2. Silver bath is a potential health hazard.
3. Not compatible with all impression materials.
4. Color contrast not as good as die stone.
5. Adaptation of wax not as good, pattern tends to lift from margins.

ELECTROFORMING

Electroforming (also known as electroplating or electrodeposition) is a process by which a thin coating of metal is deposited on the impression, after which a gypsum cast is poured. The cast thus obtained will have a metallic surface layer.

Metals used for electroforming are

○ Copper
○ Silver

Plating can be done for

○ Individual tooth impression
○ Full arch impression

Plating is done on

○ Compound impression (usually copper plated)
○ Polysulfide impression (usually silver plated)
○ Silicone impression

Other impression materials show dimensional changes when plated.

COMPONENTS OF AN ELECTROPLATING APPARATUS

A commercially available apparatus for electroplating is displayed in **Figure 17.4.**

A typical electroplating unit consists of **(Fig. 17.5)**

○ *Cathode* The impression to be coated is made the cathode.
○ *Anode* is the metal to be deposited, i.e. copper or silver.
○ Anode holder, cathode holder.
○ *Electrolyte* is a solution through which the electric current is passed. Ions are deposited from anode to cathode, e.g. silver cyanide or copper sulfate.

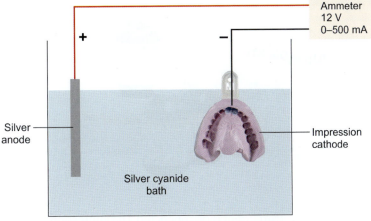

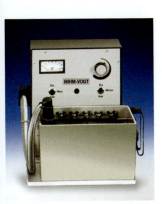

FIGURE 17.4 Electroplating unit.　　　**FIGURE 17.5** Diagrammatic representation of electroplating unit.

○ *Ammeter* registers the current in milliamperes (0–500 mA). The current passed is 10 mA per tooth area, for 12 hours.

○ *Plating tank* is made of glass or hard rubber with a well-fitting cover to prevent evaporation.

○ *Temperature* 77 to 80 °F (room temperature).

COMPOSITION OF THE ELECTROPLATING BATH

Copper forming		Silver forming	
Copper sulfate crystals	200 g	Silver cyanide	36 g
Sulfuric acid (concentrated)	30 mL	Potassium cyanide	60 g
Phenol sulfonic acid	2 mL	Potassium carbonate	45 g
Water (distilled)	1000 mL	Water (distilled)	1000 mL

PROCEDURE

○ Wash and dry the impression.

○ *Metallizing* Most impression materials do not conduct electricity. They are made conductive by applying a metallizing solution or powder with a brush.

  The metallizing agents are

  – Bronzing powder suspended in almond oil.

  – Aqueous suspension of silver powder.

  – Powdered graphite.

○ The surface of the impression tray is covered with wax 2 mm beyond the margin of the impression. This protects the tray and prevents its plating.

○ With a dropper, the impression is filled with electrolyte, avoiding air-bubbles.

○ The impression is attached to the cathode holder with an insulated wire.

○ The electrode is attached to the cathode and the impression is immersed in the electrolyte bath. Distance between the cathode (impression) and anode (metal) should be at least 4 inches.

○ Initially, current should not exceed 5 mA. Later the current is increased to 10 mA per tooth for 12–15 hours, to get a deposit of 0.5 mm (If a high current is used the surface will be granular, uneven and weak. With low currents the deposit is smooth and hard).

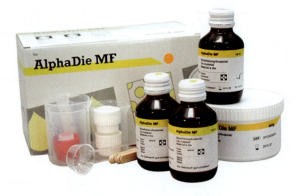

FIGURE 17.6 Polyurethane die material kit.

○ The current is disconnected. The impression is washed. The die is completed by pouring resin or dental stone to form the cast and base.

POLYURETHANE

Resin die materials were developed for applications where increased hardness and abrasion resistance is desired. One such material developed for this purpose is a polyurethane resin *(Fig. 17.6)*.

MODE OF SUPPLY

Supplied in glass bottles containing
○ Base material (200 mL)
○ Hardener (100 mL)
○ Filler (400 g)

INDICATIONS

Indicated for use with elastomers. Die separator must be applied when casting polyether impression.

Contraindication

Not indicated for use with alginates and hydrocolloid impression materials.

PROPERTIES

It is flowable, accurate in detail and dimensionally stable. It has high edge strength and abrasion resistance and is easy to trim and saw.

MANIPULATION

Briefly shake the bottles containing both the base material and hardener prior to mixing. Close the glass bottles carefully immediately after use. Do not allow the material to come into contact with water (foam).

Fill the required amount of base material in the dispensing and mixing container supplied. Then add the correct quantity of filler and thoroughly spatulate the mixture.

Add the correct quantity of hardener and spatulate the mixture again thoroughly.

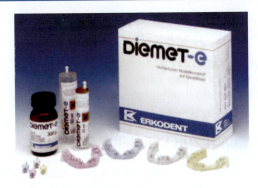

FIGURE 17.7 Epoxy resin die.

Mixing ratio   Base:hardener = 2:1. (10 g:5 g).

Approximately 15 grams filler is required for a full dental arch.

Mixing time   Approximately 30 seconds.

Pouring   After mixing the resin is poured in a thin stream into the cleaned and dried impression. The material remains flowable for approximately 2 minutes at 20 °C.

Curing   In order to prevent air voids the die may be hardened for 15 minutes, after pouring, in a dry pressure vessel at 2–4 bars. The die is sufficiently hard after 1 hour to permit trimming and grinding.

EPOXY RESIN DIE MATERIALS

Epoxy is another resin material that has been developed for die construction. They are most effective with rubber impression materials *(Fig. 17.7)*.

ADVANTAGES

Tougher and more abrasion resistant than die stone.

DISADVANTAGES

1. Slight shrinkage (0.1%).
2. Viscous, does not flow readily.
3. Setting may take up to 24 hours.

AVAILABLE AS

Two components—resin paste and hardener.

REFRACTORY CAST FOR WAX PATTERNS

A refractory cast is a special cast made from a heat resistant (investment) material. Such casts are used in the fabrication of certain large metal structures, e.g. cast removable partial dentures. Small wax structures like inlays, crowns and small FPDs can be constructed on a regular die as it can be removed from the die without significant distortion and invested separately. However, larger wax structures like that for the cast RPD, would distort if removed from the cast. RPD patterns are best constructed on a refractory cast. The pattern is invested together with the refractory cast.

Why not invest an ordinary gypsum cast?

The conventional (nonrefractory) gypsum cast cannot withstand the high temperatures involved in the casting of metal and would disintegrate under these conditions.

REFRACTORY CAST FOR CERAMICS

Refractory dies are also available for ceramic restorations [e.g. polyvest *(Fig. 17.8)* and VHT—Whipmix]. The all-porcelain restoration is directly built up on these refractory dies and fired (further detail in chapter on investments).

DIE STONE-INVESTMENT COMBINATION (DIVESTMENT)

This is a combination of die material and investing medium. A gypsum-bonded material called divestment is mixed with a colloidal silica liquid. A die is prepared from the mix and a wax pattern is constructed on it. Then the wax pattern together with die is invested in divestment.

The setting expansion of divestment is 0.9% and thermal expansion 0.6%, when heated to 677 °C.

As it is a gypsum-bonded material it is not recommended for high fusing alloys, e.g. metal-ceramic alloys.

ADVANTAGE

It is a highly accurate technique for conventional gold alloys, especially for extracoronal preparations. In this technique, removal of the wax pattern from the die is not required. Thus, possibility of distortion of wax pattern during removal from the die or during setting of the investment is minimized.

DIVESTMENT PHOSPHATE OR DVP

This is a phosphate-bonded investment that is similar to the divestment and is suitable for use with high fusing alloys.

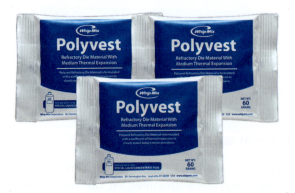

FIGURE 17.8 Refractory die material for use in the fabrication of ceramic restorations.

DIFFERENCE BETWEEN DIVESTMENT CAST AND REFRACTORY INVESTMENT CAST

Though both are quite similar, there are some fundamental differences. The investment casts are not as strong and abrasion resistant as the divestment cast. In fact, they are quite fragile and can disintegrate easily. Manufacturers have provided certain hardening solutions to compensate for this. Divestment is generally used for smaller castings, whereas investment refractory casts are used during the fabrication of larger structures, such as partial dentures frames and complete denture bases.

Gypsum Products

Chapter Outline

Products of gypsum are used extensively in dentistry. Gypsum was found in mines around the city of Paris, so it is also called *plaster of Paris*. This is a misnomer as gypsum is found in most countries. The mineral gypsum $CaSO_4 . 2H_2O$ is usually white to yellowish white in color and is found as a compact mass. Gypsum is also an industrial byproduct. For centuries gypsum has been used for construction purposes and making statues. Alabaster, a form of gypsum which is white in color, was used for building in ancient times. Besides dentistry, gypsum is also used in orthopedics for splinting fractured bones.

APPLICATIONS

1. Impression plaster was used extensively in the past for impressions of the mouth and face.
2. Various types of plasters are used to make moulds, casts and dies over which dental prostheses and restorations are made *(Figs. 18.1A to E)*.
3. To attach casts to an articulator *(Fig. 18.1D)*.
4. For bite registration (e.g., to record centric jaw relation).
5. *Dental investments* Plaster mixed with silica is known as dental investment. They are used to form refractory moulds into which molten metal is cast.

SUPPLIED AS

Powders of various colors in small preweighed sachets, in medium-sized bags or containers or in large bags, sacks or bins (bulk) *(Figs. 18.2A to C)*.

CLASSIFICATION

ISO 6873:2013

Type 1—Dental plaster for impressions

Type 2—Dental plaster

        Class 1 - for mounting

        Class 2 - for models

Type 3—Dental stone for models

Type 4—Dental stone (high strength, low expansion) for dies

Type 5—Dental stone (high strength, high expansion) for dies

TYPE 1 OR DENTAL PLASTER, IMPRESSION

Impression plaster *(Fig. 18.3A)* was one of the earliest impression materials in dentistry. Because of its rigidity (not elastic), it often had to be fractured to remove it from undercut areas in the mouth. The fractured pieces were then reassembled outside and a cast poured. Since the introduction of better materials, it is rarely used as an impression material. Currently, it is more useful as a bite registration material. Impression plaster may be flavored to make it more acceptable by the patient. It is colored to help the dentist and technician distinguish between the cast material and the impression. Impression plaster, sometimes, contains *potato*

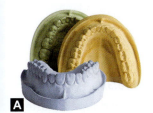

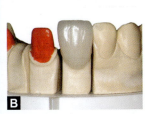 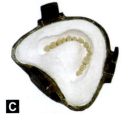 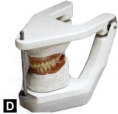 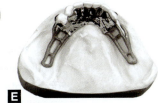

FIGURES 18.1A TO E Gypsum products are widely used in dentistry. **(A)** Orthodontic models. **(B)** A cast with removable die made from die stone. **(C)** A plaster mould used in denture construction. **(D)** Mounting plaster for mounting casts on an articulator. **(E)** Dental restoration constructed on a stone working cast.

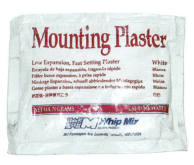 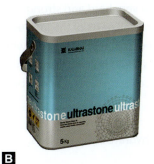 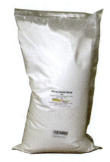

FIGURES 18.2A TO C Gypsum products are supplied in a variety of forms. as preweighed sachets, in medium sized containers or in large bags or sacks (bulk packing). **(A)** Mounting plaster. **(B)** High strength stone (die stone) in 1 to 3 kg container. **(C)** Dental stone (can range from 5 to 25 kg bulk pack).

starch to make it soluble. After the cast has hardened, the impression and cast are put in hot water. The starch swells and the impression disintegrates, making it easy to separate the cast. This type is often called *'soluble plaster'.*

USES

1. For making impressions in complete denture and maxillofacial prosthetics (not used currently for this purpose).
2. Bite registration material.

IDEAL REQUIREMENTS

1. The setting time should be under accurate control. The dentist must have sufficient time to mix, load the impression tray, carry the loaded tray to the patient's mouth and place it in position. However, once in position the plaster should harden promptly, so that there is minimum discomfort to the patient. The setting time desirable is 3 to 5 minutes.
2. For better accuracy the setting expansion should be low. Both setting time and expansion are controlled by modifiers (accelerators and retarders) added by the manufacturers.
3. The plaster should have enough strength to fracture cleanly without crumbling to facilitate removal from undercuts.

COMPOSITION

Dental plaster + K_2SO_4 + Borax + Coloring and flavoring agents.

TYPE 2 OR DENTAL PLASTER, MODEL, MOUNTING

Synonyms Model plaster, laboratory plaster, mounting plaster *(Fig. 18.3B)*.

The International Standards Organizations (ISO 6873:2013) has classified Type 2 plaster is into 2 subtypes—Class I (for mounting) and Class 2 (for models).

USES

1. For making study casts and models.
2. To make molds for curing dentures.
3. For mounting casts on articulator.

REQUIREMENTS OF AN IDEAL CAST MATERIAL

1. It should set rapidly but give adequate time for manipulation.
2. It should set to a very hard and strong mass.
3. It should flow into all parts of the impression and reproduce all the minute details.
4. It should neither contract nor expand while setting.
5. After setting, it should not warp or change shape.
6. It should not lose its strength when subjected to moulding and curing procedures.

COMPOSITION

Contains beta hemihydrate and modifiers.

TYPE 3 OR DENTAL STONE, MODEL

Synonym Class I stone or Hydrocal *(Fig. 18.3C)*.

USES

For preparing master casts and to make molds.

COMPOSITION

Ingredient	Action
Alphahemihydrate	
Coloring matter	2 to 3%
Potassium Sulphate (K$_2$SO)	Accelerator
Borax	Retarder

Some commercial dental stones contain a small amount of beta hemihydrate to provide a mix of smoother consistency.

A stone with a setting time established by the addition of proper quantities of both accelerator and retarder is called 'balanced stone'. Typical accelerators are potassium sulfate and potassium sodium tartrate (Rochelle Salts). Typical retarders are sodium citrate and sodium tetraborate decahydrate (Borax).

❍ The compressive strength varies from 3000 to 5000 psi.

❍ The setting expansion of dental stone is 0.06% to 0.12%.

❍ Hardness: 82 RHN.

TYPE 4 OR DENTAL STONE, DIE, HIGH STRENGTH, LOW EXPANSION

Synonyms Class II stone, die stone, densite, improved stone.

USES

Die stone *(Fig. 18.3D)* is the strongest and hardest variety of gypsum product. It is used when high strength and surface hardness is required. Uses include model bases, CAD/CAM dies and dies for fabricating inlay, crown and bridge wax patterns.

A thick mix is prepared as per manufacturer's instruction and vibrated into a rubber base impression. The base for such a model is poured in dental stone or dental plaster. Die stone should be left for twenty four hours to gain maximum hardness and the cast should be separated one hour after pouring. The abrasion resistance of die stone is not high as other die materials like epoxy resin.

Recent revision of the ISO (2013) have included additional requirements for Type 4 stone to reflecting the introduction of new technologies like CAD/CAM *(Table 18.1)*.

TYPE 5 OR DENTAL STONE, DIE, HIGH STRENGTH, HIGH EXPANSION

It is the most recent gypsum product *(Fig. 18.3E)* having a higher compressive strength than Type 4 stone. Improved strength is attained by making it possible to lower the w/p ratio even further. Setting expansion has been increased from a maximum of 0.10 to 0.30%. This is to compensate for the shrinkage of base metal alloys, during solidification (see Casting Alloys). Hard Rock, Jade Rock and Resinrock XL5 (by Whipmix) and Denflo-HX are examples of Type 5 stone.

USES

To prepare dies with increased expansion.

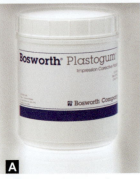

A

Type 1 - Impression plaster

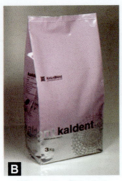

B

Type 2 - Dental plaster

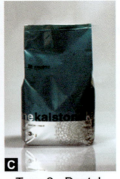

C

Type 2 - Dental plaster

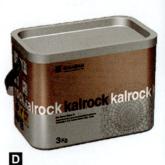

D

Type 5 - Die stone, high strength low expansion

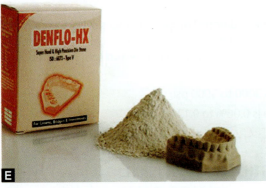

E

Type 5 - Die stone, high strength, high expansion

FIGURES 18.3A TO E The 5 types of gypsum products in dentistry.

MANUFACTURE OF GYPSUM PRODUCTS

The process of heating gypsum for the manufacture of plaster is known as *calcination*. Mined gypsum is ground and heated. When heated, gypsum (calcium sulphate dihydrate) loses part of its water of crystallization and changes to calcium sulphate hemihydrate. On further heating, the remaining water of crystallization is lost. First, hexagonal anhydrite (soluble anhydrite) is formed. Later, orthorhombic anhydrite (insoluble anhydrite) is formed.

$$CaSO_4 \cdot 2H_2O \xrightarrow{110\text{-}130\ ^\circ C} CaSO_4 \cdot \tfrac{1}{2}H_2O \xrightarrow{130\text{-}200\ ^\circ C} CaSO_4 \xrightarrow{200\text{-}1000\ ^\circ C} CaSO_4$$

(Calcium sulphate dihydrate)   (Calcium sulphate hemihydrate)   (Hexagonal anhydrite)   (Orthorhombic anhydrite)

Alpha and beta hemihydrate

Depending on the method of calcination, there are two forms of hemihydrates.

- Beta hemihydrate (plaster)
- Alpha hemihydrate (stone)
- Alpha modified hemihydrate (die stone)

Manufacture of dental plaster

Gypsum is ground and heated in an open kettle on kiln at a temperature of 110 to 130 °C. The process is called *dry-calcination*. β type of crystals are formed.

Microscopically   Fibrous aggregate of fine crystals with capillary pores. They are then ground to breakup the needlelike crystals. This improves packing.

$$CaSO_4.2H_2O \xrightarrow[\text{110-130 °C}]{\text{Heat}} CaSO_4.\tfrac{1}{2}H_2O$$
$$\text{(β hemihydrate)}$$

Manufacture of dental stone

Gypsum is calcined under steam pressure in an autoclave at 120 to 130 °C at 17 lbs/sq. inch for 5 to 7 hours. Thus, the product obtained is much stronger and harder than β hemihydrate.

$$CaSO_4.2H_2O \xrightarrow[\text{17 lbs/sq. inch pressure}]{\text{120-130 °C}} CaSO_4.\tfrac{1}{2}H_2O$$
$$\text{(α hemihydrate)}$$

Microscopically   Cleavage fragments and crystals in the form of rods and prisms.

Manufacture of high strength (α modified) stone

The gypsum is calcined by boiling it in 30% *calcium chloride solution. The* chlorides are then washed away or autoclaved in presence of *sodium succinate* 0.5%. These particles are the densest of all three types. After controlled grinding, these powders have an even higher apparent density and yield a stronger set.

Microscopically cuboidal in shape.

SETTING REACTION

When plaster is mixed with water it takes up one and a half molecules of water, i.e., it regains its water of crystallization and becomes calcium sulphate dihydrate.

$$(CaSO_4)_2.H_2O + 3H_2O \longrightarrow 2\,CaSO_4.2H_2O + \text{unreacted }(CaSO_4)_2.\tfrac{1}{2}H_2O + \text{Heat}$$

Hemihydrate + Water $\longrightarrow$ Dihydrate + Unreacted hemihydrate + Heat

The reaction is exothermic and is the same for all gypsum products. The amount of water required to produce a workable mix varies between the products. As evident from the above reaction not all of the hemihydrate converts to dihydrate. The amount of conversion is dependent on the type of stone. The highest conversion rate is seen in plaster (90%). In Type 4 and 5 stone the dihydrate content is about 50%.

THEORIES OF SETTING

Three theories have been proposed.

1. Colloidal theory
2. Hydration theory
3. Dissolution - precipitation theory

COLLOIDAL THEORY

The theory proposes that when mixed with water, plaster enters into a colloidal state through a sol-gel mechanism. In the sol state, hemihydrate combines with water (hydrates) to form dihydrate. As the water is consumed, the mass turns to a 'solid gel'.

HYDRATION THEORY

The hydration theory suggests that rehydrated plaster particles join together through hydrogen bonding to the sulfate groups to form the set material.

DISSOLUTION–PRECIPITATION THEORY (CRYSTALLINE THEORY)

This theory is *more widely* accepted. According to the theory, the plaster dissolves and reacts to form gypsum crystals which interlock to form the set solid. The setting reaction is explained on the basis of difference in solubility of hemihydrate and dihydrate. Hemihydrate is four times more soluble than dihydrate.

○ When hemihydrate is mixed in water, it forms a fluid workable suspension.

○ Hemihydrate dissolves until it forms a saturated solution.

○ Some dihydrate is formed due to the reaction. Solubility of dihydrate is much less than hemihydrate, the saturated hemihydrate is supersaturated with respect to the dihydrate. All supersaturated solutions are unstable. So the dihydrate crystals precipitate out.

○ As the dihydrate precipitates out, the solution is no longer saturated with hemihydrate and so it continues to dissolve. The process continues until no further dihydrate precipitates out of the solution.

Initially there is little reaction and thus little or no rise in temperature. This time is referred to as *induction period.* As the reaction proceeds, gypsum is formed in the form of needle-like clusters, called *spherulites (Figs. 18.4A and B)*. Continued growth and intermeshing of crystals of gypsum leads to thickening and hardening of the mass into a strong solid structure.

THE MICROSTRUCTURE OF SET GYPSUM

The set material consists of an entangled aggregate of gypsum crystals *(Figs. 18.4A and B)* having lengths of 5 to 10 μm. Two distinct types microscopic porosity can be seen in the mass.

○ Microporosity caused by residual unreacted water. These voids are spherical and occur between clumps of gypsum crystals.

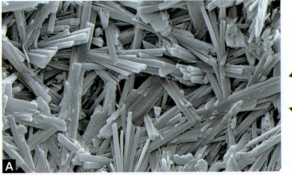
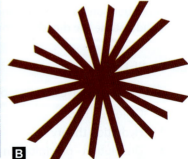

FIGURES 18.4A AND B (A) SEM of set gypsum showing needle-like clusters (x1550). **(B)** A single crystal is called a spherulite.

BOX 18.2 | Excess water

The actual amount of water necessary to mix the calcium sulphate hemihydrate is greater than the amount required for the chemical reaction (18.61 gm of water per 100 gm of hemihydrate). This is called *excess water.*

The excess water itself does not react with the hemihydrate crystals. It is eventually lost by evaporation once the gypsum is set. The excess water serves only to aid in mixing the powder particles and is replaced by voids.

○ Microporosity resulting from growth of gypsum crystals. These voids are associated with setting expansion and are smaller than the first type. They appear as angular spaces between individual crystals in the aggregate.

MANIPULATION

PROPORTIONING

To secure maximum strength a low water/powder ratio should be used. The water should be measured and the powder weighed.

Water/powder ratio

The W/P ratio is a very important factor in deciding the physical and chemical properties of the final product.

Example The higher the water-powder ratio, the longer is the setting time and weaker will be the gypsum product. Therefore, water/powder ratio should be kept as low as possible but at the same time sufficient to produce a *workable* mix.

Water requirement of a product is affected by

1. *Shape and compactness of crystals* Thus, irregular, spongy plaster particles need more water than the denser stone.
2. Small amounts of surface active materials like gum arabic plus lime markedly reduce water requirement of all gypsum products.
3. *Particle size distribution* Grinding of the powder breaks up needle like crystals. This improves packing characteristics and reduces the water needed.

Recommended w/p ratio

Impression plaster	: 0.50 to 0.75
Dental plaster	: 0.45 to 0.50
Dental stone	: 0.28 to 0.30
Die stone, Type 4	: 0.22 to 0.24
Die stone, Type 5	: 0.18 to 0.22

INSTRUMENTS

Flexible rubber/plastic bowl, stiff bladed spatula.

PROCEDURE FOR HAND-MIXING

○ Water is taken first to prevent adherence of dry powder to the sides of the bowl. Water and powder are dispensed according to the recommended W/P ratio. The powder is sifted into water in the rubber bowl. Plaster/stone dispensers are also available *(Fig. 18.5)*.

❍   It is allowed to settle for 30 seconds to minimize air entrapment.

❍   The mix is stirred vigorously. Periodically wipe the inside of the bowl with a spatula to ensure wetting of the powder and breaking up of lumps. Continue till a smooth creamy mix is obtained. Spatulation should be completed in 45 to 60 seconds.

❍   *Vibrate* the mix (using a mechanical vibrator *(Fig. 18.6)* or by repeated tapping against a bench) and pour it into the impression, taking care not to entrap air *(Fig. 18.7)*.

The mixing equipment must be meticulously clean. There should be no particles of set plaster from a previous mix sticking to the bowl or spatula. These if present will act as additional nuclei of crystallization and cause faster setting. No air must be trapped in the mixed mass. It causes loss of surface detail and weakens the cast.

MECHANICAL MIXING

Mechanical mixing under vacuum gives stronger and denser casts. However, the equipment is expensive.

SETTING TIME

The time elapsing from the beginning of mixing until the material hardens is called setting time.

Mixing time   It is the time from the addition the powder to the water until mixing is complete. A mixing time of 1 minute is usually sufficient.

Working time   It is the time available to work with the mix for the intended purpose, i.e., one that maintains an even consistency. At the end of the working period the material thickens

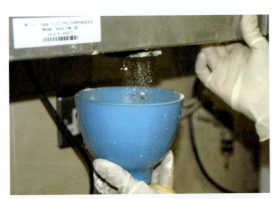

FIGURE 18.5 Stone/plaster dispenser.

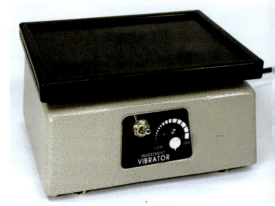

FIGURE 18.6 Stone/plaster vibrator.

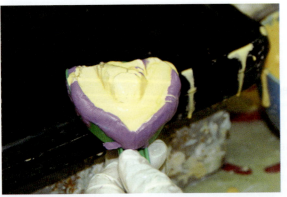

FIGURE 18.7 A vibrator improves the flow and reduces voids, thereby improving strength and accuracy.

and is no longer workable. The freshly mixed mass is semifluid in consistency and quite free flowing. A working time of 3 minutes is usually sufficient.

Initial setting time As the reaction proceeds, more hemihydrate crystals react to form dihydrate crystals. The viscosity of the mass is increased and it can no longer be poured. The material becomes rigid (but not hard). It can be carved but not moulded. This is known as *initial* setting time.

Final setting time The time at which the material can be separated from the impression without distortion or fracture.

Measurement of setting time

Usually by some type of penetration tests. Occasionally, other tests are used.

1. *Loss of gloss method* As reaction proceeds the gloss disappears from the surface of plaster mix (sometimes used to indicate initial set).
2. *Exothermic reaction* The temperature rise of the mass may also be used for measurement of setting time as the setting reaction is exothermic.
3. *Penetration tests* By using penetrometers.

Types of penetrometers

○ Vicat needle
○ Gillmore needles

Vicat needle (Fig. 18.8) It weighs 300 gm and the needle diameter is 1 mm. The time elapsing from the start of mixing till the needle does not penetrate to the bottom of the plaster is the *setting time*. The setting time obtained with the Vicat needle is similar to the initial Gillmore.

Gillmore needles Two types—small and large ***(Fig. 18.9)***. The small Gillmore needle has a 1/4 lb weight and a diameter of 1/12" (2.12 mm) while the large Gillmore has a 1 lb wt and diameter of 1/24" (1.06 mm).

Initial Gillmore The time elapsing from the start of mixing until the time when the point of the 1/4 lb Gillmore needle no longer penetrates the surface is the *initial setting time*

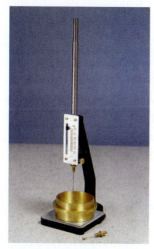

FIGURE 18.8 Vicat needle.

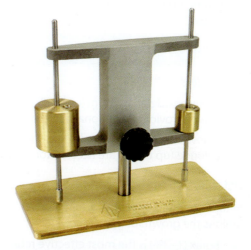

FIGURE 18.9 Gillmore apparatus. Besides dentistry, it is also used in general industry to determine initial and final set times of Portland cement, masonry cement, hydrated lime, mortars, etc.

Final Gillmore   Similarly the time elapsing from the start of mixing until the point of the 1 lb Gillmore needle leaves only a barely visible mark on the surface of the set plaster is known as the *final setting time.*

Factors affecting setting time

1.   Manufacturing process
2.   Mixing and spatulation (time and rate)
3.   Water/Powder ratio
4.   Temperature
5.   Modifiers

Manufacturing process

1.   If calcination is incomplete and excess gypsum (dihydrate) is left in the final product, the resulting plaster will set faster.
2.   If soluble anhydrite is in excess, plaster will set faster.
3.   If natural anhydrite is in excess, plaster will set slow.
4.   *Fineness*   Finer the hemihydrate particle size, the faster the set, because
     –   Hemihydrate dissolves faster, and
     –   The gypsum nuclei are more numerous and therefore, crystallization is faster.

Mixing and spatulation   Within limits the longer and faster the plaster is mixed, the faster it will set because nuclei of crystallization are broken and well-distributed within the mass.

Water/Powder ratio   More the water used for mixing, the fewer the nuclei per unit volume. Thus setting time will be prolonged.

Temperature   On increasing from a room temperature of 20 °C to a body temperature of 37 °C, the rate of the reaction increases slightly and the setting time is shortened. As the temperature is raised above 37 °C the rate of reaction decreases and the setting time is lengthened. At 100 °C the solubilities of hemihydrate and dihydrate are equal, in which case no reaction can occur and the gypsum will not set.

Modifiers (Accelerators and Retarders)   Modifiers are chemicals added in order to alter some of the properties and make it more acceptable to the dentist. If the chemical added decreases the setting time it is called an *accelerator,* whereas if it increases the setting time it is called a *retarder.*

Accelerators and retarders not only modify setting time, they also affect other properties like setting expansion and strength.

Accelerators

○   Finely powdered gypsum (up to 1%) is added by manufacturers to accelerate setting time. *Acts by* providing additional nuclei of crystallization. One source of gypsum is slurry water
○   In low concentrations, salts like sodium or potassium sulphate (2 to 3%) and sodium chloride (up to 2%) are accelerators. They *act by* making the hemihydrate more soluble

Retarders

Retarders generally act by forming a layer on the hemihydrate to reduce its solubility. It also inhibits the growth of gypsum crystals.

○   Borax (1–2%) is the most effective retarder. During setting, it forms a coating of calcium borate around the hemihydrate. Thus, the water cannot come in contact with the hemihydrate.

- In higher concentrations, sodium chloride (3.4% to 20%) and sodium sulphate act as retarders. In higher concentrations, the salt precipitates and poisons the nuclei of crystallization.
- Acetates, borates, citrates, tartrates and salts like ferric sulphate, chromic sulphate, aluminium sulphate, etc., are retarders, which *act by* nuclei poisoning by reducing the rate of solution of hemihydrate or by inhibiting growth of dihydrate crystals. Some additives react with hemihydrate, e.g., soluble tartrates and citrates precipitate calcium tartrate and citrate, respectively.
- Colloids such as gelatin, glue, agar, coagulated blood, etc. are effective retarders, presumably acting by nuclei poisoning. Contact with the gypsum during setting results in a soft, easily abraded surface.

    To avoid   The impression should be thoroughly rinsed in cold water to remove blood and saliva before pouring.

PROPERTIES

The important properties of gypsum products are

- Setting expansion
- Strength
- Hardness and abrasion resistance
- Reproduction of detail

SETTING EXPANSION

Setting expansion is measured using an extensometer. Setting expansion is of two types

1. Normal setting expansion
2. Hygroscopic setting expansion

NORMAL SETTING EXPANSION (0.05 TO 0.5%)

All gypsum products show a linear expansion during setting, due to the outward thrust of the growing crystals during setting. Crystals growing from the nuclei not only intermesh but also intercept each other during growth.

Importance of setting expansion   In dentistry, setting expansion may be both desirable and undesirable depending on the use. It is undesirable in impression plaster, dental plaster and stone as it will result in an inaccurate cast or change in the occlusal relation if used for mounting. ISO requirements for setting expansion for the various types is given in *Table 18.1*.

TABLE 18.1 Properties of various gypsum products

	* % Setting Expansion at 2 hrs.	*Comp str. (1 hr) (MPa)	Hardness (Dry) (RHN)	* (µm) Detail Reproduction
Type 1	0.15 max	4 min 8 max		75 ± 8
Type 2 (Class 1)	0.05	9		75 ± 8
Type 2 (Class 2)	0.06 min, 0.30 max	9		75 ± 8
Type 3	0.20 max	20	82	50 ± 8
Type 4	0.15 max (At 24 hr max 0.18)	35	92	50 ± 8
Type 5	0.16 min 0.30 max	35		50 ± 8

*Minimum requirement ISO 6873:2013

Increased setting expansion is desired in case of investment materials as it helps to compensate the shrinkage of the metal during casting.

Control of setting expansion

1. Mechanical mixing reduces setting expansion when compared to hand mixed stone.
2. Increase in W/P ratio reduces the setting expansion.
3. Modifiers generally reduce the setting expansion.
4. *Potassium sulphate* 4% solution reduces setting expansion from 0.5 to 0.06 %.
5. *Sodium chloride* and borax also decrease setting expansion.

For accuracy in dental procedures, the setting expansion has to be minimized. The manufacturers achieve this by addition of K_2SO_4. This, however, reduces the setting time. To counteract this, retarders like borax are also added (borax also reduces setting expansion).

HYGROSCOPIC SETTING EXPANSION

When a gypsum product is placed under water before the initial set stage, a greater expansion is seen. This is due to hygroscopic expansion. When expansion begins, externally available water is drawn into pores forming in the setting mass and this maintains a continuous aqueous phase in which crystal growth takes place freely. Under dry conditions this additional water is not available and as expansion occurs, the aqueous phase in the mix is reduced to a film over the growing crystals. It is greater in magnitude than normal setting expansion.

Importance   Used to expand some gypsum bonded investments.

STRENGTH

The strength increases rapidly as the material hardens after the initial setting. Minimum strength requirements (ISO) for various gypsum products are presented in **Table 18.1**.

Factors affecting strength

The free water content (excess water)   The greater the amount of free water in the set stone, the less the strength.

Wet strength It is the strength when excess free water (more than is necessary for reaction) is present in the set gypsum. The wet strength (1 hour compressive strength) for model plaster, dental stone, and die stone are 12.5, 31 and 45 MPa respectively.

Dry strength It is the strength of gypsum when the excess free water is lost due to evaporation. It is two or more times greater than the wet strength.

Excess water may be removed from gypsum cast by low-temperature drying. But there is no strength increase until the last 2% of free water **(Fig. 18.10)** is removed. This strength increases on drying is reversible, thus soaking a dry cast in water reduces its strength to the original level. Many products have strength values in excess of the ISO requirements. One Type 4 product claims a wet strength (1 hr) of 67 MPa and a dry strength of 121.6 MPa.

Temperature   Gypsum is stable only below about 40 °C. Drying at higher temperatures must

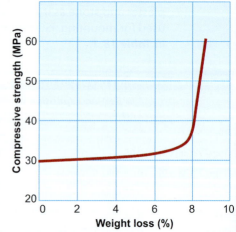

FIGURE 18.10 Effect of drying on the strength of dental stone.

be carefully controlled. Loss of water of crystallization occurs rapidly at 100 °C or higher and causes shrinkage and a reduction in strength.

Other factors affecting strength
○ *W/P ratio*   The more the water, the greater the porosity and less the strength.
○ *Spatulation*   Within limits, strength increases with increased spatulation.
○ *Addition of accelerators and retarders* Lowers strength.

TENSILE STRENGTH

Gypsum is a brittle material, thus weaker in tension than in compression.

The one hour tensile strength of model plaster is approximately 2.3 MPa. When dry, the tensile strength doubles. The tensile strength of dental stone is twice than that of plaster.

Significance   Teeth on a cast may fracture while separating from the impression. Since in practice fracture of gypsum typically occurs in tension, tensile strength is a better guide to fracture resistance.

Time at which cast can be used   The cast cannot be used as soon as it reaches its final setting (as defined by the Vicat and Gillmore tests). This is because the cast has not reached its full strength. Technically the cast can be used when it has attained at least 80% of its one hour strength. Current products are ready for use in *30 minutes.*

HARDNESS AND ABRASION RESISTANCE

Dies and casts are often used to construct restorations and prostheses. A good surface hardness and abrasion resistance is therefore essential. Hardness of some gypsum products are presented in **Table 18.1**.

Hardness is related to the compressive strength. The higher the compressive strength of the hardening mass, the higher the surface hardness. After the final setting occurs, the surface hardness remains practically constant until most of the excess water is dried, after which it increases.

The surface hardness increases at a faster rate than the compressive strength since the surface of the hardened mass reaches a dry state earlier than the inner portion of the mass. Commercial hardening solutions are available to increase the surface hardness of stone. However, surface hardness and abrasion resistance are not always related, for example, epoxy resin is more abrasion resistant than die stone, even though die stone is harder of the two.

FLOW

The flow of freshly mixed gypsum depends on the amount of water used (W/P ratio). The greater the amount of water used, the greater would be the flow. However, a correctly proportioned mix has sufficient flow. Vibrating the mix greatly improves the flow. The flow reduces as it approaches its initial set.

REPRODUCTION OF DETAIL

Gypsum products reproduce detail accurately *(Table 18.1).*

Significance
○ Impression plaster has to accurately record oral tissues.
○ Cast material has to duplicate all the detail recorded by the impression.

Factors which affect detail reproduction include compatibility with the impression material, trapped air bubbles in the mix and surface contaminants like saliva. Use of a mechanical vibrator and proper technique considerably improve detail reproduction.

SPECIALIZED GYPSUM PRODUCTS

Some gypsum products are manufactured for specific uses in dentistry. Each type is developed with specific physical properties suitable for the particular purpose.

DENTAL CASTING INVESTMENTS

Uses

To prepare refractory molds for casting dental alloys.

Adding a refractory material like silica or quartz or cristobalite to dental plaster or stone permits it to withstand high temperatures. These are called dental casting investments *(Fig. 18.11)* (detailed in Chapter on investments).

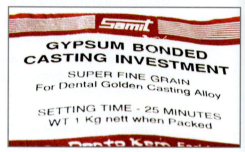

FIGURE 18.11 Gypsum bonded investment (*Courtesy:* MCODS, Manipal).

DIVESTMENT

Uses

To make refractory dies.

It is a combination of die stone and gypsum-bonded investment mixed with colloidal silica. A die is made and the wax pattern constructed on it. Then the entire assembly (die and pattern) is invested in the divestment (normally the wax pattern is removed from the die and invested separately).

The setting expansion of the material is 0.9% and thermal expansion is 0.6% when heated to 677 °C. The *advantage* of divestment is that the wax pattern does not have to be removed from the die, thus distortion of the pattern can be avoided.

SYNTHETIC GYPSUM

It is possible to make alpha and beta hemihydrate from the byproducts during the manufacture of phosphoric acid.

The synthetic product is usually more expensive than that made from natural gypsum, but when the product is properly made, its properties are equal to or exceed the latter. However, manufacture is difficult and a few have succeeded (e.g., Japan and Germany).

ORTHODONTIC STONE

For orthodontic study models, many orthodontists prefer to used white stone or plaster *(Fig. 18.12)*. These products have a longer working time for pouring of multiple models. To produce a glossy surface, finished models may be treated with 'model glow' model soap.

RESIN MODIFIED STONES

A new resin fortified die stone (e.g., ResinRock, Whipmix corporation) is available. It is a blend of synthetic resin and alpha gypsum. These stones are less brittle, have improved surface smoothness and increased resistance to abrasion. When mixed, it forms a creamy, thixotropic mix which flows more easily under vibration. Their compressive strength can be as high as 79 MPa.

MOUNTING PLASTER

Plaster used for attaching the cast to the articulator **(Fig. 18.1D)** is known as mounting plaster **(Fig. 18.13)**. Regular plaster (type II, class 1) has higher setting expansion and should be avoided for mounting. However, plasters with lower setting expansion (described by ISO 6873:2013 as Type II, Class 1) specialized for this purpose are available commercially. Important properties for these products include a low setting expansion (0 to 0.05 %) which is important for the accuracy of the mounting, low strength (12 MPa) which allows easy separation from the cast and fast setting time (3 minutes).

FAST SETTING STONE

These are exceptionally fast setting stones (2 minutes) with an early high compressive strength (1 hour - 41 MPa) which allows separation of the cast from the impression in 5 minutes. An example includes *Snap stone* (Whipmix).

CARE OF GYPSUM

CARE OF THE CAST

If the gypsum cast has to be soaked in water it must be placed in a water bath in which plaster debris is allowed to remain constantly on the bottom of the container to provide a saturated solution of calcium sulfate at all times. This is known as *'slurry water'.* If the cast is washed in ordinary water, surface layer may dissolve, hence slurry water is used to preserve surface details. Such a procedure also causes a negligible expansion. All gypsum casts must be handled carefully as any departure from the expected accuracy may result in a poorly fitting appliance.

STORAGE OF THE POWDER

1. As plaster is hygroscopic, it should be kept in *air-tight containers.* When the relative humidity is more than 70%, plaster starts taking up moisture initiating a setting reaction. This produces small crystals of gypsum which act as nuclei of crystallization. Thus in the early stages, moisture contaminated plaster *sets faster.* In later stages, as the hygroscopic action continues, the entire hemihydrate mass is covered by more crystals of gypsum. The water penetrates the mass with difficulty, thereby delaying setting. Thus heavily moisture

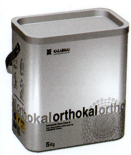
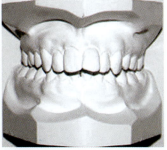

FIGURE 18.12 Orthodontic stone (Kalabhai) and model.

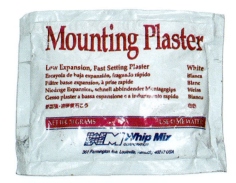

FIGURE 18.13 Mounting plaster.

contaminated stone or plaster *sets slower.* The humidity factor is a major consideration in parts of India with high atmospheric humidity.

2. It should be kept clean with no dirt or other foreign bodies.

INFECTION CONTROL

There has been an increased interest over possible cross-contamination to dental office personnel through dental impressions. If an impression has not been disinfected, it is wise to disinfect the stone cast.

Gypsum products may be disinfected by

1. Immersing cast in a disinfection solution.
2. Addition of disinfectant into the stone.
3. Overnight gas sterilization while treating patients known to have an infection (impractical for routine use).

DIFFERENCES BETWEEN DENTAL PLASTER AND DENTAL STONE

Though chemically identical, their differences are detailed in **Table 18.2**.

TABLE 18.2 Comparison of plaster and stone		
	Plaster	*Stone*
Manufacture	Dry calcination	Wet calcination
Particle size/shape	Larger, irregular porous	Smaller, regular and dense
W/P ratio	Requires more water	Requires less water
Porosity	Porous	More dense
Properties	Lower strength and hardness	Greater strength and hardness
Application	Used when strength is not of primary importance (e.g., diagnostic casts)	Used when greater strength and hardness is required (e.g., dies, master casts)

Waxes in Dentistry

During construction of a denture and many other appliances, wax is used as a modeling material. Different types of waxes are used to prepare patterns for alloy castings.

There are many varieties of waxes used, both in the clinic and laboratory. Each has particular properties depending on what it is used for. Their basic constituents are essentially similar, their exact proportion is different.

COMPONENTS OF DENTAL WAXES

Dental waxes contain natural waxes, synthetic waxes and additives *(Table 19.1)*.

CHEMICAL NATURE OF WAXES

Natural waxes are long chain, complex combinations of organic compounds of reasonably high molecular weight. The two principal groups of organic compounds contained in waxes are—

○ Hydrocarbons, e.g. saturated alkanes, and
○ Esters, e.g. myricyl palmitate (bees wax).

Some waxes, in addition, contain free alcohol and acids.

Ester—formed from union of higher fatty acids (e.g. carboxylic acid) with higher aliphatic alcohol with elimination of water.

$$\text{Alcohol} + \text{Fatty acid} \longrightarrow \text{Ester} + \text{Water}$$

TABLE 19.1 Wax components

	Natural waxes	Synthetic waxes	Additives
Minerals	Paraffin	Acrawax C	Fats
	Microcrystalline	Aerosol, OT	- Stearic acid
	Barnsdall	Castorwax	- Glyceryl tristearate
	Ozokerite	Flexowax C	
	Ceresin	Epolene N-10	
	Montan	Albacer	Oils
		Aldo 33	Turpentine
		Durawax 1032	Color
Plants	Carnauba		Natural resins
	Ouricury		Rosin
	Candelilla		- Copal
	Japan wax		- Dammar
	Cocoa butter		- Sandarac
			- Mastic
			- Shellac
			- Kauri
Insect	Beeswax		
Animal	Spermaceti		Synthetic resins
	Lanolin		- Elvax
			- Polyethylene
			- Polystyrene

MINERAL WAXES

Paraffin and microcrystalline waxes   These are distillation products of petroleum. They are both hydrocarbons. Paraffin (melts 40–70 °C) tends to be brittle. Microcrystalline (60–90 °C) is more flexible and tougher.

PLANT WAXES

Carnauba   Carnauba, also called Brazil wax and palm wax, is a wax of the leaves of the palm Copernicia prunifera, a plant native to and grown only in the northeastern Brazil. In its pure state it usually comes in the form of hard yellow-brown flakes. Melting range is 84–91 °C.

Ouricury   Ouricury wax is a brown-colored wax obtained from the leaves of a Brazilian Feather Palm Syagrus coronata or Cocos coronata by scraping the leaf surface. It melts between 79–84 °C.

Both *Carnauba and Ouricury* raise melting range and hardness of paraffin.

Candelilla It is a wax derived from the leaves of the small Candelilla shrub native to northern Mexico and the southwestern United States, Euphorbia cerifera and Euphorbia antisyphilitica. It is yellowish-brown, hard, brittle, aromatic, and opaque to translucent. Melting range is 68 to 75 °C. Mainly hardens paraffin wax.

Japan wax and cocoa butter These are not true waxes but are chiefly fats. Japan wax is also known as sumac wax, China green tallow, Japan tallow, etc. It is obtained from the lacquer tree and the Japanese wax tree which are native to Japan and China. It is pale yellow, sticky, tough, malleable, has a gummy feel and melts at 51 °C. Cocoa butter is brittle. Japan wax improves tackiness and emulsifying ability of paraffin.

INSECT WAX

Beeswax (63–73 °C) Brittle at room temperature, plastic at body temperature. Its addition reduces brittleness.

Shellac wax From the lac insect Kerria lacca.

ANIMAL WAX

Spermaceti is found in the spermaceti organ inside the sperm whale's head. It is not widely used. Mainly used as a coating for dental floss.

Lanolin is a wax obtained from wool, consisting of esters of sterols.

SYNTHETIC WAXES

The natural waxes are not consistent in their composition, and thus their properties. To overcome this, synthetic waxes are used. These are carefully prepared under controlled conditions to give standardized reliable results. They are highly refined unlike natural waxes which are frequently contaminated. Their use is still limited.

Ozokerite It is an earth wax found in western US and central Europe. It improves the physical characteristics of paraffin.

Montan Montan wax is a fossilized wax extracted from coal and lignite. It is very hard, reflecting the high concentration of saturated fatty acids and alcohols. It is hard, brittle and lustrous. Although dark brown and smelly, they can be purified and bleached. It can be substituted for plant waxes.

Ceresin It is obtained from petroleum and lignite refining. They are harder and are used to raise melting range of paraffin.

Barnsdall It raises melting range and hardness, reduces flow of paraffin.

WAX ADDITIVES

Gums They are viscous, amorphous exudates from plants that harden when exposed to air. They are complex substances mainly made of carbohydrates. They either dissolve in water or form sticky, viscous liquids, e.g. gum Arabic and tragacanth.

Fats They are tasteless, odorless and colorless substances. They are similar to wax but have lower melting temperatures and are softer. Chemically they are composed of glycerides, e.g. beef tallow and butter. They can be used to increase melting range and hardness of waxes.

Oils They lower the melting point of paraffin. Hydrocarbon oils soften waxes. Silicone oils improve ease of polishing of waxes.

Resins are exudates of certain trees and plants (except shellac which is from insects). They are complex, amorphous mixtures of organic substances. They are insoluble in water. They improve toughness. They are also used to make varnishes (by dissolving in an organic solvent).

Synthetic resins They are also used.

CLASSIFICATION OF DENTAL WAXES

ACCORDING TO ORIGIN (DESCRIBED EARLIER)

- ○ Mineral
- ○ Plant
- ○ Insect
- ○ Animal

ACCORDING TO USE

Pattern waxes	Processing waxes	Impression waxes
Inlay casting	Boxing	Corrective
RPD casting	Utility	Bite registration
Base plate	Sticky	
	Carding	
	Shellac	

ISO CLASSIFICATION (ISO 15854: 2005) FOR CASTING INLAY AND BASEPLATE WAX

The ISO recognizes 2 types of waxes which are further sub-classified according to their flow characteristics that represent their hardness.

Type I (Casting wax) - for cast metal restorations

    Class 1 - Soft

    Class 2 - Hard

Type II (Baseplate wax) - for denture bases and occlusion rims

    Class 1 - Soft

    Class 2 - Hard

    Class 3 - Extra hard

GENERAL PROPERTIES

Waxes have a number of important properties in relation to their dental use. Different uses require different properties. Waxes for patterns probably require most careful balance. Some of the important properties are

1. Melting range
2. Thermal expansion
3. Mechanical properties
4. Flow
5. Residual stresses
6. Ductility

MELTING RANGE

Waxes have melting ranges rather than melting points. Mixing of waxes may change their melting range. Melting range varies depending on its use.

THERMAL EXPANSION

Waxes expand when subjected to a rise in temperature and contract as the temperature is decreased.

Coefficient of thermal expansion and its importance   Dental waxes and their components have the largest CTE among the materials used in restorative dentistry. Temperature changes in wax patterns after removal from the mouth can produce *inaccuracies* in the finished restoration.

MECHANICAL PROPERTIES

The elastic modulus, proportional limit and compressive strength of waxes are low compared to other dental materials. These properties are strongly dependent on the temperature. As temperature decreases, the properties improve.

FLOW

Flow is an important property, especially in inlay waxes. When melted, the wax should flow readily into all the parts of the die. Flow is dependent on

1. Temperature of the wax
2. Force applied
3. The length of time the force is applied.

Flow increases as the melting point of the wax is approached.

RESIDUAL STRESS

Regardless of the method used to make a wax pattern, residual stresses will exist in the completed pattern. The stress may be compressive or tensile in nature.

Example A   When a specimen is held under compression during cooling, the atoms and molecules are forced closer together. After the specimen is cooled to room temperature and the load is removed, the motion of the molecules is restricted. This restriction results in residual stress (hidden stresses) in the specimen. When the specimen is heated, release of the residual stress is added to the normal thermal expansion, and the total expansion is greater than normal.

Example B   When a specimen is cooled while under tension, the release of the residual tensile stress results in a dimensional change that is opposite to thermal expansion, i.e., it can result in overall contraction of the specimen.

DUCTILITY

Like flow, the ductility increases as the temperature of the wax is increased. In general, waxes with low melting points have greater ductility than those with high melting points.

PATTERN WAXES

Many dental restorations or prostheses are first made with pattern waxes. The wax is later replaced with the permanent material, e.g. cast gold alloys, cobalt-chromium-nickel alloys, or polymethyl methacrylate resin. All pattern waxes have two major qualities which cause serious problems in their use—thermal change in dimension and tendency to warp or distort on standing, e.g. inlay casting wax, RPD casting wax and baseplate wax.

Types

1. Casting waxes
   - Inlay
   - Removable partial denture (the metal frame)
   - Milling wax
2. Baseplate wax (used in the construction of complete and partial denture).

INLAY CASTING WAX

The inlay casting wax is among the oldest waxes in dentistry.

USES

The pattern for inlays, crowns and FPDs is first made in wax *(Figs. 19.1A to D)*, and then replaced by metal during casting.

Direct and indirect techniques If the pattern is made directly in the tooth (in the mouth), it is said to be prepared by direct technique (Class 2 wax). If it is prepared on a replica of the tooth (die), it is called indirect technique (Class 1 wax).

IDEAL REQUIREMENTS OF INLAY CASTING WAXES

1. When softened, the wax should be uniform, there should be no graininess or hard spots in the plastic material.
2. The color should contrast with the die. A definite color contrast helps in identifying and finishing of margins.
3. The wax should not flake or crumble when the wax is softened.
4. The wax should not chip, flake or tear during carving.
5. During burnout (500 °C), it should vaporize completely without residue.

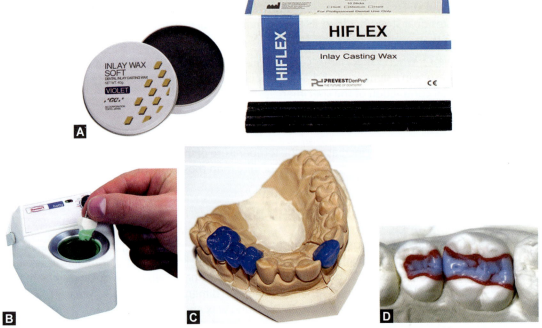

FIGURES 19.1A TO D (A) 2 forms of inlay casting waxes. **(B)** Wax bath used for the dipping technique. **(C)** Wax patterns of crowns made from inlay wax made on a die. **(D)** An inlay pattern.

TABLE 19.2 Flow requirements for inlay casting wax (Adapted from ISO 15854:2005)					
Flow in %					
	At 30 °C	*At 37 °C*	*At 40 °C*	*At 45 °C*	
Class 1	Max 1%	–	Min 50%	Min 70%	Max 90%
Class 2	–	Max 1%	Max 20%	Min 70%	Max 90%

6. The wax pattern should be completely rigid and dimensionally stable at all times until it is eliminated.
7. It should be sufficiently plastic slightly above mouth temperature and become rigid when cooled to mouth temperature (for class I waxes).
8. The wax should have good flow when heated and set rigidly when cooled (at the recommended temperature for each type see ***Table 19.2***.

CLASSIFICATION*

According to ISO 15854:2005, inlay casting waxes are classified as

○ Class 1 Soft—Extraoral or laboratory use
○ Class 2 Hard—Intraoral use

SUPPLIED AS

Blue, green or purple sticks or cakes ***(Fig. 19.1A)***. Also available as small pellets and cones. The waxes are also available in preformed shapes.

Commercial Names Harvard, Kerr, etc.

COMPOSITION

Paraffin wax, gum damar, carnauba or candelilla and coloring agents.

Paraffin wax (40–60%) This is the main ingredient. It is used to establish the melting point. Different varieties, with different melting points can be produced. Paraffin wax flakes trimmed do not give a smooth surface, so other waxes are added to modify.

Ceresin (10%) Partially replaces paraffin. Increases toughness. Easy to carve.

Gum damar (1%) Damar resin (a natural derivative from pine tree) improves the smoothness during molding and makes it more resistant to cracking and flaking. It also increases toughness of the wax and enhances the luster of the surface.

Carnauba wax (25%) This wax is quite hard and has a high melting point. It is combined with paraffin to decrease the flow at mouth temperature. It has an agreeable odor and gives glossiness to the wax surface.

Candelilla wax This wax can be added to replace carnauba wax. It contributes the same qualities as carnauba wax, but its melting point is lower and is not as hard as carnauba wax.

Synthetic waxes In modern inlay waxes, carnauba wax is often replaced partly by certain synthetic waxes (Montan). Because of their high melting point, more paraffin can be incorporated and the general working qualities are improved.

PROPERTIES OF INLAY WAX

Class 1 inlay wax is meant for use in the laboratory whereas, Class 2 wax is used in the mouth (indirect technique). Obviously, both would have slightly different properties.

---

* One popular US reference text has described this classification in reverse. However this could not be verified in current or previous ADA or ISO sources. Staff and students are advised to the use the version provided in the this text book as it is sourced from the original document (ISO 1584:2005).

Flow

Requirements according to ISO 15854:2005 *(Table 19.2)*

At 45 °C – Both Class 1 and Class 2 should have a flow between 70 to 90%.

At 37 °C – Class 2 should not flow more than 1%.

At 30 °C – Class 1 should not flow more than 1%.

It is clear that

Class 1 inlay wax This type melts and flows, when heated to around 45 °C. This temperature is tolerated by the patient. Good flow at this temperature ensures good reproduction of the inlay cavity. The wax cools down and hardens at 37 °C (mouth temperature), allowing the operator to carve and shape it in the mouth.

Class 2 inlay wax This type on the other hand hardens at 30 °C (room temperature). This wax is more suitable for the laboratory. The flow characteristics are not suitable for use in the mouth.

Thermal properties

Thermal conductivity The thermal conductivity of these waxes is low. It takes time to heat the wax uniformly and to cool it to body or room temperature.

Coefficient of thermal expansion Inlay wax has a high CTE. It has a linear expansion of 0.7% with increase in temperature of 20 °C. Its thermal changes are higher than any other dental material.

Importance This property is more significant in direct technique because contraction of the pattern can occur when it is taken from mouth to room temperature (especially in air conditioned rooms or in cold climates).

Factors affecting If the wax is allowed to cool under pressure, its thermal properties are changed. When reheated, the linear CTE is increased. The temperature of the die and the method used to apply pressure on the wax as it solidifies also influences the CTE.

Wax distortion

Wax distortion is the most serious problem in inlay wax. It is due to *release of stresses* in the pattern caused due to

1. Contraction on cooling
2. Occluded gas bubbles
3. Change of shape of the wax during molding
4. From manipulation—carving, pooling, removal, etc.

Thus the amount of residual stress is dependent on

o The method of forming the pattern

o Its handling, and

o Length of time and temperature of storage of the wax pattern

Causes of distortion Distortion is due to any method of manipulation that creates inhomogeneity of wax involving the intermolecular distance *(Figs. 19.2A and B)*.

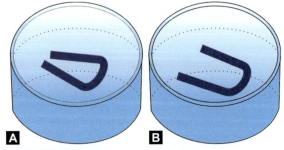

FIGURES 19.2A AND B Demonstration of wax distortion. **(A)** Bent stick of wax kept in water at room temperature. **(B)** Straightened appreciably after 24 hours.

Factors causing distortion under control of the operator *cannot be* totally eliminated. Distortion of the wax can occur

○ If wax is not at uniform temperature when inserted in the cavity, some parts of the wax pattern may thermally contract more than others when stresses are introduced.
○ If wax is not held under uniform pressure during cooling.
○ If fresh wax is melted and added in an area of deficiency, the added wax will introduce stresses during cooling.
○ During carving, some molecules of wax will be disturbed and stresses will result.

To avoid

1. Minimal carving and change in temperature.
2. Minimal storage of pattern. Invest immediately.
3. Store it in a refrigerator if necessary.

Some relaxation and distortion of pattern occurs regardless of the method used. It cannot be totally eliminated. It can only be reduced to a point which is not of clinical importance.

RESIDUE ON IGNITION

Waxes vaporize during burnout. ISO 15854:2005 limits the nonvaporizable residue to a maximum of 0.1%. Excess residue can result in an incomplete casting.

MANIPULATION OF INLAY WAX

Direct technique

Hold the stick of wax over the visible flame and *rotate it* rapidly until it becomes plastic taking care not to volatilize the wax. The softened wax is shaped approximately to the form of the prepared cavity.

After the wax is inserted into the cavity, it is held under *finger pressure* while it solidifies. The wax should be allowed to *cool gradually* to mouth temperature. Cooling rapidly by application of cold water results in differential contraction and development of internal stresses.

Localized reheating of wax with warm carving instruments has a similar effect and more distortion may occur. A cold carving instrument should be used for direct wax pattern. Withdraw the wax pattern carefully in the long axis of the preparation. The pattern should be touched as little as possible with the *hands* to avoid temperature changes.

Indirect technique

Inlay pattern is prepared over a *lubricated die*. If molten wax is used, very little residual stresses occur.

○ *Dipping method* In case of full crowns, the die can be dipped repeatedly, into hot liquid wax. The wax is allowed to cool, carved, and removed from the die.
○ *Softening in warm water* This technique is not recommended because
  – Soluble constituents may leach out and the properties of wax will change
  – Water gets into the wax causing splattering on the flame, interference with the softening of the wax surface and distortion of the pattern on thermal changes.
○ *Addition* The wax is melted and added in layers using a spatula or a brush.

Polishing

Polishing is done by rubbing with a silk cloth.

Note

1. Invest all wax patterns as soon as possible to avoid distortion.
2. Waxes oxidize on heating. Prolonged heating causes it to evaporate. There will also be darkening and precipitation of gummy deposits. To avoid this, use the lowest temperature needed for melting.

RPD CASTING WAX

The partial denture casting waxes are quite unlike the inlay casting waxes in appearance and handling properties. Currently, no ADA or ISO specification have been formulated for these waxes. However, a US federal specification (U-W-140) has been formulated to cover these waxes. These specifications are different from those of inlay waxes.

USES

To make patterns of the metallic framework and sprues of removable partial dentures.

SUPPLIED AS

It is available in different forms *(Fig. 19.3A)*.

○ Sheets 0.40 and 0.32 mm thickness
○ Preformed shapes
  – Round (10 cm), half round and half pear-shaped rods
  – Reticular, grid or mesh form
  – Clasp shapes
  – Other forms
○ Bulk wax as blocks or in containers
○ Rolls or coils of various diameters ranging for 2 to 5 mm for forming sprues.

PROPERTIES

These waxes are *tacky* and highly *ductile* as they must adapt easily and stick onto the refractory cast. They should copy accurately the surface against which they are pressed. The pattern for the RPD frame is made on a special cast known as the *refractory cast (Fig. 19.3B)*. Since the wax comes in preformed shapes, it is quite easy to assemble. The wax forms are sticky and

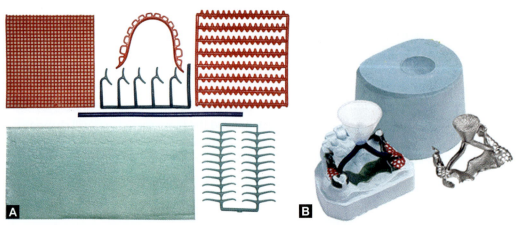

FIGURES 19.3A AND B RPD casting wax. **(A)** Preformed casting waxes save valuable laboratory time and give more consistent results. **(B)** RPD pattern formed from preformed waxes are used in the construction of removable partial dentures.

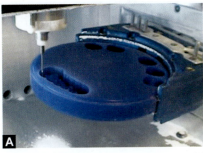
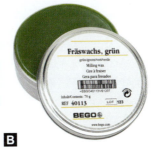
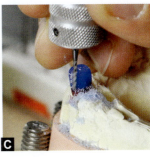

FIGURES 19.4A TO C Machinable wax. **(A)** CAD/CAM milling. **(B)** Milling wax in cake form. **(C)** Milling with handpiece.

pliable and can be adapted easily onto the cast. After the pattern is completed, it is invested and ignited. Like inlay wax, they too must vaporize with *little residue* during burnout.

MILLING WAX

Synonyms   Machinable wax

Milling or machinable wax is wax that can be shaped by milling or machining using CAD/CAM **(Fig. 19.4A)** or dental drills **(Fig. 19.4C)**. Machinable wax is an extremely hard wax with high melting temperature that is formulated to deliver machining properties including high resolution detail. The wax pattern formed after machining is invested and cast like regular casting waxes.

AVAILABLE AS

Machinable wax is available as

- Blocks
- Cylinders
- Discs **(Fig. 19.4A)**
- Cakes in containers **(Fig. 19.4B)**

PROPERTIES

It is harder and has a higher melting temperature than most other waxes. It powders or flakes on milling.

Hardness	: 53 (Shore "D" Scale)
Specific Gravity	: 0.92
Melting Point	: 115 °C
Burnout Residue	: 0.0066%
Flexural Modulus	: 45,250 PSI

Coefficient of Thermal Expansion: 7.5×10^{-5} (cm/cm/°C)

BASEPLATE WAX

Most students would be familiar with this wax. It is sometimes referred to as modeling or Type 2 (ISO 15854) wax. They are classified under pattern waxes because they are used to create the form of dentures and appliances made of acrylic and like materials. Ideally, these waxes should be easy to carve, should not chip and break at try-in and should boil out without leaving any oily residue. Flow requirements as per ISO specifications are given in **Table 19.3**.

TABLE 19.3 Flow requirements of Baseplate wax*

Temperature	Type 2 Baseplate wax					
	Class 1		Class 2		Class 3	
	Min.	Max.	Min.	Max.	Min.	Max.
°C	%	%	%	%	%	%
23,0 ± 0,1	–	1,0	–	0,6	–	0,2
30,0 ± 0,1	–	–	–	–	–	–
37,0 ± 0,1	5,0	90,0	–	10,0	–	1,2
40,0 ± 0,1	–	–	–	–	–	–
45,0 ± 0,1	–	–	50,0	90,0	5,0	50,0

* ISO 15854:2005

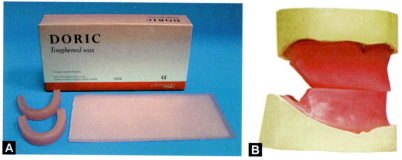

FIGURES 19.5A AND B **(A)** Baseplate wax. **(B)** Occlusion rims.

USES

These waxes are used for the following

1. To make occlusion rims **(Fig. 19.5B)**.
2. To form the contour of the denture after teeth are set.
3. To make patterns for orthodontic appliances and other prostheses which are to be constructed of plastics.

CLASSIFICATION (ISO 15854:2005)

Type I	Soft	—	for building veneers
Type II	Hard	—	to use in mouths in normal climates
Type III	Extra-hard	—	for use in tropical climates

SUPPLIED AS

Sheets of pink or red color **(Fig. 19.5A)**.

COMPOSITION

Component	Percent
Paraffin or ceresin	80.0
Beeswax	12.0
Carnauba	2.5
Natural or synthetic resins	3.0
Microcrystalline	2.5

PROCESSING WAXES

These are those waxes used mainly as accessory aids in the construction of a variety of restorations and appliances, either clinically or in the laboratory, e.g. boxing wax, beading wax, utility wax, blockout wax, carding wax and sticky wax.

BOXING WAX AND BEADING WAX

USES

Used to build up vertical walls around the impression, in order to pour the stone and make a cast. The procedure is known as *boxing (Fig. 19.6)*.

SUPPLIED AS

Boxing wax as sheets, beading wax as strips *(Figs. 19.7A and B)*.

ADVANTAGES OF BEADING AND BOXING

1. Preserves the extensions and landmarks.
2. Controls the thickness of the borders.
3. Controls the form and thickness of the base of the cast.
4. Conserves the artificial stone.

PROPERTIES

They are pliable and can be adapted easily. A slight tackiness allows it to stick to the impression.

Note The terms carding wax and boxing wax have been used interchangeably. Carding wax was the original material on which porcelain teeth were fixed when received from the manufacturer. Boxing wax is a more acceptable term.

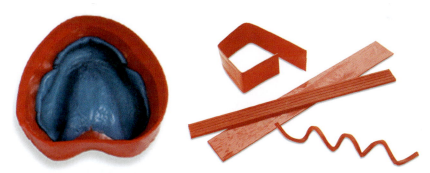

FIGURE 19.6 Boxed impression ready for pouring stone.

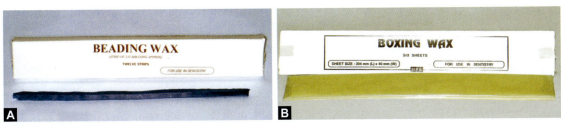

FIGURES 19.7A AND B **(A)** Beading wax. **(B)** Boxing wax.

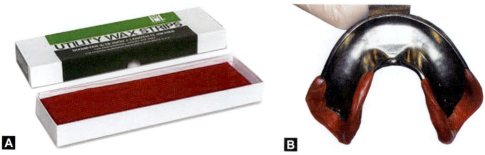

FIGURES 19.8A AND B **(A)** Utility wax is often used for tray extension **(B)**.

TECHNIQUE

Beading wax is adapted around the periphery. This wax should be approximately 4 mm wide and 3–4 mm below the borders of the impression. The height is adjusted until a boxing wax strip extends approximately 13 mm above the highest point on the impression. Stone is vibrated into the boxed impression.

UTILITY WAX

COMPOSITION

Consists mainly of beeswax, petrolatum, and other soft waxes in varying proportions.

SUPPLIED AS

It is available in the form of sticks and sheets **(Figs. 19.8A and B)**.

USES

It is *used* to adjust contour of perforated tray for use with hydrocolloids (e.g. to raise flange height, to extend the tray posteriorly, to raise palatal portion of the tray in cases of deep palate, etc.). It is pliable and can be easily molded. It is adhesive and can stick to the tray.

STICKY WAX

COMPOSITION

It consists mainly of yellow beeswax, rosin, and natural resins such as gum dammar.

PROPERTIES

It is sticky when melted and adheres closely to the surfaces to which it is applied. At room temperature, it is firm, free from tackiness, and brittle **(Fig. 19.9)**.

USES

Used for joining (assembling) metal parts before soldering and for joining fragments of broken dentures before repair procedure. A variety of other uses, mainly joining, are possible with this wax.

CARDING WAX

Carding wax is used by manufacturers for the packaging of acrylic or porcelain teeth **(Fig. 19.10)**. They are soft, tacky and pliable at room temperatures. The are available as sheets or strips.

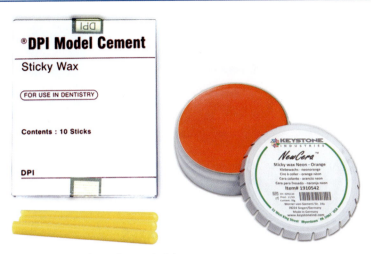

FIGURE 19.9 Different forms of sticky wax.

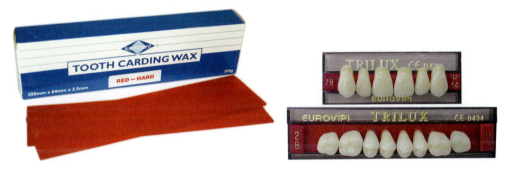

FIGURE 19.10 Carding wax.

SHELLAC

Shellac was once extensively used in dentistry to fabricate temporary denture bases and custom trays. It is also used for bite registration.

COMPOSITION

It contains *shellac wax* which is a wax from the lac insect Kerria lacca, plasticizers like stearin and stearic acid and fillers like mica (strength), talc. Some contain *aluminum* which is also used as a filler to adjust viscosity. It may be white (bleached), brown (natural color) and pink or bronze (dye) *(Figs. 19.11A and B)*.

Heating of the shellac in water above 70 °C causes leaching of the plasticizers. Heating over flame above 100 °C results in polymerization with release of water (characterized by bubbling). This results in a marked increase in its viscosity (becomes stiffer).

MANIPULATION

Being a thermoplastic material, it is manipulated by softening with heat to adapt, cut and shape it *(Fig. 19.11C)*.

DRAWBACKS

Again being a thermoplastic material, it is affected by heat and is, therefore, potentially unstable and subject to distortion. It is now largely replaced by resins which are more stable.

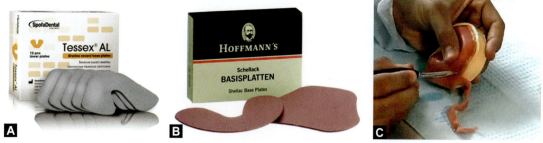

FIGURES 19.11A TO C (A) White shellac. (B) Brown shellac. (C) Fabrication of shellac baseplate.

IMPRESSION WAXES

These are used to record non-undercut edentulous portions of the mouth, and are generally used in combination with other impression materials such as polysulfide rubber, ZOE, or dental impression compound, e.g. corrective impression wax, bite registration wax.

CORRECTIVE IMPRESSION WAX

Waxes were used widely in the past for making dental impressions. Waxes are highly unstable and susceptible to distortion and are, therefore, not particularly suited for conventional impressions. However, they may be used in certain situations.

TYPES

1. Aluwax *(Fig. 19.12A)*
2. Korecta wax (No. 4) (extra soft - orange) *(Fig. 19.12B)*
3. Iowa wax—Available as 6 inch sticks or in a small container *(Fig. 19.12C)*
4. H-L physiologic paste (yellow-white)
5. Adaptol (green) *(Fig. 19.12D)*

USES

It is used as a wax veneer over an original impression to contact and register the details of the soft tissues.

1. To make functional impression of free end saddles (Class I and II removable partial dentures).
2. To record the posterior palatal seal in dentures.
3. Functional impression for obturators.

COMPOSITION AND PROPERTIES

They *consist of* paraffin, ceresin and beeswax. It may also contain metal particles like copper or aluminium. One product (Aluwax, *Fig. 19.12A*) uses aluminum particles. The flow at 37 °C is 100%. These waxes are subject to distortion during removal from the mouth. They should be *poured immediately*.

Each grade is designed for a specific purpose.

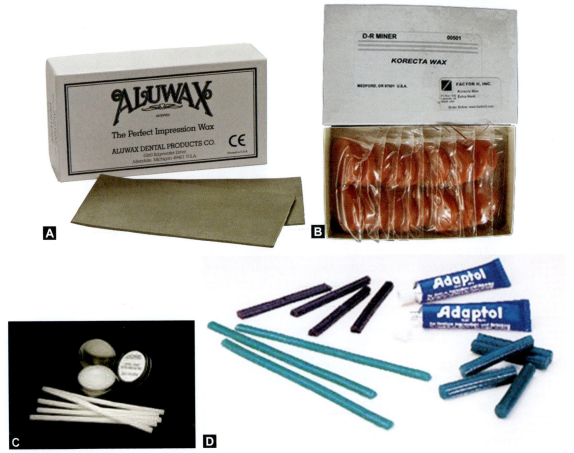

FIGURES 19.12A TO D Impression waxes. **(A)** Aluwax. **(B)** Korecta wax orange. **(C)** Iowa wax. **(D)** Adaptol Green.

BITE REGISTRATION WAX

USES

It is used to record the relationship between the upper and lower teeth. This is necessary in order to mount the casts correctly in the articulator.

SUPPLIED AS

U-shaped rods or wafers **(Figs. 19.13 and 19.14).** A thin metallic foil may be present on the undersurface or between the wax layers.

COMPOSITION

Beeswax or paraffin or ceresin. Some contain aluminum or copper particles.

PROCEDURE

The wax is softened in warm water. The soft wax is then placed between the teeth and the patient is asked to bite. After the wax hardens, it is then taken out and placed in chilled water.

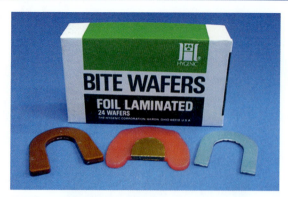

FIGURE 19.13 Bite registration wax.

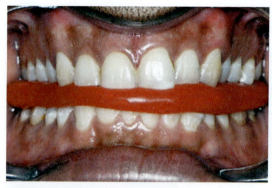

FIGURE 19.14 Bite registration process.

It is replaced back in the mouth and the patient asked to occlude for a final check. The casts of the patient is placed in the indentations formed by the teeth in the wax. It is then mounted with plaster on the articulator. Mounting should not be delayed as wax distortion can lead to inaccurate results. Bite registration can be done with other materials like zinc oxide, eugenol and silicones.

Dental Investments and Refractory Materials

A refractory is a nonmetallic material that can withstand high temperatures without degrading, softening, or losing its strength.

An investment can be described as a ceramic material which is suitable for forming a mold into which molten metal or alloy is cast *(Fig. 20.1)*. The procedure for forming the mold is described as 'investing'. These materials can withstand high temperatures. For this reason, they are also known as refractory materials. Investment materials are covered by ISO 15912:2006. This standard also covers, brazing investments and refractory die materials.

REQUIREMENTS OF AN INVESTMENT MATERIAL

1. The investment mold must expand to compensate for the alloy shrinkage, which occurs during the cooling of the molten alloy.
2. The powder should have a fine particle size to give a smooth surface to the casting.
3. The manipulation should be easy. It should have a suitable setting time.
4. The material should have a smooth consistency when mixed.
5. The set material should be porous enough to permit air in the mold cavity to escape easily during casting.
6. At higher temperatures, the investment must not decompose to give off gases that may corrode the surface of the alloy.
7. It must have adequate strength at room temperature to permit handling, and enough strength at higher temperatures to withstand the impact force of the molten metal.

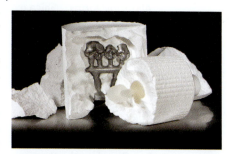

FIGURE 20.1 Cross-section through a mould.

8. Casting temperatures should not be critical.
9. After casting, it should break away readily from the surface of the metal and should not react chemically with it.
10. The material should be economical.

CLASSIFICATION OF REFRACTORY MATERIALS IN DENTISTRY (ISO 15912:2006)

The classification covers all refractory materials in dentistry including casting investment, brazing investments and refractory dies.

A. Classification based on application (ISO 15912:2006)

Type 1: for the construction of inlays, crowns and other fixed restorations

Type 2: for the construction of complete or partial dentures or other removable appliances

Type 3: for the construction of casts used in brazing procedures

Type 4: for the construction of refractory dies

B. Sub-classification based on method of burnout (ISO 15912:2006)

Class 1: recommended for burn-out by a slow- or step-heating method

Class 2: recommended for burn-out by a quick-heating method

C. Classification based on type of binder used

There are three types of investment materials based on the binder used. They all contain silica as the refractory material. The type of binder used is different.

1. *Gypsum bonded investments*   They are used for casting gold alloys. They can withstand temperature up to 700 °C.
2. *Phosphate bonded investments*   For metal ceramic and cobalt-chromium alloys. They can withstand higher temperatures.
3. *Ethyl silica bonded investments*   They are an alternative to the phosphate bonded investments, for high temperature casting. They are principally used in the casting of base metal alloy partial dentures.

GENERAL COMPOSITION OF INVESTMENTS

All investment materials contain a refractory, a binder and modifiers.

REFRACTORY

A refractory is a material that will withstand high temperatures without decomposing or disintegrating, e.g. silica.

Allotropic forms   Silica exists in at least four allotropic forms.

○ Quartz
○ Tridymite
○ Cristobalite
○ Fused quartz

They serve two functions

1. Act as a material that can withstand high temperatures.
2. Regulate the thermal expansion.

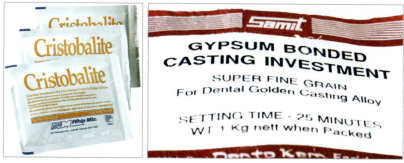

FIGURE 20.2 Representative gypsum bonded investments.

BINDER

A material which will set and bind together the particles of refractory substance, e.g. gypsum, phosphate and silicate. The common binder used for *gold alloys* is dental stone (alpha-hemihydrate). The investments for casting *cobalt chromium alloys* use ethyl silicate, ammonium sulphate or sodium phosphate.

CHEMICAL MODIFIERS

Chemicals such as sodium chloride, boric acid, potassium sulfate, graphite, copper powder or magnesium oxide are added in small quantities to modify properties.

GYPSUM BONDED INVESTMENTS

CLASSIFICATION

The ISO (15912:2006) classification for refractory materials applies to gypsum bonded investments and phosphate bonded investments. Thus, there are four types based on application—Type 1, 2, 3 and 4 and two subclasses—Class 1 and 2 based on method of burnout. (See ISO classification at beginning of chapter for details).

USES

For casting of inlays, fixed partial dentures, removable partial denture frameworks using gold alloys and other low-fusing alloys.

SUPPLIED AS

Powder in bulk or preweighed packs *(Fig. 20.2)*.

Representative commercial products Cristobalite, Novocast (Whipmix), etc.

COMPOSITION

Component	Proportion
Silica	60 to 65%
Alpha-hemihydrate (dental stone)	30 to 35%
Chemical modifiers	5%

* The original name for the standard was 'gypsum bonded investments for gold alloy casting investments.' In the 2001 revision, the limitation to 'gold alloys' was removed.

FUNCTIONS OF CONSTITUENTS

Alpha hemihydrate

- It binds and holds the silica particles together.
- Permits pouring of the mix into the mold.
- It imparts strength to the mold.
- Contributes to mold expansion (by setting expansion).

Silica quartz or cristobalite

- Acts as a refractory during heating.
- Regulates thermal expansion.
- Increases setting expansion of stone.
- Silica in the investment eliminates contraction of gypsum and changes it to an expansion during heating.

Modifiers

- Coloring matter
- *Reducing agents* They reduce any oxides formed on the metal by providing a nonoxidizing atmosphere in the mold when the mold alloy enters, e.g. carbon or copper powder.
- *Modifying chemicals* They regulate setting expansion and setting time and also prevent shrinkage of gypsum when heated above 300 °C, e.g. boric acid and sodium chloride.

MANIPULATION

The measured quantity of powder and water is mixed manually using a flexible rubber bowl and spatula or in a vacuum investment mixing machine.

SETTING REACTION

The setting reaction is similar to dental stone. When the water is mixed, the hemihydrate reacts to form dihydrate which sets to form a solid mass which binds the silica particles together.

SETTING TIME

According to ADA Sp. No. 2 for inlay investments, setting time should not be less than 5 minutes and not more than 25 minutes. The modern inlay investments set initially in 9 to 18 minutes. This provides sufficient time for mixing and investing the pattern.

Factors controlling setting time

1. Manufacturing process
2. Mixing time and rate
3. Water-powder ratio
4. Temperature
5. Modifiers—accelerators and retarders

PROPERTIES OF GYPSUM INVESTMENTS

THERMAL BEHAVIOR OF GYPSUM

When gypsum is heated to a high temperature, it shrinks and fractures. At 700 °C, it shows slight expansion and then great amount of contraction. The shrinkage is due to decomposition and release of sulfur dioxide. It contaminates the casting with the sulfides of silver and copper. So the gypsum bonded investments should not be heated above 700 °C.

THERMAL BEHAVIOR OF SILICA

When heated, quartz or cristobalite changes its *crystalline* form. This occurs at a *transition temperature*, characteristic of the particular form of silica.

○ Quartz when heated, inverts from a 'low' form known as *alpha-quartz* to a 'high' form called as *beta-quartz* at a temperature of 375 °C.

○ Cristobalite similarly when heated, inverts from 'low' or *alpha-cristobalite* to 'high' or *beta-cristobalite* at a temperature between 200 °C and 270 °C.

The beta forms are stable only above the transition temperature. It changes back to the low or alpha-form occurs upon cooling in each case. The density changes (decreases) as alpha-form changes to beta-form, with a resulting increase in volume and a rapid increase in linear expansion.

EXPANSION

Expansion aids in enlarging the mold to compensate for the casting shrinkage of the gold alloys.

Three types of expansions may be seen

1. Normal setting expansion
2. Hygroscopic setting expansion
3. Thermal expansion

Normal setting expansion

A mixture of silica and dental stone results in a setting expansion which is greater than when the gypsum product is used alone. The silica particles probably interfere with the intermeshing of the crystals as they form. Thus, the thrust of the crystals is outward during growth.

ADA Sp. No. 2 for Type-I investment permits a maximum setting expansion in air of 0.5%. Modern investments show setting expansion of 0.4%. It is regulated by retarders and accelerators.

Hygroscopic setting expansion (HSE)

When gypsum products are allowed to set in contact with water, the amount of expansion exhibited is much greater than the normal setting expansion. The increased amount of expansion is because water helps the outward growth of crystals. This expansion is known as hygroscopic setting expansion. The investment should be immersed in water before initial set is complete.

ADA Sp. No. 2 for Type-II investments requires a minimal 1.2% and maximum 2.2% expansion.

Factors affecting hygroscopic setting expansion
1. *Composition*   The finer the particle size of the silica, the greater is the HSE. Alpha-hemihydrate produces a greater expansion than beta-hemihydrate. Higher the silica content, greater is the expansion.
2. *W-P ratio*   The higher the W-P ratio of the original investment water mixture, the less is the HSE.
3. *Temperature*   Higher the temperature of the immersion water, less is the surface tension and hence, greater is the expansion.
4. *Effect of time of immersion*   Immersion before the initial set results in greater expansion.

5. *Spatulation* Shorter the mixing time, the less is the HSE.
6. *Effect of shelf-life of the investment* The older the investment, the less is the hygroscopic expansion.
7. *Confinement* of the investment by the walls of the container or the wax pattern reduces HSE. This effect is much more pronounced on the HSE than on the normal setting expansion.
8. *Effect of the amount of added water* More amount of water added during the setting period, more is the expansion.

Thermal expansion

In case of gypsum investments, thermal expansion (TE) is *achieved by* placing the mold in a furnace at a temperature not greater than 700 °C (the investment breaks down if it exceeds this temperature releasing gases which can contaminate the gold alloys). The thermal expansion behavior of one investment is shown in **Fig. 20.3**.

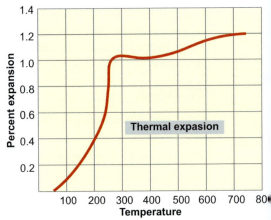

FIGURE 20.3 Thermal expansion of a gypsum bonded investment (Novocast, *Courtesy:* Whipmix Corporation).

The amount of thermal expansion required depends on which method is used for casting shrinkage compensation. If hygroscopic expansion technique is used, then TE of 0.5 to 0.6% is sufficient. But if the compensation is by TE together with normal setting expansion, then the TE should be 1 to 2%.

Type-I investments should have a TE not less than 1 nor greater than 1.6%.

Factors affecting thermal expansion
1. TE is related to the amount and type of silica used.
2. *Effect of the W-P ratio* more the water, less the TE.
3. *Effect of chemical modifiers* Small amounts of sodium chloride, potassium chloride and lithium chloride increases TE and eliminates the contraction caused by gypsum.

STRENGTH

According to ISO 15912:2006, the compressive strength for investments should not be less than 2 MPa when tested 2 hours after setting.

Factors affecting strength
1. Use of alpha-hemihydrate increases compressive strength (than beta-hemihydrate).
2. Use of chemical modifiers increases the strength.
3. More water used during mixing, less is the strength.
4. Heating the investment to 700 °C may increase or decrease strength as much as 65% depending on the composition. The greatest reduction in strength upon heating is found in investments containing sodium chloride.
5. After the investment has cooled to room temperature, its strength decreases considerably because of fine cracks that form during cooling.

POROSITY

The more the gypsum crystals present in the set investment, the less is its porosity. The less the hemihydrate content and greater the amount of gauging water, the more is its porosity. A mixture of coarse and fine particles exhibits less porosity than an investment composed of a uniform particle size (a certain amount of porosity is essential in the mold in order to allow escape of gases during casting).

FINENESS

A fine particle size is preferable to a coarse one. The finer the investment, the smaller will be the surface irregularities on the casting.

STORAGE

Investments should be stored in airtight and moisture proof containers. Purchase in small quantities.

HYGROSCOPIC THERMAL INLAY CASTING INVESTMENT

Investment that can be used as a hygroscopic or thermal type is available (e.g. Beauty cast - Whipmix). The investment contains a blend of quartz and cristobalite as the refractory. For the hygroscopic expansion technique, the investment is heated only up to 482 °C. When the thermal casting technique is used the investment (is not immersed in water but) is heated to 649 °C to achieve expansion.

INVESTMENTS FOR CASTING HIGH MELTING ALLOYS

The metal-ceramic alloys and the cobalt-chromium alloys have high melting temperatures. They are cast in molds at 850 to 1100 °C. At these temperatures, the gypsum bonded investments disintegrates. Hence, investments which can withstand higher temperatures are required. The binders used (phosphate and silicate) in these investments can withstand these high temperatures.

The investments used for this purpose are

o   Phosphate bonded investments
o   Silica bonded investments
o   Magnesia/alumina/zirconia based investments for titanium

PHOSPHATE BONDED INVESTMENT

Phosphate bonded investments are perhaps the most widely utilized investment in dentistry. This is because a substantial amount of cast dental structures today use high fusing noble or base metal alloys.

USES

For casting high fusing alloys, e.g. high fusing noble metal alloys, metal ceramic alloys and base metal alloys like nickel-chromium and cobalt-chromium.

CLASSIFICATION

The ISO (15912:2006) classification for refractory materials applies to phosphate bonded investments also. Thus, there are four types based on application—Type 1, 2, 3 and 4 and two subclasses—Class 1 and 2 based on method of burnout. (See ISO classification at beginning of chapter for details).

SUPPLIED AS

Powder in packets of varying weight with special liquid (*Fig. 20.4*).

COMPOSITION

Powder

Ammonium diacid phosphate $NH_4H_2PO_4$

○ It gives strength at room temperature.

○ It is soluble in water and provides phosphate ions.

○ It reacts with silica at high temperatures to increase strength at casting temperatures.

FIGURE 20.4 Representative phosphate bonded investment. They are mixed with a special liquid.

Silica in the form of quartz or cristobalite (80%) functions as refractory.

Magnesium oxide Reacts with phosphate ions.

Carbon Some investments contain carbon while others are carbon free. Carbon helps to produce clean castings and helps in easier divestment from the mold. For noncompatible alloys carbon free investments are preferred.

Liquid

The phosphate bonded investments are mixed with a special liquid supplied by the manufacturer. This liquid is a form of silica sol in water, which gives higher thermal expansion

SETTING REACTION

At room temperature ammonium diacid phosphate reacts with magnesium oxide to give the investment green strength or room temperature strength.

$$NH_4H_2PO_4 + MgO + 5H_2O \longrightarrow NH_4MgPO_4.H_2O$$

The ammonium diacid phosphate is used in a greater amount than is necessary for the reaction, so that the additional amount can react with silica at an elevated temperature. At higher temperatures, there is probably a superficial reaction between P_2O_5 and SiO_2 to form silicophosphate, which increases the strength of investment at higher temperature.

MANIPULATION

Powder/liquid ratio - 16 to 23 ml/100 gm.

(The liquid is usually diluted with water. The amount of liquid to water ratio varies with the particular brand of investment and type of alloy used. The amount of water used ranges from 0 to 50% depending on the expansion required).

The powder is mixed with a measured amount of liquid using a bowl and spatula. Following hand mixing for 20 seconds mechanical mixing under vacuum is done for a further 90 seconds (*Fig. 20.5*). Working time is around 8-9 minutes. The mixed material is vibrated into the casting ring or agar mold (RPD framework). The material is allowed to bench set for a minimum 30-45 minutes depending

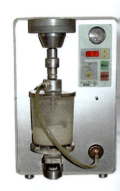

FIGURE 20.5 Vacuum investment mixer.

on the particular investment. Following this the glaze on top of the investment is scraped to allow air escape and reduce back pressure porosity during casting.

Factors affecting setting time

1. Temperature of the mix and environment. Warmer temperatures accelerate the setting. Cooling the liquid prolongs the working time.
2. Increasing the mixing time accelerates the set.
3. An increased L-P ratio delays setting and gives more working time.

PROPERTIES

EXPANSION

As mentioned earlier, expansion of the mold is desirable to compensate for casting shrinkage. Phosphate investments get their expansion from three sources.

1. *Wax pattern expansion*   The heat during setting allows a significant expansion of the wax pattern.
2. *Setting expansion*   This is around 0.7 to 1%.
3. *Thermal expansion*   Ranges from around 1 to 1.5%.

The amount of expansion is adjusted by the manufacturer for each product depending on the alloy it is intended for.

Factors affecting expansion

1. *Special liquid to water ratio*   The liquid has a considerable influence on the setting and thermal expansion of the investment. The greater the concentration of special liquid to water, the greater the thermal and setting expansions *(Fig. 20.6)*.
2. *Powder to liquid ratio*   A greater powder to liquid ratio increases expansion.

Strength

Regular investments are generally materials of low strength. *Wet strength* ranges from 4–10 MPa. Wet strength is important for handling the set material prior to casting. *Dry strength* is the strength of the investment under high temperatures. The investment should have sufficient strength to withstand the casting force of the molten alloy at high temperatures. Studies have shown that there is no correlation between wet and dry strength of phosphate bonded investments. One study indicates that investments exhibit plastic behavior at high

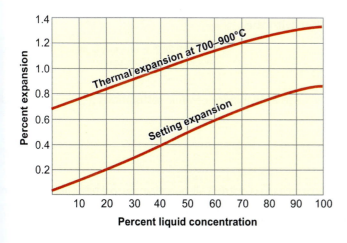

FIGURE 20.6 Influence of liquid to water concentration on the setting and thermal expansion of a phosphate bonded investment (*Courtesy:* Whip-mix Corporation).

temperatures which, under casting pressure, may be a source of inaccurate casting, a hitherto unrecognized source of error.

Thermal reactions

Phosphate bonded investments undergo thermochemical reactions when heated to high temperatures. The silica portion remains essentially unchanged. However the binder goes through various phases. On heating, the material initially dehydrates to $(NH_4MgPO_4.H_2O)_n$. Subsequently, it degrades into polymeric $(Mg_2P_2O_7)_n$, crystalline $Mg_2P_2O_7$; then the latter reacts with excess MgO present to form the final product, $Mg_3(PO_4)_2$.

Flow

Investments appear to have low flow when mixed. However, they flow readily and envelope the pattern when poured into the mold under vibration. Therefore, use of a vibrator is recommended. Surface tension reducing agents are available and should be used on the wax pattern to improve wetting.

Surface smoothness

Early phosphate investments produced rough castings when compared to gypsum based investments. Current investments have improved and now approach surface smoothness comparable to that of gypsum bonded investments.

SPECIALIZED REFRACTORY MATERIALS

PHOSPHATE BONDED REFRACTORY CASTS FOR RPDS (TYPE 2)

A refractory cast is a special cast made from a heat resistant (investment) material. Such casts are used in the fabrication of certain large metal structures like cast removable partial dentures. Small wax structures like inlays, crowns and small fixed dental prostheses (FDP) can be constructed on a regular die as it can be removed from the die without significant distortion and invested separately. However, larger wax structures like that for the cast RPD, would distort if removed from the cast. RPD patterns are best constructed on a refractory cast *(Fig. 20.7)*. The pattern is invested together with the refractory cast.

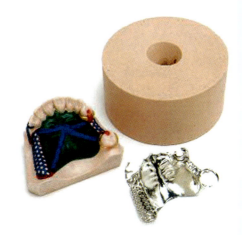

FIGURE 20.7 Refractory casts with pattern and metal casting of the same.

INVESTMENTS FOR CERAMICS

Phosphate based investments are also available for ceramic restorations (e.g. Polyvest and VHT - Whipmix, *Fig. 20.8)*.

Types

Two types are available

1. Those used as refractory dies or casts to construct all-porcelain restorations like porcelain veneers and porcelain jacket crowns (ISO 11245). Two varieties are seen based on expansion.

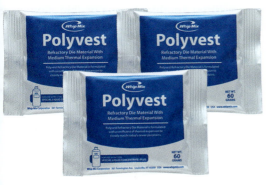
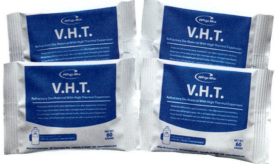

FIGURE 20.8 Representative phosphate bonded investment used for construction of ceramic restorations.

- – *Medium expansion*—Originally used for the cast glass technique. Currently used with medium expanding porcelains like Finesse, Ceramco Veneer, Duceram (Dentsply), Vita-VMK 68, Halo (3M), Noritake EX 3, etc. Example Polyvest.
- – *High expansion*—The second type is used with high expansion porcelains like Optec-HSP/VP (Jeneric/Pentron Inc.), Wil-Ceram (Williams Dental Co.), Excelco (Ney), Creation (Jensen).

2. The second type is used with heat pressed ceramics **(Figs. 20.9A to C)**. *It is not used as a die, rather,* it is used to surround the wax pattern for the heat pressing process.

Properties

These are fine-grained phosphate investment with a working time of 2–5 minutes. Unlike regular refractory materials, these can withstand repeated firings at furnace temperatures of up to 1200 °C without disintegrating. They can be used with high-expanding porcelains because of their compatible CTEs.

INVESTMENTS FOR TITANIUM CASTINGS

Conventional silica (SiO_2) based dental casting investments are used for the casting of pure titanium using casting machines specifically developed for this metal. Highly reactive molten

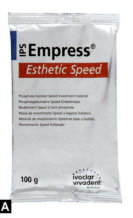
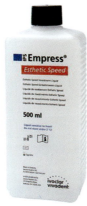
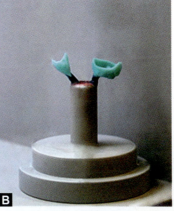
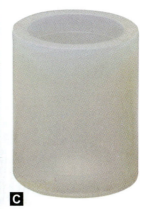

FIGURES 20.9A TO C (A) Phosphate bonded investment for heat pressed ceramics. **(B)** Wax pattern attached to sprue former. **(C)** Wax pattern is placed inside the silicone mould former into which the investment is poured.

titanium reduces SiO_2 and titanium is, in turn, oxidized. For this reason possible alternative to SiO_2 have been studied in the past decade and *MgO* (magnesia) and Al_2O_3 (alumina) are the most common in current commercial investments released for titanium casting. The surface of titanium castings presents a layered structure and its evaluation in relation to clinical performance requires further study especially in relation to the setting and thermal behavior of newly developed investments for successful compensation of metal shrinkage.

SILICA BONDED INVESTMENTS

The silica is the binder. It is derived from ethyl silicate or aqueous dispersion of colloidal silica or sodium silicate. These are less commonly used.

TYPES

Based on the binder used two types may be seen. One such investment consists of silica refractory, which is bonded by the hydrolysis of ethyl silicate in the presence of hydrochloric acid. The product of the hydrolysis is the formation of a colloidal solution of silicic acid and ethyl alcohol.

$$Si(OC_2H_5)_4 + 4H_2 \xrightarrow{HCl} Si(OH)_4 + 4C_2H_5OH$$

Ethyl silicate has the disadvantage of containing inflammable components which are required for manufacture.

Sodium silicate and *colloidal silica* are more commonly used as binders because of the above disadvantage. These investments are supplied along with *two bottles* of special liquid. One bottle contains dilute water-soluble *silicate solution* such as sodium silicate. The other bottle usually contains diluted acid solution such as *hydrochloric acid (Fig. 20.10)*.

MANIPULATION

The content of each bottle can be stored indefinitely. Before use, equal volume of each bottle is mixed so that hydrolysis can take place and freshly prepared silicic acid is formed. The powder/liquid ratio is according to manufacturer's instruction.

BRAZING (SOLDERING) INVESTMENT

In the process of assembling the parts of a restoration by soldering *(Fig. 20.11)*, such as clasps on a removable partial denture, it is necessary to surround the parts with a suitable ceramic or investment *(Figs. 20.12A and B)*.

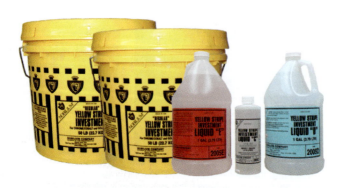

FIGURE 20.10 Ethyl silicate bonded investment by Nobilium.

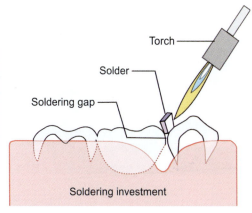

FIGURE 20.11 Soldering procedure.

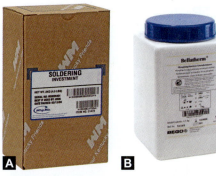

FIGURES 20.12A AND B Soldering investments.
(A) Gypsum bonded. **(B)** Phosphate bonded.

USES

1. Joining segments of fixed partial dentures *(Fig 20.11)*.
2. Fixing clasps on cast RPDs.
3. Attaching precision attachments.

TYPES

Based on the type of binder used brazing investments are of two types.

1. Gypsum-bonded (for low melting alloys, e.g. Hi Heat, Whipmix, etc.) *(Fig. 20.12A)*
2. Phosphate-bonded (for high melting alloys), e.g. Bellatherm (Bego) *(Fig. 20.12B)*.

COMPOSITION

The investment for soldering purpose is similar to casting investments containing quartz and a calcium sulfate hemihydrate/or phosphate binder.

PROPERTIES

Soldering investments are designed to have *lower setting (0.2%) and thermal expansions (0.6–1%)* than casting investments, a feature that is desirable so that the assembled parts do not shift position. Soldering investments do not have as fine a particle size as the casting investment, since the smoothness of the mass is less important. The compressive strength is generally low (between 2 to 10 MPa). Water-powder ratio ranges from 0.24 to 0.28. Setting time ranges from 15 to 20 minutes.

PROCEDURE

The parts are temporarily held together with sticky wax until they are surrounded with the appropriate investment material, after which the wax is removed. The portion to be soldered is left exposed and free from investment to permit removal of the wax and effective heating before being joined with solder *(Fig. 20.11)*. After setting, the material must be completely dry before soldering. Recommended drying temperature varies between 400 to 450 °C.

Dental Casting and Metal Fabrication Procedures

The process of casting has been known since ancient times *(Box 21.1)*. Casting is the most commonly used method for the fabrication of metal structures (inlays, crowns, partial denture frames, etc.) outside the mouth. A pattern of the structure is first made in wax. This is then surrounded by an investment material. After the investment hardens, the wax is removed (burnt out) leaving a space or mould. Molten alloy is forced into this mould. The resulting structure is an accurate duplication of the original wax pattern. However, casting is not the only way of fabricating restorations and prostheses in dentistry.

METAL RESTORATIONS IN DENTISTRY

There are many ways of fabricating a metallic restoration in dentistry.

1. Direct restorations (e.g. direct filling gold and amalgam)
2. Casting (e.g. cast crowns, posts, inlays, partial denture frames, etc.)
3. Foil adaptation and sintering * (e.g. CAPTEK crowns)
4. Electroforming

* Refer chapter on dental ceramics also

BOX 21.1   Evolution of casting process

Since its discovery, metal casting has played a critical role in the development and advancement of human cultures and civilization. The art of casting metal has been known to man since 4000 BC. Mesopotamia is generally accepted as the birthplace of castings. The first metal to be cast was copper because of its low melting point.

Furnaces The earliest furnace were simple and easy to operate, with beeswax used for patterns and bellows for blowing air into the furnace. In the iron age probably ceramic ovens were used to melt the metals. Crucible and later flame ovens were available for the melting of copper, tin and lead alloys.

Molds Different types of molds made from sand, stone, limestone and sun-baked clay were known from the early times.

Patterns The lost form technique was also prevalently used from the early times. The first patterns of casting were made probably 4000 years in Mesopotamia from beeswax. The oldest known examples of the lost-wax technique are the objects discovered in the Cave of the Treasure (Nahal Mishmar) hoard in southern Israel, and which belong to the Chalcolithic period (4500–3500 BCE).

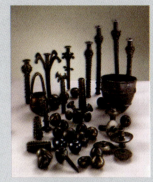

Objects from Cave of Treasure (Nahal Mishmar), Southern Israel, c. 3700 BCE.

The lost-wax method is well documented in ancient Indian literary sources. The Shilpa shastras, a text from the Gupta Period (c. 320-550 CE), contains detailed information about casting images in metal.

9000 BCE	Earliest metal objects of wrought native copper Near East
5000–3000 BCE	Chalcolithic period: melting of copper; experimentation with smelting in the Near East
3000–1500 BCE	Bronze Age: Copper and tin bronze alloys—Near East and India
2400–2200 BCE	Copper statue of Pharoah Pepi I Egypt
2000 BCE	Bronze Age Far East
1500 BCE	Iron Age (wrought iron) Ganga valley, India
1100 BCE	Discovery of wrought steel 11th century BCE
600 BCE	Iron cast in China
500 CE	Steel casting in India
400 CE	Zinc extraction in India. Distillation technique developed in 1200 CE in India (Zawar, Rajasthan.)

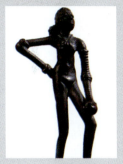

Bronze dancing girl, Indus valley, (c. 3300–1300 BCE)

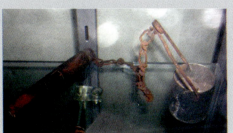

A 19th century hand powered centrifugal casting machine

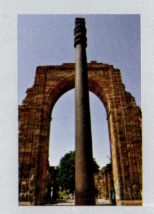

Oldest iron pillar (circa 400 BCE) Ashoka's Pillar, New Delhi, India remains unrusted for 24 centuries

5. Machining (subtractive fabrication)
    – Prefabricated posts
    – CAD/CAM
    – Copy milling
    – Electrical discharge machining.
6. Three-dimensional printing (additive fabrication).

CASTING

Many dental restorations are made by casting, e.g., inlays, crowns, removable partial denture frameworks, etc.

Casting can be *defined as* the act of forming an object in a mold *(GPT-8)*. The object formed is also referred to as 'a casting'.

STEPS IN MAKING A SMALL CAST RESTORATION

Casting is a complex process involving a number of steps and equipment. A restoration having a perfect fit is possible only if we have a good understanding of the techniques and materials used in casting. Given below are the series of steps involved in the fabrication of a simple full metal crown.

- Tooth/teeth preparation
- Impression
- Die preparation
- Wax pattern fabrication
- Attachment of sprue former
- Ring liner placement
- Assembly of casting ring
- Investing
- Burn out or wax elimination
- Casting
- Sand blasting and recovery
- Finishing and polishing.

The procedures vary slightly depending on the type of restoration. Construction of larger structures like a removable partial denture frame involve additional steps like duplication.

TOOTH/TEETH PREPARATION

The teeth are prepared by the dentist to receive a cast restoration. Care is taken to avoid undercuts in the preparation that may prevent seating. An accurate impression of the tooth/teeth is made, usually with elastomers.

DIE PREPARATION

A die is prepared from die stone or a suitable die material or the impression is electroformed.

DIE SPACER

A die spacer is coated or painted over the die which provides space for the luting cement *(Figs. 21.1A and B)*. The relief provided also improves seating of the casting.

WAX PATTERN

A pattern of the final restoration is made with type II inlay wax *(Fig. 21.2A)* or other casting waxes with all precautions to avoid distortion. Before making the pattern, a die lubricant is applied to help separate the wax pattern from the die.

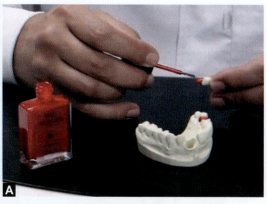
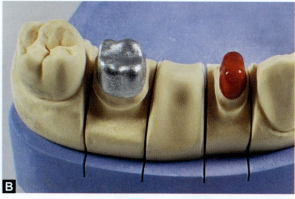

FIGURES 21.1A AND B (A) Application of die spacer. **(B)** Close-up view of the spacer coated die. Two types of spacers are visible.

SPRUE FORMER

A sprue former is made of wax, plastic or metal. The thickness is in proportion to the wax pattern. A reservoir is attached to the sprue or the attachment of the sprue to the wax pattern is flared. The length of the sprue is adjusted so that the wax pattern is approximately 1/4″ from the other end of the ring *(Fig. 21.3)*.

FUNCTIONS OF SPRUE FORMER/SPRUE

1. To form a mount for the wax pattern.
2. To create a channel for the elimination of wax during burnout.
3. Forms a channel for entry of molten alloy during casting.
4. Provides a reservoir of molten metal which compensates for alloy shrinkage during solidification.

CASTING RING LINING

A ring liner is placed inside of the casting ring. It should be short at one end. Earlier asbestos liners were used. Its use has been discontinued due to health hazard from breathing its dust.

TYPES OF NONASBESTOS RING LINERS

1. Fibrous ceramic aluminous silicate
2. Cellulose (paper)
3. Ceramic-cellulose combination *(Fig. 21.2B)*.

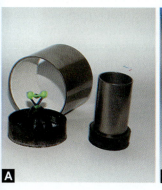
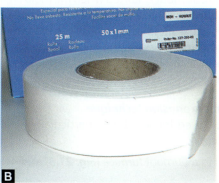

FIGURES 21.2A AND B (A) A rubber crucible former with attached wax pattern and casting rings. **(B)** Ring liner.

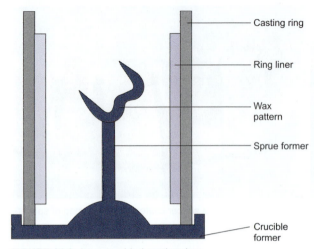

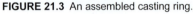

FIGURE 21.3 An assembled casting ring.

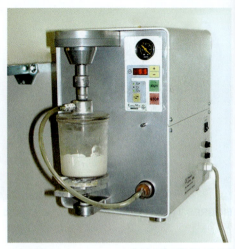

FIGURE 21.4 A vacuum investment mixer.

FUNCTIONS OF THE RING LINER

1. Allows for mold expansion (cushion effect).
2. When the ring is transferred from the furnace to the casting machine it reduces heat loss as it is a thermal insulator.
3. Permits easy removal of the investment after casting.

INVESTING

Apply wetting agent (to reduce air bubbles) on the wax pattern. Seat the casting ring into the crucible former taking care that it is located near the center of the ring *(Fig. 21.3)*. Mix the investment (in a vacuum mixer, *Fig. 21.4*) and vibrate. Some investment is applied on the wax pattern with a brush to reduce trapping air bubbles. The ring is reseated on the crucible former and placed on the vibrator and gradually filled with the remaining investment mix. It is allowed to set for 1 hour.

WAX ELIMINATION (BURNOUT) AND THERMAL EXPANSION

The *purpose* of burnout is

1. To eliminate the wax (pattern) from the mold.
2. To expand the mold (thermal expansion).

The crucible former is separated from the ring. If a metallic sprue former is used, it should be removed before burnout. Burnout is started when the mold is *wet*. If burnout has to be delayed the mold is stored in a humidor. The heating should be *gradual*. Rapid heating produces steam which causes the walls of the mold cavity to flake. In extreme cases an explosion may occur. Rapid heating can also cause cracks in the investment due to uneven expansion. It is very important to follow the investment manufacturer's technique regarding time and temperature for burnout and expansion.

Two stage burnout and expansion technique
This technique may be used for wax but is particularly indicated if the patterns or sprue formers contain plastic.

○ The ring is placed in a *burnout furnace (Fig. 21.5)* and heated gradually to 400 °C in 20 minutes.

○ Maintain it for 30 minutes.

○ Over the next 30 minutes, the temperature is raised to 700 °C and maintained for a further 30 minutes.

Single stage burnout and expansion (Rapid technique)

This technique is followed only if patterns and sprues are wax

○ Place molds directly into preheated oven at 700–850 °C (if higher temperature is warranted, place mold in preheated oven at 370 °C and then raise to final temperature).

○ Hold for 30–40 minutes and cast.

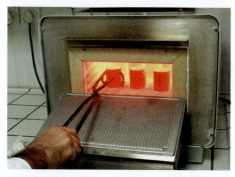

FIGURE 21.5 Wax elimination and thermal expansion of mold

The casting should be completed as soon as the ring is ready. If casting is delayed the ring cools and the investment contracts. The crown becomes smaller.

CASTING-PROCESS AND EQUIPMENT

It is the process by which molten alloy is forced into the heated investment mold.

CASTING MACHINES

Based on method of casting the machines are

1. Centrifugal force type
2. Air pressure type

Centrifugal machines may be spring driven or motor driven (*Fig. 21.6*). The main advantage of the centrifugal machines is the simplicity of design and operation, with the opportunity to cast both large and small castings on the same machine.

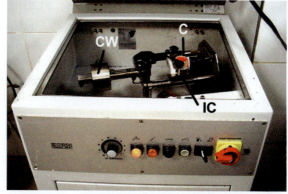

FIGURE 21.6 An induction casting machine. The molten metal is driven into the mold by centrifugal force. One arm of the machine has a counter weight (CW) which balances the weight of the arm carrying the crucible and mold as it rotates. The red hot crucible (C) and the casting ring is visible in the machine. The induction coil (IC—copper colored) is half visible and is used to melt the metal.

In air pressure type of machine, either compressed air or gases like carbon dioxide or nitrogen, can be used to force the molten metal into the mold. This type of machine is satisfactory for making small castings. This machine does not have vibration and high noise levels owing to the pressure casting and water cooling method. Some systems use argon gas to protect the alloy from oxidation (especially useful for melting titanium, *Fig. 21.10*).

Attached vacuum system   Casting machines (both centrifugal and gas pressure type) with attached vacuum system are available. The vacuum creates a negative pressure within the mold, which helps to draw the alloy into the mold.

Casting machines can also be grouped based on heating system employed

1. Torch melted (*Fig. 21.7*)
2. Induction melted (*Fig. 21.6*)
3. Arc melted.

Numerous combinations of these principles are employed in different machines.

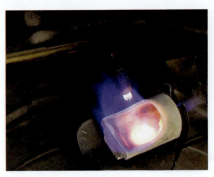

FIGURE 21.7 Flame melting.

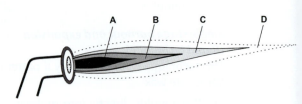

FIGURE 21.8 Parts of the flame **(A)** Mixing zone. **(B)** Combustion zone. **(C)** Reducing zone. **(D)** Oxidizing zone.

Torch melting

The fuel used is a combination of

o Natural or artificial gas and air, or

o Oxygen and acetylene gas (high fusion alloys).

The flame has four zones **(Fig. 21.8)**

A. *Mixing zone*   Air and gas are mixed here. No heat is present. It is dark in color.

B. *Combustion zone*   This surrounds the inner zone. It is green in color. It is a zone of partial combustion and has an oxidizing nature.

C. *Reducing zone*   It is a blue zone just beyond the green zone. It is the hottest part of the flame. This zone is used for the fusion of the casting alloy.

D. *Oxidizing zone*   Outermost zone in which final combustion between the gas and surrounding air occurs. This zone is not used for fusion.

The air and gas mixture is adjusted to get a reducing flame, which is used to melt the alloy **(Fig. 21.7)**. A reducing flame is preferred as it does not contaminate the alloy and is the hottest part of the flame.

Induction melting

Heating through induction is a common method of melting dental alloys today **(Figs. 21.6 and 21.9)**. Induction heating is the process of heating an electrically conducting object (usually a metal) by electromagnetic induction, where eddy currents are generated within the metal and resistance leads to Joule heating of the metal. An induction heater consists of an electromagnet, through which a high-frequency alternating current (AC) is passed. Induction melting is useful for melting high fusing alloys like metal-ceramic and base metal alloys.

Arc melting

Alloys may also be melted by a process known as arc melting. Arc melting is used to melt industrial alloys like steel. Direct current is passed between two electrodes—a tungsten electrode and the alloy. Arc melting produces very high temperatures and is used to melt high fusion metals like titanium **(Fig. 21.10)**. Arc melting may be done under vacuum or in an inert atmosphere like argon.

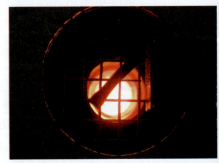

FIGURE 21.9 Induction melting. White hot molten alloy in crucible surrounded by the induction coil.

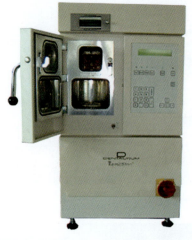

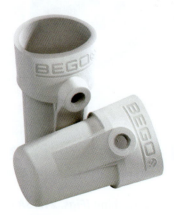

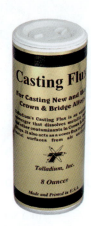

FIGURE 21.10 Titanium casting machine (Dentaurum).   **FIGURE 21.11** Casting crucible.   **FIGURE 21.12** Casting flux.

Crucibles

The crucible is a heat resistant container *(Fig. 21.11)* in which the alloy is melted prior to casting. Four types of casting crucibles are available. These are clay, carbon, quartz and ceramic. In dentistry, quartz or ceramic crucibles are commonly preferred as some alloys may be sensitive to carbon contamination. These include palladium-silver and nickel or cobalt based alloys.

Casting

The alloy is melted with the suitable heat source. *Flux powder (Fig. 21.12)* may be sprinkled over the molten metal to reduce the oxides and increase fluidity for casting. When the alloy is molten it has a *mirror-like* appearance and shifts like a ball of mercury. The hot casting ring is shifted from the burnout furnace to the casting machine. The ring is placed in the casting cradle so that the sprue hole adjoins the crucible. The crucible is solid and placed against the ring to avoid spilling of molten metal. The arm is released and allowed to rotate. This creates a centrifugal force which forces the liquid metal into the mold cavity. The arm is allowed to rotate till it comes to rest. The ring is allowed to cool for 10 minutes till the glow of the metal disappears.

QUENCHING (FOR GOLD ALLOYS)

The ring is then immersed into water. This leaves the cast metal in an annealed (softened) condition and also helps to fragment the investment. Metal-ceramic alloys and base metal alloys are not quenched.

RECOVERY OF CASTING

The investment is removed and the casting recovered. A *pneumatic* (compressed air driven) *chisel* may be used to remove the investment. Final bits of investment is removed by sandblasting.

SANDBLASTING

Sandblasting is the process by which particles of an abrasive (usually aluminum oxide) is projected at high velocity using compressed air in a continuous stream. The casting is held

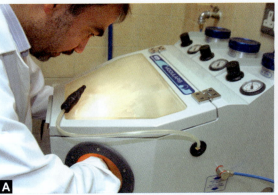
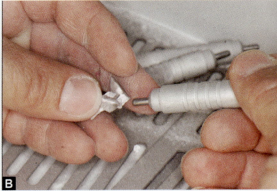

FIGURES 21.13A AND B (A) Sandblasting in progress. (B) Close-up of sandblasting.

in a sandblasting machine *(Figs. 21.13A and B)* to clean the remaining investment from its surface.

PICKLING

Surface oxides (e.g. black castings) from the casting are removed by pickling in 50% hydrochloric acid. HCl is heated but not boiled with the casting in it (done for gold alloys). Pickling is not a routine procedure and is performed only when indicated. Care should be exercised when handling strong acids.

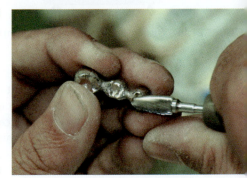

FIGURE 21.14 Casting trimmed with a carbide bur

TRIMMING

The sprue is sectioned off with a cutting disc. The casting is trimmed, shaped and smoothed with suitable burs or stones *(Fig. 21.14)*.

POLISHING

Minimum polishing is required if all the procedures from the wax pattern to casting are followed meticulously (see abrasives chapter).

CASTING DEFECTS

A casting defect is an irregularity in the metal casting process that is very undesired. Errors in the procedure often results in defective castings. The casting in such a case may not fit or may have poor esthetic and mechanical properties.

TYPES OF CASTING DEFECTS

The casting should be a replica of the pattern created in size, texture and form. Casting failures usually result from a failure to observe proper technique. Casting defects are difficult to classify because the causes and effects can often overlap.

The casting defects may be classified as
A. Metal excess (nodules, fins, larger castings, etc.)
B. Metal deficiency (smaller casting, incomplete casting, porosity, etc.)

C.   Distortion of the casting

D.   Chemical contamination of the casting

Trapped bubbles on the mold surface or cracks in the investment usually result in nodules or fins on the casting. Trapped air or shrinkage within the metal result in various types of porosity or voids in the metal.

Casting defects may be described as follows

1.   Casting size mismatch
2.   Distortion
3.   Surface roughness
4.   Nodules
5.   Fins
6.   Porosity
7.   Incomplete casting
8.   Contaminated casting

CASTING SIZE MISMATCH

The restoration should retain its dimensions after casting. Thus the casting may be

1.   Too small
2.   Too large

Casting size problems affect the fit of the restoration. Dimension related problems are usually related to improper technique and a failure to understand the properties of the materials involved in fabricating the restoration. Dimensional changes can occur at almost every stage of the restorative process starting with the impression procedure itself. Metal inherently shrinks on cooling and should be compensated for by proper matching of the alloy to the investment and technique.

DISTORTION

Distortion of the casting is usually due to distortion of wax pattern.

❍   Some distortion of wax occurs when the investment hardens or due to hygroscopic and setting expansion. It does not cause serious problems.

❍   Some distortion occurs during manipulation due to the release of stresses.

Wax distortion is minimized by

❍   Manipulation of wax at high temperature.

❍   Investing pattern within one hour after finishing.

❍   If storage is necessary, store in refrigerator.

SURFACE ROUGHNESS

Surface irregularities can range from surface roughness *(Fig. 21.15)* to larger nodules and fins.

Causes of surface roughness

1.   *Type of investment*   Phosphate bonded investments tend to have greater surface roughness when compared to gypsum bonded investments.

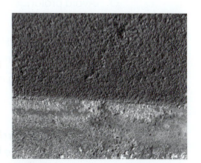

FIGURE 21.15 Surface roughness.

2. *Composition of the investment*   Proportion of the quartz and binder influences the surface texture of casting. Coarse silica produces coarse castings.
3. *Particle size of investment*   Larger particle size of investment produces coarse castings.
4. *Improper W-P ratio*   A higher W-P ratio gives rougher casting.
   - *Minimized by* using correct W/P ratio and investment of correct particle size.
5. Prolonged heating causes disintegration of the mold cavity.
   - *Minimized by* complete the casting as soon as the ring is heated and ready.
6. Overheating of gold alloy has the same effect. It disintegrates the investment.
7. Too high or too low casting pressure.
   - *Minimized by* using 15 lbs/sq inch of air pressure or three to four turns of centrifugal casting machine.
8. Foreign body inclusion shows sharp, well-defined deficiencies. Inclusion of flux shows as bright concavities.

SURFACE NODULES

Nodules *(Fig. 21.16)* on the inner surface of a casting can affect the fit of the restoration. They are usually caused by air or gas bubbles trapped on the wax pattern.

Minimized by

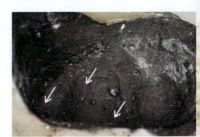

○ Proper mixing of investment
○ Vibration of mix
○ Vacuum investing
○ Painting of a think layer of investment on the pattern
○ Application of wetting agent

FIGURE 21.16 Nodules on the inner surface of a crown.

FIN

Fins are narrow raised areas on a casting usually corresponding to a crack in the investment *(Fig. 21.17)*. Molten alloy fills and solidifies in these cracks resulting in fins. Cracks are usually caused by weak investment or too rapid a heating of the investment.

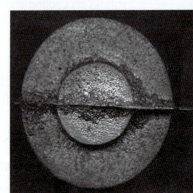

Minimized by

○ Proper water powder ratio for improved strength of investment.

FIGURE 21.17 Fins in casting.

○ Avoid prolonged and rapid heating of the mold. Heat the ring gradually to 700 °C (in at least 1 hour).
○ Proper spruing so as to prevent direct impact of the molten metal at an angle of 90°.
○ Allow the investment adequate time to set properly. Avoid premature use.
○ Careful handling of the mold to prevent it from dropping or impacting.

POROSITY

Porosity may be internal or external. External porosity can cause *discoloration* of the casting. Severe porosity at the tooth restoration interphase can even cause *secondary caries*. Internal porosity *weakens* the restoration.

Types of porosities

1. Those caused by solidification shrinkage
   - Localized shrinkage porosity
   - Suck back porosity (Irregular in shape)
   - Microporosities
2. Those caused by gas
   - Pin hole porosity
   - Gas inclusions (Usually spherical in shape)
   - Subsurface porosity
3. Those caused by air trapped in the mold (back pressure porosity)

Shrink-spot or localized shrinkage porosity

These are large irregular voids usually found near the sprue-casting junction *(Fig. 21.18)*. It occurs when the cooling sequence is incorrect and the sprue *freezes before* the rest of the casting. During a correct cooling sequence, the sprue should freeze last. This allows more molten metal to flow into the mold to compensate for the shrinkage of the casting as it solidifies. If the sprue solidifies before the rest of the casting no more molten metal can be supplied from the sprue. The subsequent shrinkage produces voids or pits known as shrink-spot porosity.

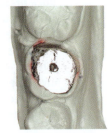

FIGURE 21.18 Localized shrink-spot porosity.

Avoid by

○ Using sprue of correct thickness.

○ Attach sprue to thickest portion of wax pattern.

○ Flaring the sprue at the point of attachment or placing a reservoir close to the wax pattern.

Suck back porosity

It is a variation of the shrink spot porosity. This is an external void usually seen in the inside of a crown opposite the sprue. A hot spot is created by the hot metal impinging on the mold wall near the sprue which causes this region to freeze last. Since the sprue has already solidified, no more molten material is available and the resulting shrinkage causes a type of shrinkage called suck back porosity *(Figs. 21.19A to C)*. It is avoided by reducing the temperature difference between the mold and the molten alloy.

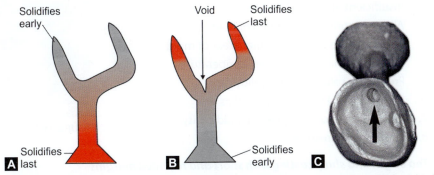

FIGURES 21.19A TO C Suck back porosity. **(A)** Correct sequence of hardening. **(B)** Suck back porosity caused by incorrect sequence of solidification. **(C)** Suck back porosity in a casting.

Microporosity

These are fine irregular voids within the casting. It is seen when the casting cools too rapidly. Rapid solidification occurs when the mold or casting temperature is too low.

Pin hole porosity

Many metals *dissolve gases* when molten. Upon solidification the dissolved gases are expelled causing tiny voids, e.g. platinum and palladium absorb hydrogen. Copper and silver dissolve oxygen.

Gas inclusion porosities

Gas inclusion porosities are also spherical voids but are larger than the pin hole type. They may also be due to dissolved gases, but are more likely due to gases carried in or trapped by the molten metal. A poorly adjusted blow torch can also occlude gases.

Back pressure porosity

This is caused by inadequate venting of the mold. Air is trapped in the mold and is unable to escape. The sprue pattern length should be adjusted so that there is not more than 1/4" thickness of the investment between the bottom of the casting ring and the wax pattern. When the molten metal enters the mold, the air inside is pushed out through the porous investment at the bottom. If the bulk of the investment is too great, the escape of air becomes difficult causing increased pressure in the mold. The gold will then solidify before the mold is completely filled resulting in a *porous* casting with *rounded short margins*.

Avoided by

○ Using adequate casting force.
○ Use investment of adequate porosity.
○ Place pattern not more than 6 to 8 mm away from the end of the ring.
○ Providing vents in large castings.

Casting with gas blow holes

If there is any *wax residue* remaining in the mold, it gives off a large volume of gas as the molten alloy enters the mold cavity. This gas can cause deficiencies in the casting and blow holes in the residue button. To help eliminate wax completely from the mold, the burnout should be done with the sprue hole facing downwards for the wax to run down.

INCOMPLETE CASTING

An incomplete casting **(Fig. 21.20)** may result when

1. Insufficient alloy used.
2. Alloy not sufficiently molten or fluid.
3. Alloy not able to enter thinner areas of mold.
4. Mold is not heated to proper temperature.
5. Premature solidification of alloy.
6. Sprue blocked with foreign bodies.
7. Back pressure due to gases in mold cavity.
8. Low casting pressure.

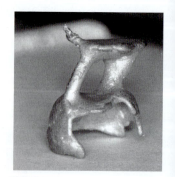

FIGURE 21.20 Incomplete casting.

Too bright and shiny casting with short and rounded margins

When the wax is not completely eliminated, it combines with oxygen or air in the mold cavity forming carbon monoxide which is a reducing agent. The gas prevents the oxidation of the surface of the casting gold with the result that the casting which comes out from the investment is bright and shiny. The formation of gas in the mold is so rapid that it also has a back pressure effect.

Small casting
If compensation for shrinkage of alloy is not done by adequate expansion of mold cavity, then a small casting will result. Another reason is the shrinkage of the impression material.

CONTAMINATION

A casting can be contaminated due to

1. Oxidation, caused by
   - Overheating the alloy
   - Use of oxidizing zone of flame
   - Failure to use flux
2. Sulfur compounds, formed by the breakdown of the investment when the ring is overheated (see black casting below).
   Avoid by
   - Not overheating alloy
   - Use reducing zone of the flame
   - Use flux

Black casting
Can be due to two reasons.

1. Overheating the investment above 700 °C causes it to decompose liberating sulfur or sulfur compounds. They readily combine with the metals in gold alloy forming a sulfide film. This gives a dark casting which cannot be cleaned by pickling.
2. A black casting can be also due to incomplete elimination of the wax pattern, as a result of heating the mold at too low temperature. A carbonized wax remains which sticks to the surface of the casting. It can be removed by heating over a flame.

OTHER METHODS OF FABRICATING RESTORATIONS AND PROSTHESES

1. Capillary casting (foil adaptation and sintering)
2. Electroforming
3. Machining (subtractive fabrication)
4. CAD/CAM
5. Copy milling
6. Electrical discharge machining
7. Three-dimensional printing (additive fabrication).

CAPILLARY CASTING TECHNIQUE (CAPTEK)

Adapting and sintering gold alloy foils (Renaissance and Captek) is a novel way of making a metal frame without having to cast it. The system was developed by Shoher and Whiteman and introduced to the dental community in 1993. Captek is an acronym for 'capillary casting technique'.

MODE OF SUPPLY

They are supplied as thin metal impregnated wax like elastic strips in two forms called Captek P and Captek G *(Figs. 21.21A to E)*. Captek P is platinum-colored strips. Captek G contains 97.5% Gold and 2.5% Silver. Captek P contains platinum, palladium and gold powder.

CAPILLARY CASTING

Captek P (Platinum/Palladium/Gold) has a porous structure and serves as the internal reinforcing skeleton.

On heating in a furnace, the Captek P acts like a metal sponge and draws in (capillary action) the hot liquid gold completely into it. Captek G provides the characteristic gold color of this system. The final coping can be described as a composite structure *(Figs. 21.22A and B)*.

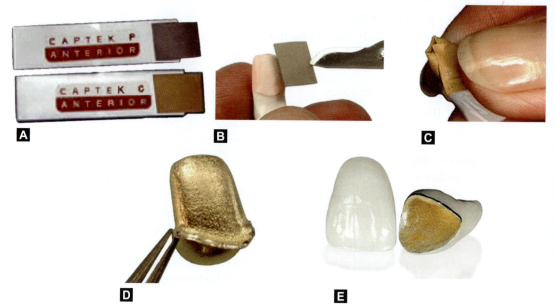

FIGURES 21.21A TO E Fabrication of Captek restorations. **(A)** Captek P and G. **(B)** Adapting captek P. **(C)** Adapting captek G. **(D)** Completed coping. **(E)** Completed crowns.

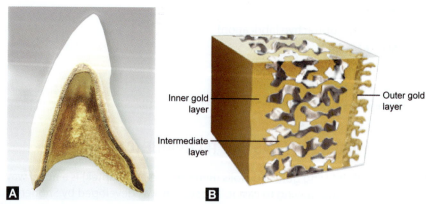

FIGURES 21.22A AND B Captek crown. **(A)** Cross-section through a Captek crown showing the composite structure. **(B)** Closeup of composite structure of Captek coping.

OVERALL COMPOSITION AFTER CAPILLARY CASTING

Captek—88.2% Gold, 4% platinum, 5% palladium, 2.8% silver

COPING THICKNESS

Anterior — 0.25 mm

Posterior — 0.35 mm.

COPING MICROSTRUCTURE

After sintering each coping is structured of three layers *(Figs. 21.22 A and B)*.

○ Inner and outer layers are 25 μm thick with a bright gold color.

○ Intermediate layer is a gold-platinum composite structure.

TECHNIQUE (FIG. 21.21)

1. A refractory die is made after duplicating the original die.
2. An adhesive is painted on to the die.
3. Strips of Captek P are cut and adapted to the die by hand instruments and light pressure. Care should be taken while adapting as the material tears and breaks easily.
4. The Captek P layer is fused in a furnace at 1075°C. This eliminates the adhesive and binders and fuses the platinum and palladium to form a porous interconnected structure.
5. Next the Captek G layer is adapted and again heated in the furnace to induce melting and infusion.
6. The composite coping is divested and trimmed.
7. Capfil and Capcon are used to form the connector when making Captek bridges.
8. A thin layer of gold slurry called Capbond - (composition similar to Captek G) is coated on to the coping. Capbond is a ceramometal bonder. It improves bonding to ceramic and also replenishes areas of the coping that have been trimmed away.
9. Opaquer and the various layers of porcelain are then condensed and fired to form the final crown.

Advantages

1. The thinner foil alloy coping allows a greater thickness of ceramic, thereby, improving the esthetics.
2. The gold color of the alloy improves the esthetics of the restoration.
3. Less reduction of tooth structure.
4. The nonesthetic high intensity high value opaquer layer seen with conventional metal ceramics is eliminated.

CAD/CAM MILLING

Dental copings, crowns and FDP frameworks also can be machined from metal blanks *(Fig. 21.23 and 21.24)* via computer-aided designing and computer-aided machining (CAD/CAM). The process is similar to that described for ceramics.

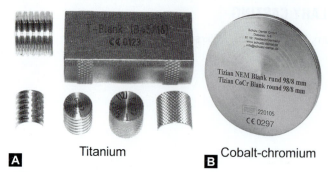

Titanium Cobalt-chromium

A **B**

FIGURES 21.23A AND B CAD/CAM blanks.

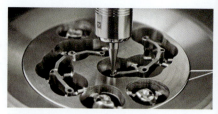

FIGURE 21.24 CAD/CAM milling process.

ADVANTAGES OF CAD/CAM

1. Improved fit.
2. Possibility of one visit restorations especially in case of smaller all restorations like inlays and crowns.
3. Complex castings like full arch FDPs, overdenture frames, partial dentures frames, etc. can be fabricated with greater ease and accuracy as compared to lost wax based castings. Reassembling the casting and soldering processes can be eliminated for these castings.
4. Structures are homogenous with minimum porosity and defects.

An image (scan) is taken of the prepared tooth and the surrounding teeth. This image, called a digital impression, draws the data into a computer. Proprietary software then creates a virtual restoration or structure. The data is sent to a milling machine where the part is milled out of a solid block of the metal *(Fig. 21.24)*. Multiple units can be milled out of a single block. Metal blanks of different compositions, shapes and sizes are available *(Fig. 21.23)*.

Milling machines currently available are capable of multiaxis milling and multiple tool changes.

COPY MILLING

Copy milling of metal structures is similar to that described for ceramics. It is based on the principle of scanning or tracing of a resin or *wax pattern* of the restoration milling a replica out of the metal blank. (Refer chapter on dental ceramics for additional information).

ELECTROFORMING

Electroforming is another method of forming a metal coping for metal ceramic systems *(Figs. 21.25A to D)*. Some examples of electroforming systems are Preciano (Heraeus Kulzer) and Microvision (Weiland).

A die spacer is applied on to the die of the prepared tooth/teeth. The dies are duplicated with gypsum product having a slight expansion of 0.1 to 0.2 %. The duplicated die is coated with a conducting silver lacquer metallizing powder *(Fig. 21.25C)* and then connected to the electrodes and immersed in to the electroplating bath *(Fig. 21.25A)*. The bath is a nontoxic cyanide-free gold-sulfite solution. Electroforming time varies according to the thickness desired and the current.

○ 0.2 mm layer thickness—240 min.

○ 0.3 mm layer thickness—329 min.

The coping formed *(Fig. 21.25D)* is separated and used to fabricate a metal-ceramic restoration.

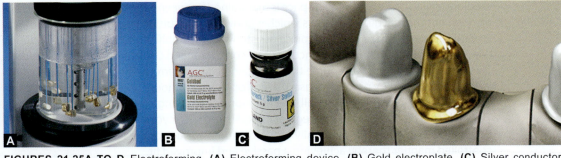

FIGURES 21.25A TO D Electroforming. **(A)** Electroforming device. **(B)** Gold electroplate. **(C)** Silver conductor. **(D)** Electroformed coping.

Electroforming is also used to replenish the worn-out telescopic prostheses that have lost their friction fit.

ELECTRICAL DISCHARGE MACHINING

The electrical discharge machining (EDM) unit *(Fig. 21.26)* was invented by the Russian Lazerenko brothers in 1943. Electrical discharge machining (EDM), sometimes colloquially also referred to as spark machining, spark eroding, burning, die sinking, wire burning or wire erosion, is a subtractive manufacturing process whereby a desired shape is obtained using electrical discharges (sparks). One of the electrodes is called the tool-electrode or tool, while the other is called the workpiece-electrode, or workpiece. Material is removed from the workpiece by a series of rapidly recurring current discharges between two electrodes, separated by a dielectric liquid and subject to an electric voltage. EDM is useful for difficult to machine alloys such as tungsten and titanium. The advent of computer-aided EDM in the early seventies, helped it gain significance in manufacturing processes. In 1982, it was introduced into dentistry by Rubeling to fabricate precision attachments. Since 1990 it has been used widely in implant prostheses.

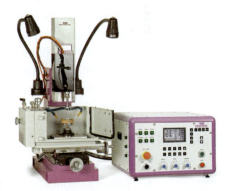

FIGURE 21.26 Electrical discharge machine.

APPLICATIONS

EDM is used in dentistry for the precise and accurate fabrication of precision attachment removable partial dentures, fixed-removable implant prostheses, and titanium-ceramic crowns. By improving the fit, a passive seating of the restoration on the implant is obtained thereby minimizing stresses to the bone.

TECHNIQUE

The tool electrode is connected to the implant abutments. The workpiece-electrode is connected to the restoration framework *(Fig. 21.27)*. Both electrode and workpiece are maintained in a liquid

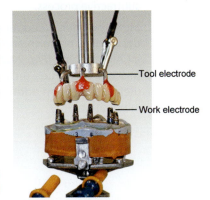

FIGURE 21.27 Assembly being readied for spark erosion.

medium (called dielectric fluid). A space is maintained between the electrode and work piece through out the machining process which is known as the cutting gap. The electrode moves towards and away from the work piece assisted by a hydraulic ram connected to it during the process. The dielectric fluid functions as a conductor and coolant during the procedure. This whole unit has a power source that maintains a direct current. The power level selection is dictated by the alloy properties used, size of object and amount of erosion required. When the cutting gap is sufficiently small, the fluid ionizes allowing electric discharges to occur. These electric discharges occur at regular intervals and such cycles takes place about 250,000 times a second. The sparks gradually erode the inner surface of the restoration in a precise controlled manner thereby achieving a passive and improved fit.

ADVANTAGES

1. Passive fit of restorations is achieved.
2. Complex structures can be shaped regardless of metal hardness.
3. Extremely thin work piece can be machined without distortion as it does not involve mechanical forces.
4. There is decreased stress on the work piece due to the cooling action of the dielectric fluid.
5. Smooth finish of final restoration is ensured.
6. There is decreased oxidation of metals during the procedure (especially useful in titanium to porcelain bonding).
7. It is rapid, efficient and accurate (within 0.0254 mm).
8. Frameworks with porcelain can be spark eroded without any stress on the porcelain due to the cooling action of the dielectric fluid.

DISADVANTAGES

1. Eroding tends to affect the corrosion resistance of titanium.
2. Skilled personnel and specialized lab equipment is mandatory.
3. The high cost of the technique limits its usage.

ADDITIVE MANUFACTURING

Additive manufacturing (AM) or three-dimensional printing is finding increasing use in dentistry. It is an additive manufacturing process in contrast to milling which is a subtractive process.

Metal powder is sequentially layered on to a gradually descending platform and fused using laser *(Fig. 21.28)* in a CAM machine *(Fig. 21.29)*. This deposition and sintering process continues until the desired object is created. (Refer chapter on additive manufacturing for additional information).

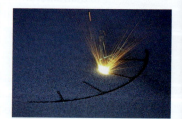

FIGURE 21.28 Laser sintering in progress.

TYPES OF METAL IN ADDITIVE MANUFACTURING TECHNOLOGIES

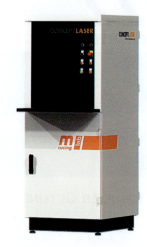

A. **Powder bed technologies**
   1. Laser beam melting
      - Selective laser melting
      - Laser melting
      - Direct metal laser sintering (DMLS)
   2. Electron beam melting (EBM)
   3. Material jetting process
B. **Powder deposition technologies**
   1. Laser engineered net shaping (LENS)
   2. Direct metal deposition (DMD)
   3. Laser cladding

FIGURE 21.29 3D laser sintering machine.

APPLICATIONS

Three-dimensional printing is used in the fabrication of metal structures in dentistry both directly and indirectly.

1. Indirect - machine prints patterns which are then cast to form metal structures.
2. Direct fabrication of metallic fixed and removable partial denture frames by laser sintering or melting *(Figs. 21.28 to 21.31)*.

METALS AVAILABLE FOR 3D PRINTING

All the metals generally available for fixed and removable dental prostheses are available in powder form for 3D printing. This includes cobalt-chromium, titanium and gold alloys.

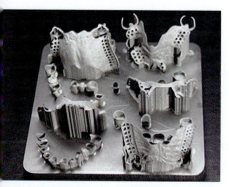

FIGURE 21.30 Dental prostheses including crowns, RPDs and FDPs made via direct metal sintering using 3D Systems' ProX 3D printer. *(Courtesy:* 3D Systems).

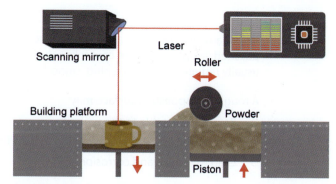

FIGURE 21.31 Representation of direct metal laser sintering process from a metal powder bed.

Abrasion and Polishing

Before any restoration or appliance is placed permanently in the mouth it should be highly polished. In spite of all the care taken during processing, many restorations and prostheses usually require further trimming, smoothing and finally polishing.

A rough or unpolished surface may

○ Be uncomfortable to the patient
○ Cause food and other debris cling to it and makes it unhygienic
○ Lead to tarnish and corrosion.

ABRASION

It occurs when a hard, rough surface slides along a softer surface and cuts a series of grooves

DEFINED AS

The wearing away of a substance or structure through a mechanical process, such as grinding, rubbing or scraping (*GPT-8*).

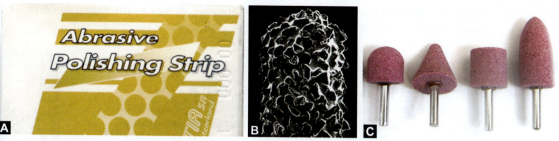

FIGURES 22.1A TO C Abrasive and polishing materials come in a wide variety of shapes and forms. **(A)** Abrasive polishing strip; **(B)** Electroplated diamond; **(C)** Bonded stone.

TYPES OF ABRASION

Abrasion may be

○ *A two body process,* e.g. action of a diamond bur on enamel.

○ *A three body process,* e.g. pumice applied with a bristle brush.

SUPPLIED AS

In dentistry the abrasive is applied to the work by a variety of tools *(Figs. 22.1A to C)*.

○ *Paper/plastic coated* The abrasive particles may be glued on to a paper or plastic disk that can be attached to a handpiece. Sand paper falls in this group.

○ *Coated strips* The abrasive (e.g. diamond) may be attached to stainless steel or plastic strips *(Fig. 22.1A)* (used for proximal stripping of teeth). This category is similar to the above.

○ *Electroplating bonding* In case of diamond rotary instruments the diamond chips are attached to steel wheels, disks and cylinders by electroplating with nickel based matrix.

○ *Bonded stones* In grinding wheels and dental stones *(Figs. 22.1B and C)*, the abrasive particles are mixed with a bonding agent that holds the particles together. Before hardening, the matrix material with the abrasive is moulded to form tools of desired shapes.

○ *Powder form* An abrasive may also be mixed with water or glycerine to form a paste or slurry. It is applied with felt cone, rubber cup or brush and used for smoothening irregularities, e.g. pumice powder *(Fig. 22.2A)*.

○ *Cake form* They are also available in the form of cakes *(Fig. 22.2B)*.

○ *Rubber impregnated* Abrasives can be incorporated into rubber or shellac disks or cups for 'soft grade' abrasion.

○ *Paste form* The abrasive is made into a paste and supplied in a tube, e.g. Ivoclar polishing paste, tooth paste, etc.

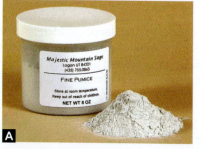
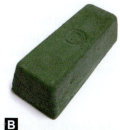

FIGURES 22.2A AND B Forms of abrasives. **(A)** Pumice powder; **(B)** Polishing abrasive in cake form.

Abrasion is affected by the properties of the abrasive as well as the target material. The important properties include hardness, strength, ductility, thermal conductivity, etc.

MECHANISM OF ABRASIVE ACTION

In a cutting tool, e.g. carbide or steel bur **(Fig. 22.3)**, the blades or cutting edges are regularly arranged and the removal of material corresponds to this regular arrangement. An abrasive tool on the other hand has many abrasive points that are not arranged in an ordered pattern. Thus, innumerable random scratches are produced.

The action of an abrasive is essentially a *cutting action*. Each tiny particle presents a sharp edge that cuts through the surface similar to a chisel. A shaving is formed which crushes to a fine powder. This powder clogs the abrasive tool and frequent cleaning is required.

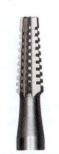

FIGURE 22.3 Steel bur. Unlike diamond these burs remove material by cutting or shaving.

STRESS, STRAIN AND HEAT PRODUCTION DURING ABRASION

While abrading metals, the crystalline structure of the metal is disturbed to depth of 10 μm. The grains become disoriented and strain hardening may occur. Thus, the surface hardness increases.

In denture resins too, rigorous abrasion introduces stresses. The generation of heat during abrasion partially relieves such stresses but if it is too great, it may relieve processing stresses and a warpage may result. The resin surface may even melt.

Similarly high speed cutting of tooth structure generates excessive heat which can lead to pulpal damage. Therefore, it is very important to control the heat by air/water spray and intermittent cutting (rather than continuous cutting).

RATE OF ABRASION

The rate of abrasion of a given material by a given abrasive is determined primarily by three factors.

1. Size of the abrasive particle.
2. The pressure of the abrasive agent.
3. Speed at which the abrasive particle moves across the surface being abraded.

SIZE OF THE PARTICLES

Larger particles cause deeper scratches in the material and wear away the surface at a faster rate. The use of course abrasive is indicated on a surface with many rough spots or large nodules. The scratches caused by the coarse abrasive must then be removed by finer ones.

PRESSURE

Heavy pressure applied by the abrasive will cause deeper scratches and more rapid removal of material. However, heavy pressure is not advisable as it can fracture or dislodge the abrasive from the grinding wheel, thus reducing the cutting efficiency. In addition, operator has less control of the abrasion process because removal of material is not uniform.

SPEED

The higher the speed, the greater the frequency per unit of time the particles contacts the surface. Thus increasing the speed increases the rate of abrasion. In a clinical situation it is easier to control speed than pressure to vary the rate of abrasion. Varying the speed has the additional advantage that low pressure can be used to maintain a high cutting efficiency.

Rotational Speed and Linear Speed

Rotational speed and linear speed should be differentiated. The speed with which the particles pass over the work is its linear speed or it is the velocity with which the particles pass over the work. Rotational speed is measured in revolutions per minute (RPM or r/min), whereas, linear speed is measured in meters per second

Linear speed is related to rotational speed according to the following formula

$V = CR$, where V = linear speed

C = circumference of the bur or disc

R = revolutions per minute

CLASSIFICATION

   A.   Finishing abrasives
   B.   Polishing abrasives
   C.   Cleansing abrasives

FINISHING ABRASIVES

Finishing abrasives are hard, coarse abrasives which are used initially to develop contour and remove gross irregularities, e.g. coarse stones.

POLISHING ABRASIVES

Polishing abrasives have finer particle size and are less hard than abrasives used for finishing. They are used for smoothening surfaces that have been roughened by finishing abrasives, e.g. polishing cakes, pumice, etc.

CLEANSING ABRASIVES

Cleansing abrasives are soft materials with small particle sizes and are intended to remove soft deposits that adhere to enamel or a restorative material.

TYPES OF ABRASIVES

EMERY

Emery consists of a natural oxide of aluminum called corundum. There are various impurities present in it, such as iron oxide, which may also act as an abrasive. The greater the content of alumina, the finer the grade of emery.

ALUMINUM OXIDE

Pure alumina is manufactured from bauxite, an impure aluminum oxide. It can be produced in fine grain sizes and has partially replaced emery for abrasive purpose. Pure alumina is also used as a polishing agent. Alumina is used in sandblasting machines (*Figs. 22.7 and 22.8*).

GARNET

It is composed of different minerals which possess similar physical properties and crystalline form. The mineral comprises of silicates of aluminium, cobalt, magnesium, iron and manganese. Garnet is coated on paper or cloth with glue. It is used on disks, which are operated on handpieces.

PUMICE

It is a highly siliceous material of volcanic origin and is used either as an abrasive or polishing agent depending on particle size. Its use ranges from smoothening dentures to polishing teeth in the mouth.

KIESELGUHR

It consists of siliceous remains of minute aquatic plants known as diatoms. The coarser form (diatomaceous earth) is used as a filler in many dental materials. It is excellent as a mild abrasive and polishing agent.

TRIPOLI

This mild abrasive and polishing agent is often confused with kieselguhr. True tripoli originates from certain porous rocks, first found in North Africa near Tripoli.

ROUGE

Rouge is a fine red powder composed of iron oxide. It is used in cake form. It may be impregnated on paper or cloth known as 'crocus cloth'. It is an excellent polishing agent for gold and noble metal alloys but is likely to be dirty to handle.

TIN OXIDE

Putty powder used as polishing agent for teeth and metallic restorations in the mouth. It is mixed with water, alcohol or glycerin and used as paste.

CHALK

It is calcium carbonate prepared by precipitation method. There are various grades and physical forms available for different polishing techniques. It is sometimes used in dentifrices.

CHROMIC OXIDE

A relatively hard abrasive capable of polishing a variety of metals. It is used as a polishing agent for stainless steel.

SAND

Sand as well as other forms of quartz is used as sand paper or as powder in sandblasting equipment.

CARBIDES

Silicon carbide and boron carbide are manufactured by heating silicon and boron at a very high temperature to effect their union with carbon. The silicon carbide is sintered or pressed with a binder into grinding wheels or disks. Most of the stone burs used for cutting tooth structure are made of silicon carbide.

DIAMOND

It is the hardest and most effective abrasive for tooth enamel. The chips are impregnated in a binder or plated on to a metal shank to form the diamond 'stones' and disks so popular with the dental profession.

ZIRCONIUM SILICATE

The mineral zircon is ground to various particle sizes and used as a polishing agent. It is used in dental prophylactic pastes and in abrasive impregnated polishing strips and disks.

ZINC OXIDE

Zinc oxide in alcohol can be used for polishing amalgam restorations.

DESIRABLE CHARACTERISTICS OF AN ABRASIVE

1. It should be irregular in shape so that it presents a sharp edge. Round smooth particles of sand are poor abrasives. Sand paper with cubical particles present flat faces to the work, and so they are not effective. Irregular and jagged particles are more effective.
2. Abrasive should be harder than the work it abrades. If it cannot indent the surface to be abraded, it cannot cut it and the abrasive dulls or wears out.
3. The abrasive should possess a high impact strength. The abrasive particle should fracture rather than dull out, so that a sharp edge is always present. Fracture of an abrasive is also helpful in shedding the debris accumulated from the work. A diamond does not fracture, it loses substances from the tip. They become clogged when used on ductile metals. They are most effective when used on brittle tooth enamel.
4. They should have attrition resistance, so that it does not wear.

GRADING OF ABRASIVE AND POLISHING AGENTS

Abrasives are graded according to the number of the last sieve it passed through. Examples silicon carbide is graded as 8, 10, 12, 14, 16, 20, 24, etc. Finer abrasives are designated as powder or flours and are graded in increasing fineness as F, FF, FFF, etc. and impregnated papers as 0,00,000, etc.

BINDER

The abrasives on a disk and wheel are held together by a binder.

Commonly used binders in dentistry are

- Ceramic bonding is used for silicon carbide or corundum in a mounted abrasive point.
- Electroplating with nickel is often used to bind the diamond chips on to the diamond rotary instruments *(Fig. 22.4)*.
- For soft grade abrasion, rubber *(Fig. 22.5)* or shellac may be used. These wear rapidly, but they are useful in some dental operations in which delicate abrasion is required.

The type of binder is related to the life of the tool in use. In most abrasives the binder is impregnated throughout with an abrasive of a certain grade so that, as a particle is removed from the binder during use another takes its place as the binder wears. Furthermore, the abrasive should be so distributed that the surface of the tool wears evenly, particularly if the disk or wheel is used for cutting along its periphery.

DIAMOND BURS

Either synthetic or natural diamond chips are employed for dental rotary instruments *(Fig. 22.4)*. The cutting efficiency of diamond rotary instruments depends on whether the diamonds used are natural or synthetic, the grit size, the distribution and the extent of plating that

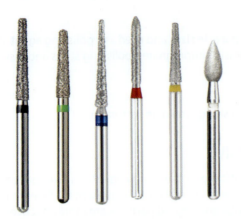

FIGURE 22.4 Diamond burs of various grits. The color indicates grit size. Black - extra coarse, Green—course, Blue—medium, Red—fine, Yellow—extra fine, and White—ultra fine.

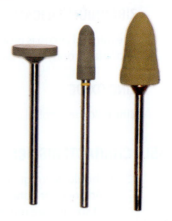

FIGURE 22.5 Rubber-bonded abrasives.

attaches the particles to the instrument shank. The larger the grit size the greater the abrasion. Some companies indicate the grit size by color coding *(Fig. 22.6)*. Adequate water spray is essential not only to minimize heat but also to reduce clogging.

POLISHING

It is the production of a smooth mirror like surface without much loss of any external form. If the particle size of an abrasive is reduced sufficiently, the scratches become extremely fine and may disappear entirely. The surface then acquires a smooth shiny layer known as a polish.

The polishing agents remove material from the surface molecule by molecule. In the process fine scratches and irregularities are filled in by powdered particulates being removed from the surface. The microcrystalline layer is referred to as polish layer or *Beilby layer*. A polishing agent is employed only after an abrasive obliterates or eliminates most of the fine scratches, leaving a smooth finish.

◯	white	15 ultra-fine
🟡	yellow	30 extra-fine
🔴	red	50 fine
🔵	blue	70-130 middle
🟢	green	160 coarse
⚫	black	180 extra-coarse

FIGURE 22.6 Color coding and corresponding grit size.

DIFFERENCE BETWEEN ABRASION AND POLISHING

The difference between an abrasive agent and a polishing agent is difficult to define. The terms are generally interchangeable.

○ *Particle size*   A given agent having a large particle size acts as an abrasive, producing scratches. The same abrasive with a smaller particle size is a polishing agent.

○ *Material removed*   Very little of the surface is removed during polishing—not more than 0.005 mm (0.002 inch).

○ *Speed*   The optimum speed for polishing is higher than that for abrading. Linear speed as high as 10000 ft/min may be used. It varies with the polishing agent. Average speed is approximately 7500 ft/min.

NONABRASIVE POLISHING

Polishing is usually achieved by an abrasive process. However a smooth shiny surface can also be achieved through nonabrasive means. These include

1. Application of a glaze layer, e.g.
   - Glazing of composites
   - Glazing of ceramics
2. Electrolytic polishing
3. Burnishing.

COMPOSITE GLAZING

A layer of glaze or gloss (a clear transparent liquid made of unfilled resin) is applied over the restoration and cured. This results in a smooth glossy surface.

GLAZING CERAMICS

Ceramics are difficult to polish conventionally. The finished restoration is subjected to high temperatures. At this temperature the surface layer melts and flows to produce a smooth glass-like surface (refer ceramics chapter for more details). Alternatively a glaze layer can be applied and fired to obtain a shiny surface.

ELECTROLYTIC POLISHING

Electrolytic polishing *(Fig. 22.7)* is not true abrasion. Although material is removed, it is removed through an *electrochemical process* rather than abrasive process.

This is the reverse of electroplating. The alloy to be polished is made the anode of an electrolytic cell. As the current is passed, some of the anode is dissolved leaving a bright surface. This is an excellent method for polishing the fitting surface of a cobalt–chromium alloy denture. So little material is removed, that the fit of the denture is virtually unaltered.

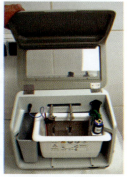

FIGURE 22.7 Electrolytic polishing unit.

BURNISHING

It is related to polishing in that the surface is drawn or moved. Instead of using many tiny particles, only one large point is used.

If a round steel point is rubbed over the margins of a gold inlay, the metal is moved so that any gap between the inlay and the tooth can be closed. A special blunt bur revolving at high speed can also be used.

Note The burnishing instrument should not adhere to or dissolve in the surface of the burnished metal, e.g. brass instruments impregnate copper into the surface of a gold inlay.

TECHNICAL CONSIDERATIONS (PROCEDURE)

METHODS OF ABRASION

Abrasion may be carried out

1. *Manually*, e.g. proximal stripping of enamel using abrasive strips.
2. *Rotary instruments*, e.g. burs, wheels, cups, discs, cones, etc.

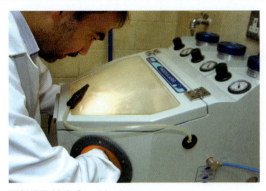

FIGURE 22.8 Sandblasting.

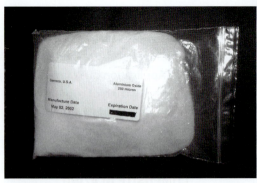

FIGURE 22.9 The term sandblasting is misleading. The process actually uses 250 micron alumina (Al_2O_3).

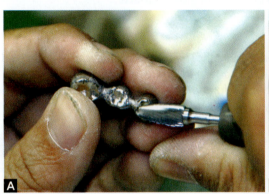

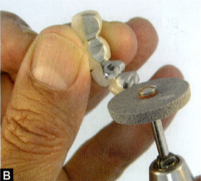

FIGURES 22.10A AND B Sequence of finishing is important. One should proceed from coarse to fine.

3. *Blasting* The object is blasted with a steady stream of abrasive, e.g. prophy-jet polishing of enamel, sandblasting *(Figs. 22.8 and 22.9)* to remove investment of castings, shell blasting, etc.

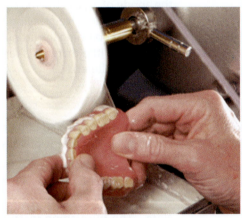

FIGURE 22.11 Canvas buff wheel with pumice is used for polishing complete dentures.

   – Smoothen work with a coarse abrasive or bur *(Fig. 22.10A)* which leaves large scratches. These scratches are removed with finer abrasives but the difference in fineness should not be too great *(Fig. 22.10B)*. The use of too fine an abrasive after a relatively coarse abrasive wastes time and may cause streaking.
   – After changing to a finer abrasive, the direction of abrasion should be changed each time if possible, so that new scratches appear at right angles to the coarser scratches, for uniform abrasion.
   – When the scratches are no longer visible to the eye, the preliminary polishing can be accomplished with pumice flour applied with a canvas buff wheel [used for resin dentures *(Fig. 22.11)*].
   – The work is cleaned to remove all traces of abrasives and the particles of the material removed by the abrasive.

- A paste is formed of pumice and water to a sticky 'muddy' consistency. The buff wheel is turned at high speed. Apply the paste to the work and carry it to the buff. Hold the work firmly but without excessive pressure. Repeat this over the entire surface till the surface is bright and well polished.
- Clean the work with soap and water. Change to a flannel buff wheel. Rotate at high speed. A polishing cake with grease is held against the buff wheel to impregnate with the agent. The work is held against the wheel and turned, so that all of the surfaces are polished uniformly. A light pressure is used to avoid excess heat generation (especially in resins).

DENTIFRICES

Popularly known as toothpastes these are agents used with a toothbrush to cleanse and polish natural teeth. They should have maximum cleansing efficiency with minimum tooth abrasion. Highly abrasive dentifrices should not be used especially when dentin (abrades 25 times faster) or cementum (35 times faster) is exposed.

FUNCTION

1. Assists the toothbrush to mechanically remove stains, debris and soft deposits from the teeth.
2. To impart a polished surface to the tooth.

Thus, they help reduce caries, maintain healthy gingiva, improve esthetics and reduce mouth odors.

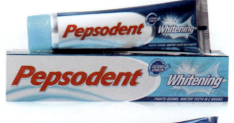
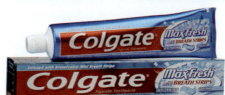

AVAILABLE AS

Pastes, powders, liquid and gels *(Fig. 22.12)*.

FIGURE 22.12 Some popular dentifrices.

CLASSIFICATION OF DENTIFRICES

Dentifrices may classified based on their primary function.

1. Caries prevention and treatment
   - Fluoride concentrations up to 1000 ppm
   - Fluoride concentrations from 1000 to 2000 ppm
   - Fluoride concentrations from 2500 to 5000 ppm
2. Periodontal disease prevention and treatment
   - Natural antibacterial and antiseptic agents
   - Synthetic antibacterial and antiseptic agent
3. Desensitizing pastes
   - Analgesic
   - Dentine tubules blocking
4. Whitening pastes
   - Abrasive
   - Bleaching

5. Pastes for specific purposes
   – Toothpastes for xerostomia (e.g. olive oil, betaine and xylitol)
   – Antiviral pastes (e.g. larifan for herpetic infection or aphthae)

COMPOSITION

The basic component of a dentifrices is the abrasive. However, pastes today contain numerous other components. Specialized dentifrices contain medicaments for various problems, such as sensitivity and gum diseases. Composition of a typical dentifrices is presented in **Table 22.1**.

HERBAL TOOTHPASTES

Some toothpastes are marketed as natural or herbal-based toothpastes **(Fig. 22.13)**. These contain extracts which are claimed to be beneficial to the gums and teeth. Some of these include extracts from the neem tree, miswak tree (salvadore persica), zanthoxylum alatum (Tomar beej - Dabur red), propolis (resinous extract collected by bees), etc.

TABLE 22.1 Components of toothpaste

Ingredient		Action
Abrasives	Dibasic calcium phosphate (dihydrate) Calcium pyrophosphate Insoluble sodium metaphosphate Hydrated silica (most efficient) Alumina, titanium oxide Calcium carbonate, sodium bicarbonate Perlite (70–75% silica dioxide) Magnesium oxide, etc.	Physically removes matter
Water		Vehicle and moisturizing
Humectants	Glycerin, sorbitol, propylene glycol	Prevents drying of paste
Detergents and foaming agents	Sodium lauryl sulfate	Decreases surface tension
Binders	Carboxymethyl cellulose Xanthan gum	
Artificial sweeteners	Sorbitol, saccharin	
Therapeutic	Sodium monofluorophosphate (Na_2PO_3F) Stannous fluoride (SnF_2) Sodium fluoride (NaF) Aminofluorides	Anticariogenic agents
	Triclosan, chlorhexidine, hydrogen peroxide, baking soda, povidone iodine, zinc citrate.	Bacteriostatic and bactericidal
	Dibasic ammonium phosphate	Acid neutralizing
	Potassium nitrate, Potassium citrate Strontium chloride, Strontium acetate Arginine, Hydroxyapatite, Calcium sodium phosphosilicate.	Desensitizing and dentin occluding
Coloring and flavoring	Mint, menthol Various fruit flavors	Flavoring

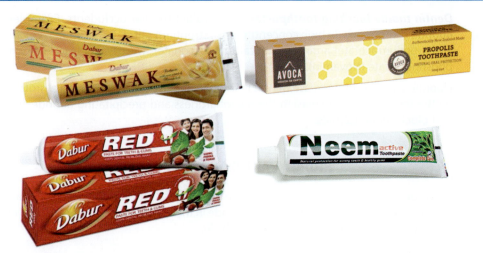

FIGURE 22.13 Dentifrices containing herbal and other natural extracts.

WHITENING AND BLEACHING TOOTHPASTES

Although in several studies whitening toothpastes have shown the ability to improve tooth color, they have several side effects. The most significant is enamel and dentin abrasion, which in turn leads to increased tooth sensitivity. A key indicator of toothpaste abrasiveness is relative dentin abrasion (RDA) *(Box 22.1)*. The larger the number, the greater the potential of dentin abrasiveness. Dentin abrasion significantly increases when the concentration of abrasive substances in toothpaste is increased. Teeth have a natural defence mechanism against abrasion, called the pellicle*. Its presence on tooth surfaces reduces the abrasive effect of toothpaste on enamel. Therefore, it is best to avoid mechanical tooth cleaning after consuming acidic foods or drinks, as they may dissolve the pellicle and can combine abrasive and erosive defects.

BOX 22.1	RDA table
A0 - 70	Low abrasive
70 - 100	Medium abrasive
100 - 150	Highly abrasive
150 - 250	Regarded as harmful limit

Bleaching toothpastes   Bleaching toothpastes contain chemicals, most commonly hydrogen peroxide or calcium peroxide. When peroxides touch the tooth surface, they break down the stain molecule, providing a bleaching effect. Various bleaching systems for home or professional use also contain these substances.

When adding peroxides to a toothpaste it should be noted that the concentration is small (usually 1% hydrogen peroxide or 0.5–0.7% calcium peroxide), and the exposure time short. Therefore, there is a lack of evidence about whether such toothpastes can improve the internal tooth color. They certainly bleach the pellicle on the tooth surface.

DESENSITIZING PASTES

Desensitizing pastes work through two methods—analgesic action and blocking of dentinal tubules.

Analgesic toothpastes   Toothpastes containing potassium salts maintain a high K^+ extracellular level, thus preventing repolarization of the nerve cell membrane and inhibiting the transmission of impulses without causing changes in the pulp. Toothpaste containing 5% or 10% potassium nitrate, can decrease tooth sensitivity for up to 4 weeks.

---

* Dental pellicle is a protein film that forms on the surface enamel by selective binding of glycoproteins from saliva that prevents continuous deposition of salivary calcium phosphate. It forms in seconds after a tooth is cleaned or after chewing. It protects the tooth from the acids produced by oral microorganisms after consuming carbohydrates.

Dentin tubule blocking toothpastes Also called tubular occludents. Examples include fluoride compounds (in high concentrations), strontium salts [10% strontium chloride (SrCl$_2$) and strontium acetate], arginine (with calcium carbonate), hydroxyapatite and calcium sodium phosphosilicate (Novamin).

Fluoride compounds increase dentin resistance against acids by forming a protective layer on the tooth surface, increasing the microhardness and precipitating fluoride compounds that block dentin tubules.

PROPHYLACTIC ABRASIVES

Oral prophylaxis is a widely used procedure in the dental office. Prophylactic polishing agents may be available commercially or can be made in the dental office. They are usually employed in paste form by mixing with a suitable vehicle.

FUNCTION

1. They remove extrinsic stains, pellicle, materia-alba and oral debris.
2. Impart a polished and esthetic appearance.

Different types of abrasives may be employed, e.g. zirconium silicate, silica, pumice, etc. In addition, some may contain fluoride in order to reduce caries.

They are applied onto the teeth with the help of rubber cups or bristle brushes *(Fig. 22.14)* which are attached to a rotary instrument.

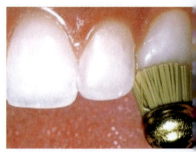

FIGURE 22.14 Prophylaxis in a dental office.

PROPHYJET

The Prophyjet *(Fig. 22.15A)* is a relatively new dental prophylaxis system of removing intraoral stains. An abrasive blasting process *(Fig. 22.15C)* is used to mechanically remove extrinsic (tobacco) stains as well as light supragingival adherent plaque and calculus. The powder is loaded into the device, which then directs the abrasive through a small nozzle in a steady *stream* of air and water.

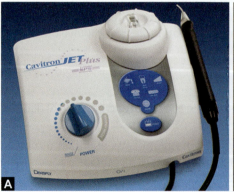 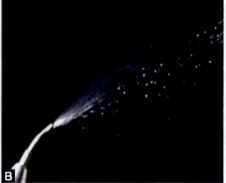 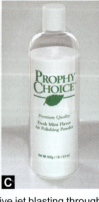

FIGURES 22.15A TO C **(A)** Prophyjet unit (Cavitron). **(B)** Prophyjet powder. **(C)** High pressure abrasive jet blasting through the nozzle.

Composition   It contains sodium carbonate, hydrophobic modified silica and a flavoring agent. It is supplied as powder in sachets or containers *(Fig. 22.15B)*.

Clinical considerations   The Prophyjet is directed at 45° angles to the tooth surface. For obvious reasons, it is less effective in proximal areas. The chances of soft tissue injury exist especially if the tissue is inflamed and friable.

DENTURE CLEANSERS

Dentures collect deposits in the same manner as natural teeth during their use. These can be removed by two ways.

- ○ Professional repolishing in the laboratory or clinic.
- ○ Soaking or brushing the dentures daily at home.

BRUSHING

The dentures may be brushed using a soft bristle brush *(Fig. 22.16)* and gentle abrasive or cream. Hard abrasives and stiff bristles should be avoided, because they may produce scratches on the denture surface.

SOAKING

Chemical cleaners *(Fig. 22.17)* are an alternative to brushing especially among very old or handicapped persons.

- ○ Alkaline perborates
- ○ Alkaline peroxides
- ○ Alkaline hypochlorites
- ○ Dilute acids

The dentures are soaked in these chemical solutions for a prescribed period of time. Their main requirements are that they should be nontoxic, non-irritant and should not attack the materials used in denture construction.

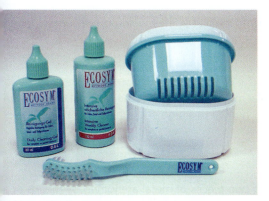

FIGURE 22.16 A home cleansing kit for dentures.

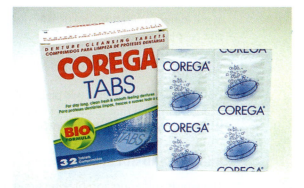

FIGURE 22.17 A commercially available chemical cleanser for soaking.

Metal Joining and Dental Lasers

It is often necessary to construct a dental appliance as separate parts and then join them together either by a soldering or welding process. Dental brazing is covered by ISO 9333.

TERMS AND DEFINITIONS

Metal joining operations are usually divided into four categories: welding, brazing, soldering and cast-joining.

WELDING

The term welding is used if two pieces of similar metal are joined together without the addition of another metal that is, the metal pieces are heated to a high enough temperature so they join together by melting and flowing.

BRAZING AND SOLDERING

The words soldering and brazing are used if two pieces of metal are joined by means of a third metal called as filler.

BRAZING

During soldering, metal parts are joined together by melting a filler metal between them at a temperature below the solidus temperature of the metal being joined and below 450 °C.

In dentistry, the joining of metal parts are done at temperatures above 450 °C, and therefore the operation should ideally be called *brazing*. This is also the term used by the ISO. However, most dentists still prefer to use the word soldering. The term 'brazing material' is often used interchangeably with the term 'solder'.

SUBSTRATE METAL

Substrate metal or parent metal refers to the metal parts to be joined. In dentistry alloys that can be soldered or welded include alloys of gold, silver, palladium, nickel, cobalt, titanium, etc.

IDEAL REQUIREMENTS OF A BRAZING MATERIAL (DENTAL SOLDER)

1. It should melt at temperatures below the solidus temperature of the parent metal.
2. When melted, it should wet and flow freely over the parent metal.
3. Its color should match that of metal being joined.
4. It should be resistant to tarnish and corrosion.
5. It should resist pitting during heating and application.

TYPES OF SOLDERS OR BRAZING MATERIALS

They may be divided into two major groups.

1. Soft solders
2. Hard solders

SOFT SOLDERS

Soft solders have low melting range of about 260 °C. They can be applied by simple means like hot soldering iron. They lack corrosion resistance and so are not suitable for dental use, e.g. lead-tin alloys (plumbers solders).

HARD SOLDERS

These have a higher melting temperature and greater strength and hardness. They are melted with the help of gas blowtorches or occasionally in an electric furnace. Hard solders are more commonly used in dentistry. They are also used for industrial purposes and in the jewelry trade, e.g. gold solders and silver solders *(Fig. 23.1)*.

PRESOLDERING AND POSTSOLDERING

The term presoldering (prebrazing) refers to soldering operation performed on metal-ceramic alloys prior to ceramic firing. Postsoldering (postbrazing) refers to soldering performed on the alloy after ceramic firing. Obviously properties required of the two solders would be different. Solders used in presoldering would be required to permit ceramic bonding as well as withstand the high porcelain firing temperatures.

APPLICATIONS OF SOLDERING

In dentistry they are used as follows.

1. For soldering various types of wires in orthodontics.
2. In pedodontics, to construct various types of space maintainers.
3. In fixed prosthodontics
   – For joining of various components of fixed partial prostheses *(Box 23.1)*.
   – Repair of perforations in crowns and bridges.
   – To develop contact points in crowns.
   – For cutting and rejoining an ill-fitting distorted bridge.
4. In removable partial prosthodontics for soldering of clasps.

COMPOSITION

GOLD SOLDERS

In the past solders were referred to by a karat number. The numbers did not describe the gold content of the solder but rather the carat of gold alloys for which the solder was to be used. In recent years the term fineness has been substituted for karat. The composition of gold solders *(Fig. 23.1A)* vary considerably depending on its fineness.

Component	Percent
Gold	45 to 81%
Silver	8 to 30%
Copper	7 to 20%
Tin	2 to 4%
Zinc	2 to 4%

SILVER SOLDERS

Silver solders *(Fig. 23.1B)* are less commonly used in dentistry. They are used when a low fusing solder is required for soldering operations on stainless steel or other base metal alloys.

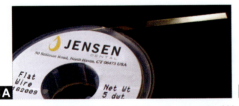
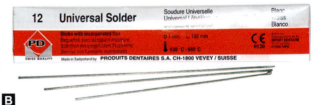

FIGURES 23.1A AND B Dental brazing metals. **(A)** Gold solder. **(B)** Silver solder.

BOX 23.1 | Improving the fit of a fixed partial denture (FPD) through soldering

The fit of a FDP is often improved when it is cast as two separate pieces. Long span FDPs are especially prone to poor fit because of distortion. The two parts of the prosthesis are tried separately in the mouth. After the operator is satisfied with the individual fit of the castings, the two pieces are assembled in the mouth and their relationship is recorded and transferred with the help of a suitable index material (impression plaster or zinc oxide eugenol or elastomers). The pieces are reassembled in the laboratory and invested using soldering investment. The parts are then joined with solder. If done correctly this technique can give superior fitting fixed partial dentures.

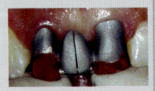

Component	Percent
Silver	10 to 80%
Copper	15 to 50%
Zinc	4 to 35%
Cadmium or phosphorous	may be present in small amounts

PROPERTIES OF DENTAL BRAZING MATERIALS

FUSION TEMPERATURE

The fusion temperature of the solder should be at least 50 °C lower than the parent metal.

- Gold solders – 690 to 870 °C
- Silver solders – 620 to 700 °C.

FLOW

A good flow and wetting (low wetting angle) of the parent metal by the solder is essential to produce a good bond.

Factors affecting flow

1. *Melting range*   Solders with short melting ranges have better flow.
2. *Composition of parent metal*   Gold and silver based alloys have better flow than nickel based alloys.
3. *Oxides*   Presence of an oxide layer on the parent metal reduces the flow.
4. Surface tension of solder.

COLOR

The color of gold solders varies from deep yellow to light yellow to white. In practice, most dental solders are able to produce an inconspicuous joint.

TARNISH AND CORROSION RESISTANCE

Tarnish resistance increases as the gold content increases. However, lower fineness gold alloys also perform well clinically without any serious tendency to discolor. Silver solders have reduced tarnish resistance when compared to gold alloy solders.

MECHANICAL PROPERTIES

Gold solders have adequate strength and hardness and are comparable to dental cast gold alloys having a similar gold content.

Silver solders also have adequate strength and are similar to the gold solders.

Tensile strength of brazed joint

According to ISO 9333:2006, the tensile strength of the brazed joint should exceed 250 MPa. If the 0,2 % proof strength of either one or both of the metallic materials to be joined by the brazing material is below 250 MPa, the tensile strength should exceed the lower of the two.

MICROSTRUCTURE OF SOLDERED JOINTS

Microscopic examination of an ideal well-formed soldered joint shows that the solder alloy does not combine excessively with the parts being soldered. There is a well-defined boundary between the solder and the soldered parts. If the heating is prolonged a diffusion takes place and the new alloy formed has inferior properties.

FLUXES

The Latin word 'flux' means flow. For a solder to wet and flow properly, the parent metal must be free of oxides. This is accomplished with the help of a flux.

FUNCTION OF FLUX

1. To remove any oxide coating on the parent metal.
2. To protect the metal surface from oxidation during soldering.

TYPES

Fluxes may be divided into three activity types.

Protective

This type covers the metal surface and prevents access to oxygen so no oxide can form.

Reducing

This reduces any oxide present to free metal and oxygen.

Solvent

This type dissolves any oxide present and carries it away. Most fluxes are usually combination of two or more of the above.

COMMONLY USED DENTAL FLUXES

The commonly used fluxes are

1. Boric and borate compounds
2. Fluoride fluxes

Boric and Borate Compounds

Boric acid and borax are used with noble metal alloys. They act as protective and reducing fluxes.

Fluorides

Fluoride fluxes *(Fig. 23.2)* like potassium fluorides are used on base metal alloys and are usually combined with borates. They help to dissolve the more stable chromium, nickel and cobalt oxides. Fluoride fluxes should be used carefully around porcelain as it can attack the porcelain.

Note Excess flux should be avoided as it can get entrapped within the filler metal and result in a weak joint.

FLUXES MAY BE SUPPLIED AS

○ Liquid (applied by painting)
○ Paste

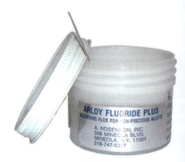

FIGURE 23.2 A fluoride flux for base metal alloys.

- ○ Powder
- ○ Fused onto the solder
- ○ Prefluxed solder in tube form.

ANTIFLUX

There are times when the operator desires that the solder should not flow out of a specific area. The flow can be controlled by use of an antiflux material. Solder will not flow into an area where antiflux has been applied. It is applied before the flux or solder is applied. Examples of antiflux are graphite (soft lead pencil), rouge (iron oxide) or whiting (calcium carbonate) in an alcohol and water suspension.

TECHNICAL CONSIDERATIONS

HEAT SOURCE

The heat source is a very important part of brazing. In dentistry, two heat sources may be used

1. Flame
2. Oven

FLAME BRAZING OR SOLDERING

The most commonly used heat source is a gas-air or gas-oxygen torch. The flame must provide enough heat not only to melt the filler metal but also to compensate for heat loss to the surroundings. Thus, the flame should not only have a high temperature but also a high heat content. Low heat content of fuels lead to longer soldering time and more danger of oxidation. Heat content is measured in Btu per cubic foot of gas.

Types of gas fuel

1. *Hydrogen*   It has the lowest heat content (275 Btu) and therefore heating would be slow **(Figs. 23.3A and B)**. It is not indicated for soldering of large FDPs.
2. *Natural gas*   It has a temperature of 2680 °C and heat content is four times that of hydrogen (1000 Btu). However, normally available gas is nonuniform in composition and frequently contains water vapor.

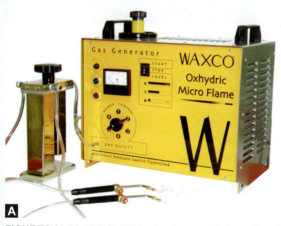
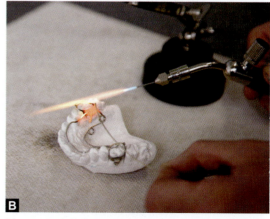

FIGURES 23.3A AND B (A) A microflame soldering unit such as this uses hydrolysis to split water into hydrogen and oxygen which is then used as fuel for the flame. **(B)** Micro flame soldering.

3. *Acetylene* It has the highest flame temperature (3140 °C) and a higher heat content than H_2 or natural gas. However, it has certain problems. Temperature from one part of its flame to another may vary by more than 100 °C. Therefore, positioning the torch is critical and proper part of the flame should be used. It is chemically unstable and decomposes readily to carbon and hydrogen. The carbon may get incorporated into the Ni and Pd alloys, and hydrogen may be absorbed by the Pd alloys.

4. *Propane* It is the best choice. It has the highest heat content (2385 Btu) and a good flame temperature (2850 °C).

5. *Butane* It is more readily available in some parts of the world and is similar to propane. Both propane and butane are uniform in quality and water-free.

OVEN BRAZING (FURNACE BRAZING)

An electric furnace with heating coils may be used for brazing. The furnace also provides heated surroundings, so less heat is lost to other parts of the fixed partial denture and the atmosphere.

TECHNIQUE OF SOLDERING

Two techniques of dental soldering are employed to assemble dental appliances

A. Free hand soldering
B. Investment soldering

FREE HAND SOLDERING

In free hand soldering, the parts are assembled and held in contact manually while the heat and solder are applied.

INVESTMENT SOLDERING

In investment soldering, the parts to be joined are mounted in a soldering type of investment. The hardened investment holds it in position while the heat and solder are applied **(Fig. 23.4)**.

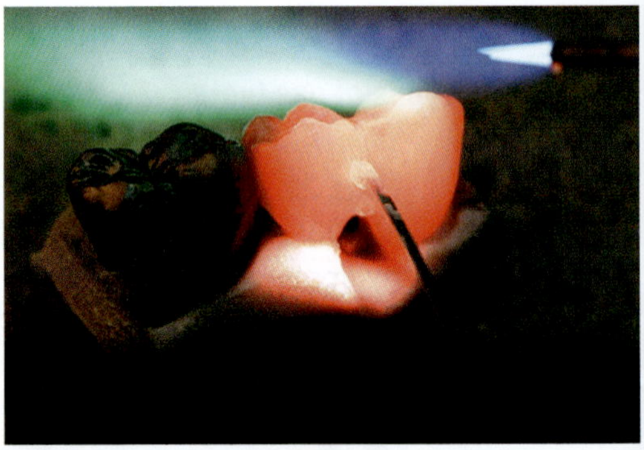

FIGURE 23.4 Investment soldering.

STEPS IN SOLDERING PROCEDURE

1. Selection of solder
2. Cleaning and polishing of components
3. Assembly of the prosthesis in soldering investment
4. Application of flux
5. Preheating the bridge assembly
6. Placement of solder
7. Application of hot gas flame to joint and solder
8. Cooling of assembly followed by quenching in water

TECHNICAL CONSIDERATIONS FOR SUCCESSFUL SOLDERING

o Cleanliness - Metal should be free of oxides
o Gap between parts
o Selection of solder - Proper color, fusion temperature and flow

○ Flux-type and amount
○ Flame - Neutral or reducing in nature
○ Temperature
○ Time

Gap   The liquid solder is drawn into the joint through capillary action. Therefore, an optimum gap is necessary for proper flow, strength of the joint and to avoid distortion of the assembly. Gap width ranging from 0.13 to 0.3 have been suggested.

If the gap is too narrow, strength is limited due to

○ Porosity caused by incomplete flow
○ Flux inclusion

If the gap is too great

○ The joint strength will be the strength of the solder.
○ There is a tendency for the parts to draw together as the solder solidifies.

Flame   The flame has multiple zones **(Fig. 23.5)**. The portion of the flame that is used should be neutral or slightly reducing. An improperly adjusted or positioned flame can lead to oxidation and/or carbon inclusion. Once the flame has been applied to the joint area, it should be not removed until brazing is complete. Due to its reducing nature, the flame gives protection from oxidation.

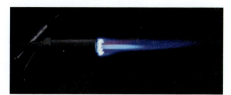

FIGURE 23.5 A neutral or reducing flame is used.

Temperature   The temperature used should be the minimum required to complete the brazing operation. Prior to the placement of the solder, the parent metal is heated till it is hot enough to melt the filler metal as soon as it touches. A lower temperature will not allow the filler to wet the parent metal. A higher temperature increases the possibility of diffusion between parent and filler metal.

Time   The flame is held until the filler metal has flowed completely into the connection and a moment longer to allow the flux or oxide to separate from the fluid solder. Insufficient time increases chances of incomplete filling of joint and possibility of flux inclusion in the joint. Excessive time increases possibility of diffusion. Both conditions cause a weaker joint.

PITTED SOLDER JOINTS

Pits or porosities in the solder joint often become evident during finishing. They are due to

○ *Volatilization* of the lower melting components due to heating at higher temperatures and for longer time.
○ Improperly melted or excess *flux* that is *trapped* in the solder joint. To avoid such pitting, less flux is applied and the heating should be discontinued as soon as the flux and solder are well melted and flowed into position.

ADVANTAGES AND DISADVANTAGES

Advantages

1. Low cost.
2. Relative effectiveness.

Disadvantages

1. Problems such as oxidation of the parts joined by weld.
2. Joint porosity and overheating of the union during the welding process can promote small structural defects and failure of the rehabilitation treatment.

WELDING

The term welding is used if two pieces of similar metal are joined together *without* the addition of another metal. It is usually used to join flat structures such as bands and brackets.

INDICATIONS

1. In orthodontics, to join flat structures like bands and brackets.
2. In pedodontics, to weld bands and other appliances.
3. In prosthodontics, to join wrought wire clasps and repair of broken metal partial dentures.

TYPES

Welding processes used in dentistry are

1. Resistance spot welding
2. Laser welding
3. Plasma arc welding (PAW)
4. Tungsten inert gas (TIG) welding

RESISTANCE SPOT WELDING

Welding is done by passing an *electric current* through the pieces to be joined. These pieces are also simultaneously *pressed* together. The resistance of the metal to flow of current causes *intense localized heating* and fusion of the metal. The combined heat and pressure *fuses* the metals into a single piece.

Welding is done in an *electric spot welding* apparatus *(Figs. 23.6A and B)*. The wires or the band to be welded is placed between the two copper electrodes of the welder. A flexible spring attached to the electrode helps to apply pressure on the metals. A hand controlled switch is

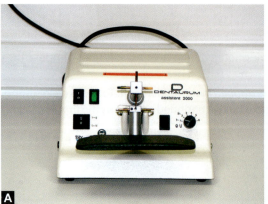
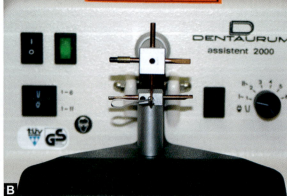

FIGURES 23.6A AND B **(A)** An electric orthodontic spot welder. **(B)** Close up of the spot welder.

used to operate the welder. On pressing the switch a large current passes through the wires or band between the copper electrodes. The combined heat and pressure fuses the metal pieces at that point and joins them. This kind of welding may also be referred to as 'spot welding'.

Prosthodontic appliances are welded in a larger machine. The parts to be joined are held together in a clamp. A hand or foot controlled switch controls the current.

Weld joints are susceptible to corrosion because of precipitation of chromium carbide and consequent loss of passivation.

TUNGSTEN INERT GAS (TIG) WELDING AND PLASMA ARC WELDING (PAW)

Plasma Arc Welding (PAW) *(Fig. 23.7)* and Tungsten Inert Gas (TIG) welding *(Fig. 23.8)* are techniques in which a union is obtained by heating materials by an arc established between a nonconsumable tungsten electrode and the part to be welded.

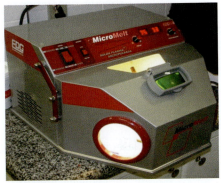

The electrode and the area to be welded are protected by using an inert gas, usually argon or a mixture of inert gases (argon and helium). The basic equipment consists of a power supply, a torch with a tungsten electrode, a shielding gas source, and an opening system for the arc. The main difference between TIG and plasma welding is the use of a constrictor torch that concentrates the electric arc in plasma welding.

FIGURE 23.7 A dental plasma arc welding machine.

PROCEDURE

The equipment allows for the adjustment of both the pulse and current which is required for welding. After adjusting the machine, screw into one of the claws a structure without use and position the parts to be welded with hands or through specific equipment, which position the parts to be joined. The argon activation is done by a foot pedal. The foot pedal is pressed until the argon flows. The buzzer will indicate when contact is made. Quickly release the pedal. The weld will be made, and the flow of argon will continue for a few seconds. It is possible that in the first few attempts, the electrode will stick to the piece making it necessary to regrind the same.

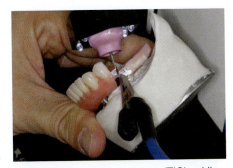

FIGRUE 23.8 Tungsten inert gas (TIG) welding.

ADVANTAGES AND DISADVANTAGES

Advantages

1. This allows execution of welds of high quality and excellent finishing, particularly in small joints.
2. The thickness of the joint allows for welding in any position, e.g. repairing removable partial prosthesis.
3. Excellent control of the weld pool, i.e. the region being welded.

4. Less time needed.
5. It can be executed directly in the working model.
6. The equipment is affordable compared to that of laser welding.
7. Allows welding in regions near the resins and porcelains.
8. Allows welding with the frameworks in close contact or with minimal space for welding, using filler metal.

Disadvantages

1. Large amount of heat to achieve fusion can cause microstructure transformations. These transformations occurring in the 'heat affected zone' can cause material distortion, residual stresses, generation of fragile microstructures, grain growth, cracks, fissures, and changes in mechanical, physical, and chemical properties, among others.
2. Insufficient weld penetration in butt type joints.
3. Porosities caused by inclusion of argon gas shield may occur in the weld region. These bubbles can initiate fractures leading to failure of welded structures.

LASER WELDING

A laser is a device that emits light through a process of optical amplification based on the stimulated emission of electromagnetic radiation. The term "laser" originated as an acronym for *"light amplification by stimulated emission of radiation"*. The first laser was built in 1960 by Theodore H. Maiman at Hughes Laboratories.

Laser is finding increasing applications in dentistry *(Box 23.2)* including welding. The laser used is a pulsed neodymium laser with a very high power density.

Among their many applications, lasers are used in optical disc drives, laser printers, and barcode scanners; fiber-optic and free-space optical communication; laser surgery and skin treatments; laser pointers; cutting and welding materials; military and law enforcement devices for marking targets and measuring range and speed; and laser lighting displays in entertainment.

BOX 23.2 | **Laser use in dentistry**

Lasers have been used in dentistry since 1994 to treat a number of dental problems. But, despite FDA approval, no laser system has received the American Dental Association's (ADA) Seal of Acceptance. That seal assures dentists that the product or device meets ADA standards of safety and efficacy, among other things. The ADA, however, states that it is cautiously optimistic about the role of laser technology in the field of dentistry. These lasers are different from the cold lasers used in phototherapy for the relief of headaches, pain, and inflammation.

Dental Applications of Laser

Tooth decay   Lasers are used to remove decay within a tooth and prepare the surrounding enamel to receive the filling.

Curing   Lasers are also used to "cure" or harden composite fillings.

Gum disease   Lasers are used to reshape gums and eliminate pockets.

Pulpectomy   Remove bacteria during root canal procedures.

Biopsy or lesion removal   Lasers can be used to remove a small piece of tissue (called a biopsy) so that it can be examined for cancer. Laser are also used to remove lesions in the mouth.

Pain relief   Used to relieve the pain of canker sores.

Surgical procedures   Like frenectomy, gingivectomy *(Fig. 23.10)*, healing abutment exposure, incisions, etc.

Teeth whitening   Lasers are used to speed up the in-office teeth whitening procedures. A peroxide bleaching solution, applied to the tooth surface, is "activated" by laser energy *(Fig. 23.9C)*, which speeds up of the whitening process.

Gum lightening Laser is used to remove the surface layer of mucosa containing the dark melanin pigment in patient with dark gums. On healing the new mucosa is lighter in color.

Welding For joining of metal parts.

How Do Lasers Work in Dentistry?

All lasers work by delivering energy in the form of light *(Fig. 23.9B and 23.10)*. When used for surgical and dental procedures, the laser acts as a cutting instrument or a vaporizer of tissue that it comes in contact with. When used for "curing" a filling, the laser takes the role of an intense curing light. When used in teeth whitening procedures, the laser acts as a heat source and enhances the effect of tooth bleaching agents.

Advantages

Compared to the traditional dental drill, lasers have certain advantages

1. They cause less pain in some instances, therefore, reducing the need for anesthesia.
2. They may reduce anxiety in patients uncomfortable with the use of the dental drill.
3. They minimize bleeding and swelling during soft tissue treatments.
4. They may preserve more healthy tooth during cavity removal.

Disadvantages

1. Lasers cannot be used on teeth with fillings already in place.
2. Lasers cannot be used in many commonly performed dental procedures. For example, lasers cannot be used to fill cavities located between teeth, around old fillings, and large cavities that need to be prepared for a crown. In addition, lasers cannot be used to remove defective crowns or silver fillings, or prepare teeth for fixed prostheses.
3. Traditional drills may still be needed to shape the filling, adjust the bite and polish the filling, even when a laser is used.
4. Lasers do not fully eliminate the need for anesthesia.
5. Laser treatment is more expensive since the cost of the laser is much higher than a dental drill. Lasers can cost between 6 to 7 times the cost of a standard drill.

Different Types of Dental Lasers Used

Many different types of lasers are used in dentistry *(Fig. 23.9A to D)*. They can be used in a wide range of power, ranging, from a fraction of a watt to 50 watts or even more.

1. The Erbium YAG laser *(Fig. 23.9A)* possesses the potential of replacing the drill. This laser is also used to alter pigmentation in the gingival tissues, providing the patient with pink gums. This laser is commonly used to prepare the patient for a cavity filling.
2. The carbon dioxide laser can be used to perform gingivectomy and to remove small tumors. As a laser that does not require local anesthesia, it poses no discomfort for the patient and is practically a bloodless procedure.
3. The argon laser is used in minor surgery. Its gas laser releases blue-green light through a fiberoptic cable to a handpiece or microscope.
4. The Nd:YAG laser is used in tissue retraction, endodontics and oral surgery. This laser usually does not require anesthesia. For procedures regarding the gingival pockets, the fiber is inserted between the gingiva and the tooth to sterilize and stimulate the tissue, causing the gingiva to adhere to the neck.
5. The Diode laser *(Fig. 23.9D)* introduced in the late 1990s has been effective for oral surgery and endodontic treatment. This laser also helps treat oral diseases and correct esthetic flaws. The diode is a compact laser.
6. Low level lasers are less well known, smaller and less expensive. Sometimes referred to as "soft lasers" the therapy performed by these lasers is called "low level laser therapy." Low level lasers improve blood circulation and regenerate tissues.

Waterlase (from Biolase)

The Waterlase combines a laser with an ultra-fine stream of water, which is capable of cutting into tooth, bone and soft tissues. As the stream of water flows into the laser beam, the water molecules become laser energized and create tiny explosions on impact with teeth or soft tissue.

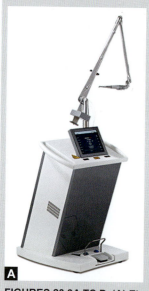
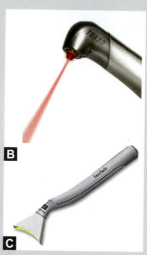
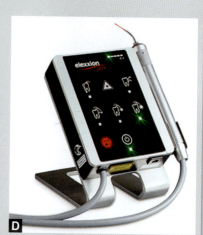

FIGURES 23.9A TO D **(A)** Elexxion duros Er:YAG hard tissue laser. **(B)** Laser handpiece. **(C)** Laser handpiece for tooth whitening. **(D)** A 15 watt table top diode laser unit.

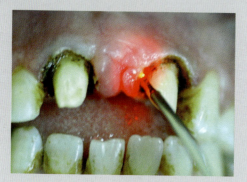

FIGURE 23.10 Laser gingivectomy.

COMMERCIAL NAMES

- Elexion Duros, Claros, Nano, Pico (Elexxion AG, Germany)
- Dental laser DL 2002 (Dentaurum, Germany)
- Haas laser LKS (Haas Laser GmbH, Germany)
- Heraeus Haas laser 44P (Heraeus Kulzer GmbH, Germany)
- Bego laserstar (Bego, Germany)

The unit **(Figs. 23.11A and B)** consists of a small box that contains the laser tip, an argon gas source and a stereo microscope with lens crosshairs for correct alignment of the laser beam with the components. The maximum depth the laser can penetrate is 2.5 mm. The heat generated is small, so the parts can be hand held during welding and it can be done close to the ceramic or even resin facings without damaging it.

INDICATIONS

Laser welding is used mainly to join titanium components. This is because the commercially pure titanium (cpTi) used in dentistry for fixed and removable partial denture frameworks

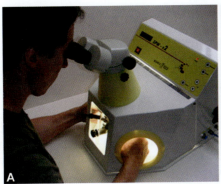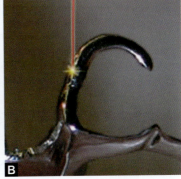

FIGURES 23.11A AND B (A) A Laser welding unit in operation. **(B)** Close-up of laser welding of a RPD clasp.

is highly reactive in air. Ordinary soldering procedures result in a weak joint because of the formation of thick layer of titanium oxide (especially when heated above 850 °C). Laser welding or plasma welding can be done at lower temperatures.

MECHANISM

When the light beam reaches the surface of the metal, the metal absorbs its energy, converting it into heat that penetrates into the interior of the metal by conduction. Owing to a high concentration of heat, the metal is taken to its melting point, and a series of events culminates in the formation of a keyhole or spots that will be filled with the melted metal.

ADVANTAGES OF LASER WELDING

Advantages

1. Lower heat generation.
2. It can be executed directly in the working model.
3. Allows welding in regions near the resins and porcelain portions without fear of damage to these materials.
4. No oxide formation because of the inert argon atmosphere.
5. Joint made of the same pure titanium as the components, thus reducing the risk of galvanic corrosion.
6. It produces a keyhole that concentrates the energy absorbed in a small region, resulting in high penetration and formation of a narrow heat affected zone (HAZ) that results in less distortion compared to conventional welding methods;
7. Less time expended
8. Allows welding with the structures in close contact or with minimal space for brazing using filler metal.

Disadvantages

1. Residual stress introduced into welding joints is a consequence of heating and cooling cycles of the welding process. This affects the mechanical behavior of laser-welded structures.
2. Argon gas can cause porosities which can lead to the failure of welded structures.
3. Insufficient penetration of the laser beam can cause a big defect or internal failure if equipment not adjusted properly.
4. High cost of the equipment.

CAST-JOINING

Cast-joining is an alternative method of joining metals parts that are difficult to solder such as base metal alloys. The two parts are joined by a third metal which is cast into the space between the two. The two parts are held together purely by mechanical retention which is achieved by proper flow of the new metal during casting. Therefore, if the cast metal is poorly adapted it can result in a weak joint.

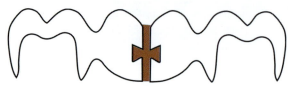

FIGURE 23.12 A mechanical interlocking design between two parts joined by cast-metal.

The joint area is ground to make a space of at least 1 mm. Mechanical undercuts are prepared at the interphase *(Fig. 23.12)*. The parts to be joined are assembled with the help of an index. Hard inlay casting wax is flowed into the space and a sprue is attached. The structure is then invested in a casting ring using suitable casting investment. The wax is burnt out and molten metal is cast into the space.

RADIOGRAPHIC ASSESSMENT OF JOINTS

Most prosthodontic structures are usually fabricated in commercial laboratories. The quality of the structure especially that of the joints can be assessed through a radiograph. The structure is placed on a film and exposed. It is turned 90 degrees and exposed a second time on a new film. The structure is assessed for defects like porosity and cracks especially in the joints. Porosity and other defects in the joints can weaken the restoration causing it to fail in the mouth during function. The best joints are those that are cast as one piece, followed by soldered and cast-joined.

Additive Manufacturing in Dentistry

Additive manufacturing is finding increasing use in dentistry. More popularly known as 'three-dimensional printing', it is an *additive* manufacturing process in contrast to conventional CAD/CAM which is a *subtractive* process. The first 3D printer was invented by Hideo Kodama of Nagoya, Japan. In 1984, Chuck Hull of 3D Systems Corporation further refined the process and named it stereolithography. The process involved the sequential laying down of photocured polymer to produce a three-dimensional plastic object.

As the technology developed it encompassed a wider variety of technologies and materials including metals, waxes, polymers, paper, ceramics, etc. By 2000, the umbrella term additive manufacturing (AM) technologies was used to describe all processes involving the CAD based production of objects through sequential layering.

Synonyms Other terms include three-dimensional printing, desktop manufacturing, rapid manufacturing, additive fabrication, additive layer manufacturing, layer manufacturing, and freeform fabrication, rapid prototyping, etc.

APPLICATIONS

Using data from oral scans and CAD designs, 3D printing can be used to produce

1. Surgical guides *(Fig. 24.1)*.
2. Veneers for try-in.
3. Study models *(Fig. 24.2)*.
4. Orthodontic appliances (aligners).

5. Surgical planning and mock surgeries using models designed with the aid of CT or MRI scan data.

6. Wax patterns *(Fig. 24.3)* for casting dental restorations like inlays, crowns and FDPs *(Fig. 24.4)*.

7. Restorations and removable denture frames can be directly fabricated from the raw metal (Co-Cr, titanium or gold alloy in powder form).

8. Maxillofacial prostheses.

9. Bioprinting can potentially engineer living organs, bone, skin and other tissues for plastic and reconstructive surgery, drug testing, etc.

FUNDAMENTALS OF 3D PRINTING

The fundamentals of additive manufacturing includes

1. Scan data input
2. Computer-aided design
3. Computer aided (additive) manufacturing

3D printable models may be created with a computer-aided design (CAD) package or via a 3D scan of the mouth, impression or model. CT or MRI data can also be used. The computer corrects errors in the scan data called fix-up. The 3D model which is in .skp, .dae, .3Ds or some other format that needs to be converted to either a .STL or a .OBJ format, to allow the printers software to be able to read it. Once that is done, the .STL file needs to be processed by a piece of software called a "slicer" which converts the model into a series of thin layers and produces

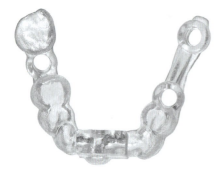

FIGURE 24.1 3D printed surgical guide for implants.

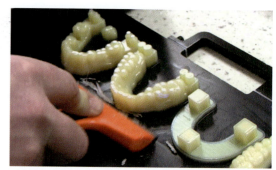

FIGURE 24.2 Dental models made from light cured photopolymerized resin.

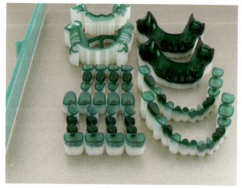

FIGURE 24.3 3D printed wax patterns of crowns, FDPs and removable partial dentures.

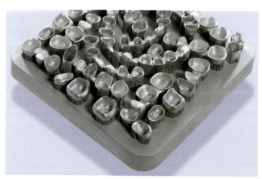

FIGURE 24.4 3D printed metal crowns and FDPs.

a G-code file containing instructions for the specific type of 3D printer used. The 3D printer follows the G-code instructions to lay down successive layers of liquid, powder, binder, paper or sheet material to build the model from a series of cross sections.

CLASSIFICATION OF ADDITIVE MANUFACTURING (AM) TECHNOLOGIES

The different types of 3D printers each employ a different technology that processes different materials in different ways. It is important to understand that one of the most basic limitations of 3D printing, in terms of materials and applications is that there is a no 'one solution fits all'. For example some 3D printers process powdered materials (nylon, plastic, ceramic, metal), which utilize a heat source (laser, electron beam) to sinter/melt/fuse layers of the powder together in the defined shape. Others process liquid resin and again utilize a light/laser to solidify the resin layer by layer. Jetting of fine droplets is another 3D printing process, reminiscent of 2D inkjet printing, but with a binder to fix the layers. Perhaps the most common and easily recognized process is deposition, and this is the process employed by the majority of entry-level 3D printers. This process extrudes plastics, commonly PLA or ABS, in filament form through a heated extruder to form layers and create the predetermined shape. The various types of additive manufacturing technologies currently available are summarized in *Table 24.1* and *Boxes 24.1 to 24.8*.

TABLE 24.1 Overview of additive manufacturing technologies

Type	Technologies	Materials
Material extrusion	Fused filament fabrication (FFF) also called fused deposition modelling (FDM)	Thermoplastics (e.g. PLA, ABS, HIPS, nylon), HDPE, metals, edible materials, rubber (Sugru), modelling clay, plasticine, RTV silicone, porcelain, metal clay, etc
	Robocasting	Ceramics, metal alloy, cermet, metal matrix composite, ceramic matrix composite
Powder bed fusion	Direct metal laser sintering (DMLS)	Almost any metal alloy
	Electron beam melting (EBM)	Almost any metal alloy including titanium
	Selective laser melting (SLM)	Titanium, cobalt chromium, stainless steel,
	Selective laser sintering (SLS)	Thermoplastics, metals, ceramics, glass
	Selective heat sintering (SHS)	Thermoplastics
Binder jetting	Binder jetting	Polymer, ceramic materials, metals
	Plaster-based 3D printing (PP)	Plaster
Material jetting	Material jetting (U-V)	Wax, plastics (PMMA)
Sheet Lamination	Laminated object manufact-uring (LOM)	Paper, metal foil, plastic film
VAT-based photopolymerization	Stereolithography (SLA)	Photopolymer
	Digital light processing (DLP)	Photopolymer
	Continuous liquid interface production	Photopolymer
Directed Energy Deposition	Electron beam free form fabrication (EBF3)	Almost any metal alloy in wire form
	Laser cladding	Almost any metal alloy in powder form
	Laser engineered net shaping (LENS)	Almost any metal alloy in powder form
	Direct metal deposition (DMD)	Almost any metal alloy in powder form

DESCRIPTION OF SOME ADDITIVE MANUFACTURING (AM) TECHNOLOGIES

BOX 24.1 | Material jetting

Material jetting is a 3D printing process whereby the actual build materials (in liquid or molten state) are selectively jetted through multiple jet heads (with others simultaneously jetting support materials). However, the materials tend to be liquid photopolymers, which are cured with a pass of UV light as each layer is deposited.

Material jetting is the only additive manufacturing technology that can combine different print materials within the same 3D printed model in the same print job.

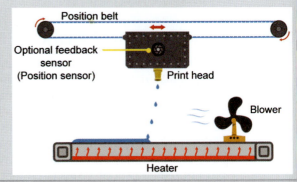

BOX 24.2 | Binder jetting

In binder jetting, the material being jetted is a binder. It is selectively sprayed into a powder bed to fuse it a layer at a time to create the required part. As is the case with other powder bed systems, once a layer is completed, the powder bed drops incrementally and a roller or blade smooths the powder over the surface of the bed, prior to the next pass of the jet heads.

Advantages of this process like with SLS, include the fact that the need for supports is negated because the powder bed itself provides this functionality. Furthermore, a range of different materials can be used, including ceramics and food. A further distinctive advantage of the process is the ability to easily add a full color palette which can be added to the binder. The parts resulting directly from the machine, however, are not strong and may require post-processing to ensure durability.

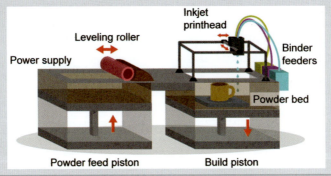

BOX 24.3 | Digital light processing (DLP)

DLP or digital light processing is a similar process to stereolithography in that it is a 3D printing process that works with photopolymers. The major difference is the light source. DLP uses a more conventional light source, such as an arc lamp, with a liquid crystal display panel or a deformable mirror device, which is applied to the entire surface of the of photopolymer resin in a single pass, generally making it faster than SL.

However, one advantage of DLP over SL is that only a shallow vat of resin is required to facilitate the process, which generally results in less waste and lower running costs.

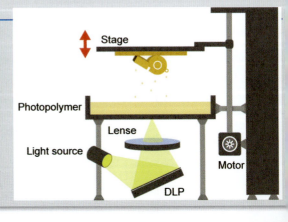

BOX 24.4 Fused deposition modeling

3D printing utilizing the extrusion of thermoplastic material is probably the most common and recognizable 3D printing process. The popular name for the process is fused deposition modeling (FDM), however this is a trade name, registered by Stratasys, the company that originally developed it. Other manufacturers generally referred to it as Fused Filament Fabrication (FFF).

The process works by melting plastic filament that is deposited, via a heated extruder, a layer at a time, onto a build platform. Each layer hardens as it is deposited and bonds to the previous layer. Systems have evolved and improved to incorporate dual extrusion heads.

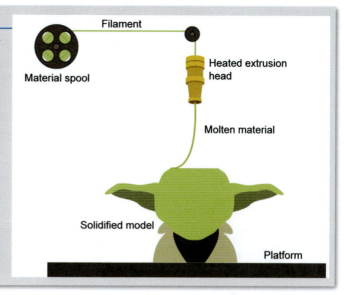

BOX 24.5 Robocasting

Robocasting or Direct Ink Writing (DIW) is an additive manufacturing technique in which a filament of 'ink' is extruded from a nozzle, forming an object layer by layer. The technique was first developed in the United States in 1996 as a method to allow geometrically complex ceramic green bodies to be produced. A fluid (typically a ceramic slurry), referred to as an 'ink', is extruded through a small nozzle, drawing out the shape of each layer of the CAD model. The ink exits the nozzle in a liquid-like state but retains its shape immediately, exploiting the rheological property of shear thinning. It is distinct from fused deposition modeling (FDM) as it does not rely on the solidification or drying to retain its shape after extrusion.

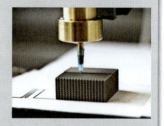

To date the most researched application for robocasting is in the production of biologically compatible tissue implants (bioprinting). Lattice structures can be formed quite easily which allow bone and other tissues in the human body to grow and eventually replace the transplant. With various medical scanning techniques the precise shape of the missing tissue is established and input into 3D modeling software and printed.

BOX 24.6 Electron beam melting (EBM)

The Electron Beam Melting 3D printing technique is a proprietary process developed by Swedish company Arcam. This metal printing method is very similar to the Direct Metal Laser Sintering (DMLS) process in terms of the formation of parts from metal powder. The key difference is the heat source, which, as the name suggests is an electron beam, rather than a laser, which necessitates that the procedure is carried out under vacuum conditions.

EBM has the capability of creating fully-dense parts in a variety of metal alloys, even to medical grade, and as a result the technique has been particularly successful for a range of production applications in the medical industry, particularly for implants. However, other hi-tech sectors, such as aerospace and automotive have also looked to EBM technology for manufacturing fulfilment.

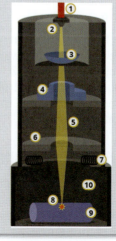

1. High voltage cable
2. Incandescent cathode
3. Bias cup
4. Primary anode
5. Electron beam
6. Focusing coil
7. Deflection coil
8. Weld bead
9. Work piece
10. Vacuum chamber

BOX 24.7   Laser sintering technique

Laser sintering and laser melting are interchangeable terms that refer to a laser-based 3D printing process that works with powdered materials. The laser is traced across a powder bed of tightly compacted powdered material. As the laser interacts with the surface of the powdered material it sinters, or fuses, the particles to each other forming a solid. As each layer is completed the powder bed drops incrementally and a roller smooths the powder over the surface of the bed prior to the next pass of the laser for the subsequent layer to be formed and fused with the previous layer.

The build chamber is completely sealed as it is necessary to maintain a precise temperature during the process. Once finished, the excess powder is removed to leave the 'printed' parts. One of the key advantages of this process is that the powder bed serves as an in-process support structure for overhangs and undercuts, and therefore complex shapes that could not be manufactured in any other way are possible with this process.

However, on the downside, because of the high temperatures required for laser sintering, cooling times can be considerable. Furthermore, porosity has been a issue with this process, and while there have been significant improvements towards fully dense parts, some applications still necessitate infiltration with another material to improve mechanical characteristics.

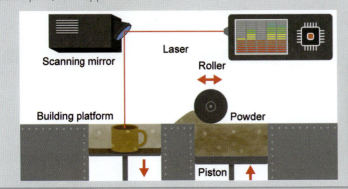
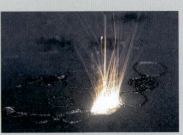

BOX 24.8   Sheet lamination and Directed energy deposition

Sheet Lamination

Sheet lamination processes include ultrasonic additive manufacturing (UAM) and laminated object manufacturing (LOM). The Ultrasonic Additive Manufacturing process uses sheets or ribbons of metal, which are bound together using ultrasonic welding.

Directed Energy Deposition

Directed energy deposition (DED) covers a range of terminology like laser engineered net shaping, directed light fabrication, direct metal deposition, 3D laser cladding'It is a more complex printing process commonly used to repair or add additional material to existing components. In this class of technology metal or alloy powder is actually deposited on the work surface and sintered or melted using various means.

3D DENTAL PRINTERS

3D printers for dental applications are manufactured by a range of companies *(Figs. 24.5A to D)*. These include Invision wax printer, Objet Eden 260V, Varseo Dental 3D Printing System (BEGO), Projet 3510DPPro, 3Z LAB 3D wax printer (solidscape), Stratasys Crownworx and Frameworx, Renishaw AM 250 (for metal), etc. They range in size from small desktop models to larger floor machines. The technology they employ also varies according to the objects they fabricate.

SUPPORT STRUCTURES FOR 3D PRINTED OBJECTS

Some printing techniques require external or internal supports to be built for undercut areas, cantilevers and other overhanging features for greater stability and strength during the manufacturing process. These supports are later mechanically removed or dissolved upon completion of the print.

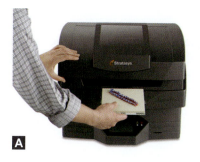

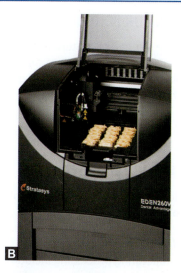

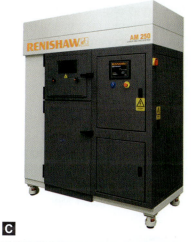

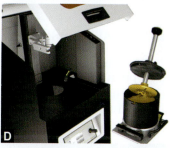

FIGURES 24.5A TO D 3D printers for dental applications. **(A)** A 3D wax printer (FrameWorx by Stratasys). **(B)** A 3D printer for dental models and casts. **(C)** A 3D metal printer dental for alloys.. **(D)** The Bego (Varseo) uses LED based stereolithography technology to make RPD and other pattens for casting.

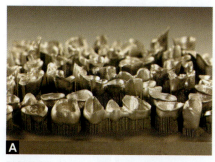

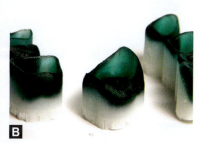

FIGURES 24.6A AND B Support structures. **(A)** 3D printed metal crowns and FDPs showing support structures. **(B)** 3D printed wax crowns showing support structures.

1. In metal and plastic printing, multiple supports are printed connecting the restoration to the base *(Fig. 24.6A)*.
2. Some 3D printers print wax patterns along with a second water soluble support material *(Fig. 24.6B)*. This material is removed after completion by dissolving in water *(Figs. 24.7A and B)*.
3. In powder bed systems, the unused powder surrounding the object functions as a support structure *(Box 24.7)*.

RAW MATERIALS FOR 3D PRINTING

A wide variety of materials are available for 3D printing. These include thermoplastics, granulated alloys (titanium alloys, metal alloys), foil, paper, photopolymers, liquid resins, rubber-like materials, silicones, glass, ceramic slurry, foods, medication, bioink make of cells and stem cells for tissue generation. etc.

These materials are in various forms like thermoplastic filaments, wire, granules, powder, photopolymerizing liquid resin, paste, liquid, etc (*Figs. 24.8A to C*).

POST-MANUFACTURING PROCESSING

Following the fabrication, the objects produced may require some form of processing for improved properties and finish. Objects manufactured may have layer lines and other artefacts of the printing process. Some of the products are produced in the green state and require to be sintered. Metals may require various forms of heat treatment. Thus post-manufacturing processing include support material removal, finishing and polishing, sealing, chemical treatment, sintering, heat treatment, etc.

3D PRINTED MAXILLOFACIAL PROSTHESES

British company Fripp Design and Research has developed 3D-printed prosthetic eyes that could be produced much faster than existing handmade versions, reducing the cost by 97 percent. The company which is also working on 3D-printed ears and noses for patients with facial disfigurements, has collaborated with Manchester Metropolitan University to

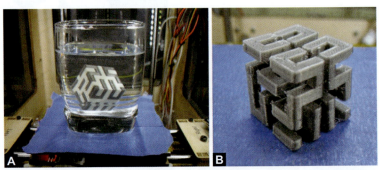

FIGURES 24.7A AND B (A) Dissolution of support material (white) by immersing in water. **(B)** Same object after removal of support material.

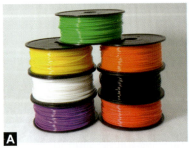 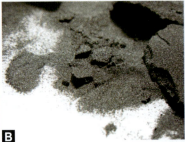 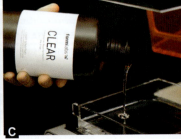

FIGURES 24.8A TO C Materials for Additive manufacturing. **(A)** Thermoplastic filaments for FFD. **(B)** Metal granules fo laser sintering. **(C)** Photopolymerizing liquid resin for stereolithography.

develop ocular prosthetics that are 3D-printed in batches, with intricate coloured details including the iris and blood vessels already included.

Currently, prosthetic eyes are moulded in acrylic and painted by hand to match the patient's eye color. This process is time-consuming and expensive, whereas producing the eyes using a 3D printer *(Fig. 24.9)* enables up to 150 eyes to be made in an hour. All of the components are printed from powder in full color using a Z-Corp 510 machine before the resulting form is encased in resin. Compared to the existing handmade production method, this helps to remove any variation in quality and significantly reduces the cost of each eye. (Refer also chapter on maxillofacial prosthetic materials).

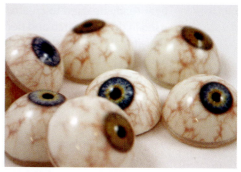

FIGURE 24.9 3D printed eyes.

3D PRINTING TECHNOLOGY IN SURGICAL PLANNING

Hospitals around the world are increasing turning to 3D technology to plan complex surgeries. In January 2015, doctors at London's St Thomas' Hospital had used images obtained from a magnetic resonance imaging (MRI) scan to create a 3D printing replica of the heart of a two-year-old girl with a complex hole in it. They were then able to tailor a Gore-Tex patch to effect a cure. 3D printing means surgeons can go into an operation with a much better idea of what they would find.

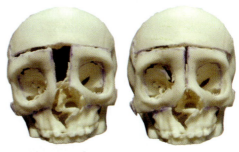

FIGURE 24.10 3D printed skull of a patient with hypertelorism.

Similarly plastic and maxillofacial surgeons in Bengaluru, Karnataka, India, used a 3D printed model *(Fig. 24.10)* for a surgical procedure to plan and correct orbital hypertelorism using both a box osteotomy as well as a facial bipartition technique with the aid of Osteo 3D, a company that is focused on 3D printing for the healthcare industry.

Similar processes are now being used in hospitals and universities to plan complex surgeries, for patient education and as teaching aids for medical students.

TISSUE ENGINEERING

Several terms have been used to refer to this field of research including organ printing, bioprinting, computer-aided tissue engineering, etc. The term *regenerative medicine* is often used synonymously with tissue engineering, although those involved in regenerative medicine place more emphasis on the use of *stem cells* or progenitor cells to produce tissues.

San Diego based Organovo, a regenerative medicine company, was the first company to commercialize 3D bioprinting technology. The company utilizes its NovoGen MMX Bioprinter *(Fig. 24.11)* for 3D bioprinting. The printer is optimized to be able to print skin tissue, cartilage, heart tissue and blood vessels among other basic tissues that could be suitable for surgical therapy and transplantation. It is hoped bioprinting technology will eventually be used to create fully functional human organs for transplants. They could be used in drug research and perhaps eliminate the need for testing in animals. The possibility of using 3D tissue printing to create soft tissue architectures for reconstructive and plastic surgery is also being explored.

Though scientists have been able to engineer artificial organs such as livers and kidneys, these organs lack crucial elements required for full and independent functioning, such as working blood vessels, tubules for collecting urine, etc. Without these the body has no way to get the essential nutrients and oxygen deep within the tissues. Fully functional printed organs may yet be possibility in the future.

HOW BIOPRINTING WORKS

In the bioprinting process, layers of living cells are deposited on to a gel medium or sugar matrix and slowly built up to form three-dimensional structures or scaffolds including vascular systems *(Box 24.9)*. Another process uses an extracellular matrix (ECM) protein as scaffold. As Organovo have demonstrated, it is not necessary to print all of the details of an organ with a bioprinter, as once the relevant cells are placed in roughly the right place nature completes the job. This point is illustrated by the fact that the cells contained in a bioink spheroid are capable of rearranging themselves after printing. For example, experimental blood vessels bioprinted using bioink spheroids comprising of an aggregate mix of endothelial, smooth muscle and fibroblast cells, once placed in position by the bioprint head demonstrated migration and reorganization. With no technological intervention, the endothelial cells migrate to the inside of the bioprinted blood vessel, the smooth muscle cells move to the middle, and the fibroblasts migrate to the outside.

INCUBATING THE NEW TISSUE

Scientists hope to be able one day to print some types of replacement parts directly into patients' bodies. Currently, tissues must spend a few days to few weeks maturing in a type of incubator called a bioreactor.

BIOINK

BioInk *(Fig. 24.12)* is a chemically defined hydrogel used to print 3D tissue models in bioprinters. It supports growth of different cell types. It allows cell adhesion, migration, and

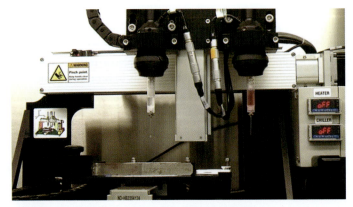

FIGURE 24.11 Organovo's NovoGen MMX bioprinter.

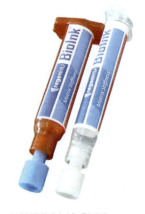

FIGURE 24.12 Bioink.

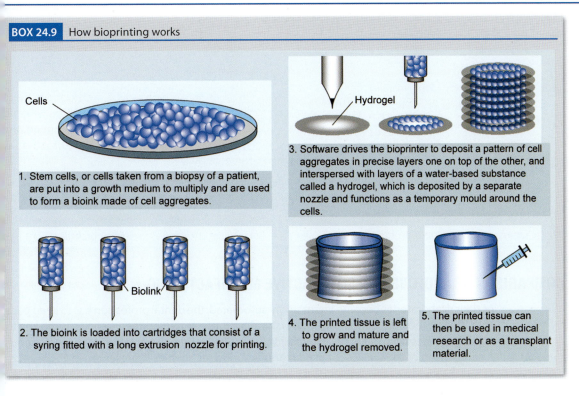

BOX 24.9 How bioprinting works

Cells

1. Stem cells, or cells taken from a biopsy of a patient, are put into a growth medium to multiply and are used to form a bioink made of cell aggregates.

Biolink

2. The bioink is loaded into cartridges that consist of a syring fitted with a long extrusion nozzle for printing.

Hydrogel

3. Software drives the bioprinter to deposit a pattern of cell aggregates in precise layers one on top of the other, and interspersed with layers of a water-based substance called a hydrogel, which is deposited by a separate nozzle and functions as a temporary mould around the cells.

4. The printed tissue is left to grow and mature and the hydrogel removed.

5. The printed tissue can then be used in medical research or as a transplant material.

differentiation. It mimics the natural extracellular matrix and is biodegradable. This material was developed by researchers at the University of Missouri, Columbia.

To make bioink, scientists create a slurry of cells that can be loaded into a cartridge and inserted into a specially designed printer, along with another cartridge containing a gel known as biopaper. After inputting the standards for the tissue, the printer lays down alternate layers to build a three-dimensional structure, with the biopaper creating a supportive matrix that the ink can thrive on. The individual droplets fuse together, eventually latticing upwards through the biopaper to create a solid structure.

One potential use for bioink is in skin grafting. By creating grafts derived from the patient's own cells, it could reduce the risk of rejection and scarring. Although initial bioink developments began with skin regeneration, the technology has advanced to also incorporate bone and muscle. This makes bioinks a total regenerative technology. Bioink could also be used to make replacements for vascular material removed during surgeries, allowing people to receive new veins and arteries. Eventually, entire organs could be constructed from this material. Bioprinted tissue could potentially remove the anxiety of finding donors as well as also allay fears about contaminated organ supplies or unscrupulous organ acquisition methods. These will enable medical researchers to test drugs on bioprinted models of the liver and other organs, thereby reducing the need for animal tests.

OSTEOINK

Osteoink is a ready-to-use calcium phosphate paste for structural engineering dedicated to regenHU's BioFactory and 3D Discovery printers. Osteoink is a highly osteoconductive biomaterial close to the chemical composition of human bone. Dedicated for hard tissue engineering, such as bone, cartilage or structural scaffold manufacturing, Osteoink can be combined with regenHU's biomaterial product portfolio (e.g. BioInk) to create complex 3D tissue mimetic models.

TABLE 24.2 Comparison of additive and subtractive manufacturing

	3D printing	CAD milling
1.	Computer aided	Computer aided
2.	Creates objects by adding material	Creates objects by removing material
3.	Does not require burs	Requires burs
4.	Can produce complex shapes without requiring special strategies or changing tools	Special strategies and parameters required to compensate for the size of the cutting tool
5.	Can print multiple parts at the same time	Can machine only one object at a time
6.	Can combine multiple raw materials in a single object (depending on the system)	Can use only one type of raw material at a time
7.	Little waste produced	Machining produces considerable waste
8.	There is nothing to break or change	Burs require changing as they break or wear

COMPARISON OF ADDITIVE AND SUBTRACTIVE MANUFACTURING

As dental laboratories become increasingly automated, the dental profession has to keep pace with the fast moving technology. Understanding these emerging technologies is the key to making choices on what is best suited for the individual dentist or laboratory professional. A comparison of the two CAD-based manufacturing techniques is presented in *Table 24.2.*

ADVANTAGES OF 3D PRINTING

1. Reduction fabrication times.
2. Reduced fabrication costs.
3. Clean, safe and efficient process.
4. Less waste as only the required amount of material is used (unlike CAD milling).
5. No need to store bulky models as they can be stored digitally and reproduced on demand.
6. Hollow objects can be created with greater ease.
7. Possible to print complex shapes and structures.
8. Possibility of using multiple materials in a single object.
9. Less stresses introduced in the object (compared to machining which may introduce microcracks in the object).
10. Rapid prototyping.

PART-6

Alloys in Dentistry

Dental Casting Alloys

Metal restorations and prostheses are an integral part of dentistry. Metals are among the strongest materials and provide strength and durability to any structure. There are two ways of constructing a metal restoration—direct and indirect. Direct techniques have been used in modern dentistry since the introduction of direct filling gold and amalgam in the 19th century. Indirect dental restorations were introduced into the dental profession with the patenting of the centrifugal casting machine and the lost wax technique by William H. Taggart in 1907.

TERMINOLOGY

ALLOY

An alloy is defined as a metal containing *two or more* elements, *at least one* of which is *metal* and all of which are mutually soluble in the molten state.

NOBLE METALS

Noble metals have been used for inlays, crowns and FDPs because of their resistance to corrosion in the mouth. Gold, platinum, palladium, rhodium, ruthenium, iridium, osmium and silver are the eight noble metals. However, in the oral cavity, silver can tarnish and therefore is not considered a noble metal.

PRECIOUS METALS

The term precious indicates the intrinsic value of the metal. The eight noble metals are also precious metals and are defined so by major metallurgical societies and federal government agencies, e.g. National Institute of Standards and Technology and National Material Advisory Board.

All noble metals are precious but all precious metals are not noble. Of the eight noble metals, four are very important in dental casting alloys, i.e. gold, platinum, palladium and silver. All four have a face-centered cubic crystal structure and all are white colored except for gold.

Gold   Pure gold is a soft and ductile metal with a yellow 'gold' hue. It has a density of 19.3 g/cm^3 and a melting point of 1063 °C. Gold has a good luster and takes up a high polish. It has good chemical stability and does not tarnish and corrode under normal circumstances.

Silver   Sometimes described as the 'whitest' of all metals. It has the lowest density (10.4 g/cm^3) and melting point (961°C) among the precious casting alloys. Its CTE is 15.7×10^{-6}/°C which is comparatively high.

Palladium   Density is 12.02 g/cm^3. Palladium has a higher melting point (1552°C) and lower CTE (11.1×10^{-6}/°C) when compared to gold.

Platinum   It has the highest density (21.65 g/cm^3) highest melting point (1769°C) and the lowest CTE among the four precious metals.

SEMIPRECIOUS METALS

There is no accepted composition which differentiates 'precious' from 'semiprecious'. Therefore, the term semiprecious should be avoided.

BASE METALS

These are non-noble metals. They are important components of dental casting alloys because of their influence on physical properties, control of the amount and type of oxidation and their strengthening effect. Such metals are reactive with their environment and are referred to as 'base metals'. Some of the base metals can be used to protect an alloy from corrosion by a property known as passivation. Although they are frequently referred to as nonprecious, the preferred term is base metal.

Examples   Chromium, cobalt, nickel, iron, copper, manganese, etc.

HISTORY AND CLASSIFICATION OF DENTAL CASTING ALLOYS

At the beginning of the twentieth century when dental casting techniques were evolving, the alloys were predominantly gold based. Taggart in 1907 was the first to describe the *lost wax technique* in dentistry. The existing jewelry alloys were quickly adopted for dental purposes. Initially, copper, silver and platinum were the main alloying elements. As the alloys evolved it was felt that a classification was needed. In 1932, the National Bureau of Standards classified the alloys according to their hardness (Type I, Type II, etc.).

At that time it was felt that gold alloy with less than 65% gold, tarnished too easily in the oral cavity. By 1948, metallurgists experimenting with various alloys were able to decrease the gold content while maintaining their resistance to tarnish. This breakthrough was due to *palladium*. It counteracted the tarnish potential of silver.

The main requirements of the original dental casting alloys were simple

1. They should not tarnish in the mouth.
2. They should be strong (for use as bridges).

This soon changed with the introduction of special alloys (metal-ceramic alloys) that could bond to porcelain in the late 1950s. The composition and requirements of these alloys became more complex. For example, they had to contain elements that could enhance bond to porcelain, they had to have a higher melting temperature (because porcelain had high fusion temperatures), etc.

Another important development were the rapid increase in gold prices in the 1970s. As gold became more expensive, people began to look for less expensive metals for dental castings. Manufacturers began experimenting with base metal alloys like nickel-chromium and cobalt-chromium. These alloys were already in use since the 1930s for the construction of cast partial denture frameworks. Prior to this, the Type IV gold alloys were used extensively for this purpose. These base metals soon replaced the Type IV gold alloys for partial denture use because of their light weight, lower cost and tarnish resistance. When the gold prices shot up, these base metal partial denture alloys were quickly adapted for use in fixed prosthodontics. Subsequently, newer formulations allowed their use as metal-ceramic alloys.

Today there is such a wide variety of alloys in the market that classifying them is not easy. A number of different classifications are mentioned below.

ACCORDING TO USE

A. Alloys for all metal and resin veneer restorations* (e.g. inlays, posts, resin and composite veneered crowns and FDPs).
B. Alloys for metal-ceramics restorations (e.g. PFM crowns and FDPs).
C. Alloys for removable dentures ** (e.g. RPD frames and complete denture bases).

BASED ON YIELD STRENGTH AND PERCENT ELONGATION (ADA SP. 5)

Type I   Soft

Type II   Medium

Type III   Hard

Type IV   Extra-hard

(This 1934 classification was *originally intended for gold alloys* and were based on hardness. Since 1989, it was relaxed to include any dental alloy as long as they met the new yield strength and percentage elongation criteria. Types I and II are known as 'inlay alloys' and Types III and IV are known as 'crown and bridge alloys'. Type IV is occasionally used for RPD frames).

---

*Some authors classify this as crown and bridge alloys. Unfortunately, this can create confusion; for example, metal-ceramic alloys are also crown and bridge alloys.
**Also known as RPD alloys, which again unfortunately is not fully accurate as they can be used for other structures. However, until a more suitable terminology is found, this classification will be continued.

ACCORDING TO NOBILITY (ADA 1984)

A. High noble metal alloys (HN)   Contains ≥ 40 wt% Au and ≥ 60 wt% noble metals

B. Noble metal alloys (N)   Contains ≥ 25 wt% of noble metals

C. Predominantly base metal alloys (PB)   Contains < 25 wt% of noble metals

D. Base metal

This classification is popular among manufacturers.

BASED ON MECHANICAL PROPERTIES (ISO 22674:2006)

The current ISO classification supersedes all previous classifications and covers all metals used in dentistry for restorations and prostheses. It makes no distinction between noble and base metal. ISO 22674:2006 classifies all metallic materials into six types according to its mechanical properties.

Type 0 - Intended for low stress bearing single-tooth fixed restorations, e.g. small veneered one-surface inlays, veneered crowns.*

Type 1 - Intended for low stress bearing single-tooth fixed restorations, e.g. veneered or unveneered one-surface inlays, veneered crowns.

Type 2 - Intended for single tooth fixed restorations, e.g. crowns or inlays without restriction on the number of surfaces.

Type 3 - Intended for multiple unit fixed restorations, e.g. bridges.

Type 4 - Intended for appliances with thin sections that are subject to very high forces, e.g. removable partial dentures, clasps, thin veneered crowns, wide-span bridges or bridges with small cross-sections, bars, attachments, implant retained superstructures.

Type 5 - Intended for appliances in which parts require the combination of high stiffness and strength, e.g. thin removable partial dentures, parts with thin cross-sections, clasps.

ACCORDING TO MAJOR ELEMENTS

A. Gold alloys

B. Silver alloys

C. Palladium alloys

D. Nickel alloys

E. Cobalt alloys

F. Titanium alloys

ACCORDING TO THE THREE MAJOR ELEMENTS

A. Gold-palladium-silver

B. Palladium-silver-tin

C. Nickel-chromium-molybdenum

D. Cobalt-chromium-molybdenum

E. Iron-nickel-chromium

F. Titanium-aluminum-vanadium

ACCORDING TO THE NUMBER OF ALLOYS PRESENT

A. Binary—two elements

---

* also includes metal-ceramic restorations produced by electroforming or sintering.

B. Ternary—three elements

C. Quaternary (and so forth)—four elements

CLASSIFICATION ACCORDING TO USE OF DENTAL CASTING ALLOYS

The huge choice of alloys in the market makes the process of identification a difficult task. They are similar in some aspects, but yet, each have their own distinct features. These alloys vary not only in the type of metal but also the percentage of each within the alloy. In spite of their wide variation in composition, they must meet the requirements of their intended use. For example, all metal-ceramic alloys regardless of whether they are noble or base must meet the requirements of porcelain bonding. For this reason, the classification according to use is recommended and will be the basis of the subsequent discussion of alloys.

A. Alloys for all metal and resin veneer restorations
   - High noble
   - Noble
   - Predominantly base metal
   - Base metal

B. Alloys for metal-ceramics restorations
   - High noble
   - Noble
   - Predominantly base metal
   - Base metal

C. Alloys for casting large structures
   - High noble
   - Noble
   - Predominantly base metal
   - Base metal

GENERAL REQUIREMENTS OF CASTING ALLOYS

All cast metals in dentistry have some basic common requirements.

1. They must not tarnish and corrode in the mouth.
2. They must be sufficiently strong for the intended purpose.
3. They must be biocompatible (nontoxic and nonallergenic).
4. They must be easy to melt, cast, cut and grind (easy to fabricate).
5. They must flow well and duplicate fine details during casting.
6. They must have minimal shrinkage on cooling after casting.
7. They must be easy to solder.

Not all of them meet all the requirements. Some have shown a potential for allergic reactions (nickel containing alloys) and other side effects when used without proper precautions. Some are quite difficult to cast. Some are so hard (base metal alloys) that they are difficult to cut, grind and polish. All alloys shrink on cooling. Some (base metal alloys) show more shrinkage than others. The shrinkage cannot be eliminated, but it can be compensated for (see investments). Besides these general requirements, alloys intended for a certain specific use must meet requirements for that. For example, metal-ceramic alloys must have additional requirements in order to be compatible with porcelain. The requirements for metal-ceramic alloys will be described later.

ALLOYS FOR ALL METAL RESTORATIONS

These alloys were among the earliest alloys available to dentistry. The early alloys were mostly gold alloys. Since they were intended for all-metallic and later for resin veneered restorations, they just had to meet the basic requirements (see general requirements). No special requirements are needed for veneering with resin.

Currently, the use of these alloys are slowly declining because of

- ❍ Increased esthetic awareness has reduced the trend for metal display.
- ❍ Increasing popularity of all-ceramic and metal-ceramic restorations.
- ❍ Reducing popularity of resin and composite as veneering material. Resin facings have a number of disadvantages.
  - – They wear rapidly (poor wear resistance).
  - – They may change color (color instability and stain absorption).
  - – They are porous. They tend to absorb food material and bacteria. This makes it unhygienic and gives it a bad odor.

CLASSIFICATION (ANSI/ADA SP. NO. 5)

(As mentioned before this 1934 classification was *originally intended for gold alloys* and was based on hardness. In 1989, it was relaxed to include any dental alloy as long as they met the new yield strength and percentage elongation criteria).

TYPE I SOFT

Small inlays, Class III and Class V cavities which are not subjected to great stress. They are easily burnished.

TYPE II MEDIUM

Inlays subject to moderate stress, thick 3/4 crowns, abutments, pontics, full crowns, and sometimes soft saddles.

TYPE III HARD

Inlays, crowns and bridges, situations where there may be great stresses involved. They usually can be age hardened.

TYPE IV EXTRA-HARD

Inlays subjected to very high stresses, partial denture frameworks and long span bridges. They can be age hardened.

Types I and II are generally called 'inlay alloys' and Types III and IV are known as 'crown and bridge alloys'. Because of the increased use of composite and ceramic inlays, the Type I and II inlay alloys are rarely used currently. Most of the discussion will focus on the Types III and IV alloys.

USES

These alloys are *not intended* for porcelain bonding. They may be used as an *all-metal* restoration or with a *resin veneer*.

1. Inlays and onlays *(Figs 25.1A)*
2. Crowns and FDPs *(Fig. 25.1B)*

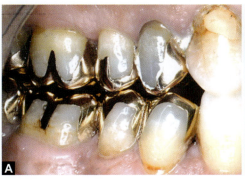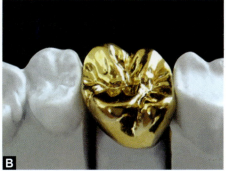

FIGURES 25.1A AND B **(A)** Gold onlays. **(B)** A gold crown.

3. Partial denture frames (only the Type IV)
4. Post-cores *(Fig. 25.2)*

TYPES

These alloys will be discussed under the following categories.

High noble — Gold alloys

Noble — Silver palladium alloys

Base metal — Nickel-chrome alloys

Cobalt-chrome alloys

Titanium and its alloys

Aluminum-bronze alloys

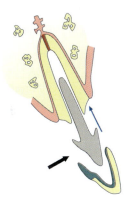

FIGURE 25.2 Post-core.

GOLD ALLOYS (FOR ALL-METAL RESTORATIONS)

Synonyms Traditional gold alloys, Au-Ag-Cu alloys.

Why do we alloy gold?
Pure gold is a soft and ductile metal and so is not used for casting dental restorations and appliances in its pure state. It is alloyed commonly with copper, silver, platinum, nickel and zinc. Alloying gold with these metals not only improves its physical and mechanical properties but also reduces its cost.

The display of metal particularly gold was once acceptable and probably was even a symbol of social status. The current trend is to avoid the display of metal. At the same time, increase in the platinum, palladium and silver content of modern alloys have resulted in whiter colored gold alloys. Thus, there are *'yellow gold alloys'* and *'white gold alloys'.* The rise in gold prices have also led to the availability of alloys with low gold content. These are the *'low golds'.*

The gold alloys discussed here are high noble alloys because of their high noble metal content (see classification according to nobility).

GOLD CONTENT

Traditionally, gold content of dental casting alloys was called

○ Karat

○ Fineness

KARAT

It refers to the parts of pure gold present in 24 parts of alloy, e.g.

- 24 karat gold is pure gold.
- 22 karat gold is 22 parts pure gold and 2 parts of other metal.

Note In current dental alloys, the term karat is rarely used.

FINENESS

Fineness of a gold alloy is the parts per thousand of pure gold. Pure gold is 1000 fine. Thus, if 3/4 of the gold alloy is pure gold, it is said to be 750 fine.

Note The term fineness also is rarely used to describe gold content in current alloys (however, it is often used to describe gold alloy solders).

PERCENTAGE COMPOSITION

The percentage composition of gold alloys is preferred over karat and fineness. Since 1977, ADA requires manufacturers to specify the percentage composition of gold, palladium and platinum on all their dental alloy packaging.

$$\frac{Karat \times 100}{24} = \% \, gold$$

Fineness is 10 times the percentage gold composition, i.e. fineness $\times$ 10 = %gold.

COMPOSITION OF GOLD ALLOYS

Type	% Au	% Cu	% Ag	% Pd	% Pt	% In, Sn, Fe, Zn, Ga
I	83	6	10	0.5	—	Balance
II	77	7	14	1	—	Balance
III	75	9	11	3.5	—	Balance
IV	69	10	12.5	3.5	3	Balance

FUNCTIONS OF CONSTITUENTS

Gold

It provides tarnish and corrosion resistance and has a desirable appearance. It also provides ductility and malleability.

Copper

It is the principal hardener. It reduces the melting point and density of gold. If present in sufficient quantity, it gives the alloy a reddish color. It also helps to age harden gold alloys. In greater amounts, it reduces resistance to tarnish and corrosion of the gold alloy. Therefore, the maximum content should not exceed 16 percent.

Silver

It whitens the alloy, thus helping to counteract the reddish color of copper. It increases strength and hardness slightly. In larger amounts, however, it reduces tarnish resistance.

Platinum

It increases strength and corrosion resistance. It also increases melting point and has a whitening effect on the alloy. It helps reduce the grain size.

Palladium

It is similar to platinum in its effect. It hardens and whitens the alloy. It also raises the fusion temperature and provides tarnish resistance. It is less expensive than platinum, thus reducing the cost of the alloy.

The minor additions are

Zinc

It acts as a scavenger for oxygen. Without zinc, the silver in the alloy causes absorption of oxygen during melting. Later during solidification, the oxygen is rejected producing gas porosities in the casting.

Indium, tin and iron

They help to harden ceramic gold-palladium alloys, iron being the most effective.

Calcium

It is added to compensate for the decreased CTE that results when the alloy is made silver free (the elimination of silver is done to reduce the tendency for green stain at the metal-porcelain margin).

Iridium, ruthenium, rhenium

They help to decrease the grain size. They are added in small quantities (about 100–150 ppm).

Note   All modern noble metal alloys are fine grained. Smaller the grain size of the metal, the more ductile and stronger it is. It also produces a more homogeneous casting and improves the tarnish resistance. A large grain size reduces the strength and increases the brittleness of the metal. Factors controlling the grain size are the rate of cooling, shape of the mold and composition of the alloy.

PROPERTIES OF GOLD ALLOYS

COLOR

Traditionally, the gold alloys were gold colored. The color of modern gold alloys can vary from gold to white. It depends on the amount of whitening elements (silver, platinum, palladium, etc.) present in the alloy.

MELTING RANGE

Ranges between 920–960 °C. The melting range of an alloy is important. It indicates the type of investment required and the type of heating source needed to melt the alloy.

DENSITY

It gives an indication of the number of dental castings that can be made from a unit weight of the metal. In other words, more number of cast restorations per unit weight can be made from an alloy having a lower density, than one having a higher density. Gold alloys are lighter than pure gold (19.3 g/cm^3).

- Type III — 15.5 g/cm^3
- Type IV — 15.2 g/cm^3

The castability of an alloy is also affected by density. Higher density alloys cast better than lower density alloys.

YIELD STRENGTH

The yield strength is   Type III — 207 MPa
                        Type IV — 275 MPa

HARDNESS

The hardness indicates the ease with which these alloys can be cut, ground or polished. Gold alloys are generally more user friendly than the base metal alloys which are extremely hard.

The hardness values   Type III — 121 MPa
                      Type IV — 149 MPa

ELONGATION

It indicates the ductility of the alloy. A reasonable amount is required especially if the alloy is to be deformed during clinical use, e.g. clasp adjustment for removable partial dentures, margin adjustment and burnishing of crowns and inlays. Type I alloys are easily furnished. Alloys with low elongation are very brittle. Age hardening decreases ductility.

○ Type III—30–40%
○ Type IV—30–35%.

MODULUS OF ELASTICITY

This indicates the stiffness/flexibility of the metal. Gold alloys are more flexible than base metal alloys (Type IV—90×10^3 MPa).

TARNISH AND CORROSION RESISTANCE

Gold alloys are resistant to tarnish and corrosion under normal oral conditions. This is due to their high noble content. Noble metals are less reactive.

CASTING SHRINKAGE

All alloys shrink when they change from liquid to solid. The casting shrinkage in gold alloys is less (1.25–1.65%) when compared to base metal alloys.

The shrinkage occurs in three stages:

1. Thermal contraction of the liquid metal.
2. Contraction of the metal while changing from liquid to solid state.
3. Thermal contraction of solid metal as it cools to room temperature.

Shrinkage affects the fit of the restoration. Therefore, it must be controlled and compensated for in the casting technique.

BIOCOMPATIBILITY

Gold alloys are relatively biocompatible.

CASTING INVESTMENT

Gypsum-bonded investments may be used for low fusing gold alloys.

HEAT TREATMENT OF GOLD ALLOYS

Heat treatment of alloys is done in order to alter its mechanical properties. Gold alloys can be heat treated if it contains sufficient amount of *copper*. Only Type III and Type IV gold alloys can be heat treated.

There are two types of heat treatment.

1. Softening heat treatment (solution heat treatment).
2. Hardening heat treatment (age hardening).

SOFTENING HEAT TREATMENT

Softening heat treatment increases ductility, but reduces strength, proportional limit and hardness.

Indications

It is indicated for appliances that are to be ground, shaped or otherwise cold worked in or outside the mouth.

Method

The casting is placed in an electric furnace for 10 minutes at 700 °C and then it is quenched in water. During this period, all intermediate phases are changed to a *disordered solid solution* and the rapid quenching prevents ordering from occurring during cooling. Each alloy has its optimum temperature. The manufacturer should specify the most favorable temperature and time.

HARDENING HEAT TREATMENT (OR AGING)

Hardening heat treatment increases strength, proportional limit and hardness but decreases ductility. It is the copper present in gold alloys which helps in the age hardening process.

Indications

For strengthening metallic dentures, saddles, FDPs and other similar structures before use in the mouth. It is not employed for smaller structures, such as inlays.

Method

It is done by 'soaking' or aging the casting at a specific temperature for a definite time, usually 15–30 minutes. It is then water quenched or cooled slowly. The ageing temperature depends on the alloy composition but is generally between 200 and 450 °C. During this period, the intermediate phases are changed to an *ordered solid solution* (the proper time and temperature for age hardening an alloy is specified by its manufacturer).

Ideally, before age hardening an alloy, it should first be subjected to a softening heat treatment in order to relieve all strain hardening (stresses which occurs during finishing). Starting the hardening treatment when the alloy is in a disordered solid solution allows better control of the aging process.

LOW GOLD ALLOYS

Also known as 'economy golds'. They are crown and FDP alloys having gold content below 60% (generally in the 42–55% range). However, gold must be the major element.

This is a *gold colored base metal alloy* which was frequently misused in India to make all-metal crowns and FDPs since many years. They are also sometimes referred to as *Japanese gold* or *K-metal*. These alloys *do not contain any gold* or precious metal. The alloy is absolutely *contraindicated* for any intraoral dental use because of its low strength, low wear resistance and tendency to tarnish. It has a high initial gold-like luster and patients are deliberately misled by unscrupulous practitioners into believing it was gold. Thanks to the availability of better materials its use has declined considerably. Unfortunately, one does come across restorations made from this alloy even to this day. Some practitioners still offer this material as a lower cost alternative, in addition to the regular alloys.

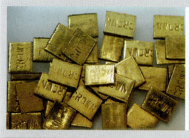 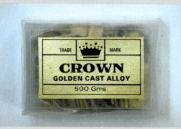 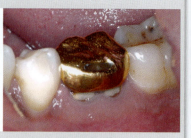

The low gold alloys were developed because of the increase in gold prices. However, reducing gold content increased tarnish and corrosion. This problem was overcome by two discoveries.

❍ Palladium made the silver in gold alloy more tarnish resistant. 1% palladium was required for every 3% of silver.

❍ The silver-copper ratio had to be carefully balanced to yield a low silver rich phase in the microstructure.

ADVANTAGES

Because of this research numerous low gold alloys were introduced into the market. Thus, these alloys were not only less expensive but also had good tarnish and corrosion resistance. Their properties are comparable to Types III and IV gold alloys.

SILVER-PALLADIUM ALLOYS

These alloys were introduced as a cheaper alternative to gold alloys. It is predominantly silver in composition. Palladium (at least 25%) is added to provide nobility and resistance to tarnish. They may or may not contain copper and gold. They are white in color.

Type	Component	Proportion	
Ag-Pd (non-copper)	Ag	0–72%	Properties are like Type III gold alloys
	Pd	25%	
Ag-Pd-Cu	Ag	60%	Properties are like Type IV gold alloys
	Pd	25%	
	Cu	15%	

The properties of the silver-palladium alloys are similar to the Types III and IV gold alloys. However, they have lower ductility and corrosion resistance. They also have a significantly lower density than gold alloy. This may affect its castability.

A major difference between Types III and IV Ag-Pd alloys is that the latter can be significantly age hardened because of its gold and copper content.

NICKEL-CHROME AND COBALT-CHROMIUM ALLOYS

These are known as base metal alloys and are extensively used in many of the developing countries. In India, because of their relatively low cost many of the laboratories use these alloys along with resin facings.

These metals are very strong and hard. Because of this, they are generally difficult to work with (cutting, grinding, polishing, etc.). They are dealt in more detail in subsequent sections.

TITANIUM AND TITANIUM ALLOYS

These metals can be used for all-metal and metal-ceramic restorations, as well as partial dentures. They are described later under metal-ceramic restorations.

ALUMINUM-BRONZE ALLOY

Bronze is an alloy known to man since ancient times. Traditional bronze is copper alloyed with tin. The ADA approved bronze (**Fig. 25.3**) does not contain tin. The composition is as follows:

Component	Proportion
Copper	81–88%
Aluminum	8–10%
Nickel	2–4%
Iron	1–4%

Being relatively new, the information on these alloys is relatively scanty.

PROPERTIES*

Color	Yellow gold
Melting range	1012–1068 °C
Density	7.8 g/cm³
Brinell harness number	104
Yield strength	30,000 psi
Elongation	29%

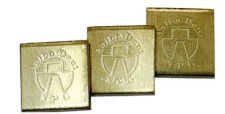

FIGURE 25.3 Aluminum bronze alloys (*Courtesy:* BDCH, Davangere).

METAL-CERAMIC ALLOYS

Metal-ceramic alloys are those alloys that are compatible with porcelain and capable of bonding to it. A layer of porcelain is fused to the alloy to give it a natural tooth-like appearance. Porcelain being a brittle material fractures easily, so these alloys are used to reinforce the porcelain.

Several types of alloys are used to cast substructures for porcelain-fused-to-metal crowns and FDPs. They may be noble metal alloys or base metal alloys (see classification). All have coefficient of thermal expansion (CTE) values which match that of porcelain.

Note CTE has a reciprocal relationship with melting point, i.e. the higher the melting point of a metal, lower is its CTE.

---

* Properties (as provided by the manufacturer)

Synonyms

Porcelain-fused-to-metal (PFM), ceramometal alloys, porcelain-bonded-to-metal (PBM). The preferred term, however, is metal ceramic or PFM.

EVOLUTION OF METAL-CERAMIC ALLOYS

The metal-ceramic alloys evolved from resin-veneered crown and bridge alloys. Resin facing faced the problem of gradual wear and had to be replaced over time. Besides resin could not be used on the occlusal surface. To retain a resin veneered restoration undercuts had to be provided. The early metal-ceramic alloys were high gold alloys (88% gold). They were not strong enough for FDP use. In the early days before porcelain-metal bonding was clearly understood, porcelain had to be retained by mechanical means with the help of undercuts. Later, it was discovered that adding 1% of base metals like iron, tin, indium, etc. induced chemical bonding by the formation of an oxide layer. This significantly improved the bond strength between porcelain and metal.

REQUIREMENTS OF ALLOYS FOR PORCELAIN BONDING

In addition to the general requirements of alloys mentioned earlier, metal-ceramic alloys have certain specific requirements in order to be compatible with porcelain veneering.

1. Its melting temperature should be higher than porcelain firing temperatures.
2. It should be able to resist creep or sag at these temperatures.
3. Its CTE should be compatible with that of porcelain.
4. They should be able to bond with porcelain.
5. It should have a high stiffness (modulus of elasticity). Any flexing of the metal framework may cause porcelain to fracture or delaminate.
6. It should not stain or discolor porcelain.

USES OF METAL-CERAMIC ALLOYS

1. As the name implies these alloys are intended for porcelain veneered restorations (crowns and FDPs—*Fig. 25.4*).
2. They can also be used for all-metal restorations.

TYPES (CLASSIFICATION) OF METAL-CERAMIC ALLOYS

Alloys for metal ceramics restorations may be categorized as

1. High noble (commonly referred to as gold alloys) *(Fig. 25.5)*
   - Gold-palladium-platinum alloys
   - Gold-palladium-silver alloys
   - Gold-palladium alloys
2. Noble (commonly referred to as palladium alloys)
   - Palladium-silver alloys
   - Palladium-gallium-silver alloys
   - Palladium-gold alloys
   - Palladium-gold-silver alloys
   - Palladium-copper alloys
   - Palladium-cobalt alloys

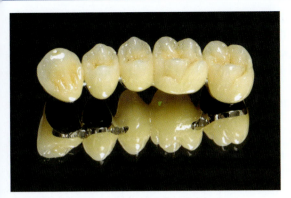

FIGURE 25.4 Metal-ceramic fixed partial denture.

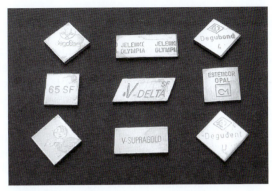

FIGURE 25.5 Gold-based metal-ceramic alloys (1 g). Most are white gold alloys. V supra gold (Bottom row middle) has a light gold color. SF denotes silver free.

3. Base metal
   - Nickel-chromium alloys
   - Nickel-chromium-beryllium alloys
   - Cobalt-chromium alloys
   - Pure titanium
   - Titanium-aluminum-vanadium

THE HIGH NOBLE (GOLD-BASED) METAL-CERAMIC ALLOYS

The high noble alloys contain more than 40 wt% gold and are therefore also referred to as gold alloys or gold based alloys *(Fig. 25.5)*.

COMMON FEATURES OF HIGH NOBLE (GOLD BASED) ALLOYS

Cost These are the most expensive crown and bridge alloys. However, in spite of the cost, these alloys are user friendly and are preferred in practices where the clientele can afford the cost.

Color The color can range from white to gold depending on the gold content. The whitening alloys are palladium and platinum. The gold color when present can enhance the vitality of the porcelain thus improving the esthetics.

Melting range Porcelain is fired at a temperature of 900–960 °C. Thus obviously these alloys must have melting temperatures much higher than the temperatures at which porcelain is fired. Pure gold has a melting temperature of 1063 °C. The melting temperature is raised by the addition of platinum (1769 °C) and palladium (1552 °C).

The melting temperatures of these alloys range from 1149–1304 °C.

Density Ranges from 13.5 to 18.3 g/cm^3 (depending on the gold content). Because of the high gold and noble metal content, these alloys have a high density. The density reduces as more palladium is added.

Castability The high density of these alloys make them easy to cast. If done well one can expect most of the fine features to be accurately duplicated.

Yield strength Ranges from 450 to 572 MPa.

Hardness and workability Ranges from 182 to 220 VHN. These alloys are relatively softer when compared to the base metal alloys and so are extremely easy to work with. They are easy to cut, grind and polish.

Percent elongation Ranges from 5 to 20%. This gives an indication of the ductility of the alloy. The higher the value, the more ductile it is.

Porcelain bonding The presence of an oxide layer on the surface of metal ceramic alloys assists in chemical bonding of porcelain to the alloy. Pure noble metal alloys rarely form an oxide layer. To induce the formation of an oxide layer, 1% of base metals like *tin, indium, iron*, etc. are added to the alloy. This significantly improved the bond strength between the porcelain and the metal.

Sag resistance During porcelain firing, the metal frame has to withstand temperatures as high as 950 °C. At these temperatures, there is a danger of the metal substructure sagging under its own weight, thereby deforming. The longer the span, the greater the risk. The ability of a metal to resist sag is known as sag resistance. Compared to base metal alloys, gold alloys are less sag resistant.

Tarnish and corrosion Because of their high noble metal content, these alloys are extremely stable in the oral environment. Noble metals have low reactivity to oxygen and therefore do not tarnish easily.

Biocompatibility High noble alloys have had a good and safe track record. They are not known to cause any problems in the mouth.

Reusability These alloys are stable and so scrap from these alloys can be recast at least two or three times. However, the more volatile base metals like zinc, indium, tin, etc., may be lost. To compensate for this, *equal amounts* of new alloys should be mixed. The scrap should be cleaned by sandblasting and ultrasonic cleaning before use. Alloys from different manufacturers should not be mixed as it may change its composition and properties.

Scrap value The high noble alloys have good scrap value. Many suppliers and manufacturers accept used alloy scrap.

Soldering Gold-based alloys are quite easy to solder.

TYPES

The following three types will be briefly described:
1. Gold-palladium-platinum alloys
2. Gold-palladium-silver alloys
3. Gold-palladium alloys

Commercial names Some of the available alloys are presented in *Table 25.1.*

GOLD-PALLADIUM-PLATINUM ALLOYS

COMPOSITION

Component	Proportion
Gold	80–88 wt%
Palladium	5–11 wt%
Platinum	6–8 wt%
Silver	0–4.9 wt% (rarely present)
Base metals	Balance (around 1%)

TABLE 25.1 Commercial names of some noble and high noble alloys

High noble alloys (Au > 40%)	Gold-palladium-platinum	Jelenko'O' (Jelenko) SMG-3
	Gold-platinum	Willbond Bio 88 PF (Willkinson)*
	Gold-platinum-palladium	Degudent H (Degussa)
	Gold-palladium-silver	Wilbond 75 (Willkinson)** Cameo (Jelenko) RxWCG (Jeneric/Pentron) Special white (Degussa)
	Gold-palladium	Olympia (Jelenko) Orion (Ney) Deva 4 (Degussa) Willbond 65SF(Willkinson)***
Noble alloys (Au < 40%)	Palladium-gold	Nobilium 30 NS
	Palladium-gold-gallium	Olympia II (Jelenko)
	Palladium-gold-silver	Rx SWCG (Jeneric) Regent (Sterngold) Shasta (Willkinson)
	Palladium-silver-gallium-gold	Wilpal 76 (Willkinson) Integrity (Jensen) Protocol (Williams)
	Palladium-silver	Jelstar (Jelenko) Pors On (Degussa) Will-Ceram W-1 (Williams)
	Palladium-copper-gallium-gold	Spirit (Jensen) Wilpal 76SF (Willkinson)
	Palladium-gallium-cobalt	PTM-88 (Jelenko)
	Palladium-cobalt-gallium	APF (Jeneric)
	Palladium-cobalt	Bond-on (Aderer)

* Rich yellow colored   ** Yellow colored   *** SF denotes silver free

Sag resistance   These alloys have a slightly lower sag resistance. Therefore, long span FDPs should be avoided with this alloy.

GOLD-PALLADIUM-SILVER ALLOYS

COMPOSITION

Component	Proportion
Gold	39–77 wt%
Palladium	10–40 wt%
Silver	9–22 wt%
Base metals	Balance (around 1%)

The silver has a tendency to discolor some porcelains.

GOLD-PALLADIUM ALLOYS

COMPOSITION

Component	Proportion
Gold	44–55 wt%
Palladium	35–45 wt%
Base metals	Balance (around 1%)

The absence of silver eliminates the discoloration problem.

NOBLE (PALLADIUM-BASED) METAL-CERAMIC ALLOYS

By definition, these alloys must contain at least 25% of noble metal alloy. Currently, the noble metal-ceramic alloys are mostly palladium-based. The high cost of gold prompted the development of the cheaper base metal alloys. Unfortunately, many soon became disillusioned because of the difficulty to work with these alloys (poor castability and high hardness). The palladium based alloys were developed during this period. Their properties were between that of the high noble alloys and the base metal alloys. They also had good scrap value.

COMMON FEATURES OF PALLADIUM-BASED (NOBLE) ALLOYS

Cost   Their cost range between that of the gold alloys and the base metal alloys.

Color   They are white in color.

Density   They are less denser than the gold alloys (10.5–11.5 g/cm³).

Castability These alloys have a lower density than the gold alloys and so do not cast as well. However, they are better than the base metal alloys in this regard.

Workability   Like the gold alloys these alloys are extremely easy to work with. They are easy to cut, grind and polish.

Melting range   A typical melting range is 1155–1304 °C. The melting range of these alloys like the gold ceramic alloys are high. This is desirable to ensure that these alloys do not melt or sag during porcelain firing.

Yield strength Ranges from 462 to 685 MPa. These compare favorably with the high noble ceramic alloys which in turn compare favorably to the Type IV alloys.

Hardness   Ranges from 189 to 270 VHN. They tend to be slightly harder than the high noble metal-ceramic alloys.

Percent elongation   Ranges from 10 to 34%. This gives an indication of the ductility of the alloy. The higher the value the more ductile it is.

Porcelain bonding   Like the gold alloys, base metals like tin, indium, etc. are added to enhance porcelain bonding.

Tarnish and corrosion   Because of their high noble metal content, these alloys are extremely stable in the oral environment.

Scrap value   The palladium based alloys have good scrap value. Many suppliers and manufacturers accept used alloy scrap.

Biological considerations   These alloys are very safe and biocompatible. Some concerns have been expressed over the copper content.

TYPES

The following are the palladium-based alloys.

- Palladium-silver alloys
- Palladium-copper alloys
- Palladium-cobalt alloys
- Palladium-gallium-silver alloys
- Palladium-gold alloys
- Palladium-gold-silver alloys

Brand names   The representative alloys are presented in *Table 25.1.*

PALLADIUM-SILVER ALLOYS

These alloys were introduced in the 1970s as an alternative to gold and base metal alloys. Their popularity has declined a little because of the *greening* problem.

COMPOSITION

Component	Proportion
Palladium	53–60 wt%
Silver	28–40 wt%
Base metals	Balance (1–8%)

Esthetics (greening)   The high silver content causes the most severe *greening* (greenish-yellow discoloration) problem among all the metal-ceramic alloys. This must be kept in mind when using it for anterior teeth. Some manufacturers have provided special agents to minimize this effect (gold metal conditioners and coating agents). Another alternative is to use special *non-greening porcelain*.

PALLADIUM-COPPER ALLOYS

These are relatively new alloys. Little information is available regarding their properties.

COMPOSITION

Component	Proportion
Palladium	74–80 wt%
Copper	5–10 wt%
Gallium	4–9 wt%
Gold	1–2 wt% (in some brands)
Base metals	around 1 wt%

Esthetics   Copper can cause a slight discoloration of the porcelain, but is not a major problem. During the oxidation firing the metal acquires a dark brown almost black oxide layer. Care should be taken to mask this completely with opaquer. Also of concern is the dark line which develops at the margins.

Castability   These alloys are technique sensitive. Slight errors can lead to faulty castings.

PALLADIUM-COBALT ALLOYS

COMPOSITION

Component	Proportion
Palladium	78–88 wt%
Cobalt	4–10 wt%
Gallium	up to 9 wt% (in some brands)
Base metals	around 1 wt%

Esthetics Cobalt can cause some insignificant discoloration. However, more care should be taken for masking the dark oxide layer with opaquer.

Sag resistance They are the most sag resistant of all the noble alloys.

PALLADIUM-GALLIUM ALLOYS

There are two groups of these alloys, viz. the palladium-gallium-silver and the palladium-gallium-silver-gold.

COMPOSITION

Component	Proportion
Palladium	75 wt%
Gallium	6 wt%
Silver	5–8 wt%
Gold	6 wt% (when present)
Base metals	around 1 wt%

Esthetics The oxide layer though dark is still somewhat lighter than the palladium copper and palladium cobalt alloys. The silver content does not cause any greening.

BASE METAL ALLOYS FOR METAL-CERAMIC RESTORATIONS

Alloys which contain little or no noble metals are known as base metal alloys. As mentioned earlier, these alloys were introduced as a cheaper alternative to the more expensive noble metal-ceramic alloys. In countries like the USA, Western Europe and the oil rich Middle-Eastern states, there is a preference for noble and high noble metal-ceramic alloys. In contrast, developing countries have shown a preference for base metal-ceramic alloys. This is because the economic concerns far outweigh the advantages of the more user-friendly high noble alloys.

The first base metal alloys were the cobalt-chromium alloys primarily used for removable partial denture alloys. The nickel-chrome alloys were introduced later. The latest in the series are titanium and its alloys.

Like the gold alloys, the base metal alloys can be used for many purposes. However, one must differentiate between the ones used for all-metal and the metal-ceramic restorations. Obviously, the metal-ceramic alloys would be formulated with specific properties since they are to be used with ceramics.

Base metal alloys used for metal-ceramics include

- ❍ Nickel-chromium (nickel based) alloys
- ❍ Cobalt-chromium (cobalt based) alloys
- ❍ Pure titanium
- ❍ Titanium-aluminum-vanadium alloys

Commercial names Trade names of some metal-ceramic alloys are presented in ***Table 25.2.***

NICKEL-CHROMIUM ALLOYS

Although cobalt chromium alloys are used for metal-ceramic crowns and FDPs, many laboratories prefer to use nickel-chromium alloys. For this reason, the discussion will focus mostly on these alloys. Cobalt-chromium will be discussed later under alloys for removable dentures. Representative commercial alloys are shown in ***Figure 25.6***.

COMPOSITION

Basic elements

Component	Proportion
Nickel	61–81 wt%
Chromium	11–27 wt%
Molybdenum	2–9 wt%

(Some alloys occasionally contain one or more minor elements).

TABLE 25.2 Commercial names of some base metal-ceramic alloys

Nickel-based alloys	Ni-Cr-Mo	Wiron 99 (Bego) Wirocer (Bego)
	Ni-Cr-Mo-Be	Litecast B (Williams) Rexillium III (Pentron)
Cobalt-based alloys	Co-Cr-Mo	Wirobond C (Bego)
	Co-Cr	Remanium LFC

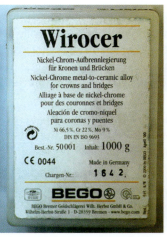

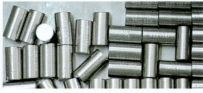

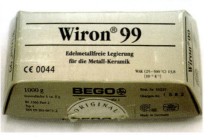

FIGURE 25.6 Representative nickel chromium alloys for metal-ceramic restorations (*Courtesy:* CODS, Davangere).

The minor additions include

Component	Proportion
Beryllium	0.5–2.0 wt%
Aluminum	0.2–4.2 wt%
Iron	0.1–0.5 wt%
Silicon	0.2–2.8 wt%
Copper	0.1–1.6 wt%
Manganese	0.1–3.0 wt%
Cobalt	0.4–0.5 wt%
Tin	1.25 wt%

(Function of the ingredients are described under removable partial denture alloys).

GENERAL PROPERTIES OF NICKEL-BASED ALLOYS

Cost They are the cheapest of the casting alloys.

Color They are white in color.

Melting range A typical melting range is 1155–1304 °C. The melting range of these alloys like the gold ceramic alloys are high.

Density Ranges from 7.8 to 8.4 g/cm³. They have just half the density of the gold alloys making them much lighter. One can get more castings per gram compared to the gold alloys.

Castability They are extremely technique sensitive. One reason may be their lower density compared to the gold alloys.

Hardness and workability Ranges from 175 to 360 VHN. They tend to be much harder than the high noble metal ceramic alloys. Unlike the gold alloys these alloys are extremely difficult to work with in the laboratory. Their high hardness makes them very difficult to cut (sprue cutting), grind and polish. In the mouth, more chair time may be needed to adjust the occlusion. Cutting and removing a defective crown or FDP can be quite demanding. The high hardness results in rapid wear of carbide and diamond burs.

Yield strength Ranges from 310 to 828 MPa. These alloys are stronger than the gold and palladium based alloys.

Modulus of elasticity Ranges from 150 to 218 GPa. This property denotes the stiffness of the alloy. Base metal alloys are *twice as stiff* as the gold ceramic alloys. Practically, this means that we can make thinner, lighter castings or use it in long span FDPs where other metals are likely to fail because of flexing. Gold alloys require a minimum thickness of at least 0.3–0.5 mm, whereas base metal alloys copings can be reduced to 0.3 mm (some even claim 0.1 mm).

Percent elongation Ranges from 10 to 28%. This gives an indication of the ductility of the alloy. Though they may appear to be ductile, these alloys, however, are not easily burnishable. This may be related to additional factors like the high hardness and yield strength.

Porcelain bonding These alloys form an adequate oxide layer which is essential for successful porcelain bonding. However, occasionally the porcelain may delaminate from the underlying metal. This has been blamed on a poorly adherent oxide layer which occurs under certain circumstances which have not been fully understood.

Sag resistance These materials are far more stable at porcelain firing temperatures than the gold based alloys. They have a higher sag resistance.

Esthetics A dark oxide layer may be seen at the porcelain metal junction.

Scrap value As may be expected these alloys have poor scrap value because of the low intrinsic value of the elements.

Tarnish and corrosion resistance These alloys are highly resistant to tarnish and corrosion. This is due to the property known as *passivation*. Passivation is the property by which a resistant oxide layer forms on the surface of chrome containing alloys. This oxide layer protects the alloy from further oxidation and corrosion. These alloys can maintain their polish for years. Other self passivating alloys are *titanium* and *aluminum*.

Soldering Soldering is necessary to join bridge parts. Long span bridges are often cast in two parts to improve the fit and accuracy. The parts are assembled correctly in the mouth and an index made. The parts are then reassembled in the laboratory and joined together using solder. Base metal alloys are much more difficult to solder than gold alloys.

Casting shrinkage These alloys have a higher casting shrinkage than the gold alloys. Greater mould expansion is needed to compensate for this. Inadequate compensation for casting shrinkage can lead to a poorly fitting casting.

Etching Etching is necessary for resin-bonded restorations (e.g. Maryland bridges) to improve the retention of the cement to the restoration. Etching of base metal alloys is done in a electrolytic etching bath.

Biological considerations Nickel may produce allergic reactions in some individuals. It is also a potential carcinogen.

Beryllium which is present in many base metal alloys is a potentially toxic substance. Inhalation of beryllium containing dust or fumes is the main route of exposure. It causes a condition known as 'berylliosis'. It is characterized by flu-like symptoms and granulomas of the lungs.

Precautions Adequate precautions must be taken while working with base metal alloys. Fumes from melting and dust from grinding alloys should be avoided (wear mask). The work area should be well-ventilated. Good exhaust systems should be installed to remove the fumes during melting.

CASTING INVESTMENTS FOR METAL CERAMIC ALLOYS

Due to the high melting temperature of these alloys, only phosphate-bonded or silica-bonded investments are used. However, in case of gold-based metal-ceramic alloys, carbon containing phosphate-bonded investments are preferred.

TITANIUM AND ITS ALLOYS FOR METAL-CERAMIC APPLICATIONS

Titanium in the form of the oxide rutile, is abundant in the earth's crust. The ore can be refined to metallic titanium using a method called the Kroll's process.

Titanium and its alloys have been available to the dental profession since the 1970s. Historically, titanium has been used extensively in aerospace, aeronautical and marine applications, because of its high strength and rigidity, its low density and corresponding low weight, its ability to withstand high temperatures and its resistance to corrosion.

The use of titanium for medical and dental applications has increased dramatically in recent years. Over the past three decades, the development of new processing methods-like computer-aided machining and electric discharge machining, has expanded titanium's useful range of applications in biomedical devices.

Titanium has become available for use in metal-ceramics. It is also used for removable partial denture alloy frames and of course commercial implants. It has been adopted in dentistry, because of its excellent biocompatibility, light weight, good strength and ability to passivate.

USES

In dentistry

1. Metal-ceramic restorations.
2. Dental implants.
3. Partial denture frames *(Fig. 25.7)*.
4. Complete denture bases.
5. Bar connectors.
6. Titanium mesh membranes (Tiomesh) are used in bone augmentation.

(In dentistry, it is especially useful as an alternative alloy to those who are allergic to nickel).

In surgery

1. Artificial hip joints.
2. Bone splints.
3. Artificial heart pumps.
4. Artificial heart valves parts.
5. Pacemaker cases.

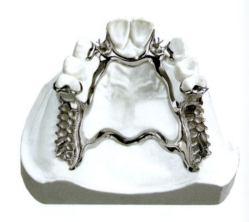

FIGURE 25.7 A titanium removable partial denture frame.

ASTM GRADES OF TITANIUM

ASTM International (the American Society for Testing and Materials) recognizes four grades of *commercially pure* titanium (CpTi) and three titanium alloys (Ti-6Al-4V, Ti-6Al-4V extra-low interstitial [low components] and Ti-Al-Nb).

SUPPLIED AS

Ingots weighing 18–40 g (height of 11.8–16.8 mm) in 1 kg boxes *(Fig. 25.8)*.

Representative products Rematitan M (Dentaurum) — Grade 4

Tritan (Dentaurum) — Grade 1

PROPERTIES OF COMMERCIALLY PURE TITANIUM

Phases In its metallic form at ambient temperature, titanium has a hexagonal, close-packed crystal lattice (α phase), which transforms into a body-centered cubic form (β-phase) at 883 °C. The phase is susceptible to oxidation.

Color It is a white color metal.

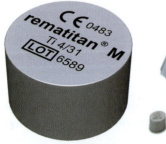
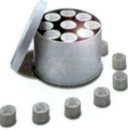

FIGURE 25.8 Grade 4 titanium (Rematitan by Dentaurum).

Density   It is a light weight metal (density 4.5 g/cm³) when compared to nickel chrome (8 g/cm³) and gold alloys (15 g/cm³).

Modulus of elasticity   Its modulus of elasticity is 110 Gpa which makes it only half as rigid as base metal alloys. However, this appears to be sufficient for most dental uses.

Melting point   Its melting point is quite high (1668 °C). Special equipment is needed for casting titanium.

Yield strength   Varies from 460 to 600 MPa.

Tensile strength   Varies from 560 to 680 MPa.

Coefficient of thermal expansion   This is an important property when it is used as a metal ceramic alloy. When used as a metal ceramic alloy the CTE (8.4 × 10⁻⁶/ °C) is far too low to be compatible with porcelain (12.7 to 14.2 × 10⁻⁶/°C). For this reason special *low fusing porcelains* have been developed to get around this problem.

Tarnish and corrosion   Titanium has the ability to *self-passivate*. The metal oxidizes almost instantaneously in air to form a tenacious and stable oxide layer approximately 10 nanometers thick. The oxide layer protects the metal from further oxidation. In addition, the oxide layer allows for bonding of fused porcelains, adhesive polymers or, in the case of endosseous implants, plasma-sprayed or surface-nucleated apatite coatings.

Biocompatibility   It is nontoxic and has excellent biocompatibility with both hard and soft tissues.

FABRICATION OF TITANIUM RESTORATIONS

Titanium structures can be made by

1.   Casting or
2.   Machining.

Casting

Casting of titanium is a challenge because of its high melting temperature, low density and high reactivity to atmospheric air. Machines for casting titanium are generally more expensive than that for other dental casting alloys.

Dental castings are made via pressure-vacuum or centrifugal casting methods. The metal is melted using an electric plasma arc or inductive heating in a melting chamber filled with inert gas or held in a vacuum. The inert gas prevents surface reaction with the molten metal. Investments with high setting expansion are used to compensate for the high casting shrinkage of titanium.

Machining

Dental implants generally are machined from billet stock of pure metal or alloy. Dental crowns and FDP frameworks also can be machined from metal blanks *(Fig. 25.9)* via CAD/CAM. Abrasive machining of titanium, however, is slow and inefficient, which greatly limits this approach. Another method for fabricating dental appliances is electric discharge machining, which uses a graphite die (often reproduced from the working die) to erode the metal to shape via spark erosion.

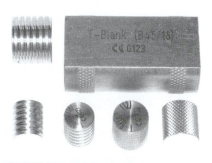

FIGURE 25.9 Titanium blanks for CAD-CAM.

CERAMIC VENEERING

Special low fusing porcelains with fusing temperatures below 800 °C are used with titanium. This is because titanium changes to the β-form (at 883 °C) which is susceptible to oxidation.

ADVANTAGES AND DISADVANTAGES OF TITANIUM

Advantages

1. High strength.
2. Light weight.
3. Binary.
4. Low tarnish and corrosion because of ability to passivate.
5. Can be laser welded.
6. Limited thermal conductivity.

Disadvantages

1. Poor castability.
2. Highly technique sensitive.
3. Requires expensive machines for casting and machining.
4. Low fusing porcelains (below 800 °C) required to prevent β phase transformation.

REMOVABLE DENTURE ALLOYS

Larger structures like complete denture bases and partial denture frames are also made from dental alloys. Being larger structures they require more quantities of alloy, which can make them quite heavy and expensive (if gold were to be used). Thus it became necessary to develop lighter and more economical alloys. Most of the large castings today are made from base metal alloys, occasionally Type IV gold alloys are used.

ADDITIONAL REQUIREMENTS FOR PARTIAL DENTURE ALLOYS

Besides all the earlier mentioned general requirements of casting alloys, RPD alloys have a few special requirements.

1. They should be light in weight. Being much larger structures, the lighter weight aids in retention in the mouth.
2. They should have high stiffness. This aids in making the casting more thinner. This is important especially in the palate region, where having a thin palatal portion makes it more comfortable to the patient. The high stiffness prevents the frame from bending under occlusal forces.
3. They should have good fatigue resistance. This property is important for clasps. Clasps have to flex when inserted or removed from the mouth. If they do not have good fatigue resistance they may break after repeated insertion and removal.
4. They should be economical. Large structures would require more metal and therefore the cost of the alloy should be low.
5. They should not react to commercial denture cleansers.

TYPES

The alloys for removable denture use are

1. Cobalt-chromium alloys

2. Nickel-chromium alloys
3. Aluminum and its alloys
4. Type IV noble alloys
5. Titanium

COBALT-CHROMIUM ALLOYS

Cobalt-chromium alloys have been available since the 1920s. They possess high strength. Their excellent corrosion resistance especially at high temperatures, makes them useful for a number of applications.

These alloys are also known as *'stellite'* because of their shiny, star-like appearance. They are bright lustrous, hard, strong and possess nontarnishing qualities.

SUPPLIED AS

Small ingots (cuboidal, cylindrical shapes) in 1 kg boxes *(Fig. 25.10)*.

Representative products   Wironium plus (Bego), Sheralit imperial (Shera).

APPLICATIONS

1. Denture base
2. Cast removable partial denture framework *(Fig. 25.11)*
3. Crowns and fixed partial dentures
4. Bar connectors.

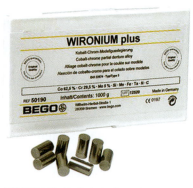

FIGURE 25.10 Cobalt-chromium alloy.

COMPOSITION

Component	Proportion
Cobalt	35–65%
Chromium	23–30%
Nickel	0–20%
Molybdenum	0–7%
Iron	0–5%
Carbon	up to 0.4%
Tungsten, manganese, silicon and platinum	traces

According to ADA Sp. No. 14 a minimum of 85% by weight of chromium, cobalt, and nickel is required.

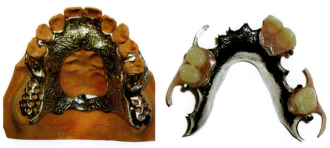

FIGURE 25.11 Cast RPD frame can be made from cobalt-chromium.

FUNCTIONS OF ALLOYING ELEMENTS

Cobalt

Imparts hardness, strength and rigidity to the alloy. It has a high melting point.

Chromium

Its passivating effect ensures corrosion resistance. The chromium content is directly proportional to tarnish and corrosion resistance. It reduces the melting point. Along with other elements, it also acts in solid solution hardening. 30% chromium is the upper limit for attaining maximum mechanical properties.

Nickel

Cobalt and nickel are interchangeable. It decreases strength, hardness, MOE and fusion temperature. It increases ductility.

Molybdenum or tungsten

They are effective hardeners. Molybdenum is preferred as it reduces ductility to a lesser extent than tungsten. Molybdenum refines grain structure.

Iron, copper and beryllium

They are hardeners. In addition, beryllium reduces fusion temperature and refines grain structure.

Manganese and silicon

Primarily oxide scavengers to prevent oxidation of other elements during melting. They are also hardeners.

Boron

Deoxidizer and hardener, but reduces ductility.

Carbon

Carbon content is most critical. Small amounts may have a pronounced effect on strength, hardness and ductility. Carbon forms carbides with the metallic constituents which is an important factor in strengthening the alloy. However, excess carbon increases brittleness. Thus, control of carbon content in the alloy is important.

PROPERTIES

The cobalt-chromium alloys have replaced Type IV gold alloys, especially for making RPDs, because of their lower cost and good mechanical properties.

Density

The density is half that of gold alloys, they are lighter in weight (8 to 9 g/cm³).

Fusion temperature

Thus casting temperature of this alloy is considerably higher than that of gold alloys (1250 °C to 1480 °C).

ADA Sp. No. 14 divides it into two types, based on fusion temperature, which is defined as the liquidus temperature.

○ Type-I (high fusing)—liquidus temperature greater than 1300 °C.
○ Type-II (low fusing)—liquidus temperature not greater than 1300 °C.

Yield strength

It is higher than that of gold alloys (710 MPa).

Elongation

Their ductility is lower than that of gold alloys. It depends on composition, rate of cooling and the fusion and mould temperature employed. The elongation value is 1–12%.

Caution These alloys work harden very easily, so care must be taken while adjusting the clasp arms of the partial denture. They may break if bent too many times.

Modulus of elasticity

They are twice as stiff as gold alloys (225×10^3 MPa). Thus, casting can be made thinner, thereby, decreasing the weight of the RPD.

Hardness

These alloys are 50% harder than gold alloys (432 VHN). Thus, cutting, grinding and finishing are difficult. It wears off the cutting instrument. Special hard, high speed finishing tools are needed.

Tarnish and corrosion resistance (passivation)

Formation of a layer of chromium oxide on the surface of these alloys prevents tarnish and corrosion in the oral cavity. This is called 'passivating effect'.

Caution Hypochlorite and other chlorine containing compounds that are present in some denture cleaning solutions will cause corrosion in base metal alloys. Even the oxygenating denture cleansers will stain such alloys. Therefore, these solutions should not be used to clean chromium based alloys.

Casting shrinkage

The casting shrinkage is much greater (2.3%) than that of gold alloys. The high shrinkage is due to their high fusion temperature.

Porosity

As in gold alloys, porosity is due to shrinkage of the alloy and release of dissolved gases. Porosity is affected by the composition of the alloys and its manipulation.

TECHNICAL CONSIDERATIONS FOR CASTING ALLOYS

Based on the melting temperatures of the alloys, we can divide the alloys into high fusing and low fusing alloys.

LOW-FUSING ALLOYS

The gold alloys used for all-metal restorations may be considered as low fusing. Obviously, the technical requirements of these alloys would be different from the high-fusing alloys.

Investment material Gypsum bonded investments are usually sufficient for the low-fusing gold alloys.

Melting The regular gas-air torch is usually sufficient to melt these alloys.

HIGH-FUSING ALLOYS

The high-fusing alloys include noble metal-ceramic alloys (gold and palladium alloys) as well as the base-metal alloys (all-metal, metal-ceramic alloys and partial denture alloys).

Investment material for noble metal alloys The high melting temperatures prevent the use of gypsum-bonded investments. Phosphate bonded or silica bonded investments are used for these alloys.

Investment material for base-metal alloys Phosphate-bonded or silica-bonded investments are also used for these alloys. However, there is one difference. These alloys are very sensitive to a change in their carbon content. Therefore, *carbon containing investments* should be avoided when casting base-metal alloys.

Burnout A slow burnout is done at a temperature of 732–982 °C. It is done two hours after investing.

Melting The high fusion temperature also prevents the use of gas-air torches for melting these alloys. Oxygen-acetylene torches are usually employed. Electrical sources of melting such as carbon arcs, argon arcs, high frequency induction, or silicon-carbide resistance furnaces may also be used.

TECHNIQUE FOR SMALL CASTINGS

The wax pattern is usually constructed on a die stone model. The wax pattern is removed and then invested (for more details see chapter on casting techniques).

TECHNIQUE FOR LARGE CASTINGS

The procedure for large castings like RPD frames is slightly more complex. Unlike the crown or FDP pattern, the RPD pattern is difficult to remove from the model without distortion and damage. Therefore, a modification in the technique is required. A duplicate of the model is made using investment material (this is called refractory cast). The wax pattern is constructed on the refractory cast **(Fig. 25.12A)**. The pattern is not separated from the refractory cast, instead the refractory cast is invested along with the pattern **(Fig. 25.12C)**.

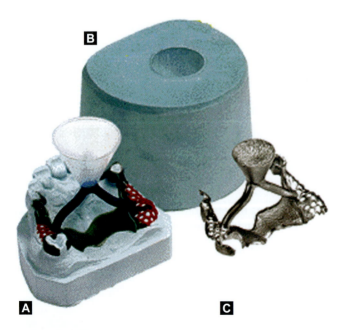

FIGURES 25.12A TO C (A) Partial denture wax patterns are constructed directly on the refractory cast. **(B)** The whole cast together with the pattern is invested to form a mold. The completed casting is also shown **(C)**.

ADVANTAGES AND DISADVANTAGES OF BASE METAL ALLOYS

ADVANTAGES OF BASE METAL ALLOYS

1. Lighter in weight.
2. Better mechanical properties (exceptions are present).
3. As corrosion resistant as gold alloys (due to passivating effect).
4. Less expensive than gold alloys.

DISADVANTAGES

1. More technique sensitive.
2. Complexity in production of dental appliance.
3. High fusing temperatures.
4. Extremely hard, so requires special tools for finishing.
5. The high hardness can cause excessive wear of restorations and natural teeth contacting the restorations.

COMPARISON OF A GOLD ALLOY AND A BASE METAL ALLOY

A comparison of the 2 alloys are shown in ***Table 25.3.***

TABLE 25.3 Comparison of cobalt-chromium and type IV gold alloy		
Properties	*Cobalt-chromium*	*Gold Type - IV*
Strength	Adequate	Adequate
Density (g/cm)	8 (lighter)	15 (heavier)
Hardness	Harder than enamel	Softer than enamel
Stiffness	Stiff	More flexible
Melting temperature	1300°C	900°C
Casting shrinkage	2.25%	1.25–1.65%
Heat treatment	Complicated	Simple
Tarnish resistance	Adequate	Adequate
Cost	Economical	High for large castings
Workability	Difficult to cut, grind and polish	Cutting and polishing easy
Investment	Phosphate bonded (non-carbon)	Gypsum bonded
Heat source for melting	Oxyacetylene torches	Gas-air torch
Solderability	Difficult	Easier

Dental Implant Materials

Chapter Outline

- Definition
- History and Development of Implants
- Types of Implants
- Materials Used
- Titanium
- Surface Coated Titanium
- Ceramics
- Stainless Steel
- Polymers and Composites
- Other Materials
- Implant Parts
  - Basic Implant Design
  - Implant Fixture

- Implant Abutments
- Implant Motor
- Implant Drills
- Cover Screw
- Healing Abutment
- Implant Abutment Connection
- Platform Switching
- Biointegration and Osseointegration
- Titanium Allergy
- Zirconia Implants
- Zirconia Anatomic Root-form Implants

- Implant Surfaces and Coatings
  - Grit Blasting
  - Acid Etching
  - Anodization
  - Shot/Laser Peening
  - Hydroxyapatite Coated Implants
  - Plasma Sprayed HA
  - Electrophoretic Deposition (EPD) of HA
  - Biomimetic Coating Technique

Implanting a foreign material directly into the bone in order to replace missing teeth has been a goal sought since ancient times. Though many materials have been tried, currently, the vast majority of implant systems use titanium in some form.

DEFINITION

A dental implant is a material or device placed in and/or on oral tissues to support an oral prosthesis *(GPT-8)*.

History and Development of Implants

Man has been searching for ways to replace missing teeth for thousands of years. Ancient Egyptians used tooth shaped shells and ivory to replace teeth. The Etruscans living in what is now modern Italy, replaced missing teeth with artificial teeth carved from the bones of oxen.

Further evidence of tooth replacement was found in 1931 by an archeological team excavating in Honduras. A mandible of Mayan origin was discovered that had tooth-shaped pieces of shells placed in the sockets of three missing lower incisor teeth.

Modern implant dentistry began in the early 19th century. A lot of experiments were conducted on what material would work best. Attempts were first made

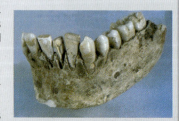
Mayan mandible with shell implant

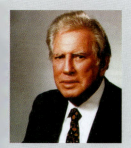

Leonard Linkow

at implanting natural teeth from another person's mouth, but these implants failed due to infection or were rejected by the host tissue. Implants made of gold, porcelain, silver and even lead were being tried, with only a fair measure of success and little or no predictability.

As early as 1918, Greenfield devised the Iridoplatinum root form basket implant. Other early implants were those of Chercheve, Formiggini and others. An interesting design was the Tripodal pin implant of Scialom. Interestingly some of these early designs were ahead of their times. Their failure to gain widespread popularity could probably be attributed to the fact that prosthetic techniques, antibiotic use, infection control, instrumentation and impression materials had not yet advanced far enough.

One of the early pioneers in this field *Dr. AE Strock* in 1931, suggested using Vitallium, a metal alloy for dental implants. In 1947, Manlio Formiggini of Italy developed an implant made of tantalum. At the same time, Raphael Chercheve was using implants made of a chrome-cobalt alloy. By 1964, commercially pure titanium was accepted as the material of choice for dental implants. Ever since almost all dental implants are made of titanium. The body does not recognize titanium as a foreign material, resulting in less host rejection of the implant. Other areas of medicine recognize this fact and use titanium for other implants such as joint replacements and heart valves.

In the 1950s an important discovery was made which had great implications for tooth replacement therapy. During an experiment involving the study of blood circulation in animals, Dr. Per-Ingvar Branemark discovered that the hollow titanium rod used in the study was not retrievable when the experiment was complete. Further studies showed that the animals' bone had directly attached to the titanium surface. This phenomenon was called osseointegration, defined by the American Academy of Implant Dentistry as "the firm, direct and lasting biological attachment of a metallic implant to vital bone with no intervening connective tissue." This firm anchor is what makes dental implants a wonderful option for replacing teeth.

Experimentation with implant designs, not just those that were shaped like the tooth root, was also being done. In 1941, Dr. Gustav Dahl of Sweden provided a retentive mechanism for jaws that were completely edentulous. This was the introduction of the subperiosteal implant. Dr. Leonard Linkow of New York introduced the blade form implant *(Fig. 26.1)* in 1967. These blades came in a variety of sizes and forms and were the most widely used type of implant until the 1980s.

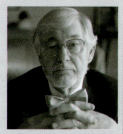

Per-Ingvar Branemark

Implants are no longer restricted to the mouth. They have been successfully used all over the body for various roles. Whether implants are here to stay is no longer a question, but research into perfecting materials, procedures and training will continue in this exciting field of dentistry.

TYPES OF IMPLANTS

A. *Subperiosteal*—a framework that rests upon the bony ridge but does not penetrate it *(Fig. 26.1)*.

B. *Transosteal*—penetrates completely through the mandible *(Fig. 26.2)*.

C. *Endosseous*—partially submerged and *anchored within the bone (Figs. 26.3 and 26.4)*.

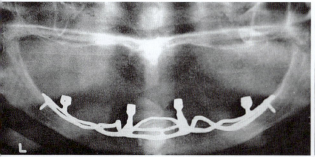
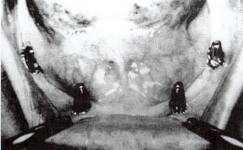

FIGURE 26.1 Subperiosteal implant radiograph (left). Intraoral view (right).

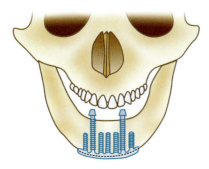

FIGURE 26.2 Transosteal implant.

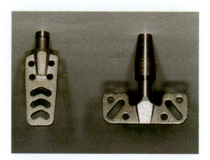

FIGURE 26.3 Linkow's blade vent endosseous implants were widely used prior to the era of cylindrical implants.

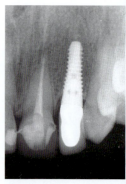

FIGURE 26.4 Radiograph showing an endosteal implant

MATERIALS USED

1. *Metals* — Stainless steel
   — Cobalt-chromium-molybdenum based
   — Titanium and its alloys
   — Surface coated titanium
2. *Ceramics* — Hydroxyapatite
   — Bioglass
   — Aluminum oxide
3. *Polymers and composites*
4. *Others* — Gold, tantalum, carbon, etc.

TITANIUM

Commercially pure titanium (cp Ti) is currently the most widely used material for implants *(Fig. 26.5)*. It has become the material of choice because of its

○ Low density (4.5 gm/cm^2) but high strength.
○ Minimal biocorrosion due to its passivating effect.
○ Excellent biocompatibility.

Titanium also has good stiffness. Although its stiffness is only half that of steel, it is still 5 to 10 times higher than that of bone.

Titanium alloys Alloyed forms of titanium are also used. Its alloyed form contains 6 wt.% aluminum and 4 wt.% vanadium.

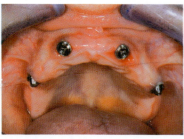
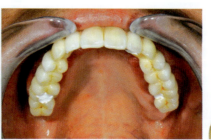
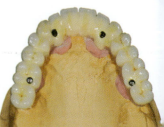

FIGURE 26.5 Four titanium screw implants in the maxillary edentulous jaw are used to support a screw retained fixed prosthesis.

Surface coated titanium

The newer implant designs use titanium that is coated with a material that bonds and promotes bone growth (bioactive). The implant is coated with a thin layer of *tricalcium phosphate* or *hydroxyapatite* that has been *plasma sprayed*.

CERAMICS

These may be *bioactive* on *bioinert*. Their applications are still limited because of their low tensile strength and ductility. Currently they are primarily used as surface coats on titanium implants.

Bioactive, e.g.,

- ○ Hydroxyapatite
- ○ Bioglass (CaO, NaO, P_2O_5 and SiO_2)

Bioinert, e.g., aluminum oxide is used either in the polycrystalline form or as a single crystal (sapphire). It is well-tolerated by bone but does not promote bone formation. They are available in screw or blade form and are used as abutments in partially edentulous mouths.

STAINLESS STEEL

18-8 or Austenitic steel had been tried as an implant material. It has high strength and ductility. Currently these materials are rarely used.

PRECAUTIONS

Since it contains nickel, it should be avoided in nickel sensitive patients. It is most susceptible to pit and crevice corrosion so the passivating layer must be preserved. Direct contact of the implant with a dissimilar metal crown is avoided to prevent galvanism.

POLYMERS AND COMPOSITES

Polymers have been fabricated in porous and solid forms for tissue attachment and replacement augmentation. However, in some implants they are mainly used within the implants as connectors for stress distribution (shock absorption).

OTHER MATERIALS

In the past, gold, palladium, tantalum, platinum and alloys of these metals have been used. More recently, zirconium and tungsten have been tried. Titanium has replaced most of these materials. Carbon compounds were used for root replacement in the 1970s. They are also marketed as coatings for metallic and ceramic devices.

IMPLANT PARTS

BASIC IMPLANT DESIGN

Since endosseous cylindrical root form implants are the most widely used design, subsequent discussions will focus on these. Implants can range from complex, having multiple components to more simple designs. Most endosseous implants can be divided into two basic parts *(Fig. 26.6).*

- ○ Fixture—embedded in bone
- ○ Abutment—supports the crown

The implant may be

○ One piece–Implant and abutment are joined together *(Fig. 26.7A)*

○ Two-piece–Implant and abutment are separate. The abutment is secured to the implant by means of an abutment screw *(Fig. 26.7B)*

IMPLANT FIXTURE

Over the years various implant designs have been developed and used. Currently, the most favored form is the cylindrical screw or the tapered screw *(Figs. 26.8A to D)*. The implant is inserted through a surgical procedure. The abutment is usually screwed onto the implant at a later date. The crown is then constructed and either screwed on or cemented onto the abutment thus completing the restoration.

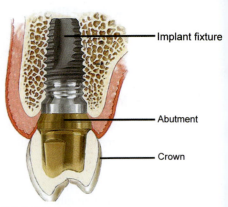

FIGURE 26.6 Components of endosseous implants

Implants are usually designed as a system and depending on the company various accessory components are also available. The components are usually specific for the particular system and are usually not interchangeable. Some of them become part of the implant itself while others aid in the various stages of implant placement and tooth restoration. These include the drills, healing caps, impression copings, implant analogue, laboratory accessories, etc.

IMPLANT ABUTMENTS

Definition

Implant abutment is that portion of a dental implant that serves to support and/or retain any fixed or removable dental prosthesis (GPT-8).

Classification of abutments

A. *According to fabrication procedure*
  1. Stock abutment   2. Custom   3. CAD/CAM

B. *According to material used*
  1. Titanium   2. Zirconia   3. Gold   4. Steel

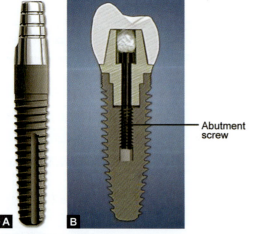

FIGURES 26.7A AND B **(A)** One piece implant-abutment. **(B)** Two-piece implant-abutment.

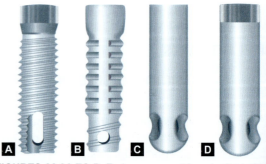

FIGURES 26.8A TO D Endosseous root form implants **(A)** Titanium screw. **(B)** Hydroxyapatite screw. **(C)** Hydroxyapatite. **(D)** Titanium plasma sprayed.

C. *According to angulation*

    1. Angled   2. Nonangled

Stock abutments   Also known as the preparable, easy, or direct abutments. They are factory produced and provide the most accurate fit to the implant. They can be modified at the chairside or in the laboratory. They come in varying sizes and emergence profiles. Some come with scalloped margins for improved marginal esthetics.

Stock abutments are of two varieties

Hollow abutments   These are abutments with a channel through which the connecting screw attaches it to the implant fixture.

Solid abutment   The abutment comes with its own built-in screw. The abutment itself is screwed onto the implant.

Custom   Cast custom abutments have long been a workhorse in implant dentistry. They were first popularized as the "UCLA" abutment design and provided a means for waxing custom emergence profiles of the subgingival portion of the abutment, flexibility in margin level placement, and for correction of angulation problems.

CAD/CAM   State of the art software and milling machines utilize the scan data from the patient's dental casts and the computer generated abutment design to enable production of an abutment specific for the patient.

Angled abutments   Angled abutments are used to correct the implant-crown alignment, e.g., upper central incisors often need angled abutments.

Zirconia abutments   Zirconia is a strong tooth colored ceramic material. These are indicated for patients demanding an increased level of esthetics.

One-piece implant-abutment   Some manufacturers do not provide separate abutments, rather the abutment is combined with the implant and is, therefore, inserted along with the implant.

EQUIPMENT AND PARTS ASSOCIATED WITH IMPLANT SURGERY

Implant motor

These are high torque motors with foot control and saline stand *(Fig. 26.9)*. The handpiece is contra-angled and has a nozzle for saline irrigation. Torque ranges from 50–70 Ncm. Speed ranges from 300 to 40,000 rpm. Having low speed but high torque is important for implant drilling.

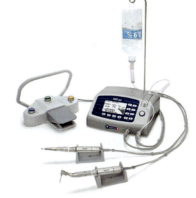

FIGURE 26.9 Implant motor with saline irrigation.

Implant drills

The pilot drill is the first drill used. It helps to establish direction of the subsequent drilling and implant placement. Subsequent drills are introduced in series of increasing size *(Fig. 26.10)*. Drills are usually made of stainless steel.

Cover screw

Implant surgery is usually done in two stages. In the first stage the implant is inserted in the bone and left to integrate for a period of 2 months. After the

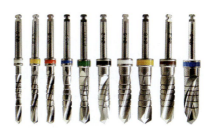

FIGURE 26.10 Implant drills.

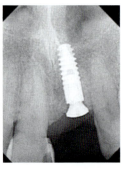

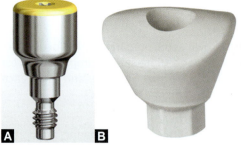

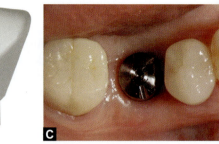

FIGURES 26.12A TOC (A) Regular healing abutments. **(B)** Anatomic healing abutment. **(C)** Healing abutment in position.

FIGURE 26.11 Cover screw.

implant is placed, a cover screw *(Fig. 26.11)* is used to cover the coronal end of the abutment. The cover screw prevents bony ingrowth and keeps the abutment chamber patent while the implant is integrating.

Healing abutment

The healing abutment is usually placed 2–3 months later at the second stage. The cover screw of the buried implant is exposed. The cover screw is removed and a healing abutment placed instead. The healing abutment exposes the implant to the oral cavity *(Fig. 26.12C)* and prepares the space for the future abutment. The healing abutment may be cylindrical or anatomic in design *(Figs. 26.12A and B)*.

Function of healing abutment

1. Allows the punched out tissue to heal.
2. Promotes the development of sulcus epithelium.
3. Helps to develop papilla and marginal gingiva, thus improving the soft tissue esthetics.
4. Helps to develop a proper emergence profile from the implant platform to the crown, thus improving the restoration esthetics (transition from the narrower implant to the broader artificial tooth).

IMPLANT ABUTMENT CONNECTION

The implant abutment connection is an important part of the implant design. It is one of the factors which help in proper functioning, stability and longevity of the implant. The abutment is secured to the implant with the help of a screw. During occlusal function considerable stress may be transferred to the screw and can lead to its early loosening or even fracture. Manufacturers have, therefore, incorporated certain design features to reduce the stress on the abutment screw.

Function of the implant abutment connection

The implant/abutment interface determines joint strength, stability, and lateral and rotational stability. It also reduces stress on the abutment screw.

Types of implant abutment connections

There are two ways the implant and abutment connect or interface.

1. External
2. Internal

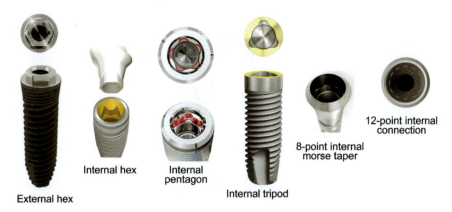

External hex

Internal hex Internal pentagon Internal tripod 8-point internal morse taper 12-point internal connection

FIGURE 26.13 Various types of implant abutment connections.

EXTERNAL HEX

The original Brånemark protocol required several externally hexed implants to restore fully edentulous arches *(Fig. 26.13)*.

INTERNAL HEX

One of the first internally connected implants was designed with a 1.7-mm-deep hex below a 0.5 mm wide, 45° bevel. Its features were intended to distribute intraoral forces *deeper* within the implant to protect the retention screw from excess loading, and to reduce the potential of microleakage. Internally connected implants also provide superior strength for the implant/abutment connection.

Since the introduction of the internal connection concept, further design enhancements have been made in an attempt to enhance the implant/abutment connection. Included in such efforts is the "Morse" taper, wherein a tapered abutment post is inserted into the nonthreaded shaft of a dental implant with the same taper. Other internal connection designs have followed, frequently with variations in the numbers of hexes, connection length, angulation, etc.

Some of the internal implant abutment connections are (Fig. 26.13)

- 3 point internal tripod — Replace select (Noble Biocare)
- 5 point internal pentagon — Tiologic (Dentaurum)
- 6 point internal hex — Frialit 2 (Friadent)
- 8 point internal morse taper — (ITI) Straumann
- 12 point conical seal — Astra (Astra Tech)

PLATFORM SWITCHING

Platform switching is a method used to preserve alveolar bone levels around dental implants. The concept refers to placing an abutment of narrower diameter on implants of wider diameter *(Figs. 26.14A and B)*, rather than placing abutments of similar diameters (referred to as platform matching - *Fig. 26.15*).

BIOINTEGRATION AND OSSEOINTEGRATION

For an implant to function, it must integrate with the oral tissues. The term osseointegration was first described by Per Ingvar Branemark and refers to the fusion of the bone with the implant.

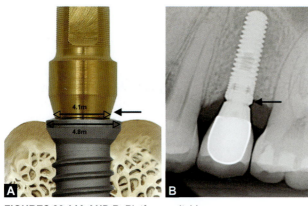

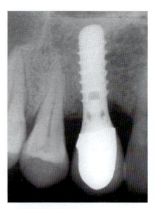

FIGURES 26.14A AND B Platform switching.

FIGURE 26.15 Platform matching.

Defined as An apparent direct connection of an implant surface and host bone without intervening connective tissue [GPT-8] (**Fig. 26.16**).

Thus a direct structural and functional connection between the bone and implant allows the implant to transmit functional stresses directly to the bone.

To achieve osseointegration, the bone must be viable, space between the implant and bone should be less than 10 nm and contain no fibrous tissue. Presence of fibrous tissue usually signifies failure.

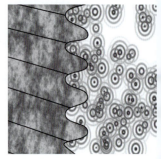

FIGURE 26.16 Representation of osseointegration.

Factors favoring osseointegration

1. Proper treatment planning
2. Atraumatic drilling of bone
3. Selection of proper implant material
4. Implant design
5. Favorable occlusal forces
6. Bone quality
7. Good oral hygiene
8. No contraindicating local or systemic factors

Other factors include the nature of the surface coating and surface configuration. Recently there has been interest in coating titanium with certain materials that actively promote a favorable bone response. These are referred to as 'bioactive'. Examples of bioactive materials are hydroxyapatite, tricalcium phosphate and bioactive glasses. Commercially available bioactive glasses include Bioglass, Ceravital, Biogran and glass ceramic A-W. These materials are generally too weak and brittle to stand alone. However, when used as a coating (50 to 75 µm) on the surface of titanium, it combines the strength of titanium with its bioactive qualities.

If successful, the ceramic coating becomes completely fused with the surrounding bone. In this case the interphase is termed 'biointegration' because there is no intervening space between the bone and the implant.

Implant material and design is continually evolving. With every passing year the failure rates are gradually reducing. Current implants enjoy a 95 to 98% clinical success rate. More advances in both design, material and technique may be expected in the future.

TITANIUM ALLERGY

In the last couple of year, the question if titanium allergy really exists has been raised in scientific literature. The reactions are not necessarily local, but appear in other parts of the body. One of the reasons why the existence of titanium allergy has been debated might be that the golden standard for metal allergy testing, patch testing, has not been properly developed for titanium. The patch test is a skin test, where salts of the metals tested are placed on the skin of the back under occlusion. 24–72 hours later a dermatologist evaluates the reaction and the presence of a rash is taken as evidence of a positive reaction. Unfortunately, titanium dioxide, a salt of titanium used for patch testing, does not penetrate the skin under the conditions of patch test. This is one of the reasons why patch test in its current form often gives false negative results in patients with titanium-induced inflammation in the body.

The latest available research from Europe and Japan shows that between 2–4% of all patients with titanium implants develop an allergic reaction to either titanium or to one or more of the metals used in the titanium alloy.

The symptoms most often observed after implantation with titanium-containing implants are varied, so they will be different in different patients. In addition to symptoms shown adjacent to implants on the mucosa in the mouth, or on the skin on the body, there may be other systemic symptoms. These symptoms are akin as those described after the exposure to other allergens, like nickel or mercury, in sensitised individuals. Symptoms arise because stimulated lymphocytes produce cytokines, which in turn, affect the HPA-axis. The result is multiple nonspecific symptoms such as profound fatigue, pain, cognitive dysfunction, headache, sleep problems, etc.

Allergy due to titanium might be accountable for the failure of implants in some cases (known as *cluster patients*). It has been documented that the risk of titanium allergy is more prevalent in patients having sensitivity to other metals. In such types of cases, an allergy assessment is suggested to exclude problems related with titanium implants.

ZIRCONIA IMPLANTS

Although titanium is the preferred choice for dental implants as it is an inert material, in rare circumstances it may encourage toxic or allergic type I or IV reactions. Its high strength, fracture toughness, and its white color make zirconia an interesting material for the construction of implant abutments and superstructures especially in the anterior zone.

Indications for zirconia implant

1. Esthetic considerations
2. Sensitivity or allergy to titanium

Zirconia implants *(Fig. 26.17)* should be considered in patients with known allergy to titanium. (See chapter on Dental ceramics for more information on Zirconia implants)

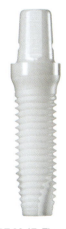

FIGURE 26.17 Zirconia one-piece implant with abutment.

ZIRCONIA ANATOMIC ROOT-FORM IMPLANTS

Synonyms Root analogue implants, anatomic implants, custom implants, bioimplant

Zirconia-based anatomic root-form implants *(Figs. 26.18A and B)* were introduced into dental implantology as an alternative to conventional cylindrical implants. Owing to its ability to be milled into the shape of the natural tooth root and be placed immediately following

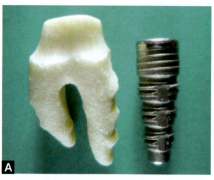
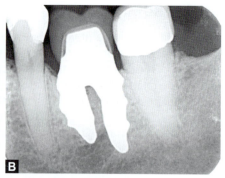

FIGURES 26.18A AND B **(A)** Zirconia root form implants. **(B)** Periapical view.

extraction, its excellent biomechanical characteristics, biocompatibility, and bright tooth-like color, zirconia has the potential to become a substitute for titanium as dental implant material.

Immediate placement of implant similar in shape and size to the extracted root has its own advantages. By adapting the root to the extraction socket instead of adapting the bone to a preformed standardized implant they reduced the bone and soft tissue trauma. Immediate custom-made root analogue implants were possible because of advances in material and CAD/CAM technology. (See chapter on Dental Ceramics for more information on Zirconia anatomic root-form implants).

Advantages

1. Esthetic
2. Biocompatible
3. Immediate placement
4. No additional drilling or surgery required
5. No complications of implant surgery
6. Shorter waiting period
7. Fits into original socket
8. Immediate placement preserves bone and soft tissue (less resorption)
9. Preserves root eminences of the alveolar bone
10. Sinus lift not required
11. Bone graft not required
12. Little or no swelling or pain
13. Faster recovery time

IMPLANT SURFACES AND COATINGS

The implant surface is critical to the proper biointegration of the implant. For this purpose various techniques have been used to modify the implant surfaces **(Fig. 26.19)** to improve its integration to the surrounding tissues. The techniques may be classified as

1. *Ablative procedures* Ablation is removal of material from the surface of an object by blasting, vaporization, chipping, or other erosive processes.
    - Grit blasting
    - Acid etching
    - Anodizing
    - Shot/ laser peening

2. *Additive procedures* It is a process of creating a layer by addition of material.
   - Plasma spraying
   - Electrophoretic deposition
   - Sputter deposition
   - Soluble gel coating
   - Soluble blast media
   - Pulsed laser deposition
   - Biomimetic precipitation

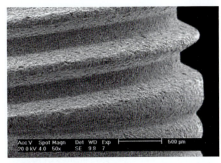

FIGURE 26.19 On closer look many implants have a rough surface. Implant surface is critical to the proper biointegration of the implant.

GRIT BLASTING

A rough surface is created by grit-blasting the machined titanium implant surface with hard particles. The particles are projected through a nozzle at high velocity by means of compressed air. This is followed by washing in nonetching acid and distilled water to remove residual blasting material. The microtextured surfaces has been shown to allow for increased bone apposition compared to machined surfaces by increasing *(Fig. 26.20A)* the surface area. Some manufacturers combine both blasting and etching *(Fig. 26.20B)*.

Grit blasting materials

1. Calcium phosphates like hydroxyapatite (HA) and beta-tricalcium phosphate
2. Titanium oxide
3. Zirconia
4. Alumina

Disadvantages

In the case of alumina, residual blasting media is often embedded into the implant surface *(Fig. 26.21)* and can interfere with integration.

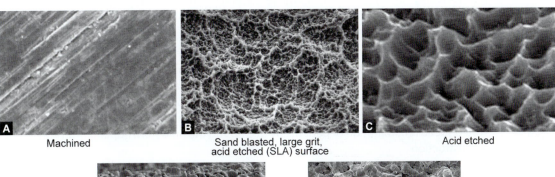

Machined | Sand blasted, large grit, acid etched (SLA) surface | Acid etched

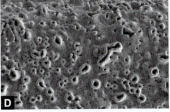
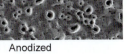

Anodized

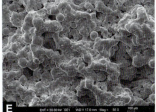

Plasma sprayed coating

FIGURES 26.20A TO E Various implant surfaces with higher magnification.

ACID ETCHING

The implant surface can be roughened through acid etching *(Fig. 26.20C)* with sulphuric or hydrochloric acids.

Advantages of acid etching

1. Produces a cleaner surface as there is no possibility of an external agent embedding onto the implant surface.
2. No possibility of loss of the layer through debonding, dissolution or wear thus avoiding concerns of long term fixation.

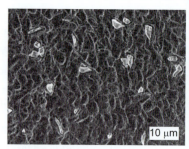

FIGURE 26.21 Embedded blast material (TiO_2) following grit blasting.

ANODIZATION

Anodizing is an electrochemical process used to increase the thickness of the natural oxide layer on the surface of the titanium (to more than 1000 nm). Anodization modifies the microstructure and crystallinity of the titanium oxide layer *(Fig. 26.20D)*. Anodization is done with the help of strong acids (e.g., sulphuric, phosphoric, nitric acids, etc.) at high current density and voltage (200 A/m^2 at 100 V).

SHOT/LASER PEENING

Shot peening is similar to sand blasting, where the surface is bombarded with small spherical particles causing small indentations to form.

Laser peening involves the use of high intensity pulses of laser to create a regular honeycomb pattern with small pores.

HYDROXYAPATITE COATED IMPLANTS

Hydroxyapatite (HA) (also called hydroxylapatite or calcium hydroxide phosphate), is a naturally occurring mineral form of calcium apatite with the formula $Ca_{10}(PO_4)_6(OH)_2$. Bone is a specialized mineralized connective tissue consisting by weight of 33% organic matrix, permeated by HA, which makes up the remaining 67% of bone. For this reason, HA is being investigated as a possible material for coatings or composites.

Rationale

The use of hydroxyapatite implants have been reported to stimulate bone healing, resulting in an improvement in the rate and strength of initial implant integration. Hence, the dense HA layer on the top of titanium substrate is mainly for biointegration to bone tissue and enhanced implant stability. Thus, it is believed that the use of HA coatings on metallic implants would speed rehabilitation of patients by decreasing the time from implant insertion to final reconstruction.

PLASMA SPRAYED HYDROXYAPATITE

Numerous methods of depositing HA on metallic implants have been reported. The current deposition process is plasma spraying or arc plasma spraying. A gas stream (pure argon or a mix of argon/hydrogen) is used to carry HA powder, which is then passed through an electrical plasma produced by a low-voltage, high-current electrical discharge. The plasma heats the hydroxyapatite, partially melting it. The semimolten HA powder is sprayed onto the titanium where it solidify. It has been reported that plasma spraying of HA results in coatings with a thickness greater than 30 μm. The bonding of the plasma-sprayed HA coatings appears to be entirely mechanical in nature.

Besides HA, other materials like titanium can also be plasma sprayed onto the titanium surface *(Fig. 26.20E)*.

Problems with plasma-sprayed coatings

Problems cited with the plasma-sprayed coatings include

1. Variation in bond strength between the coatings and the metallic substrates
2. Alterations in HA structure due to the coating process
3. Poor adhesion between the coatings and metallic substrates

ELECTROPHORETIC DEPOSITION (EPD) OF HA

EPD is a process in which colloidal particles of HA suspended in a liquid medium is deposited onto the implant under the influence of an electric field. EPD can produce coatings ranging from 1,500. A post-deposition heat treatment is required to densify the coating. A major disadvantage is the possibility of delamination of the layer in clinical use.

BIOMIMETIC COATING TECHNIQUE

Biomimetic coating technique for nucleation and growth of bone-like crystals on a pretreated substrate by immersing it in a supersaturated solution of calcium phosphate under physiological conditions (37 °C and pH = 7.4). This method can be modified for the incorporation of drugs or growth factors onto the implant surface thereby making the implants osteoinductive and osteoconductive.

The various brands and their implant surface types are outlined in *Table 26.1.*

TABLE 26.1 Different surfaces in commercially available implants

Implant	Surface modification
Ankylos Plus, XiVE, Frialit—Dentsply Friadent, GmbH	Sandblasted, large grit blasted, acid-etched
NobelActive—Nobel Biocare, Zurich, Switzerland	Phosphate enriched titanium oxide—TiUnite
GSIII—Osstem, South Korea	Resorbable blast media (RBM)—calcium phosphate hydroxyapatite
NanoTite—Biomet 3i, Palm Beach Gardens, Florida, USA	Calcium phosphate by discrete crystal deposition
Straumann Bone Level - Institute Straumann AG, Switzerland	SLActive—Sandblasted, large grit blasted followed by acid etching
Laserlok Surface—Biohorizon, Birmingham, Alabama	Laser peening
Pitt-Easy—Sybron Implant Solutions GmbH, Germany	Vacuum titanium plasma spray (V-TPS)
Tioblast—AstraTech Dental, MOIndal, Sweden Zimmer Screw Vent	Grit blasted with titanium oxide Microtextured hydroxyapatite surface

Wrought Metals and Alloys

Chapter Outline

Wrought metal is obtained from cast metal. A wrought metal or alloy is one that has been worked, drawn or shaped into a serviceable form, e.g. plates, band materials, bars, and wires. The process of forming wrought metal objects has been known since ancient times. For example, swords used in warfare were formed by subjecting a hot piece of metal to a beating process. Other things used in daily life like farming equipment and kitchen utensils are also made by a similar process.

MANUFACTURE OF WROUGHT ALLOYS

Wrought metal is usually derived from cast metal or alloy. Wrought metal is formed when the parent metal is subject to various deformative processes like drawing, extruding, machining, beating, rolling, forging, etc. Examples of some of these processes are

1. Round wires are obtained by drawing a cast alloy through a series of dies.
2. Rolling process is used to form sheets and rods.
3. Forging is a process by which an object is formed by compressing the parent metal between two dies. Stainless steel crowns are made by this process.

Manufacture of wrought alloys results in a tremendous amount of stresses (known as work hardening). These stresses are relieved by heat treatment during or after manufacture.

STRUCTURE OF WROUGHT ALLOYS

All alloys are initially formed by casting. When a cast metal is subject to any deformation, it is considered a wrought metal. Wrought alloys have a fibrous structure which result from the cold working applied during the drawing operation to shape the wire. At the atomic level the deformative processes involved in the manufacture of wrought alloys results in various types of atomic deformations and disruptions. These include dislocations, twinning and fracture.

DISLOCATIONS

On application of a shear force, dislocation of the atoms occurs along a plane called as the slip plane. The simplest type of dislocation is known as edge dislocation. The dominant slip planes are characteristic for each type of crystal structure. For example, face-centered cubic (fcc) structures have the greatest number of slip planes. Therefore, metals with a fcc structure like gold, copper, nickel, palladium, silver, platinum, etc. are highly ductile and easy to draw. Body-centered cubic (bcc) metal have intermediate levels of ductility. Hexagonal close-packed structures (hcp) have the least amount of slip systems and therefore are relatively brittle, e.g. zinc. Dislocations occur only in materials having a crystalline structure. Dislocations cannot exist in materials with a noncrystalline structure like dental ceramics and polymeric materials.

TWINNING

Another type of permanent deformation is known as twinning. The deformation occurs along either side of a plane in such a way that it mirrors each other. Twinning is favored over dislocation in metals that have relatively few slip systems.

FRACTURE

Continuation of cold working in a heavily deformed metal eventually leads to fracture. The fracture initiates from microcracks that occur at points where there is an accumulation of dislocations or at boundaries between different microstructural phases. Alloys can undergo brittle or ductile fracture depending on a variety of factors, such as composition, microstructure and strain rate. When a ductile alloy fractures under tension, there is a reduction in the diameter of the metal (necking down) at the fracture site prior to fracture. Ductile fracture sites are characterized by a dimpled morphology. Microvoids or porosities may be seen at the fracture site.

Fracture due to cold working is a cause for concern in dentistry. Examples are fractures of endodontic instruments like root canal files and reamers within the canal. Retrieval of such instruments can often be difficult. That is why it is necessary to use these instruments in the correct sequence and manner and to change these instruments at regular intervals rather than use them till it breaks.

ANNEALING

The effects of cold working like strain hardening, susceptibility to corrosion and loss of ductility can be neutralized by a heating process called *annealing*.

STAGES OF ANNEALING

Annealing takes place in three stages

1. Recovery

2. Recrystallization
3. Grain growth

The time and temperature for annealing is dependent on the melting temperature of the alloy. A commonly observed rule is to use a temperature that is approximately half the melting point of the metal or alloy on the absolute scale (K).

Recovery

In the recovery stage, there is a slight decrease in tensile strength with no change in ductility. The most important beneficial changes occur during the recovery phase. As mentioned earlier, cold worked metal contains a lot of residual stresses. The purpose of annealing heat treatment is to relieve these stresses. Maximum stress relief occurs during the recovery stage.

Recrystallization

On further heating, changes in the microstructure begin to take place. The deformed grains begin to recrystallize forming new stress free grains. The metal essentially regains its old soft and ductile condition. The metal loses its properties of resilience rendering it useless for its intended purpose. Thus recrystallization must be avoided.

Grain growth

In this phase the recrystallized grains continue to grow with larger grains consuming smaller grains. Grain growth does not proceed indefinitely, but rather ceases until a coarse grain structure is formed. There is no significant difference in ductility and tensile strength from that observed in the previous stage.

Significance It is clear from the above that annealing should be done only until the recovery stage. Uncontrolled heating of dental related appliances can result in unintended changes within the structure.

USES OF WROUGHT ALLOYS

1. Orthodontic wires
2. Prosthodontic clasps
3. Root canal instruments like files and reamers
4. Steel bands and brackets for orthodontic and pedodontic use
5. Stainless steel crowns
6. Dental instruments

ORTHODONTIC WIRES

Various types of wires are used in fixed and removable orthodontics for tooth movement and stabilization.

Classification (ISO 15841:2014)

Wires are classified on the basis of their elastic behavior.

○ Type 1 wires: Wires displaying linear elastic behavior during unloading at temperatures up to 50 °C.

○ Type 2 wires: Wires displaying nonlinear elastic behavior during unloading at temperatures up to 50 °C.

GENERAL PROPERTIES OF ORTHODONTIC WIRES

Orthodontic wires are formed into various configurations or incorporated into appliances. When activated, these wires apply forces to the teeth and move them to the desired alignment. The force is determined by the appliance design and the material properties of the wire.

The following properties are important in orthodontic treatment.

○ *Force generated* The force generated by the wire on the tooth is dependent on its composition and design. For a given design, the force generated is proportional to the wire's stiffness.

○ *Elastic deflection and working range* Biologically, low constant forces are less damaging. This is best achieved by a large elastic deflection because it produces a more constant force and has a greater 'working range'.

$$\text{Maximum elastic deflection} = \frac{\text{Proportional limit (PL)}}{\text{Modulus of elasticity (MOE)}}$$

○ *Springiness* It is a measure of how far a wire can be deflected without causing permanent deformation.

○ *Stiffness* Amount of force required to produce a specific deformation.

Stiffness = 1/springiness

○ *Resilience* It is the energy storage capacity of the wires which is a combination of strength and springiness.

○ *Formability* It represents the amount of permanent bending; the wire will tolerate before it breaks.

○ *Ductility* of the wire.

○ *Ease of joining* Most wires can be soldered or welded together.

○ *Corrosion resistance* and stability in the oral environment is important for the appliance durability as well as biocompatibility.

○ *Biocompatibility* Most orthodontic wires are biocompatible. People generally allergic to nickel may get allergic reactions from nickel containing orthodontic wires.

○ *Cost* is a factor in orthodontics. The titanium alloy wires are more expensive than the stainless steel or the cobalt chromium nickel wires.

TYPES

○ Wrought gold alloys
○ Wrought base-metal alloys
○ Stainless steel
○ Cobalt-chromium-nickel
○ Nickel-titanium
○ Beta-titanium

WROUGHT GOLD ALLOYS

USES

Primarily to make clasps in partial dentures.

CLASSIFICATION

Type I—High precious metal alloys

Type II—Low precious metal alloys

COMPOSITION

The composition varies widely.

Gold	— 25 to 70%	Copper	— 7 to 18%
Platinum	— 5 to 50%	Nickel	— 1 to 3%
Palladium	— 5 to 44%	Zinc	— 1 to 2%
Silver	— 5 to 41%		

PROPERTIES

They generally resemble Type IV casting gold alloys. Because of the cold working, wires and other wrought forms have improved mechanical properties like hardness and tensile strength when compared to cast structures.

However, care should be taken during soldering. Prolonged heating at higher temperatures can cause it to recrystallize. Recrystallization changes the properties and makes the wire brittle.

WROUGHT BASE-METAL ALLOYS

A number of wrought base-metal alloys are used in dentistry, mainly as wires for orthodontic treatment. The alloys are

○ Stainless steel (iron-chromium-nickel)

○ Cobalt-chromium-nickel

○ Nickel-titanium

○ Beta-titanium

STAINLESS STEEL

Steel is an iron-based alloy which contains less than 1.2% carbon. When chromium (12 to 30%) is added to steel, the alloy is called as stainless steel. Elements other than iron, carbon and chromium may also be present, resulting in a wide variation in composition and properties of the stainless steels.

PASSIVATION

Stainless steels are resistant to tarnish and corrosion, because of the *passivating effect* of the chromium. A thin, transparent but tough and impervious oxide layer forms on the surface of the alloy when it is exposed to air, which protects it against tarnish and corrosion. It loses its protection if the oxide layer is ruptured by mechanical or chemical factors.

TYPES

There are three types of stainless steel based on the lattice arrangement of iron.

1. Ferritic

2. Martensitic

3. Austenitic
4. Duplex
5. Precipitation Hardening

FERRITIC STAINLESS STEELS

Pure iron at room temperature has body-centered cubic (BCC) structure and is referred to as ferrite, which is stable up to 912 °C.

PROPERTIES AND USE

The ferric alloys have good corrosion resistance, but less strength and hardness. So they find little application in dentistry.

MARTENSITIC STAINLESS STEELS

When austenite (face-centered cubic structure) is cooled very rapidly (quenched), it will undergo a spontaneous, diffusionless transformation to a body-centered tetragonal (BCT) structure called martensite. This is a highly distorted and strained lattice, which results in a very hard and strong but brittle alloy.

PROPERTIES AND USES

Corrosion resistance of the martensitic stainless steel is less than that of the other types. Because of their high strength and hardness, martensitic stainless steels are used for surgical and cutting instruments. Bur shanks are also made from this steel.

AUSTENITIC STAINLESS STEELS

At temperatures between 912 °C and 1394 °C, the stable form of iron is a face-centered cubic (FCC) structure called austenite. The austenitic stainless steel alloys are the most corrosion resistant of the stainless steels.

AUSTENITE-FINISH TEMPERATURE

It is the temperature at which the metallurgical transformation from the low-temperature martensite phase to the high-temperature austenite phase is completed.

COMPOSITION

Chromium — 18%
Nickel — 8%
Carbon — 0.08-0.15%

USES

This alloy is also known as *18-8 stainless steel*. They are commonly used by orthodontists and pedodontists in the form of bands and wires *(Figs. 27.1 and 27.2)*. Type 316 L (contains carbon-0.03% maximum) is the type usually used for implants.

AVAILABLE AS

They are available as annealed and partially annealed wires. They are usually supplied as rolls of varying thickness.

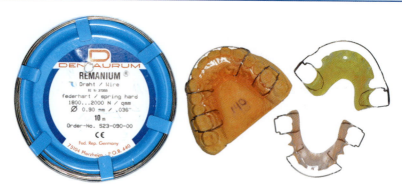

FIGURE 27.1 A stainless steel wire roll (left) and some of the appliances made from the wires.

ADVANTAGES

Austenitic steel is preferred to ferritic alloys because of some desirable properties

1. Greater ductility and ability to undergo more cold work without breaking.
2. Substantial strengthening during cold working.
3. Greater ease of welding.
4. The ability to readily overcome sensitization.
5. Less critical grain growth.
6. Comparative ease in forming.

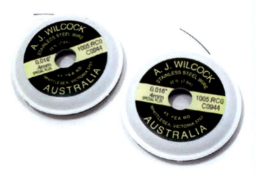

FIGURE 27.2 High tensile stainless steel wire.

PROPERTIES

Sensitization

The 18-8 stainless steel may lose its resistance to corrosion if it is heated between 400 and 900 °C (temperature used during soldering and welding).

The reason for a decrease in corrosion resistance is the precipitation of *chromium carbide* at the grain boundaries at these high temperatures. The small, rapidly diffusing carbon atoms migrate to the grain boundaries from all parts of the crystal to combine with the large, slowly diffusing chromium atoms at the periphery of the grain. When the chromium combines with the carbon in this manner, its *passivating qualities are lost* and the corrosion resistance of the steel is reduced.

Stabilization (methods to minimize sensitization)

1. From a theoretical point, the carbon content of the steel can be reduced to such an extent that carbide precipitation cannot occur. However, this is not economically practical.
2. By stabilization, i.e., some element is introduced that precipitates as a carbide in preference to chromium. Titanium is commonly used. Titanium at six times the carbon content, inhibits the precipitation of chromium carbide at soldering temperatures. These are known as *stabilized stainless steels.*

Annealed and partially annealed wires

When stainless steel wires are fully annealed, they become soft and highly formable. When it is partially annealed, the yield strength is increased and formability decreased. Stainless steel is available in different grades depending on their yield strength. Both the fully annealed and partially annealed wires are used as orthodontic wires.

Mechanical properties

In orthodontic wires, strength and hardness may increase with a decrease in the diameter because of the amount of cold working in forming the wire.

- Tensile strength — 2100 MPa
- Yield strength — 1400 MPa
- Hardness — 600 KHN

BRAIDED AND TWISTED WIRES

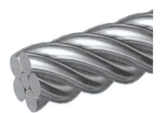

Very small diameter stainless steel wires (about 0.15 mm) can be braided or twisted together to form either *round* or *rectangular* shaped (about 0.4 to 0.6 mm in cross-section) wires *(Fig. 27.3)*. These wires are available as straight lengths or as formed archwires in the form of 3 strands or in increasing number of strands.

FIGURE 27.3 A braided wire.

These braided or twisted wires are able to sustain large elastic deflections in bending, and apply low forces for a given deflection when compared with solid stainless steel wire.

SOLDERS FOR STAINLESS STEEL

Silver solders are used. The soldering temperatures for orthodontic silver solders are in the range of 620 to 665 °C.

FLUXES

It is similar to that recommended for gold soldering with the exception of–

- The addition of the potassium fluoride. Fluoride helps to dissolve the passivating film supplied by the chromium.
- A higher boric acid to borax ratio lowers the fusion temperature.

WROUGHT COBALT-CHROMIUM-NICKEL ALLOYS

These wrought alloys were originally developed for use as watch springs (Elgiloy). Their properties are excellent also for orthodontic purposes.

COMPOSITION

Co —	40%	Mn —	2%
Cr —	20%	C —	0.15%
Ni —	15%	Be —	0.04%
Mo —	7%	Fe —	15.8%

HEAT TREATMENT

Softening heat treatment 1100 to 1200 °C followed by a rapid quench. Hardening heat treatment 260 to 650 °C, e.g. 482 °C for 5 hours.

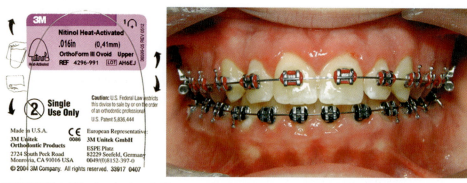

FIGURE 27.4 Nitinol arch wires (left) are used extensively in orthodontic treatment (above).

The wires are usually heat treated and supplied in several degrees of hardness (soft, ductile, semispring temper and spring temper).

PHYSICAL PROPERTIES

Tarnish and corrosion resistance is excellent. Hardness, yield, and tensile strength similar to those of 18-8 stainless steel.

NICKEL-TITANIUM ALLOYS

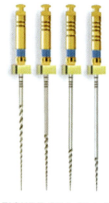

FIGURE 27.5 Nickel-titanium files.

Nickel-titanium shape memory alloys were first discovered by Buehler in the early 1960s. He was working at the Naval Ordinance Laboratory (NOL) at the time, hence the name Nitinol. His discovery formed the basis of the first commercial shape memory alloy. These nickel-titanium alloy (also called nitinol) wires have large elastic deflections or working range and limited formability, because of their low stiffness and moderately high strength. They are used extensively as arch wires in fixed orthodontic treatment *(Fig. 27.4)*. They are also used to manufacture endodontic instruments *(Fig. 27.5)*.

AVAILABLE AS

Nickel titanium alloy wires are available as springs in addition to formed arch wires. Nickel titanium wires are commercially available in martensitic (M-Niti) and austenitic (A-Niti) depending on their use in different phases of orthodontic treatment.

COMPOSITION

The primary elements are nickel and titanium. Addition of copper to nickel and titanium alloy improves the thermal reactive properties of the wire, which help in consistent and efficient orthodontic tooth movement. Other additions made to alter the phase transformation temperature are elements such as iron and chromium which lower the temperature.

PROPERTIES OF NITINOL ALLOYS

SHAPE MEMORY AND SUPERELASTICITY

This alloy exists in various crystallographic forms. At high temperature, a stable body-centered cubic lattice (austenitic phase) exists. On appropriate cooling or an application of stress, this transforms to a close-packed hexagonal martensitic lattice with associated volumetric change. This behavior of the alloy (austenite to martensite phase transition) results in two features of clinical significance called as 'shape memory' and 'superelasticity', or 'pseudoelasticity'.

The 'memory' effect is achieved by first establishing a shape at temperatures near 482 °C. The appliance, e.g. archwire is then cooled and formed into a second shape. Subsequent heating through a *lower transition temperature* (37 °C - mouth temperature) causes the wire to return to its original shape. The phenomenon of superelasticity is produced by transition of austenite to martensite by stress due to the volume change which results from the change in crystal structure.

Stressing an alloy initially results in standard proportional stress-strain behavior. However, at the stress where it induces the phase transformation, there is an increase in strain, referred to as superelasticity. At the completion of the phase, it reverts to standard proportional stress-strain behavior. Unloading results in the reverse transition and recovery. This characteristic is useful in some orthodontic situations because it results in *low forces* and a very *large working range* or springback.

These wires are useful because it is possible to achieve phase transformation at *room temperature* when force is applied. Wires with different transformation temperatures are now available, which enable the clinician to select the precise wires for different needs.

Density   Their density is approximately 6.5 g/cm^3.

Melting range   Melting temperature in the range 1240 to 1310 °C.

TITANIUM ALLOYS

Like stainless steel and nitinol, pure titanium has different crystallographic forms at high and low temperatures. At temperatures below 885°C the hexagonal close packed (HCP) or alpha lattice is stable, whereas at higher temperatures the metal rearranges into a body-centered cubic (BCC) form called β-titanium.

α-titanium is not used in orthodontic applications. The β-form is more useful in orthodontics. However, to retain the β-form as it cools to room temperature elements like molybdenum are added. This stabilizes the β-form and prevents its transformation to the α-form. For orthodontic use the titanium alloys are supplied as precut arch wires *(Fig. 27.6)* usually in a rectangular cross-sectional form *(Fig. 27.7)*.

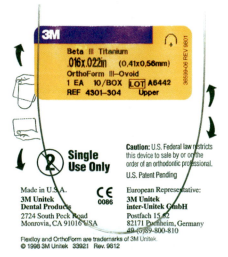

FIGURE 27.6 Titanium (Beta III by 3M) arch wire.

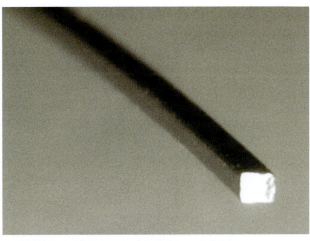

FIGURE 27.7 Wires come in different cross-sectional shapes including round, square and rectangular.

COMPOSITION

Ti	—	79%
Mo	—	11%
Zr	—	6%
Sn	—	4%

MECHANICAL PROPERTIES

1. Modulus of elasticity - 70 GPa.
2. Yield strength - 860 to 1200 MPa.
3. The high ratio of yield strength to modulus produces orthodontic appliances that can undergo large elastic activations when compared with stainless steel.
4. Beta-titanium can be highly cold-worked. It can be bent into various configurations and has formability comparable to that of austenitic steel.
5. *Welding* Clinically satisfactory joints can be made by electrical resistance welding of beta-titanium.
6. *Corrosion resistance* Both forms have excellent corrosion resistance and environmental stability.
7. Heat treatment can alter its properties, therefore, heat treatment of these wires is not recommended.

PART-7

Indirect Restorative and Prosthetic Materials

Dental Ceramics

CHAPTER OUTLINE

Dental ceramics holds the promise of a restorative material, that can realistically duplicate teeth, to the extent that the layperson may find it difficult to differentiate *(Fig. 28.1)*. One might argue that composite resins have a similar esthetic potential. However, there is a difference— dental ceramics are far more stronger, durable, wear resistant, and virtually indestructible in the oral environment. They are impervious to oral fluids and absolutely biocompatible. They do have some drawbacks which will be discussed subsequently. Because of their huge potential, it is still a fast growing area in terms of research and development. Thanks to the continuing research, these materials once restricted to restoring single crowns have now expanded to include long span fixed partial dentures.

USES AND APPLICATIONS

1. Inlays and onlays.
2. Esthetic laminates (veneers) over natural teeth.
3. Single (all ceramic) crowns.

4. Short and long span (all ceramic) FDP.
5. As veneer for cast metal crowns and bridges (metal ceramics).
6. Artificial denture teeth (for complete denture and partial denture use).
7. Ceramic post and cores.
8. Ceramic orthodontic brackets.

EVOLUTION OF DENTAL CERAMICS

Ceramics are among the oldest materials known to man. Ceramic objects dating back to 20,000 years have been found in China. The history of glass dates back to 3500 BC in Mesopotamia. The term 'glass' was first developed during the late Roman empire. Ceramics comes from Greek word keramikos, which means pottery and keramos, which means potter's clay.

An *esthetic and durable* material that could accurately reproduce missing teeth or teeth structure had always been a dream. Prior to the use of porcelain, crowns were made entirely of gold or other alloys. As demands for esthetics increased, tooth colored resin was used as a veneer over the metal in the esthetic areas. Around the early 1900s, porcelain crowns were introduced to dentistry by Charles Land (grandfather of aviator Charles Lindbergh) who coined the term *porcelain jacket crowns (PJC)*. The restoration was extensively used after improvements were made by EB Spaulding and publicized by WA Capon. While not known for its strength due to internal microcracking, the porcelain "jacket" crown (PJC) was used extensively until the 1950s. These early crowns were made of feldspathic porcelains which generally were materials of poor strength. They were also very difficult to fabricate and did not fit well (poor margins).

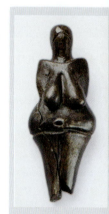

"The worlds oldest ceramic object, the Venus of Dolni Vestonice, from the Czech Republic, 26,000 years old."

To reduce the risk of internal microcracking during the cooling phase of fabrication, the porcelain-fused-to-metal (PFM) crown was developed in the late 1950s by Abraham Weinstein. The bond between the metal and porcelain prevented stress cracks from forming. This led to the era of the metal-ceramics *(Fig. 28.1)*. Prior to this, metal FDPs were veneered (covered) with tooth colored acrylic in order to hide the metal. These veneers did not last very long and had to be replaced often. Besides they could not be used to cover the occlusal surface because of their poor wear resistance. The metal-ceramic crowns and fixed dental prostheses were instantly accepted because of their superior esthetics, wear resistance and strength. The ceramic could be used to veneer the occlusal surface as well. Since the margins were in metal, the marginal fit was highly accurate.

In spite of the success of the metal-ceramic restorations, they did not represent the final solution. The underlying opaquer covered metal did not allow the natural passage and reflection of light as in natural teeth. Under certain lighting conditions these crowns appeared dense, dark and *opaque*. The margin of the restoration appeared to be *dark*, even when hidden below the gums as it sometimes showed through the gums (the gums developed a bluish discoloration).

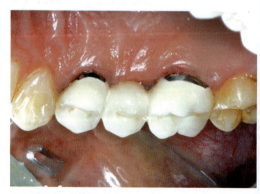

FIGURE 28.1 Porcelain-fused-to-metal fixed partial denture.

Some manufacturers did attempt to solve this problem by introducing 'shoulder porcelains'. A portion of the metal was removed from the labial margin (metal free margin) and replaced with shoulder porcelain. However, this still did not entirely solve the problem of translucency.

The first breakthrough at developing a stronger all-ceramic restoration came in 1965. McLean and Hughes introduced an alumina reinforced core material which improved the strength of the porcelain. However, they were still not strong enough for posterior use and of course the problem of marginal adaptation still remained.

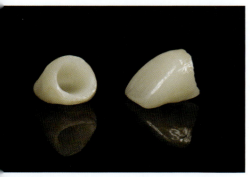

FIGURE 28.2 All porcelain (metal free) crowns.

The 1990s saw the reemergence of the *all-ceramic crown (Fig. 28.2) as well as small fixed partial dentures*. The strength of the restorations had been improved through the introduction of newer porcelains and fabrication techniques. The marginal adaptation and fit had also improved considerably when compared to the first generation all-porcelain crowns. The new generation ceramics included *castable glass* ceramics, *injection molded* ceramics, *glass infiltrated* core ceramics, *CAD/CAM* (computer-aided design, computer-aided machining) ceramics, etc. With the increase in strength the use of all ceramic restorations gradually expanded to include posterior crowns and bridges. A major reason for this was the introduction of stabilized zirconia and CAD/CAM. Ceramic technology continue to evolve because of the high demand for esthetic tooth colored restorations.

Definition

Compounds of one or more metals with a nonmetallic element, usually oxygen. They are formed of chemical and biochemical stable substances that are strong, hard, brittle, and inert nonconductors of thermal and electrical energy (*GPT- 8*).

CLASSIFICATION OF DENTAL PORCELAINS

The wide variety of ceramic systems available in the market make classification of ceramics a challenging task. The manufacturer provides equipment and material compatible for the particular system. They are usually not interchangeable.

ACCORDING TO FIRING TEMPERATURE

○ High fusing	1300 °C or above
○ Medium fusing	1101 °C to 1300 °C
○ Low fusing	850 °C to 1100 °C
○ Ultra low fusing	less than 850 °C

ACCORDING TO TYPE

○ Feldspathic porcelains

○ Leucite reinforced glass ceramics

○ Tetrasilicic fluormica based glass ceramics

○ Lithia disilicate based ceramics

○ Alumina reinforced ceramics

○ Spinel reinforced ceramics

○ Zirconia reinforced ceramics

Porcelain vs. Ceramic

The terms porcelain and ceramics are often used interchangeably. However there are subtle differences. Ceramic is a broad term that includes earthenware, bone ware, pottery, brick, stoneware and of course porcelain and any other article made of clay and hardened by heat. Porcelain is a subcategory of ceramics and is characterized by its hard, glass-like and translucent qualities. All porcelains are ceramics, but all ceramics are not porcelains.

ACCORDING TO ITS FUNCTION WITHIN THE RESTORATION

- ❍ Core ceramics – Supports and reinforces the restoration in all-ceramic restorations
- ❍ Opaquer ceramics – Masks or hides the metal or underlying core ceramic. Bonds ceramic to underlying metal
- ❍ Veneering ceramics
  - – Body or dentin – Simulates the dentin portion of natural teeth
  - – Incisal – Simulates the enamel portion of natural teeth
  - – Gingival – Simulates the darker gingival portion of teeth
  - – Translucent – Simulates translucent incisal enamel seen some times in natural teeth
- ❍ Stains – Used to color ceramics to improve esthetics
- ❍ Glaze – Imparts a smooth glossy surface to the restoration

ACCORDING TO MICROSTRUCTURE

- ❍ Glass ceramics
- ❍ Crystalline ceramics
- ❍ Crystal containing glasses

ACCORDING TO FABRICATION PROCESS

- ❍ Condensable ceramics
- ❍ Slip-cast glass-infiltrated ceramics
- ❍ Heat pressed (hot isostatic) ceramics
- ❍ Castable ceramics
- ❍ Machinable ceramics
- ❍ Various combinations of the above

BASIC CONSTITUENTS AND MANUFACTURE OF FELDSPATHIC PORCELAIN

The wide variety of ceramic products in the market, makes it virtually impossible to provide a single composition. Traditionally, porcelains were manufactured from a mineral called *feldspar*. These porcelains are referred to as *feldspathic porcelains*. As technology improved other ceramic systems were introduced, like core porcelains, glass ceramics, etc. The composition of these differ from the traditional feldspathic porcelains.

BASIC STRUCTURE

Most current ceramics consist of two phases.

- ❍ Glassy phase—acts as the matrix
- ❍ Crystalline phase—dispersed within the matrix and improves strength and other properties of the porcelain, e.g. quartz, alumina, spinel, zirconia, etc.

The structure of porcelain is similar to that of glass *(Box 28.1)*. The basic structure therefore consists of a three dimensional *network of silica* (silica tetrahedra). Pure glass melts at too high a temperature for dental use. Adding certain chemicals lowers the melting temperature by disrupting the silica network. The glass obtains porcelain-like qualities when the silica network is broken by *alkalies* like sodium and potassium. This also lowers the fusion temperature. These chemicals are known as *glass modifiers* or *fluxes*. Other substances which act as glass modifiers are alumina (Al_2O_3) and boric oxide (B_2O_3). Boric oxide forms its own separate network between

BOX 28.1	Comparison of glass and porcelain

Glass	Porcelains
Random amorphous (noncrystalline) structure	Ordered crystalline structure in glassy matrix
Transparent	Opaque
Composed mainly of silica	Contains silica and other crystalline phases

the silica network. Adding certain opacifiers reduces the transparency and completes the transformation to dental porcelain.

BASIC CONSTITUENTS

The basic constituents of feldspathic porcelains are

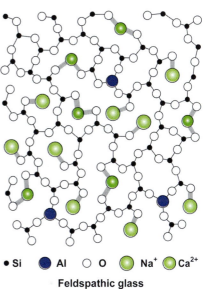

- Feldspar – Basic glass former/matrix
- Kaolin – Green stage binder
- Quartz – Filler and opacifier
- Alumina – Additional glass former and flux
- Alkalies – Glass modifiers (flux)
- Color pigments – Modifies color
- Opacifiers – Reduces transparency

• Si   ● Al   ○ O   ● Na⁺   ● Ca²⁺

Feldspathic glass

Feldspar

It is a naturally occurring mineral and forms the basic constituent of feldspathic porcelains. Most of the components needed to make dental porcelain are found in feldspar. It thus contains potash (K_2O), soda (Na_2O), alumina (Al_2O_3) and silica (SiO_2). It is the basic glass former. When fused at high temperatures (during manufacture) it forms a feldspathic glass containing potash feldspar ($K_2O.Al_2O_3.6SiO_2$) or soda feldspar ($Na_2O.Al_2O_3.6SiO_2$). Pure feldspathic glass is quite colorless and transparent. As explained earlier, various glass modifiers and opacifiers are added to alter its sintering temperature, viscosity, thermal coefficient of expansion (CTE) and appearance.

Kaolin

Kaolin also called china clay, is a white clay-like material (hydrated aluminum silicate). Kaolin is named after the hill in China (Kao-ling) from which it was mined for centuries. It acts as a binder when wet, helping to shape the green porcelain. It also gives opacity to the mass. Some manufacturers use sugar or starch instead of kaolin.

Quartz

Quartz is a form of silica. Ground quartz acts as a refractory skeleton, providing strength and hardness to porcelain during firing. It remains relatively unchanged during and after firing.

Alumina

Aluminum oxide (alumina) replaces some of the silica in the glass network. It gives strength and opacity to the porcelain. It alters the softening point and increases the viscosity of porcelain during firing.

Another glass former is boric oxide (B_2O_3) which forms its own glass network (also called lattice) interspersed between the silica network (lattice).

Glass modifiers

Alkalies such as sodium, potassium and calcium are called glass modifiers. Glass modifiers lower the fusion temperature and increase the flow of porcelain during firing. They also raise the CTE (important in metal-ceramics). However, too high a concentration of glass modifiers is not good for the ceramic because

○ It reduces the chemical durability of the ceramic

○ It may cause the glass to devitrify (crystallize)

Opacifiers

Since pure feldspathic porcelain is quite colorless, opacifiers are added to increase its opacity in order to simulate natural teeth. Oxides of zirconium, titanium and tin are commonly used opacifiers.

Color modifiers

Natural teeth come in a variety of shades. In addition, it acquires external stains from the environment. Thus, color modifiers are required to adjust the shades of the dental ceramic. Various metallic oxides provide a variety of color, e.g. titanium oxide (yellow-brown), nickel oxide (brown), copper oxide (green), manganese oxide (lavender), cobalt oxide (blue), etc. They are fused together with regular feldspar and then reground and blended to produce a variety of colors.

OTHER SPECIALIZED PORCELAINS

Glazes

It is a special type of colorless porcelain applied to the surface of the completed ceramic restoration to give it a smooth finish as well as increase the life of the restoration. Obviously they do not contain opacifiers. They must also have a lower fusion temperature and therefore must contain a lot of glass modifiers. This also makes them somewhat less chemically durable.

Stains

They are porcelain powders containing a high concentration of color modifiers (as described previously). They too have a lower fusion temperature made possible by an increased content of glass modifiers. Stains are used to provide individual color variation in the finished restoration *(Fig. 28.2)*.

Opaquer porcelains

It is a specialized type of porcelain which is used to conceal the metal core in PFM (metal-ceramic) restorations. It is the first layer applied before the addition of the regular porcelain. Obviously, it contains a high concentration of *opacifiers*. Some amount of color modifiers are also added.

Reinforced core ceramics

The low strength of traditional feldspathic porcelain prompted research into methods of reinforcing ceramics. The first reinforced ceramic (alumina reinforced) was introduced by McLean and Hughes in 1965. Subsequently other materials and techniques were introduced. Among the strongest of the core ceramics currently available are the machined zirconia cores.

MANUFACTURE

Traditionally, porcelain powders are manufactured by a process called *fritting*. Various components are mixed together and fused. While it is still hot, it is quenched in water. This causes the mass to crack and fracture, making it easier to powder it. The frit is ground to a fine powder and supplied to the consumer in bottles. Most of the chemical reaction takes place during the manufacture (pyrochemical reaction). During subsequent firing in the dental laboratory, there is not much of chemical reaction). The porcelain powder simply fuses together to form the desired restoration.

PORCELAIN/CERAMIC SYSTEMS

Currently, various ceramic systems exist which can be quite confusing to the dental student. The entire restoration may be made of just one type of porcelain (e.g. an inlay machined from a single block of ceramic) or it may be *layered* with different types of porcelains. Many crowns and FDPs are fabricated as layered restorations. A layered restoration can be divided into 2 basic parts *(Fig. 28.3)*.

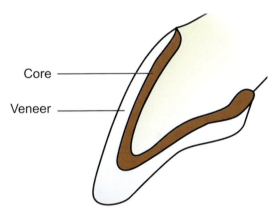

FIGURE 28.3 Simplified structure of a ceramic crown. Core is for support and may be made of metal in case of a metal ceramic crown or a dense strong ceramic in case of an all ceramic crown.

○ Core (or substructure)

○ Veneer (outer layer).

Core   The core provides support and *strength* for the crown. Early crowns were constructed entirely of a single type of feldspathic porcelain (e.g. PJC). In 1965 McLean demonstrated improved strength in crowns layered over an aluminous core. Since then other core materials and techniques have been introduced. The core functions as a supporting frame. Freshly mixed porcelain is like wet sand. It needs to be supported while it is being condensed and built up. The core is therefore usually constructed *first*. The rest of the restoration is built up on to the core.

With metal-ceramic crowns the *metal coping* or *frame* takes the role of the ceramic core. They provide the support and reinforcement. Examples of *core materials currently available are* alumina, spinel, zirconia, etc.

Veneer   The core is usually dense and opaque and generally unesthetic. The esthetics is improved by firing additional layers of ceramic known as veneer porcelains. The core is veneered with various layers of specialized porcelains called dentin, enamel, cervical and translucent. It can also be internally and externally (surface) stained to mimic natural teeth color and finally glazed.

CLASSIFICATION AND DESCRIPTION OF CERAMIC SYSTEMS

The ceramic restorations available today may be metal bonded or made completely of ceramic. Based on the substructure or core material used there are two basic groups. They are further divided based on the fabrication method.

A. *Metal-ceramic (metal bonded or PFM) restorations*

    1. Cast metal-ceramic restorations

       - Cast noble metal alloys

- Cast base metal alloys
- Cast titanium (ultra low fusing porcelain).
2. Burnished foil metal ceramic restorations
   - Capillary casting [sintered gold alloy foil coping Renaissance, Captek)]
   - Bonded platinum foil coping.

B. All ceramic restorations

1. Platinum foil matrix condensed porcelain restorations
   - Conventional feldspathic porcelain restorations
   - Porcelain restorations with aluminous core
   - Ceramic jacket crown with leucite reinforced core (Optec HSP)
2. Castable glass ceramics (Dicor)
3. Pressable glass-ceramics
   - Leucite reinforced glass-ceramics (IPS Empress)
   - Lithia disilicate reinforced glass-ceramics (IPS Empress 2)
4. Glass infiltrated core porcelains
   - Glass infiltrated aluminous core (In-Ceram)
   - Glass infiltrated spinel core (In-Ceram Spinell)
   - Glass infiltrated zirconia core (In-Ceram Zirconia)
5. Ceramic restorations from CAD/CAM ceramic blanks
   - Feldspathic porcelain blanks (Vitablocs Mark II)
   - Lithia disilicate glass ceramic blanks (IPS e max CAD, Kavo)
   - Glass infiltrated blanks (Alumina, Spinell, Zirconia)
   - Partially sintered zirconia blanks (Vita In-Ceram YZ)
   - Sintered zirconia blanks (Everest ZH blanks)
6. Ceramic restorations from copy milled ceramic blanks
   - Alumina blocks (Celay In-Ceram)
   - $MgAl_2O_4$ blocks (In-Ceram spinell).

METAL-CERAMIC RESTORATIONS

Synonyms Porcelain-fused-to-metal (PFM), metal-bonded restorations, ceramo metal, etc.

The early porcelain jacket crowns (PJC) did not use reinforcing cores and were therefore weak. The metal-ceramic restorations *(Fig. 28.4)* were developed around the same time Mclean introduced the aluminous core porcelains (1965). The cast metal core (called coping) or framework *(Fig. 28.5)* significantly strengthened the porcelain restoration and this soon became the most widely used ceramic restoration. According to a 1994 survey, 90% of all ceramic restorations were porcelain-fused-to-metal. The metal-ceramic systems are covered by *ISO 9693*.

The metal-ceramic system was possible because of some important developments.

❍ Development of a metal and porcelain that could bond to each other

❍ Raising of the CTE of the ceramic in order to make it more compatible to that of the metal.

This obviously meant that a lot of research had to go into both porcelain and metal composition before they could be used for metal-ceramics.

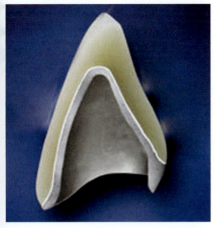

FIGURE 28.4 Cross section through a metal ceramic crown fused to nickel chromium alloy.

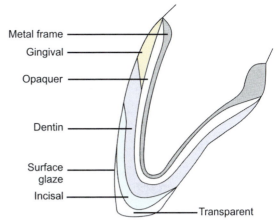

FIGURE 28.5 Parts of a metal ceramic crown. Transparent is used to duplicate the thin translucent enamel seen in some natural teeth.

TYPES OF METAL-CERAMIC SYSTEMS

As previously mentioned the metal-ceramic systems can be divided into

1. Cast metal ceramic restorations
    - Cast noble metal alloys (feldspathic porcelain)
    - Cast base metal alloys (feldspathic porcelain)
    - Cast titanium (ultra low fusing porcelain).
2. Swaged metal ceramic restorations
    - Capillary cast [sintered gold alloy foil (Renaissance, Captek)]
    - Bonded platinum foil coping.

CAST METAL-CERAMIC RESTORATIONS

The cast metal-ceramic restoration is hugely popular. Because of the strong metal frame it is possible to make long span fixed partial dentures. It can also be used in difficult situations where an all-ceramic restoration cannot be given because of high stresses and reduced preparation depth.

USES

1. Single anterior and posterior crowns.
2. Short and long span anterior and posterior FDPs.

COMPOSITION OF CERAMIC FOR METAL BONDING

Feldspathic porcelains are used for metal bonding. The basic composition is quite similar to that of feldspathic porcelain described earlier except for the higher alkali content (soda and potash). The higher alkali content was necessary in order to raise the CTE. Unfortunately this also increased the tendency of the ceramic to devitrify and appear cloudy. A typical composition is shown in *Table 28.1*.

A special opaquer porcelain is needed to mask the underlying metal so that it does not show through the ceramic *(Fig. 28.8)*. The opaquer has a high content of opacifiers. Similarly, the composition of glazes would be different. Glazes have a higher concentration of glass modifiers like soda, potash and boric oxide.

SUPPLIED AS

1. Enamel porcelain powders in various shades (in bottles) *(Fig. 28.6)*
2. Dentin porcelain powders in various shades (in bottles)
3. Liquid for mixing enamel, dentin, gingival and transparent
4. Opaquer powders in various shades/ and liquid for mixing *(Fig. 28.7)*
5. Gingival porcelain powder in various shades
6. Transparent porcelain powder
7. A variety of stain (color) powders
8. Glaze powder
9. Special liquid for mixing stains and glaze

MANIPULATION AND TECHNICAL CONSIDERATIONS

CONSTRUCTION OF THE CAST METAL COPING OR FRAMEWORK

A wax pattern of the restoration is constructed and cast in metal. Metals used for the frame or coping include noble metal alloys, base metal alloys and recently titanium (see chapter on casting alloys and casting procedures).

TABLE 28.1 A sample percentage composition of porcelain powder for metal ceramics

	Dentin porcelain	Enamel porcelain
Silica (SiO_2)	59.2	63.5
Alumina (Al_2O_3)	18.5	18.9
Soda (Na_2O)	4.8	5.0
Potash (K_2O)	11.8	2.3
Boric oxide (B_2O_3)	4.6	0.12
Zinc oxide (ZnO)	0.58	0.11
Zirconium oxide (ZrO_2)	0.39	0.13

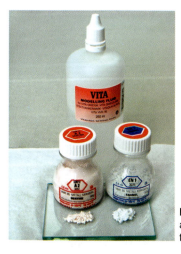

FIGURE 28.6 Enamel and dentin powders with the modelling liquid.

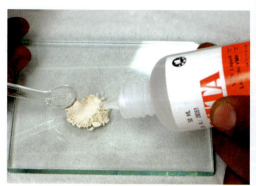

FIGURE 28.7 Opaquer powder is mixed and applied to hide the metal. It is mixed with the liquid to produce a sandy mix. A glass spatula is used for mixing as metal might abrade and contaminate the porcelain.

METAL PREPARATION

A clean metal surface is essential for good bonding. Oil and other impurities from the fingers can contaminate. The surface is finished with ceramic bonded stones or sintered diamonds. Final texturing is done by sandblasting with an alumina air abrasive, which aids in the bonding. Finally, it is cleaned ultrasonically, washed and dried.

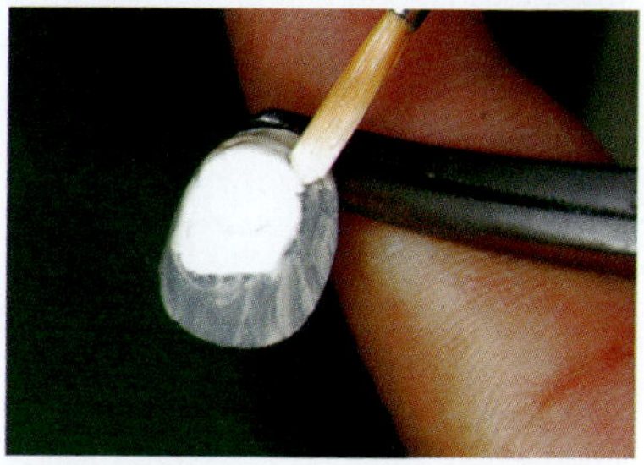

DEGASSING AND OXIDIZING

The casting (gold porcelain systems) is heated to a high temperature (980°C) to burn off the impurities and to form an oxide layer which help in the bonding. Degassing is done in the porcelain furnace.

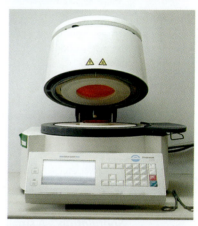

FIGURE 28.8 Application of opaquer.

OPAQUER

The opaquer is a dense yellowish white powder supplied along with a special liquid. The opaquer has *two important functions*. It is used to cover (mask) the metal frame and prevent it from being *visible*. It also aids in bonding the veneering porcelains to the underlying frame. The metal framework is held with a pair of *locking forceps*. Opaquer powder is dispensed on to a ceramic palette and mixed with the special liquid to a *paste like* consistency *(Fig. 28.7)*. It is applied on to the metal frame with a *brush* and *condensed (Fig. 28.8)*. The excess liquid is blotted with a tissue paper. The opaquer is built up to a thickness of 0.2 mm. The casting with the opaquer is placed in a porcelain furnace *(Fig. 28.9)* and fired at the appropriate temperature *(Box 28.2)*. Opaquer may be completed in two steps.

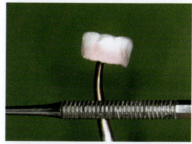

FIGURE 28.9 Ceramic furnace.

CONDENSATION

The process of packing the powder particles together and removing the excess water is known as condensation.

Purpose

Proper condensation packs the particles together. This helps minimize porosity, improve strength and reduce firing shrinkage. It also helps remove the excess water.

Condensation techniques

Vibration Mild vibration by tapping or running a serrated instrument *(Fig. 28.10)* on the forceps holding the metal frame helps to pack the particles together and bring out the excess water which is then blotted by an absorbent paper *(Fig. 28.11)*. An ultrasonic vibrator is also available for this purpose.

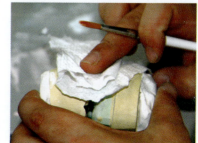

FIGURE 28.10 Condensing with mild vibration.

FIGURE 28.11 Blotting to remove excess water.

BOX 28.2 | Firing of porcelains

The process of sintering and fusing the particles of the condensed mass is known as firing. The powder particles flow and fuse together during firing. Making the restoration dense and strong. Firing is done in a porcelain furnace.

The Porcelain Furnace

Firing is carried out in a porcelain furnace. There are many companies which manufacture furnaces. Modern furnaces are computer controlled and have built-in programs to control the firing cycle. The programs can also be modified by the operator.

Firing Cycle

The entire program of preheating, firing, subjecting to vacuum, subjecting to increased pressure, holding and controlled cooling is known as a firing cycle. The firing cycles vary depending on the stage - opaquer firing, dentin firing, glaze firing, etc. The firing temperature is lowered gradually for each subsequent firing cycle. The opaquer has the highest temperature and the glaze has the lowest.

Preheating

The condensed mass should not be placed directly into the hot furnace. This can cause a rapid formation of steam which can break up the mass. Modern furnaces have a mechanism whereby the work is gradually raised into the furnace. This is known as preheating.

Vacuum Firing

During firing of the porcelain, a vacuum (negative pressure) is created in the furnace. This helps to reduce the porosity in the ceramic. The vacuum is later released raising the pressure in the furnace. The increased pressure helps to further reduce the size of any residual air bubbles not eliminated by the vacuum. The vacuum is not activated during the glaze firing.

Cooling

The cooling of the fired porcelain should be well controlled. Rapid cooling can cause the porcelain to crack or it can induce stresses inside which weaken the porcelain. Cooling is done slowly and uniformly and is usually computer controlled.

Spatulation A small spatula is used to apply and smoothen the wet porcelain. This helps to bring out the excess water.

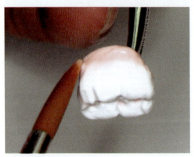

FIGURE 28.12 Building the restoration.

Dry powder Dry powder is placed on the side opposite a wet increment. The water moves towards the dry powder pulling the wet particles together.

DENTIN AND ENAMEL

The dentin powder (pink powder) is mixed with distilled water or the supplied liquid. A glass spatula should be used (ceramic powder is abrasive and can abrade the metal and contaminate the porcelain). The bulk of the tooth is built up with dentin. A portion of the dentin in the incisal area is cut back and enamel porcelain (white powder) can be added *(Fig. 28.12)* building the restoration. After the build-up and condensation is over *(Fig. 28.13)*, it is returned to the furnace for sintering.

ADDITIONS

It is not necessary to build up the restoration in one step. Large or difficult restorations may be built up and fired in two or more stages. After each firing *(Box 28.2)* the porcelain may be shaped by grinding and additional porcelain is placed in deficient areas. Each additional firing is done at a lower temperature.

Caution The restoration should not be subject to too many firings. Excessive firings can give rise to a over translucent, lifeless restoration.

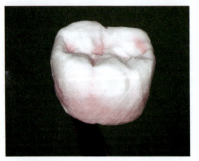

FIGURE 28.13 The built up crown.

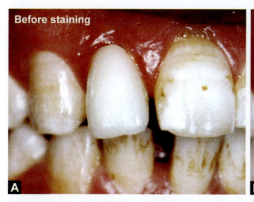
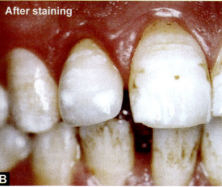

FIGURES 28.14A AND B Stained porcelain crown. Staining improves the vitality of the crown. **(A)** The lateral incisor before staining appears white and artificial. **(B)** The same tooth after applying yellow brown cervical stains and white fluorosis streaks and patches.

GINGIVAL AND TRANSPARENT PORCELAIN

The enamel of some natural teeth may appear transparent. This is usually seen near the incisal edges. If present it can be duplicated using *transparent* porcelain. The cervical portions of natural teeth may appear more darker (e.g. more yellow) than the rest of the tooth. When indicated *cervical* porcelains are used to duplicate this effect (they are also referred to as *gingival* or *neck* dentin).

SURFACE STAINING, CHARACTERIZATION AND EFFECTS

Natural teeth come in variety of hues and colors. Some of them are present at the time of eruption (intrinsic, e.g. white fluorosis stains), while others are acquired over a period of time from the environment (extrinsic, e.g. coffee, tobacco, etc.). Staining and characterization helps make the restoration look natural and helps it to blend in with the adjacent teeth *(Figs. 28.14A and B)*. The stain powders *(Fig. 28.15)* are mixed with a special liquid, applied and blended with a brush. With more and more emphasis on recreating the

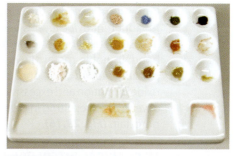

FIGURE 28.15 Porcelain stains and glazes.

natural look, *effects* are created using special techniques. This includes defects, cracks or other anomalies within the enamel.

GLAZING

Before final glazing, the restoration is tried in the mouth by the dentist. The occlusion is checked and adjusted by grinding. Final alterations can be made to improve the shape of the restoration. After all changes have been completed the restoration is ready for glazing. The restoration is smoothened with a fine stone prior to glazing to remove gross scratch marks. Glazing provides a smooth glossy surface to the restoration.

Objectives of glazing

1. Glazing enhances esthetics.
2. Enhances hygiene.
3. Improves the strength. Glazed porcelain is much stronger than unglazed ceramic. The glaze inhibits crack propagation.

4. Reduces the wear of opposing teeth. The rough surface on unglazed porcelain can accelerate wear of the opposing natural teeth.

Types

Over glaze The glaze powder is mixed with the special liquid and applied on to the restoration. The firing temperature is lower than that of the body porcelain. The firing cycle does not usually include a vacuum. Chemical durability of over glaze is lower because of the high flux content.

Self glaze A separate glaze layer is not applied. Instead the restoration is subject to a controlled heating at its fusion temperature. This causes only the surface layer to melt and flow to form a vitreous layer resembling glaze.

PORCELAIN-METAL BOND

Falls into two groups

○ Chemical bonding across the porcelain-metal interface.
○ Mechanical interlocking between porcelain and metal.

CHEMICAL BONDING

Currently regarded as the primary bonding mechanism. An adherent *oxide layer* is essential for good bonding. In base metal alloys, *chromic oxide* is responsible for the bond. In noble metal alloys, *indium and tin oxide* and possibly *iridium oxide* does this role. Both inadequate oxide formation and excessive oxide build up can lead to a weak bond resulting in delamination of the overlying porcelain *(Fig. 28.16)*.

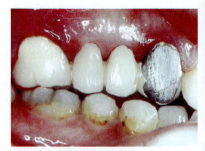

FIGURE 28.16 A failed metal-ceramic FDP. The ceramic veneer (canine) has delaminated leaving the metal exposed. In this case it was because of a poorly adherent metal oxide layer.

MECHANICAL INTERLOCKING

In some systems mechanical interlocking provides the principal bond. Sandblasting is often used to prepare the metal surface. Presence of surface roughness on the metal oxide surface improves retention, especially if undercuts are present. Wettability is important for bonding.

ADVANTAGES AND DISADVANTAGES OF METAL-CERAMIC RESTORATIONS

ADVANTAGES

1. Better fracture resistance because of the metal reinforcement.
2. Better marginal fit because of the metal frame.

DISADVANTAGES

1. Poor esthetics when compared to all-ceramic restorations because the underlying metal and opaquer reduces the overall translucency of the tooth.

2. The metal frame and the lack of translucency sometimes shows through the gingiva resulting in the characteristic dark margins.

OTHER METAL-CERAMIC SYSTEMS

CAPILLARY CAST (SINTERED GOLD ALLOY FOIL-CERAMIC) RESTORATIONS

Adapting and sintering gold alloy foils (Renaissance and Captek) is a novel way of making a metal frame without having to cast it. The system was developed by Shoher and Whiteman and introduced to the dental community in 1993. Captek is an acronym for 'capillary casting technique'. The technique is used to make crowns and fixed prostheses using proprietary materials and techniques *(Figs. 28.17A to C)*. (Refer chapter on 'casting procedures' for additional information).

Composition, mode of supply and capillary casting

They are supplied as thin strips in two forms called Captek P and Captek G. Captek P (Platinum/Palladium/ Gold) has a porous structure and serves as the internal reinforcing skeleton. Captek G is 97.5% Gold and 2.5% Silver. On heating in a furnace, the Captek P acts like a metal sponge and draws in (capillary action) the hot liquid gold completely into it. Captek G provides the characteristic gold color of this system. The final coping can be described as a composite structure.

Technique

The technique for fabrication is described in the chapter 'Casting procedures'.

Advantages

1. The thinner foil alloy coping allows a greater thickness of ceramic, thereby, improving the esthetics.
2. The gold color of the alloy improves the esthetics of the restoration.
3. Less reduction of tooth structure.
4. The nonesthetic high intensity high value opaquer layer seen with conventional metal ceramics is eliminated.

BONDED PLATINUM FOIL—CERAMIC CROWNS

A platinum foil coping is adapted on to the die. To improve the bonding of the ceramic to the platinum foil coping, an *electrodeposition technique* is used. A thin layer of tin is

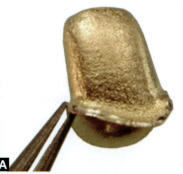
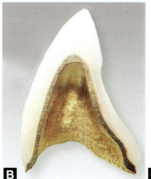
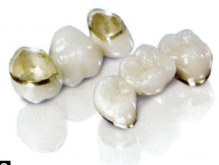

FIGURES 28.17A TO C Sintered gold alloy foil-ceramic restorations. **(A)** A Captek coping. **(B)** Cross-section through a Captek crown. **(C)** A Captek FDP.

electrodeposited on to the foil and then oxidized in a furnace. The advantages of using bonded platinum foil is similar to that for swaged gold alloy foil.

The electrodeposition technique

This is a technique used to improve both esthetics and bonding. A layer of *pure gold* is electrodeposited on to the metal. This is followed by a quick minimal deposition of *tin* over the gold.

Advantages
1. The gold color enhances the vitality of the porcelain, thereby, enhancing esthetics (the normal technique requires a heavy unesthetic opaque layer to cover the dark metal oxide surface).
2. The tin helps in chemical bonding (through formation of tin oxide).
3. Improves wetting at the gold-porcelain interface thereby reducing porosity.
4. The electrodeposition technique can be used on metals, such as stainless steel, cobalt chromium, titanium and other non-gold and low gold alloys.

ALL-CERAMIC RESTORATIONS

The all-ceramic restorations are made *without* a metallic core or sub-structure. This makes them esthetically superior to the metal-ceramic restoration. Unfortunately, all-ceramic restorations had lower strength, thus, metal-ceramics continued to be the restoration of choice for the majority of restorations till the 1990s. Continued research have led to improved all-ceramic systems with greater strength and fracture resistance. Manufacturers today claim the new generation all-ceramic materials are capable of producing not only single crowns but anterior and even posterior all-ceramic FDPs as well. Long span FDPs have also been attempted.

The all-ceramic restorations are grouped according to their type and method of fabrication

1. Condensed sintered
   - Traditional feldspathic porcelain jacket crown
   - Porcelain jacket crown with aluminous core (Hi-Ceram)
   - Ceramic jacket crown with leucite reinforced core (Optec HSP).
2. Cast glass ceramics (Dicor).
3. Injection molded (leucite reinforced) glass ceramic (IPS Empress).
4. Slip cast-glass infiltrated ceramics
   - Glass infiltrated aluminous core restorations (In-Ceram)
   - Glass infiltrated spinell core restorations (In-Ceram Spinell)
   - Glass infiltrated zirconia core (In-Ceram Zirconia).
5. Milled ceramic restoration or cores
   - CAD/CAM restorations
   - Copy milled restorations

(Blocks or blanks of various ceramics are machined to form the restoration. Examples are alumina, zirconia, lithia disilicate, etc. The various types are detailed in a subsequent section - see classification of machinable ceramics).

PORCELAIN JACKET CROWN

These are crowns made entirely of feldspathic porcelain. They are constructed on a platinum foil matrix which is subsequently removed.

TYPES

1. Porcelain jacket crown (traditional).
2. Porcelain jacket crown with aluminous core.
3. Porcelain jacket crown with leucite reinforced core (Optek HSP).

Note   The above two are generally referred to as *'porcelain jacket crowns'* or PJCs. The subsequently introduced ceramics are referred to as *'ceramic jacket crowns'* or *CJCs'* and *'glass ceramic crowns'.*

TRADITIONAL PORCELAIN JACKET CROWN

The all-porcelain crown (PJC) has been around since a century (early 1900s). These early crowns are also referred to as *traditional* or *conventional* PJCs. They were made from conventional high fusing feldspathic porcelains. As mentioned before these were very brittle and fractured easily (half moon fractures). The marginal adaptation was also quite poor. Because of these problems they gradually lost popularity and are no longer used presently.

PORCELAIN JACKET CROWN WITH ALUMINOUS CORE

The problems associated with traditional PJCs led to the development of the PJC with an *alumina reinforced core (McLean and Hughes, 1965) (Fig. 28.18)*. The increased content of alumina crystals (40 to 50%) in the core strengthened the porcelain by interruption of crack propagation. In spite of the increased strength they were still brittle and therefore not indicated for posterior teeth and their use was restricted to anterior teeth. The composition of the alumina reinforced PJC is shown in *Table 28.2*.

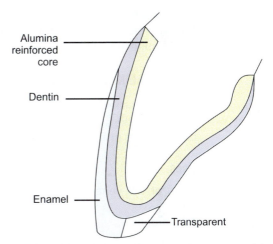

FIGURE 28.18 The porcelain jacket crown with aluminous core.

Technical considerations

The porcelain jacket crowns are made using the platinum foil matrix technique.

Platinum foil matrix

A platinum foil is adapted to the die *(Figs. 28.19A and B)* with a wooden point. The platinum foil functions as matrix. It supports the porcelain during condensation and firing.

TABLE 28.2 A sample percentage composition of aluminous porcelain			
	Aluminous core	*Dentin*	*Enamel*
Silica (SiO$_2$)	35.0	66.5	64.7
Alumina (Al$_2$O$_3$)	53.8	13.5	13.9
Calcium oxide (CaO)	1.12	—	1.78
Soda (Na$_2$O)	2.8	4.2	4.8
Potash (K$_2$O)	4.2	7.1	7.5
Boric oxide (B$_2$O$_3$)	3.2	6.6	7.3
Zirconium oxide (ZrO$_2$)			

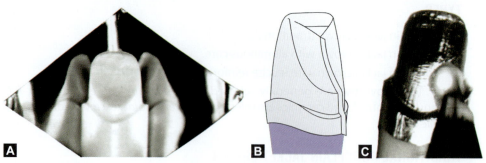

FIGURE 28.19A TO C The porcelain jacket crown with aluminous core.

Condensation and firing

The core porcelain is carefully condensed on to the foil *(Fig. 28.19C)*. The foil with the condensed porcelain is carefully removed from the die. It is then placed in the furnace and fired. After cooling, the rest of the crown is built up with conventional feldspathic porcelain.

Removing the foil

After completion of the restoration the platinum foil is gently teased out and discarded. This can be quite difficult.

LEUCITE REINFORCED PORCELAIN (OPTEC HSP)

Optec HSP is a feldspathic porcelain with a higher leucite crystal content (leucite reinforced). Its manipulation, condensation and firing is quite similar to the alumina reinforced porcelain jacket crowns (using platinum foil matrix).

Uses

Inlays, onlays, veneers and low stress crowns.

Advantages

1. They are more esthetic because, the core is less opaque (more translucent) when compared to the aluminous porcelain.
2. Higher strength.
3. No need of special laboratory equipment.

Disadvantages

1. Fit is not as good as metal ceramic crowns.
2. Potential marginal inaccuracy.
3. Not strong enough for posterior use.

CASTABLE GLASS CERAMIC

The castable glass ceramic is quite unlike the previously mentioned porcelains. Its properties are more closer to that of glass *(Box 28.4)* and its construction is quite different. This is the only porcelain restoration made by a centrifugal casting technique. The subsequent 'ceramming' process is also quite unique to this porcelain. Ceramming enhances the growth of mica crystals within the ceramic.

SUPPLIED AS

The first commercially available castable glass-ceramic for dental use was 'Dicor' developed by Corning glass works and marketed by Dentsply. They are supplied as glass ingots. A precrystallized form called Dicor MGC is also available as machinable blanks for CAD/CAM.

COMPOSITION

Dicor glass-ceramic contains 55 vol% of *tetrasilicic fluormica crystals*.

FEATURES

The Dicor glass-ceramic crown is very esthetic. This is because of its greater translucency (unlike some other porcelains which have more opaque core). It also picks up some of the color from the adjacent teeth (chameleon effect) as well as from the underlying cement. Thus the color of the bonding cement plays an important role.

USES

Inlays, onlays, veneers and low stress crowns.

FABRICATION OF A DICOR CROWN

To understand the salient features of this material, the step-by-step construction of a crown will be described

1. The pattern is first constructed in wax *(Fig. 28.20A)* and then invested in refractory material like a regular cast metal crown.
2. After burning out the wax, nuggets of Dicor glass are melted and cast into the mold in a centrifugal casting machine.
3. The glass casting *(Fig. 28.20B)* is carefully recovered from the investment by sandblasting and the sprues are gently cut away.
4. The glass restoration is then covered with an embedment material to prepare it for the next stage called ceramming.
5. Ceramming is a heat treatment process by which the glass is strengthened. Ceramming results in the development of microscopic crystals of mica, which
   - Improves the strength and toughness of the glass

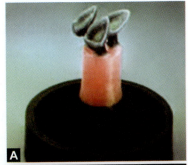
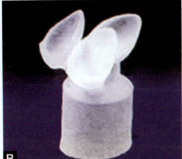

FIGURES 28.20A AND B Castable glass ceramics (Dicor). **(A)** Wax pattern. **(B)** Cast glass.

- Improves the esthetics of the restoration (it reduces the transparency of the glass making it more opaque and less glass-like).
6. The cerammed glass can be built up with special veneering porcelain and fired to complete the restoration. Surface stains may be applied to improve the esthetics.

ADVANTAGES

1. Ease of fabrication.
2. Good esthetics (greater translucency and chameleon effect).
3. Improved strength and fracture toughness.
4. Good marginal fit.
5. Very low processing shrinkage.
6. Low abrasion of opposing teeth.

DISADVANTAGES

1. Inadequate strength for posterior use.
2. Internal characterization not possible. Has to be stained externally to improve esthetics.

HEAT PRESSED (HOT-ISOSTATICALLY PRESSED) CERAMICS

This is another ceramic material which again is quite unlike the previous ceramics because of its unique way of fabrication (injection molding). It is a precerammed glass-ceramic having a high concentration of reinforcing crystals. The material supplied in the form of ingots is softened under high temperatures and forced into a mold created by a lost wax process.

Synonyms Injection moulded or Heat-pressed glass-ceramics.

TYPES AND MODE OF SUPPLY

Heat pressed ceramics are supplied as *ingots (Figs. 28.21 and 28.22)* of various compositions. These include

1. Heat pressed glass ceramics
   - Leucite or $KAlSi_2O_6$ reinforced (IPS Empress, Finesse, Optimal, Cerpress, etc).
   - Lithium disilicate reinforced (IPS empress 2, OPC 3G).
2. Heat pressed veneering ceramics [e.g. IPS ZirPress *(Fig. 28.22)*, Vita PM9] are available for use as a pressed layer over machined zirconia cores.

Compatible veneering ceramics in powder-liquid form may be provided along with the ingots or acquired separately.

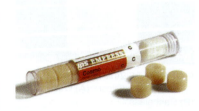

FIGURE 28.21 IPS Empress ingots.

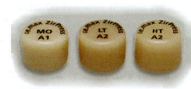

FIGURE 28.22 IPS Zir Press.

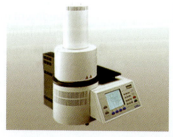

FIGURE 28.23 The pressing furnace.

USES

Inlays, onlays, veneers *(Fig. 28.25D)* and low stress crowns. Small 3 unit FDPs may be constructed with IPS Empress 2.

MICROSTRUCTURE

IPS Empress—contains 35 to 40% vol of leucite crystals *(Table 28.3)*.

IPS Empress 2—consists of 65 to 70% by volume *(Table 28.3)* of interlocked elongated lithia disilicate crystals. The crystal size varies from 0.5 to 4 µm in length.

The crystals within the structure improve the fracture resistance by reducing crack propagation.

FABRICATION

1. The wax *(Fig. 28.25B)* patterns of the restorations are invested in refractory material and heated to 850 °C in a furnace to burn off the wax and create the mold space.

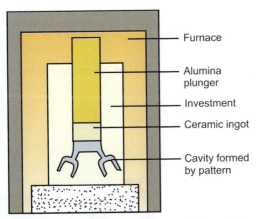

FIGURE 28.24 Schematic representation of the pressing process.

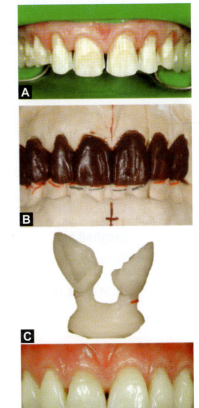

FIGURES 28.25A TO D IPS empress. **(A)** Teeth prepared for veneers. **(B)** Wax patterns. **(C)** Pressed ceramic still attached to the sprue. **(D)** The completed restorations.

TABLE 28.3 Composition of two popular hot-isostatically pressed ceramics

IPS Empress 1		IPS Empress 2	
Silica (SiO$_2$)	63	Silica (SiO$_2$)	57-80
Alumina (Al$_2$O$_3$)	17.7	Alumina (Al$_2$O$_3$)	0-5
Soda (Na$_2$O)	4.6	Potash (K$_2$O)	0-13
Potash (K$_2$O)	11.2	Phosphorous pentoxide (P$_2$O$_5$)	0-11
Boric oxide (B$_2$O$_3$)	0.6	Lithium (Li$_2$O)	11-19
Calcium oxide (CaO$_2$)	1.6	Zinc oxide (ZnO)	0-8
Titanium dioxide (TiO$_2$)	0.2	Magnesium MgO	0-5
Barium oxide (BaO)	0.7	Lanthanum oxide (La$_2$O$_3$)	0.1-6
Cerium oxide (CeO2)	0.4	Pigments	0-8
Pigments			

2. It is then transferred to the pressing furnace *(Fig. 28.23)*. A ceramic ingot and an alumina plunger is inserted in to the sprue *(Fig. 28.24)*.
3. Pressing temperature for IPS Empress—1075 to 1180 °C
4. Pressing temperature for IPS Empress 2—920 °C
5. The pressing is done under air pressure of 1,500 psi.
6. The core or restoration *(Fig. 28.25C)* is retrieved from the flask.
7. Compatible veneering porcelains are added to the core to build up the final restoration *(Fig. 28.25D)*.
8. It can also be directly fabricated as a crown in which case, the crown is stained and glazed directly.

ADVANTAGES

1. Better fit (because of lower firing shrinkage).
2. Better esthetics due to the absence of metal or an opaque core.

DISADVANTAGES

1. Need for costly equipment.
2. Potential of fracture in posterior areas.

GLASS INFILTRATED CERAMICS

These are specialized core ceramics reinforced by an unique *glass infiltration process*. They are also sometimes referred to as *slip-cast ceramics*.

Types

Currently there are three types depending on the core material used.

1. Glass infiltrated alumina core (In-Ceram Alumina).
2. Glass infiltrated spinell core (In-Ceram Spinell).
3. Glass infiltrated zirconia core (In-Ceram Zirconia).

Supplied as

Oxide powder (alumina, spinell or zirconia) with mixing liquids, glass powder and veneering ceramics *(Figs. 28.26 to 28.28)*.

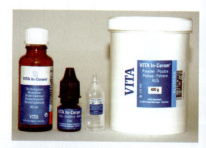

FIGURE 28.26 Alumina powder and other accessories used to make the core.

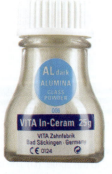

FIGURE 28.27 Glass powder.

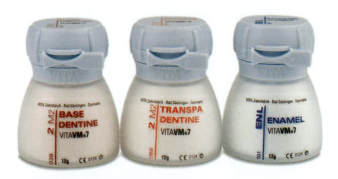

FIGURE 28.28 Vita VM7 is a veneering ceramic designed for In-Ceram.

GLASS INFILTRATED ALUMINA CORE (IN-CERAM ALUMINA)

This ceramic system has a unique *glass infiltration process* and the first of its kind claimed for anterior FDP fabrication. The glass infiltration process compensates for firing shrinkage. The final core after completion of the glass infiltration is made up of about 70% alumina and 30% (sodium lanthanum) glass.

Indications

1. Anterior and posterior crowns, and
2. Short span anterior fixed dental prostheses.

Composition

Alumina powder	
Al_2O_3	99.7
MgO	0.03

Infiltration glass powder	
La_2O_3	49.6
SiO_2	19.1
TiO_2	6.16
CaO	3.14
Others	2.0

Fabrication *(Figs. 28.29A to I)*

1. Two dies are required. One in stone and the other in *refractory die* material.
2. Preparing the slip—Measured quantity (38 g) of alumina powder is added slowly into a beaker containing 1 ampoule of mixing liquid and a drop of additive liquid. Mixing is done with the help of a special ultrasonic unit (Vitasonic). The water in the Vitasonic should be chilled using ice cubes. The prepared slip should be smooth and homogenous. The slip is applied on to the refractory die using the *slip cast* method (the water from the slurry is absorbed by the porous die leaving a dense layer of alumina on the surface). Once started the slip should not be allowed to dry out before the coping is completed. The process is continued until an alumina coping of sufficient thickness is obtained.
3. The fragile slip cast alumina coping is dried at 120 °C for 2 hours.
4. The coping is sintered (Inceramat furnace) for 10 hours at 1120 °C.
5. After sintering the copings are tested for cracks using a special dye.
6. The next step is *glass infiltration*. Glass powder is mixed with distilled water. One or two thick coats (1-2 mm) is applied on to the sintered alumina coping (outer surface only) and fired for 2-3 hours at 1110 °C on a platinum foil. The glass melts and infiltrates into the porous alumina coping through capillary action.
7. The excess glass forms a glassy layer on the surface which is trimmed off using special diamond burs, followed by sandblasting. A glass control firing (1000 °C) is carried out.
8. The coping is then built up using special veneering ceramics (Vita VM 7).

Advantages

1. Good fit and marginal adaptation.
2. Good strength when compared to the earlier all ceramic crowns. Claimed to be strong enough for posterior single crowns and anterior FDP use.

Disadvantages

1. Comparatively less esthetic because of the opacity of the alumina core.
2. Quite tedious to fabricate.
3. Not all the FDPs were successful, a few of them did fracture occasionally.

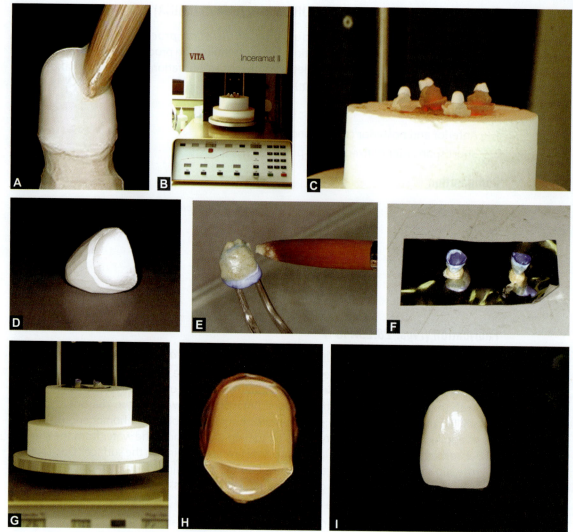

FIGURES 28.29A TO I Fabrication of an In-Ceram restoration. **(A)** Slip casting. **(B)** In-ceram furnace. **(C)** Sintering of the slip. **(D)** Sintered coping. **(E)** Glass slurry applicaion. **(F)** Embedded in investment. **(G)** Glass infiltration furnace. **(H)** Glass infiltrated coping. **(I)** The completed restoration.

Uses

1. In addition to inlays, onlays, veneers and low stress (anterior and posterior) crowns, this material can be used to construct low stress anterior FDPs. Because of its occasional tendency to fracture when used for FDP construction its use should be carefully selected.

2. For people allergic to metal based restorations.

3. Where esthetics is absolutely critical.

GLASS INFILTRATED SPINELL CORE (IN-CERAM SPINELL)

In-Ceram Spinell is an offshoot of In-Ceram Alumina. Because of the comparatively high opacity of the alumina core, a new material was introduced known as In-Ceram spinell. It uses spinel ($MgAl_2O_4$) instead of alumina. The fabrication process is quite similar to that for In-Ceram Alumina.

The In-Ceram Spinell is more translucent and therefore more esthetic compared to the In-Ceram Alumina core. Since the strength is lower, its use is limited to low stress situations.

Indications

Its high translucency makes it a material of choice for crowns and restorations in *esthetic* (anterior crowns) and stress free zones.

Contraindications

The high translucency contraindicates it in situations where the underlying tooth structure is severely discolored and needs to be masked. Its low strength also contraindicates it for posterior situations and FDPs.

GLASS INFILTRATED ZIRCONIA (IN-CERAM ZIRCONIA)

Zirconia (ZrO_2) is a naturally occurring mineral. Crystals of Zirconia are used as a substitute for diamond. In-Ceram Zirconia is the strongest of the three glass infiltrated core materials. The final glass infiltrated ICZ cores contains around 30 wt% zirconia and 70 wt% alumina.

Indications

Its high strength makes it a material of choice for posterior crowns and short span fixed partial dentures in high stress areas (posterior FDPs).

It is *not particularly suited for esthetic zones* because of its greater opacity.

However, in cases where there is severe discoloration, In-Ceram Zirconia helps mask the discolored tooth structure because of its greater opacity.

CAD/CAM CERAMICS

Constructing a dental ceramic restoration is technique sensitive, labor intensive and time consuming. Machined ceramics were introduced to overcome some of these problems. They are also known as milled or machined ceramics.

Machinable ceramic systems can be divided into two categories

1. CAD/CAM systems
2. Copy milled systems

CAD/CAM SYSTEMS

These are systems that can design and produce restorations out of *blocks* or *blanks of ceramics* with the aid of a computer. CAD/CAM is acronym for *computer aided design-computer aided manufacturing.*

HISTORY OF CAD/CAM

The major development in the field of dental CAD/CAM took place in the 1980s. They were influenced by three important pioneers. The first was Duret who fabricated crowns through a series of processes starting with an optical impression of the prepared tooth. The milling was done by a numerically controlled milling machine (the precursor of modern CAM/CAM). The second pioneer was Mörmann, developer of the CEREC system at the University of Zurich. A compact chair-side machine milled the crown from measurements of the preparation taken by an intraoral camera. At the time, the system was innovative as it allowed 'same-day restorations'. With the announcement of this system, the term CAD/CAM spread rapidly to the dental profession. The third was Andersson, the developer of the Procera system in the 1980s.

The Japanese also developed many systems in the 1980s but these were not commercially successful because of the resistance from health insurance companies. The early systems had to overcome many problems including limited computing power, poor marginal accuracy, etc. Current CAD/CAM systems have come a long way. With improvements in technology, material and software, restoration fabrication is considerably more accurate and operator friendly as well. CAD/CAM systems are now part of everyday dentistry.

Commercially available CAD/CAM systems

Many systems are currently available using a variety of techniques and materials *(Fig. 28.30)*. Some examples of commercially available CAD/CAM systems are - Cerec (Sirona), Sirona InLab, Everest (Kavo), Cercon (Dentsply), Lava (3M ESPE), Zeno (Weiland), 5-tec (Zirkonzahn), etc.

ESSENTIALS OF A CAD/CAM SYSTEM

The CAD/CAM system consists of 5 essentials

1. Scanner or digitizer   –   Virtual impression
2. Computer   –   Virtual design (CAD)
3. Milling station   –   Produces the restoration or framework
4. Ceramic blanks   –   Raw material for the restoration
5. Furnace   –   For postsintering, ceramming etc.

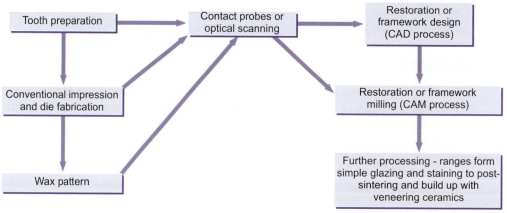

FIGURE 28.30 Schematic representation of CAD/CAM production.

BOX 28.5 Combining various porcelains and processing techniques

- In some systems the entire restoration can be made entirely from the same material. Example - An inlay or laminate may be constructed entirely with pressable ceramics or from a machined feldspathic block.
- In many systems at least 2 or more processing techniques and materials have to be combined to produce the final restoration for a variety of reasons like esthetics, ease of fabrication, need for correction, etc.

Most reinforced core ceramics are too opaque to be used to construct the entire restoration with it. These cores have to be built up with veneering ceramics, characterized with stains and then glazed to produce the final restoration. Example 1—Glass infiltrated cores are too opaque and have to be layered with condensing type veneering porcelains to produce the final restoration. Example 2—Machined alumina cores are frequently built up with condensable ceramics. Example 3—In one system machined zirconia blocks are overlayed with a pressable veneering material (Zir Cad and Zir Pres).

An important point to remember is that various ceramics should be compatible with each other when used together. Non- compatible products may have difference in CTE which can cause failure of the restoration. The manufacturers usually specify the veneering materials compatible with their products.

Scanner or digitizer

The dimensions of the prepared tooth (or die or wax pattern) are picked up and digitized in order to create a 3 dimensional image of the prepared tooth in the computer. This is achieved by scanning of the preparation or the die.

The 2 types of digitizers currently employed are

1. *Contact probes* Physically contacts the die as it moves along its surface while transmitting the information to the computer. E.g. Procera Forte contact scanner.
2. *Scanners* Unlike contact probes, scanners are optical devices. These include
    –   *Intraoral hand-held wands (Fig. 28.31A)* These are chairside scanners. The intraoral scanner reflects light (visible light, laser or LED) and captures it with a camera to create an optical impression of the prepared tooth and adjacent structures. Multiple images have to be captured to stitch together a composite 3D image in the computer. In some systems a special powder is dusted to reduce reflection and improve readability.
    –   *Laboratory scanners* These are larger devices that scan the cast or die using different technologies. Some use a camera to capture multiple images similar to the intraoral scanner (white light optical scanner). Others use 2 cameras to capture the object from multiple angles using white light (e.g. Kavo Everest - *Figs. 28.31B and 28.32*) or laser planes projected in a grid pattern. The Procera optical scanner uses a laser beam to measure distances (conoscopic holography).

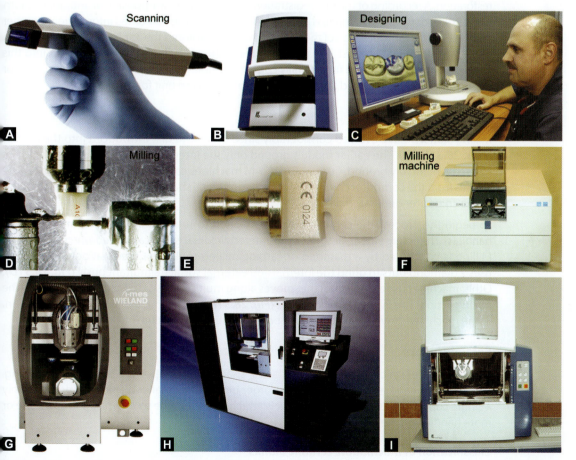

FIGURES 28.31 A TO I CAD/CAM systems **(A)** Tooth preparation may be scanned directly in the mouth with a hand held scanner. **(B)** The preparation may also be scanned from a cast (Kavo scanner). **(C)** A computer aids in designing the final restoration or coping. **(D)** The design is transferred to the milling station and a restoration is milled. **(E)** A milled laminate. **(F)** cerec 3 (Sirona) inlab. **(G)** Zeno 2100 (Weiland). **(H)** Lava (3 M Espe). **(I)** Everest (Kavo) milling station.

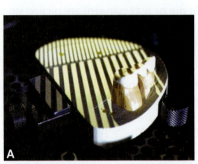
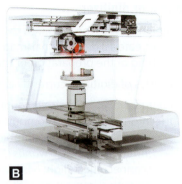

FIGURE 28.32A AND B **(A)** Light beam scanner (Kavo Everest). **(B)** Laser conoscopic holography (new Procera optical scanner).

Computer (CAD process)

The restoration or the core is designed in the computer *(Fig. 28.31C)*. Most manufacturers have their own software for the CAD process. The CAD process aids in designing either the restoration, coping or the FDP substructure. The computer can automatically detect the finish line. Some use a library of tooth shapes that is stored on the computer to suggest the shape of the proposed restoration. A recording of the bite registration (the imprint of the opposing or antagonist tooth in a wax-like or rubbery material) is also added to the data. The combined information together with the 3D optical impression of the prepared tooth establishes the approximate zone in which the new restoration can exist. The proposed restoration can then be morphed to fit into this zone in an anatomically and functionally correct position. The dentist can make corrections or modify the design if required and then send it to the milling unit for completion.

Milling station

Milling stations have evolved considerably since they were first introduced into the market *(Figs. 28.31E to I)*. The earlier models ground only the internal surface. The external surface had to be manually ground. Current CAD/CAM machines can grind the external surface also. Signals from the computer control the milling tool which shapes the ceramic block according to the computer generated design.

To begin the process the ceramic block is attached to the machine via a frame or built-in handle(s). The enlargement factor (see presintered zirconia) is also calculated where applicable. Milling is performed by a diamond or carbide milling tool. The Cerec station *(Fig. 28.31F)* uses 2 diamond burs to grind the internal and external surface simultaneously *(Fig. 28.31D)*. Other machines use a single tool that moves along multiple axis (3 to 5 axis) and performs the milling action. The Everest (Kavo) Engine *(Fig. 28.31I)* is an example of a 5 axis milling action. Some machines (Kavo Everest) can mill both ceramic and titanium.

Ceramic blanks

A variety of ceramic blanks in various sizes, shades and shapes are available for milling. Multiple units can be produced from the larger blocks. The smaller blanks may produce only a single coping or restoration. The blank is attached via a frame to the machine or by one or more handles on the blank itself.

Classification of machinable ceramic blanks
1. Feldspathic porcelain blanks [Vitablocs Mark II (Vita)].
2. Glass ceramic blanks
    —   Tetrasilicic fluormica based glass ceramic [Dicor MGC (Dentsply)]

- Leucite based [ProCad (Ivoclar), Everest G (Kavo)]
- Lithia disilicate glass ceramic [IPS e max CAD (Kavo)].
3. Glass infiltrated blanks
    - Alumina (Vita In-Ceram Alumina)
    - Spinell (Vita In-Ceram Spinell)
    - Zirconia (Vita In-Ceram Zirconia).
4. Presintered blanks
    - Alumina (Vita In-Ceram AL)
    - Ytrria stabilized Zirconia (Vita In-Ceram YZ).
5. Sintered blanks
    - Ytrria stabilized Zirconia (Everest ZH blanks).

Brief description of various materials for CAD/CAM

The fabrication process is system and material specific. The prepared tooth or teeth is scanned directly from the mouth or from a model made from a regular impression. Next the restoration or substructure is designed on the computer. The blank is attached to the milling station and the bar code scanned. The time taken for milling depends on the size and complexity of the restoration as well as the material used. For example, presintered zirconia is easier to mill than sintered zirconia. It also reduces wear of the milling tools.

After milling, the structure is separated from the blank using water cooled cutting and grinding disc or burs. Subsequent processing procedures are then initiated depending on the material and system used.

Feldspathic blanks (Fig. 28.33)   Feldspathic restorations can be milled to full contour. The restoration is glazed after milling. Optional processing includes veneering and staining. *Uses - inlays, laminates and anterior crowns.*

Leucite reinforced (Fig. 28.34)   These blanks can be milled to full contour. The restoration is glazed after milling. Optional processing includes veneering and staining. *Uses - inlays, onlays, laminates and anterior crowns.*

Lithium disilicate (Fig. 28.34)   The ceramic is machined in an intermediate crystalline state in which the material shows its characteristic bluish shade ***(Fig. 28.35A).*** In this stage the material is easier to shape and can be tried in the mouth. This is followed by a simple, quick crystallization process (30 minutes) in a conventional ceramic oven in which it reaches its final strength and the desired esthetic properties such as tooth color, translucence and brightness ***(Fig. 28.35B).*** Optional processing includes veneering and staining. *Uses - inlays, onlays, and anterior and posterior crowns.*

Glass infiltrated ceramics (Fig. 28.36)   These are usually machined as cores or FDP substructures. Subsequent processing includes glass infiltration, veneering, and glazing.

Uses   In-Ceram Spinell is recommended for anterior single crowns copings. In-Ceram Alumina is indicated for anterior and posterior crowns and 3 unit anterior FDP substructures. In-Ceram Zirconia can be used for anterior and posterior crowns and 3 unit FDP substructures.

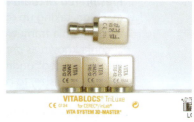

FIGURE 28.33 Feldspathic porcelain.

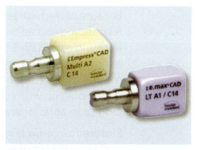

FIGURE 28.34 Glass ceramic blanks—leucite based (above) and lithia disilicate (bottom).

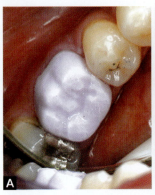
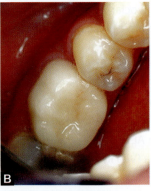

FIGURES 28.35A AND B (A) Milled lithia disilicate crown in the presintered state can be tried in the mouth. This is possible because there is no shrinkage during the subsequent ceramming process. Note the color change after heat treatment **(B)**. (*Courtesy:* Dr. Hanan Abuasi, MOH, Kuwait).

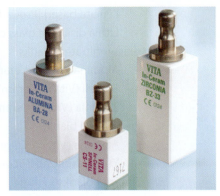

FIGURE 28.36 CAD/CAM blanks for glass infiltration method.

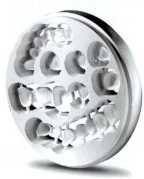

FIGURE 28.37 Presintered zirconia blank for multiple units.

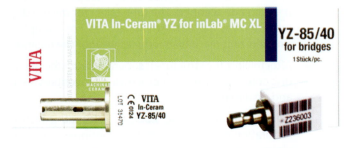

FIGURE 28.38 Presintered Zirconia. Blank with bar code is shown on the inset.

Presintered zirconia (Figs. 28.37 and 28.38) Fully dense zirconia is extremely difficult to machine, taking up to two hours just to fabricate a single unit. Therefore, most restorations with zirconia frameworks are fabricated by machining a porous or partially fired block of zirconia known as *presintered zirconia*. These are usually used as cores for crown or FDPs. In the presintered condition they are usually softer and easier to mill. They are milled to a slightly (20%) larger size, to compensate for the subsequent sintering shrinkage. Following milling they have to be sintered (called post sintering). Sintering is done in a furnace. Sintering time and temperature varies between brands.

○ Sintering time – 6 to 7.5 hours
○ Sintering temperature – 1350 to 1530 °C

Because of the high temperatures involved special furnaces are required for zirconia sintering. All grinding and adjustments should be completed prior to sintering. Adjustments following sintering especially in the connector areas weaken the structure. Any adjustments required after postsintering should be done with water cooled, vibration free, fine diamonds. The restoration may be immersed in special coloring liquid to improve the esthetics. The restoration is then built up with compatible veneering ceramics. *Uses*—core construction for crowns and long span anterior and posterior FDPs.

Sintered zirconia (Figs. 28.39 and 28.40) Since these materials are already fully sintered, *post sintering* is not required. This material is milled in 1:1 ratio as no shrinkage is expected. Because of its extreme hardness milling takes more time and causes more wear of the milling tool. Subsequent processing includes build up with compatible veneering ceramics. *Uses*—

core construction for crowns and long span anterior and posterior FDPs. (Zirconia is described in greater detail in a subsequent section).

Sintering furnaces

Furnaces are an important part of CAD/CAM dentistry. A variety of furnaces are available depending on the type of blank used. For example In-Ceram alumina blanks have to be glass infiltrated in a furnace following machining. Leucite or lithia disilicate blanks have to be cerammed to induce partial crystallization. The furnace for the sintering of zirconia is highly specialized as it involves very high temperatures. Zirconia sintering can involve temperatures greater than 1500 °C.

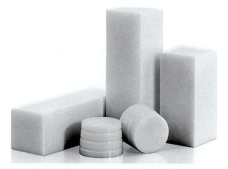

FIGURE 28.39 Sintered zirconia blanks (KAVO).

COPY MILLED (CAM) SYSTEMS

Some systems use a copy milling technique to produce ceramic cores or substructures for FDPs. In copy milling a *wax pattern* of the restoration is scanned and a replica is milled out of the ceramic blank (see **Table 28.4** for comparison of CAD/CAM and copy milling).

Commercial systems available

Examples of commercially available copy-milling systems are
1. Celay **(Figs. 28.41A to C)** (*Mikrona* AG, Spreitenbach, Switzerland).
2. Cercon (Degudent, Dentsply). Cercon has both CAD/CAM and copy-milling systems.
3. Ceramill system **(Fig. 28.42)**.

Fabrication of a copy-milled restoration substructure

The Cercon system will be described **(Figs. 28.43A to I)**.

❍ A stone die is prepared from the impression of the preparation.

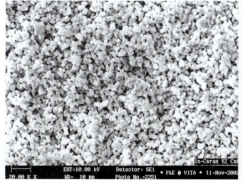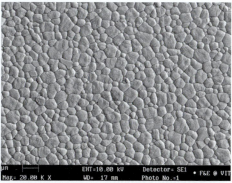

FIGURE 28.40 SEM showing microstructure of unsintered (presintered (left) and sintered (right) In-ceram Zirconia. Sintering fuses the particles to form dense ceramic.

TABLE 28.4 Comparison of CAD/CAM and copy-milling	
CAD/CAM	*Copy-milling*
Scans preparation	Scans pattern
Restoration designed virtually	Restoration designed manually
Object milled from virtual pattern	Restoration mills replica of pattern

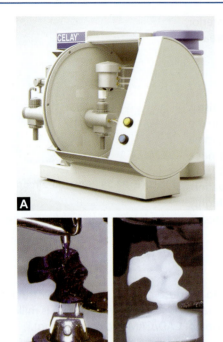

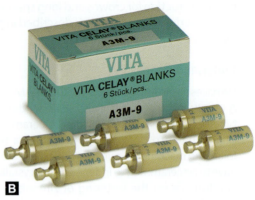

FIGURES 28.41A TO C (A) Celay copy milling system. **(B)** Celay blanks. **(C)** Close-up of copying and milling process showing the wax pattern and the milled inlay.

○ A pattern of the restoration is created using wax.

○ The pattern is fixed on the left side of the milling machine (Cercon Brain).

○ A presintered zirconia blank is attached to the right side (milling section) of the machine. The machine reads the bar code on the blank which contains the enlargement information.

○ On activation the pattern on the left side is scanned (noncontact optical scanning) while the milling tool on the right side mills out the enlarged replica (30% larger) of the pattern from the attached ceramic blank.

○ The milled structure is removed from the machine and sectioned off from the frame. Any remaining attachment stubs are trimmed and final adjustments are made.

○ The zirconia structure is then placed in a sintering furnace (Cercon Heat) and fired for 6 hours at 1350 °C to complete the sintering process.

○ The restoration is completed using compatible veneering porcelains.

Ceramill system

Unlike the earlier system, the Ceramill system *(Fig. 28.42)* is based on the pantograph type of copy milling which, according to the company, "puts the material back in the hands of the technician". To create a zirconia coping, the user applies a light-cured resin over a traditional die, attaches the resin pattern into a plastic plate and inserts it into the milling unit, side by side with a YtZP zirconia blank. The unit has two conjoined arms that hold the

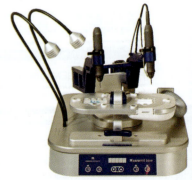

FIGURE 28.42 Ceramill.

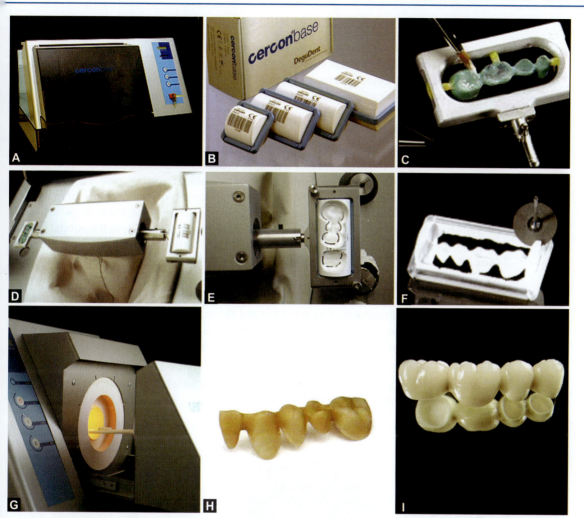

FIGURES 28.43A TO I Fabrication of a zirconia restoration with the Cercon system. **(A)** Cercon brain (milling unit). **(B)** Zirconia blanks. **(C)** Wax pattern. **(D)** Blank in position. **(E)** Milling. **(F)** Separating. **(G)** Sintering (cercon heat). **(H)** A completed substructure. **(I)** A completed prosthesis.

probe tip and the milling handpiece. The user manually traces the resin buildup with the probe tip while the other arm simultaneously mills a duplicate coping out of the zirconia block.

Networked CAD/CAM production (Procera AllCeram)

The Procera system by Nobel Biocare is a unique system where restorations are produced using information sent via internet. In this system impression is sent to a local Nobel licenced laboratory. Here the impression is poured and the conventional die is scanned by a contact scanner [Procera Forte - *(Fig. 28.44)*]. The coping is designed (CAD) and together with the dimensions of the scanned die, the information is passed via internet to a fully automated industrial scale remote production facility which may be in another country. Here an *enlarged die* is milled via CAM process. The core is produced by dry pressing on to the die and is followed by sintering. The sintered copings are individually checked for quality control and shipped to the laboratory of origin where the subsequent veneering is completed. Thus in this system the laboratory needs to invest only in the scanner and the CAD software.

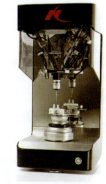

FIGURE 28.44 Procera contact scanner. Inset - contact probe.

YTTRIA STABILIZED ZIRCONIA CERAMICS

Zirconium is one of the most abundant elements in the earth's crust. *Zirconia* is the oxide of zirconium metal (ZrO_2). Zirconium oxide is a white crystalline oxide ceramic with unique properties. Its most naturally occurring form is the rare mineral, baddeleyite. A form of cubic zirconia is popularly used as a diamond simulant *(Figs. 28.45A to C)*.

Transformation toughening

It has the highest strength among the dental ceramics because of its high degree of crack resistance. This is possible because of a unique property of zirconia to undergo a process known as *transformation toughening (Fig. 28.46)*. The stable form of zirconia is the *monoclinic* form. When zirconia is heated, it changes to its *tetragonal* high-temperature phase which again reverts back to the monoclinic form on cooling. However, addition of *yttrium oxide* (3–5%) also known as *yttria* maintains the zirconia in its high temperature tetragonal form at room temperature. Thus, this form of zirconia is known as 'yttria-stabilized zirconia polycrystal' *(Box 28.6)*.

When a stress is applied to the zirconia as in the beginning of a crack formation, it reverts back to its monoclinic form locally with an accompanying increase in volume. The local increase in volume introduces compressive stresses around the crack and slows its growth. This is also known as 'tension expansion' - a phenomenon otherwise known only in the case of steel. For this reason zirconium oxide is also known as 'ceramic steel'.

The introduction of zirconia as a core material revolutionized dental ceramics. Its unique transformation toughening process, made it possible to construct relatively long span fixed partial dentures in both anterior and posterior locations.

Cubic zirconia   Baddeleyite   Zirconia powder

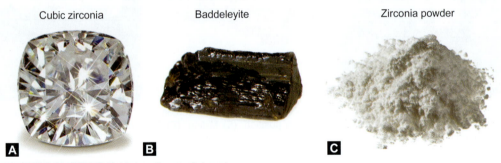

FIGURES 28.45A TO C Various forms of zirconia.

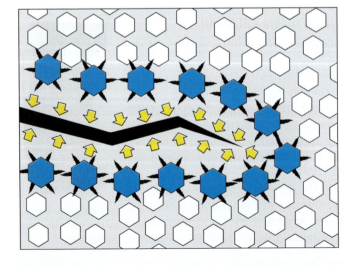

FIGURE 28.46 Representation of transformation toughening. The illustration shows the compressive forces around the crack caused by transformation and expansion of the zirconia crystals around the crack (adapted from Vita).

BOX 28.6	Yttria stabilized zirconia

The addition of minor components to the zirconia, such as yttrium, can produce a crystal that is both strong and resistant to crack generation because of the unique "transformation toughening" that occurs when zirconia goes from a tetragonal phase to a monolithic phase. It is this monolithic phase of zirconia that is resistant to breakage when used in full-coverage restorations.

Composition

Composition	Wt%
Zirconium dioxide (ZrO_2)	90-92
Yttrium oxide (Y_2O_2)	3-5
Hafnium oxide (HfO_2)	< 3
Aluminum oxide (Al_2O_3)	<0.25
Silicon dioxide (SiO_2)	< 1

Available as

Blanks of different sizes and shapes. Both sintered and presintered forms are available. Presintered form is a partially sintered form and is easier to mill. Following milling the dental laboratories complete the sintering to achieve full density. Blanks may be of a single color in which case manufacturers provide special coloring liquids for dipping or painting. Some manufacturers provide blanks in different shades (preshaded blanks).

Manufacture

Ingredients which are in powder form are compacted (isostatic or axial) to form blanks of different sizes and shapes.

Properties of zirconia

Dental zirconia is a extremely hard, dense, strong and highly opaque material. Its properties are summarized in **Table 28.5**.

Density	9 g/cm³
Melting point	2715 °C
Refractive index	2.13
Soluble in	Hydrofluoric acid and hot sulfuric acid.
Flexure strength	900 to1200 MPa
MOE	210 GPA
CTE	$10.5 \times 10^{-6}/$ °C
Esthetics	Compared to PFM restorations zirconia based restorations are more esthetic because of the elimination of metal display. However, when compared to other more translucent porcelains like lithium disilicate, zirconia appears less translucent and more opaque. Higher translucency will let more light into the restoration, and if used in conjunction with a clear cement, a more life-like appearance can often be achieved. The lower translucency is because of its higher crystalline content. When of equal thicknesses, the most translucent zirconia is only 73% as translucent as conventional lithium disilicate.

Chipping of veneering ceramic

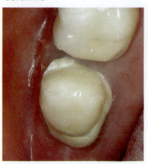

FIGURE 28.47 Chipped veneering ceramic over a zirconia crown.

Zirconia is a very strong material that can support an FDP. Nevertheless, chipping of the veneering ceramics has been reported, especially in the molar region *(Fig. 28.47)*. In several published studies, the veneer chipping rate was approximately 15% after 3 to 5 years. The chipping varied between different manufacturers of veneering ceramics. Laboratory studies have shown that low-fusing porcelains may be less resistant to cracking than high-fusing porcelains and the porcelain density is lower. Zirconia is a good thermal insulator that prevents heat transfer to the veneer porcelain, stopping it from becoming fully dense whether fast-fired or fired at a low temperature. Also, fast cooling may create stress in the porcelain, which could lead to cracking. Any surface adjustment, such as grinding, sandblasting, and even polishing, can change the phase on the surface of the zirconia and may affect the stability and strength of the zirconia as well as the veneer porcelain.

Fracture of zirconia restorations

Occasionally, total fracture of the zirconia core itself have been observed especially in the region of the second molars and over implants in the posterior region. Excessive or coarse grinding can cause cracks, which penetrate into the zirconia substructure, causing transformation that may initially hold these cracks closed. However, over time with exposure to the oral environment and reversal of the transformation stress, the cracks can begin to propagate. Furthermore, many of the "high-translucency zirconias" have low amounts of alumina, which is an important stabilizer. Lower amounts of alumina may cause excessive transformation, cracking, and tooth abrasion; however, clinical trials are expected to provide a more definitive answer.

Wear of opposing teeth

Studies using natural teeth have shown that zirconia causes excessive wear of the natural tooth structure. Glazing alone is not sufficient as the glaze wears off exposing the rough surface underneath. Ongoing studies appear to show that polished zirconia is "wear-kind". Therefore polishing, in addition to glazing is recommended currently to reduce wear of natural teeth.

CERIA STABILIZED ZIRCONIA ALUMINA CERAMICS

Ceria-stabilized zirconia-alumina nanocomposite (ZrO_2/Al_2O_3) (Ce-TZP/A) have recently become available and is even claimed to be superior to Y-TZP in clinical use. Cerium oxide (CeO_2), also known as ceric oxide, ceria, or cerium dioxide, is an oxide of the rare earth metal cerium. Its mode of action is similar to that of yttria.

ADVANTAGES AND DISADVANTAGES OF CAD/CAM CERAMIC RESTORATIONS

Advantages

1. Less waiting period. In some cases same day restorations are possible.
2. Stronger porcelain. Milled ceramic is stronger.

3. In some systems, the scanning is done directly in the mouth so there is no need to make impression.
4. Reduced porosity, therefore greater strength.
5. One visit (only in systems that mill full contour restorations with minimal subsequent processing. CAD/CAM restorations which employ core ceramics, subsequent processing like sintering or glass infiltration, ceramming, layering, etc., require more time).
6. Lab equipment can be minimized as equipment involved with metal casting and processing are not required.
7. Ability to copy the original form of the tooth can produce restorations that are duplicates of the original tooth.

Disadvantages

1. Costly equipment.
2. Scanning the preparation is technique sensitive.
3. Still not as strong as PFM restorations.
4. Problem of chipping of veneering ceramic in case of zirconium core ceramics.

GENERAL PROPERTIES OF FUSED CERAMICS

The properties of porcelain vary widely depending on type and composition.

STRENGTH

The early porcelains were weak and brittle and tended to break easily (fracture or chipping). Current porcelain systems have considerably improved in strength and toughness (**Box 28.7**). However, care still has to be taken during manufacture and fabrication of these materials to ensure that flaws that can lead to fracture are not incorporated. The strength of porcelain is usually measured in terms of flexure strength (or modulus of rupture).

Flexure strength It is a combination of compressive, tensile, as well as shear strength. The strength of various types of porcelains are given in **Table 28.5**. Flexure strength of dental ceramic restorations vary from 70 MPa for feldspathic veneering porcelains to 1200 MPa for machined zirconia core restorations.

Tensile strength Porcelains are inherently brittle materials. Tensile strength is low because of the unavoidable surface defects like porosities and microscopic cracks. When porcelain is placed under tension, stress concentrates around these imperfections and can result in brittle fractures.

TABLE 28.5 Properties of different ceramics used in dentistry

Ceramic type	Flexure strength MPa	MOE GPa	CTE × 10⁻⁶/°C	Hardness VHN	Fracture toughness MPa.m$^{1/2}$
PFM (VMK 68)	70	69	6.4–7.8		0.7
Dicor	90–124				1.2
IPS Empress	120–170	65	15–17	370	1.3
IPS Empress 2	350	95	9.7–10.6	400	3.3
In-ceram Alumina	500				4.4–4.8
In-ceram Spinell	350				2.7
In-ceram Zirconia	700				6.8
Stabilized Zirconia	900–1200	210	10.5		9

Porcelains are by nature brittle. Minute scratches, cracks, defects, porosity, etc., on the surface of the porcelain act as stress concentration points. When excessive tensile force or a sharp impact force is applied on the ceramic, the crack propagates through the crack tip until it penetrates through the entire thickness of the ceramic. This is the reason why surface glazing or polishing is important to eliminate as many of the surface defects as possible. The methods to improve the fracture resistance of ceramic materials are described.

Residual Compressive Stresses through CTE Mismatch

The method is to have layers of ceramic with slight differences in the coefficient of thermal expansion (CTE). The inner layer should have a slightly higher CTE than the outer layer. Thus on cooling to room temperature after firing the inner layer shrinks faster than the outer layer thereby pulling the outer layer inwards and creating compressive stresses within the outer layer. The principle is applied in both metal-ceramic restorations and all ceramic restorations where restorations are built up through layering. The inner metal coping usually has a higher CTE than the veneering ceramic. The innermost layers of ceramic like the opaquer will have a higher CTE than the enamel and dentin layers. Similarly in multilayered all ceramic restorations the inner core will have a higher CTE than the outer veneering ceramic. (However, one must remember that CTE differences should be precisely calculated. Extreme differences in CTE can actually lead to failure of the ceramic).

Residual Compressive Stresses through Thermal Tempering

The method is used in the automobile industry to strengthen glass. Residual compressive stresses may be created by rapidly cooling the surface of the object while it is in the hot or molten state. The outer portions cools and forms a rigid skin while the inner portion is still hot. As the inner portion cools it shrinks and creates compressive stresses within the outer portion.

Residual Compressive Stresses through Ion Exchange

The ion exchange process involves 2 ions with difference in size. When a ceramic object is placed in a bath of molten potassium salt, some of the sodium ions present in the surface glass is replaced by the potassium ions. The potassium ion is about 35% larger than the sodium ion. When the larger ion squeezes into the place formerly occupied by the smaller sodium ion large compressive stresses are created. The resulting compression leads to greater toughening of the glass than is possible by thermal strengthening. Glass thus treated is used in particular in the aircraft industry and other sectors where safety is all-important. The ion-exchange process is also sometimes referred to as chemical tempering. One commercially available product GC Tuf-Coat (GC) is used for chemical toughening. This potassium rich slurry is applied on the restoration and heated at 450 °C for 30 minutes in a furnace. However, the fracture resistance is confined to the surface of the glass to a thickness of just 100 µm.

Dispersion Strengthening

Many of the modern glass based ceramics use dispersion strengthening. The process involves the dispersion of a crystalline material within the ceramic which interrupts the formation of a crack. The crack cannot pass as easily through the crystal particle as easily as it does through the glass matrix. Dispersion strengthening is dependent on the type, size, CTE and total content of the crystal within the ceramic. Examples of crystals used for dispersion strengthening are leucite, lithia disilicate, tetrasilic fluormica, alumina, spinell, zirconia, etc.

Transformation Toughening

The transformation toughening phenomenon is primarily associated with yttria-stabilized zirconia core ceramics. The process involves stress-induced transformation of the material at the tip of the crack with accompanying volume expansion. This places the area at the tip of the crack under compression and thereby halts the progress of the crack. For further explanation see section on yttria stabilized zirconia.

Minimizing Stresses through Optimal Design

Even the strongest ceramics can fail if the restoration is not designed properly. This includes sufficient thickness (at least 2 mm) for the ceramic, avoiding sharp internal line angles and point angles, avoiding marked changes in thickness, etc. Sharp angles or points on the internal surface of the restoration can act as stress raisers. Excessive thickness of porcelain in metal-ceramic restoration may lead to fracture because of insufficient support by the metal substructure. In the case of all-ceramic FDPs, the connector should have sufficient height and width. It should be concave and should avoid sharp angles.

Strengthening by Bonding to a Stronger Substrate

The strength of porcelain can be improved considerably when it is bonded to a stronger substructure. For example in metal-ceramic restorations the inner metal coping provides a stiff and stable support which reduces the tensile forces on the overlying ceramic. In all-ceramic restorations, the alloy frame is substituted by high strength reinforced core ceramics like zirconia and alumina. The inner coping also acts as a skin, reducing the formation and propagation of internal cracks. This function is evident is ceramics bonded to platinum or gold foil. The foils obviously do not provide the same kind of high strength support as seen in cast alloy copings but rather provides a protective inner skin that reduces internal defects.

Minimizing Fabrication Defects and Stresses

The ceramic can be made stronger by proper manipulation and fabrication. Proper condensation and vacuum firing reduces porosity in the restoration. Proper cooling reduces the development of internal stresses and strains. Manufacturers instructions should be followed. Proper oxidation firing favors bond formation in metal-ceramics.

Shear strength is low and is due to the lack of ductility caused by the complex structure of porcelain.

Factors affecting strength
1. *Composition*
2. *Surface integrity* Surface imperfections like micro-cracks and porosities reduce the strength. Thus grinding should be followed by glazing or polishing.
3. *Improper condensation*   Poor condensation introduces voids and reduces density of the porcelain.
4. *Firing procedure*   Inadequate firing and overfiring weakens the structure.

MODULUS OF ELASTICITY

Porcelain has high stiffness. The stiffness values range from 69 to 210 GPa for the various ceramic systems ceramics.

SURFACE HARDNESS

Porcelain is much harder (370 to 400 VHN) than natural teeth.

ABRASIVENESS OF CERAMICS

Wear of opposing teeth is a concern when using ceramic restoration.

❍ Unglazed or unpolished porcelain can cause severe wear of natural teeth especially if dentin is exposed. This can happen in cases of occlusal interferences or when excessive masticatory forces are involved as in bruxing. Thus, ceramic restorations are contraindicated in bruxers. Porcelain restorations must always be glazed or polished after grinding.

❍ Wear of enamel occurs by the gouging action caused by asperities (projecting crystals) on the ceramic surface. The abrasiveness of the ceramic depends on the type of asperities present. Alumina and zirconia are more abrasive than plain glass.

❍ Prolonged exposure to carbonated beverages increases the wear rate of enamel. Ultralow fusing ceramics are less abrasive to enamel than conventional ceramics *(Box 28.8)*.

❍ Ceramics having smaller crystal size or finer particles show reduced enamel wear.

THERMAL PROPERTIES

Thermal conductivity   Porcelain has low thermal conductivity which is important to prevent extreme cold or heat transmission to the sensitive dentin and pulpal tissues in cases of restorations in vital teeth.

Coefficient of thermal expansion The CTE is an important property for dental ceramics especially for layered restorations. The CTE of the various layers should be closely matched. Extreme differences can induce a lot of stresses in the ceramic leading to immediate or subsequent failure. The CTE values range depending on the type of ceramic. Some of the veneering ceramics for metal-ceramic have value ranging from 6.4 to $7.8 \times 10^{-6}/°C$, which is close to that of natural teeth. The CTE values for metal-ceramic alloys have to be lowered to improve its compatibility with ceramics.

SPECIFIC GRAVITY

The true specific gravity of porcelain is 2.242. The specific gravity of fired porcelain is usually less (2.2 to 2.3), because of the presence of air voids.

DIMENSIONAL STABILITY

Fired porcelain is dimensionally stable.

CHEMICAL STABILITY

It is insoluble and impermeable to oral fluids. Also it is resistant to most solvents. However, hydrofluoric acid causes etching of the porcelain surface. A source of this is *APF (acidulated phosphate fluoride)* and stannous fluoride, which are used as topical fluorides. A 4 minute exposure of feldspathic porcelain to 1.23% *APF* or 8% stannous fluoride resulted in surface roughness which may lead to subsequent staining. The acid attacks the glassy phase rather than the crystalline phases.

Hydrofluoric acid is used to etch the porcelain. Ceramic etchants are also used for intraoral repair of fractured ceramic.

Porcelain-metal and inter-ceramic bonds

The interphase between the veneer porcelains and the supporting ceramic or metal core is an area of interest. The restoration can fail if the bond is weak. Many test methods have been used to determine bond strengths. One study (Petra et al, 2008) using a shear bond test have shown metal-ceramic systems to have a far higher bond strength than zirconia-based all-ceramic systems (12.5±3.2 for Vita In-Ceram YZ Cubes/Vita VM9, 11.5±3.4 for DC-Zirkon/ IPS e.max Ceram, and 9.4±3.2 for Cercon Base/Cercon Ceram S compared to 27.6±12.1, 26.4±13.4 MPa).

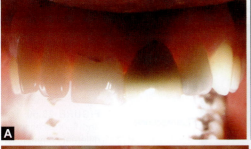
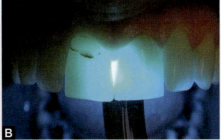
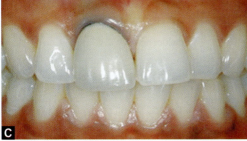

FIGURES 28.48A TO C Demonstrating of difference in translucence. **(A)** Old PFM crown that have been replaced by a more translucent ceramic crown **(B)**. **(C)** Unesthetic dark margins are sometimes associated with PFM crowns.

Esthetic properties

Esthetics is a very complex subject and is an interplay of many factors. Esthetics is dependent on the ability of the material to mimic natural teeth in 5 important fields.

1. Shape   2. Texture   3. Color   4. Translucence   5. Fluorescence

In general, they have excellent esthetic properties especially the all-ceramic restorations. The color stability is also excellent. It can retain its color and gloss for years. Different porcelains together with

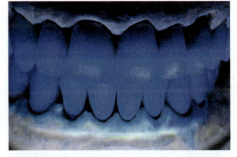

FIGURE 28.49 Fluorescence under certain artificial lighting.

internal and external stains are available to mimic almost any effect seen in natural teeth. Some of the current ceramics are also able to match the fluorescence *(Figs. 28.49 and 28.50)* of natural teeth under certain artificial lighting, e.g. in discotheques.

Translucence
The esthetic qualities of porcelain vary according to the type of ceramic. Metal-ceramic restorations do not have the same level of translucence as some of the all-ceramic restorations *(Figs. 28.48 and 28.50)*.

These concerns include

1. Darkening of the gums around the margins of the restoration *(Fig. 28.48C).*
2. Visibility of the margin as a dark line because of display of metal.
3. Certain esthetic concerns have been raised when the dense opaquer layer is visible through thin crowns (in metal-ceramic and In-Ceram crowns). However, this is more of an error in technique. The dentist must ensure an adequate depth of preparation (at least 1.2 to 1.4 mm) to ensure sufficient thickness of dentin/enamel veneer to mask the opaquer.

Not all metal free ceramic crowns have the same degree of translucence. Some porcelains are highly translucent lithia disilicate crowns whereas others are highly opaque (zirconia).

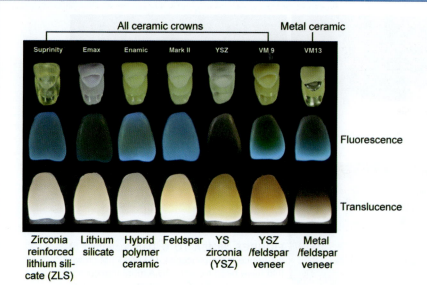

FIGURE 28.50 Translucence and fluorescence properties of different commercially available ceramics.

Role of the underlying cement

The underlying cement plays an important role in case of translucent crowns. Resin cement of various shades and translucency are the cements of choice for bonding the more translucent ceramic restorations.

Biocompatibility

Glazed porcelain is one of the most biocompatible materials in dentistry when placed in direct contact with tissues. However, ceramic dust which is produced when grinding or machining ceramics is harmful if inhaled. Proper evacuation of the dust and wearing of mouth mask is mandatory.

CEMENTING OF CERAMIC RESTORATIONS

The type of cement used depends on the type of restoration (metal ceramic or full ceramic) and its location (anterior or posterior). Both resin based cements and glass ionomer based cements have been used to bond ceramic restorations.

Because of the translucency of *some* all-ceramic restorations (e.g. glass ceramic crowns), the underlying cement may influence the esthetics (color) of the restoration. Therefore the shade of the cement used should be carefully selected.

Resin bonding agents

Many clinicians advocate resin luting cements for ceramic restorations especially those with greater translucency for a number of reasons.

1. Resin bonding generates the high bond strengths needed for such restorations to succeed.
2. Esthetics at the margins is better with resin cements.
3. Improved translucence.
4. Improved fracture resistance and long term survival.
5. Reduces water access to the inner ceramic surface.
6. Etching blunts the tips of microcracks within the ceramic thereby inhibiting crack propagation.

Bonding of the cement to the porcelain can be improved by

○ Sandblasting

○ Chemical etching

○ Use of silane primers (for silica based porcelains)

Sandblasting

The inner surface of the ceramic restoration creates minute irregularities helping the cement to retain better. However, chemical etching appears to be superior. Following sandblasting clean in distilled water in an ultrasonic bath for 10 minutes.

Etching of porcelain

Ceramic restorations which are bonded using resin cements (usually *veneers* and *inlays*) have to be etched. Etching improves the bond of the resin to the ceramic. Etching is commonly done with *hydrofluoric acid* **(Fig. 28.51)** or ammonium bifluoride (NH_4HF_2). The acid attacks and selectively dissolves the inner surface of the ceramic **(Fig. 28.52)**. The acid is available in two concentrations 5% and 9.5%. An etching time of 2 minutes is usually sufficient.

Overetching can result in the formation of a white residue on the surface of the porcelain. This is believed to be a mix acid-reaction salts and crystal fragments. Following etching the restoration is cleaned by placing in ethanol followed by a 5 minute immersion in an ultrasonic bath.

The tooth surface is also etched using phosphoric acid. Before placing the cement, a bond agent is applied to both surfaces (tooth and porcelain).

Precautions HF has the ability to readily penetrate skin tissues (often without causing an external burn), and cause extensive internal tissue damage, as well as alter blood calcium levels (due to the formation of CaF_2), which can lead to dangerous heart arrythmias. Suitable precautions should be taken while handling concentrated HF.

Bonding of alumina and zirconia based restorations

Zirconia and alumina restorations can be cemented traditionally with a range of conventional cements for a number of reasons.

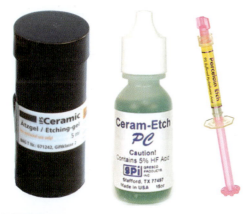

FIGURE 28.51 Ceramic etchants consists of hydrofluoric acid (5%).

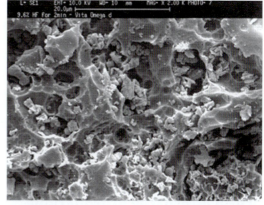

FIGURE 28.52 SEM of etched ceramic (Vita Omega) using 9.6% hydrofluoric acid for 2 minutes.

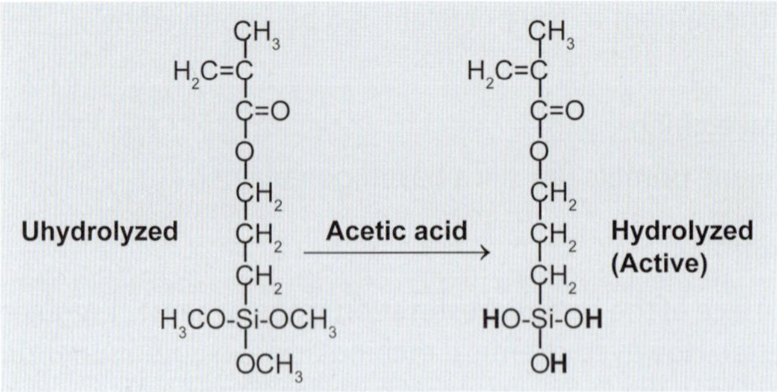

FIGURE 28.53 Acetic acid is used to activate silane (3-methacryloxypropyltrimethoxysilane).

1. Alumina and zirconia based ceramics cannot be etched or silanated that easily when compared to are silica-based ceramics.
2. They are more opaque and so the cement does not significantly affect esthetics.

Zirconia/alumina restorations with *good retention* may be cemented with glass ionomer, resin-modified glass ionomer and carboxylate cements, or with self-adhesive resin cements. However, restorations with less than ideal retention should be bonded with adhesive resin cement, enamel/dentin bonding agent, and a special zirconia primer.

Silane treatment

Silanes are a class of organic molecules that contain one or more silicon atoms. The specific silane typically used in dentistry for both intraoral repair and treatment of ceramic restorations is *3-methacryloxypropyltrimethoxysilane* **(Fig. 28.53)**. This silane is a difunctional molecule. One side of this molecule is nothing more than a methacrylate group capable of copolymerization with methacrylate-based adhesives and resins routinely used for dental procedures. The other side, after hydrolysis, has the potential to form chemical bonds to the porcelain surface.

To be able to function as a coupling agent and interact chemically with porcelain surfaces, silane must first be hydrolyzed or activated with acetic acid. This is done with acetic acid **(Fig. 28.53)**.

The silane comes in 2 forms

1. Single bottle (active or hydrolyzed form) **(Fig. 28.54)**
2. Two bottle (nonhydrolyzed form)

Two-bottle silane systems typically consist of a nonhydrolyzed silane/ethanol solution in one container and an acetic acid/water solution in the other.

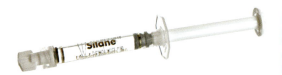

FIGURE 28.54 Silane primer.

The single bottle hydrolyzed or active form is less stable and has a shorter shelf life.

CEMENTING METAL-CERAMIC CROWNS AND FIXED PARTIAL DENTURES

These are cemented like conventional restorations. The cement does not affect the esthetics because it is not visible through the restoration. Any conventional cement may be used.

REPAIR OF CERAMIC RESTORATIONS

Ceramic restorations are difficult to repair intraorally primarily because of poor bond strength of the repaired fragment. However, in certain situations intraoral repair may be undertaken

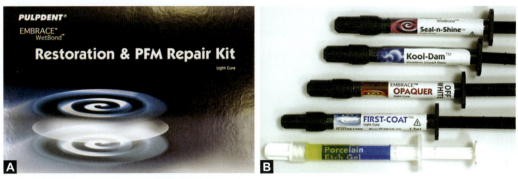

FIGURES 28.55A AND B A representative porcelain repair kit.

as a temporary or intermediate procedure before a new restoration is fabricated. Intraoral repair is carried out using composite.

A typical intraoral repair kit *(Figs. 28.55A and B)* consists of a porcelain etching gel (HFI acid), a bonding agent, and opaquer to mask the metal and a glaze. The gingival tissues are first protected with a protective gel (Kool Dam). Next the ceramic is etched with the gel. The bonding agent is applied and light cured followed by the opaquer (usually in case of metal-ceramic restorations). For the bulk of the repair a regular light cured composite is used of the appropriate shade. After trimming and shaping the final glaze coat is applied (super shine).

PORCELAIN DENTURE TEETH

Porcelain denture teeth *(Figs. 28.56A and B)* are more natural looking than acrylic teeth. They have excellent biocompatibility and are more resistant to wear. Porcelain denture teeth also have the advantage of being the only type of denture teeth that allow the denture to be rebased.

Porcelain teeth are made with high fusing porcelains. Two or more porcelains of different translucencies for each tooth are packed into metal molds and fired on large trays in high temperature ovens. The retention of porcelain teeth on the denture base is by mechanical interlocking. Anterior teeth have projecting metal pins that get embedded in the denture base resin during processing *(Figs. 28.56A and B)*. Posterior teeth on the other hand are designed with holes (diatoric spaces) in the underside into which the denture resin flows.

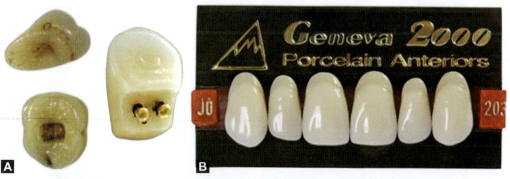

FIGURES 28.56A AND B Porcelain denture teeth. Porcelain teeth are similar in appearance to resin teeth. However, unlike resin teeth they are retained with projecting pins (anterior teeth). Posterior teeth have channels in them into which the resin flows and locks (*Courtesy:* Vijay Dental, Chennai).

The disadvantages of porcelain denture teeth are

1. They are brittle and make a clicking sound during contact.
2. They require a greater interridge distance as they cannot be ground as thin as acrylic teeth in the ridge-lap areas without destroying the diatoric channels or pins that provide their only means of retention.
3. The higher density increases their weight.

MONOLITHIC RESTORATIONS

A monolithic restoration is a restoration made entirely of the same material throughout. A monolithic crown eliminates the layer of a weaker porcelain over the crown thereby making the crown much stronger.

The two examples of monolithic ceramics are

1. Monolithic lithium disilicate
2. Monolithic zirconia.

MONOLITHIC LITHIUM DISILICATE

IPS e.max lithium disilicate is a monolithic glass ceramic restoration. It offers dentists improved fit, improved esthetics, and improved durability (400 Mpa). It can be pressed or milled using a CAD/CAM system into full contour. It has no interface, and no layered veneer. And because the ceramic ingots are blended with dentin colored and translucent ceramics, these posterior crowns match posterior dentition with slight translucency in cusp tips. They are customized with paint-on shades and then a layer of glaze for a final shine.

MONOLITHIC ZIRCONIA

A monolithic zirconia restoration is a restoration made entirely of the same material throughout *(Figs. 28.57A and B)*.

Advantage   Because there is no layering porcelain, monolithic zirconia posterior crowns have the advantage over layered restorations like the layered zirconia restorations and PFM because there is no porcelain to delaminate, chip, or fracture. This makes the crown much stronger.

Indications   The material was originally intended to provide a durable, more esthetic alternative to posterior metal occlusal PFMs or cast gold restorations for demanding situations like bruxers, implant restorations and areas with limited occlusal space.

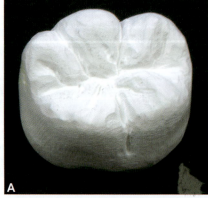 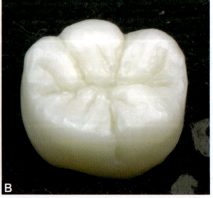

FIGURES 28.57A AND B (A) Restoration in the just milled stage. Note the chalky appearance. **(B)** Restoration after sintering with suitable glaze and stain.

Commercial names
BruxZir, Lava Plus High Translucency Zirconia, etc.

Esthetic considerations

Because they are made of the same material throughout they do not have the opaquer core show-through seen in layered zirconia core restorations.

The color of early restorations, though close to the desired shade, the final restoration was usually too high in value. Current MZ crowns have improved esthetics thanks to improvements of the dyeing liquids over the past 2 years and likely will continue to evolve. Recent changes in coloration protocol for MZ restorations have seen the introduction of a three-zone coloring system and special effects stains. More translucent zirconia restorations have also been introduced.

Technical considerations

Monolithic zirconia restorations begin as chalky white blocks *(Fig. 28.57A)*. They are milled to their designed shape and then dyed to the required shade *(Fig. 28.57B)*.

Staining
Staining is done in one of 2 ways

1. Monochrome technique
2. Gradient shading

In the monochrome technique *(Fig. 28.58A)* the restoration is soaked in a dyeing liquid for 2 minutes to approximate the desired shade. Being chalky and porous the restoration absorbs the stain.

In the three-zone gradient shading *(Fig. 28.58B)* technique

1. The unsintered restoration is first brushed with the desired final color around the cervical zone of the crown.
2. Next, the body of the crown is brushed with the desired body shade.
3. Finally, effect shades are used to characterize the occlusal area of the crown.

Sintering
After the milled crown has been shade-adjusted in the coloring solution, it is sintered in an oven for 6.5 hours at 1,560 °C. Sintering drives the tetragonal zirconia to its monoclinic phase and the gives the milled crown its great resistance to fracture and breakage. During the sintering process, the zirconia shrinks and becomes much more dense. A computer program is used to increase the size of the crown during the milling process to compensate for the shrinkage that occurs during the sintering process.

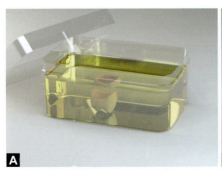
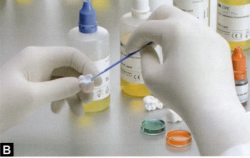

FIGURES 28.58A AND B **(A)** Monochrome staining. **(B)** Gradient shading.

CERAMIC POSTS

With the increasing use of more translucent crowns color of the underlying restorative materials is a concern. Metallic post and cores can sometimes reduce the esthetics of ceramic restorations by

1. Blocking the passage of light through the restoration.
2. Producing a grayish zone near the gingival margins.

With the increasing demand for esthetic restorations, ceramic posts may be used instead metallic post and cores.

Types of ceramic post and core systems

1. Prefabricated ceramic posts with composite resin cores.
2. Prefabricated ceramic posts with pressed ceramic cores (CosmoPost - Ivoclar).
3. Copymilled ceramic (zirconia) post and core *(Fig. 28.59)*.

CosmoPost

The CosmoPost (Ivoclar Vivadent) is a parallel ceramic post composed of ZrO_2, HfO_2, Y_2O_3 and Al_2O_3. The CosmoPost in combination with the Cosmo Ingot which is a pressable ceramic is used to fabricate esthetic post and core foundations on which crowns may be fabricated. However, care must be exercised in selecting cases as these posts are susceptible to fracture.

According to one study, the fracture load of copy-milled zirconia ceramic posts is significantly lower than that of prefabricated zirconia ceramic posts of the same size.

PEDIATRIC ZIRCONIA CROWNS

Prefabricated zirconia crowns have become available for deciduous teeth *(Fig. 28.60)*. These have provided a treatment alternative to polycarbonate crowns to address the esthetic concerns and ease of placement of extra-coronal restorations on primary anterior teeth. The placement technique is similar to the polycarbonate crowns. The treatment is simple and effective and represents a promising alternative for rehabilitation of decayed primary teeth.

ZIRCONIA IMPLANTS AND ABUTMENTS

Its high strength, fracture toughness, and its white color make zirconia an interesting material for the construction of implant abutments and superstructures especially in the anterior zone.

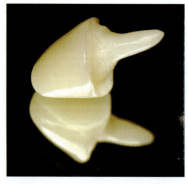

FIGURE 28.59 Zirconia post and core.

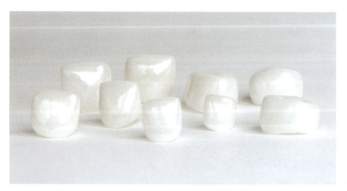

FIGURE 28.60 Prefabricated pediatric zirconia crowns.

Indications

Two factors which favour the choice of zirconia as an abutment or implant material.

1. Esthetic considerations.
2. Sensitivity or allergy to titanium.

Although titanium is the preferred choice for dental implants as it is an inert material. In rare circumstances it may encourage toxic or allergic type I or IV reactions. Allergy due to titanium might be accountable for the failure of implants in some cases (known as *cluster patients*). It has been documented that the risk of titanium allergy is more prevalent in patients having sensitivity to other metals. In such types of cases, an allergy assessment is suggested to exclude problems related with titanium implants.

Zirconia abutments and implants should be considered in patients with known allergy to titanium.

Problems encountered

The abutment is connected to the implant by means of a fixation screw *(Fig. 28.61A)*. Being a brittle material, friction between the fixation screw and the internal surface of the ceramic abutment could produce high internal stresses that could lead to occasional unexpected fracture. One way of getting around this problem is using a one piece abutment-implant *(Fig. 28.61B)*.

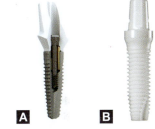

FIGURES 28.61A AND B (A) Zirconia abutment-titanium implant. **(B)** One-piece zirconia abutment-implant.

ZIRCONIA ANATOMIC ROOT-FORM IMPLANTS

Synonyms Root analog implants, anatomic implants, custom implants, bioimplant.

Zirconia-based implants were introduced into dental implantology as an alternative to titanium implants. Owing to its ability to be milled into the shape of the natural tooth root and be placed immediately following extraction, its excellent biomechanical characteristics, biocompatibility, and bright tooth-like color, zirconia has the potential to become a substitute for titanium as dental implant material.

Immediate placement of implant similar in shape and size to the extracted root has its own advantages (see advantages below). By adapting the root to the extraction socket instead of adapting the bone to a preformed standardized implant they reduced the bone and soft tissue trauma. Immediate custom-made root analog implants were possible because of advances in material and CAD/CAM technology.

Technique

Following atraumatic extraction, the extracted tooth is digitally scanned and a root-abutment analog *(Figs. 28.62A and B)* is constructed using CAD/CAM. The surface of the implant is made rough for osteoconductivity as well as designed to provide immediate stabilization. Implant milling and sintering takes a couple of hours to complete. The patient is recalled the next day for implant placement *(Fig. 28.62B)*.

Recovery time is very fast as neither soft nor hard tissue is traumatized. After a 8-12 week healing period the final restoration is constructed *(Figs. 28.62C and D)*.

Advantages

1. Esthetic
2. Biocompatible

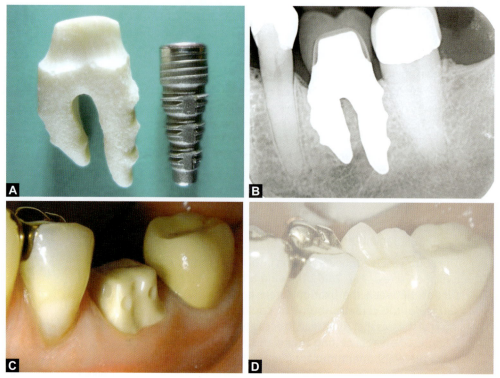

FIGURES 28.62A TO D (A) Zirconia root form implants. **(B)** Periapical view. **(C)** Intraoral view of abutment before crown placement. **(D)** After crown placement.

3. Immediate placement
4. No additional drilling or surgery required
5. No complications of implant surgery
6. Shorter waiting period
7. Fits into original socket
8. Immediate placement preserves bone and soft tissue (less resorption)
9. Preserves root eminences of the alveolar bone
10. Sinus lift not required
11. Bone graft not required
12. Little or no swelling or pain
13. Faster recovery time

Author queries:

1. Please provide citation for Box 29.1 in the text.
2. Please provide the citation for Fig. 29.21B in the text.

29
CHAPTER

Denture Resins and Polymers

CHAPTER OUTLINE

- History of False Teeth
- Earlier Denture Materials
- Classification of Denture Base Materials
- Synthetic Resins
  - Classification of Resins
  - Ideal Requirements
  - Uses of Resins
- Nature of Polymers
- Polymerization—Chemistry
- Acrylic Resins
- Poly (Methyl Methacrylate) Resins
- Heat Activated Denture Base Acrylic Resins
  - Compression Molding Technique
  - Separating Medium
  - Finishing and Polishing
  - Injection Molding Technique
- Chemically Activated Denture Base Acrylic Resins
  - Sprinkle on Technique

- Adapting Technique
- Fluid Resin Technique
- Light Activated Denture Base Resins
- Microwave Cured Denture Resins
  - Specialized Poly (Methyl Methacrylate) Materials
  - High Impact Strength Materials
  - Rapid Heat—Polymerized Resins
  - Resin Teeth
  - Special Tray Acrylic Resins
  - Pattern Resins
- Methyl Methacrylate Monomer
- Poly (Methyl Methacrylate)
- Processing Errors
  - Porosity
  - Internal Porosity
  - External Porosity
  - Crazing
  - Denture Warpage

- Repair of Dentures
- Infection Control
- Care of Acrylic Dentures
- Denture Cleansers
- Denture Reliners
- Heat Cured Acrylic Resin
- Chairside Reliners
- Soft or Resilient Denture Liners
  - Vinyl Resins
  - Silicone Rubbers
  - Tissue Conditioners
- Rebasing of Dentures
- Provisional Materials
  - Preformed Crowns
  - Polycarbonate
  - Cellulose Acetate Crown Formers
  - Custom Made Crowns
  - Polymethyl Methacrylate
  - Polyethyl (Isobutyl) Methacrylate Resins
  - Epimines

History of Dentures

Replacements for decaying or lost teeth have been made for thousands of years. Skillfully designed dentures were made as early as 700 B.C.E using ivory and bone. During Medieval times, dentures were seldom considered. Gaps between teeth were expected, even nobles had them. Queen Elizabeth I filled the holes in her mouth with cloth to improve her appearance in public. When dentures were installed, they were hand-carved and tied in place with silk threads. Retention of false teeth became more difficult as the number of teeth diminished in the mouth and those that wore full sets of dentures had to remove them before eating. Upper and lower plates fit poorly, and were held together by steel springs *(Fig. 29.1)*. Many including George Washington suffered from tooth loss and unfit dentures.

The major reason that the level of technology didn't increase is because suitable materials for false teeth were hard to find. In ancient times, the most common material for false teeth were animal bone or ivory, especially from

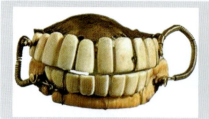

FIGURE 29.1 George Washington's dentures 1795 made by his dentist John Greenwood.

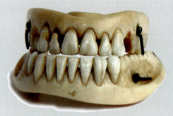

FIGURE 29.2 Ivory dentures inlaid with natural human teeth.

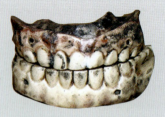

FIGURE 29.3 18th century porcelain dentures retrieved from a grave in France.

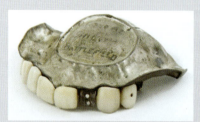

FIGURE 29.4 Metal denture base made from German silver which belonged to a soldier from the Battle of Shiloh 1862.

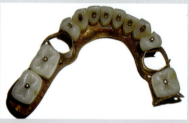

FIGURE 29.5 1860 partial denture constructed from metal and vulcanite held by anchoring studs. The two metal loops were fitted to remaining teeth.

elephants or hippopotamus. Human teeth were also used; pulled from the dead or sold by poor people from their own mouths *(Fig. 29.2)*. These teeth soon rotted or decayed. Rich people got dentures made of silver, gold, mother of pearl, or agate. In 1774, Duchateau and Dubois de Chemant designed a full set of dentures that would not rot *(Fig. 29.3)*. They were the first porcelain dentures. Giuseppangelo Fonzi created a single porcelain tooth held in place by a steel pin in 1808. Claudius Ash made an improved porcelain tooth in 1837. Porcelain dentures moved to the United States in the 1800s. They were marketed on a large scale. Porcelain dentures were prone to chip and also tended to appear too white to be convincing. Porcelain was tolerated by denture bearing mucosa but was difficult to fabricate and easily broken.

In the 1700s plaster of Paris was introduced as an impression material. It was used to make a mold of the patient's mouth. This helped the shape of the dentures to be more precise. Swaged gold was used as denture base for those who could afford it. Other metals like German silver were also used as denture base *(Fig. 29.4)*. There was a real breakthrough when vulcanized rubber was discovered by Charles Goodyear in 1839 *(Fig. 29.5)*. This is a cheap, easy to work with material that could be shaped to fit the mouth and hold the denture. The casting machine was invented by Bean in 1870 and aluminum bases with teeth set in vulcanite were used. Vulcanite and other dental products were supplied in India under British rule primarily by the Bombay Burma Trading company which was set up in 1863 by the Wallace Brothers *(Fig. 29.6)*. After independence the company was taken over by the Wadia group, the dental branch of which continues today as the Dental Product of India (DPI). A little later plastics were introduced and celluloid and phenol formaldehyde resins were tried in place of rubber. The discovery of acrylic resins in the early 20th century and improved impression techniques have since revolutionized denture treatment.

Prior to 1937, the materials used for denture bases were vulcanite, nitrocellulose, phenol formaldehyde, vinyl plastics and porcelain.

Vulcanite

Vulcanite was discovered by Charles Goodyear in 1839. It was the first material that could be molded rather than the traditional method of swaging or carving *(Figs. 29.5 to 25.7)*. It contains rubber with 32% sulphur and metallic oxides for color.

Advantages

- Nontoxic and nonirritating
- Excellent mechanical properties
- Easy to mold and fabricate

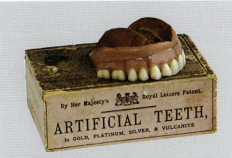

FIGURE 29.6 Vulcanite dentures.

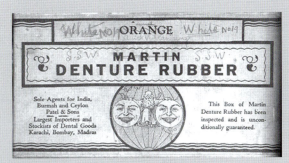

FIGURE 29.7 Vulcanite denture material were available in India under British rule (*Courtesy:* CODS, Manipal).

Disadvantages

- It absorbs saliva and becomes unhygienic due to bacterial proliferation. Unpleasant odor, when processed.
- Poor esthetics due to opacity of rubber.
- The material is quite hard to polish.
- Dimensional changes occur due to
  - Thermal expansion during heating in the vulcanizer
  - Contraction of 2 to 4% by volume during addition of the sulphur to the rubber.

Nitrocellulose

Celluloid was invented by Hyatt in 1868 and used as a denture base material from about 1890. Its color was better than vulcanite. It used camphor as a plasticizer which gave it an unpleasant taste and odor. Though short-lived, this material indicated a general evolution towards plastics as the denture base material of choice. Some of their disadvantages are enumerated below.

- Dimensionally unstable and distorted in service
- High water absorption
- Poor color stability (turns from pink to green with time)
- Contains unpleasant tasting plasticizers (Camphor)
- Highly flammable.

Phenol Formaldehyde

Phenol-formaldehyde resin (also known as Bakelite) was discovered in 1909. By 1929 they were introduced to dentistry and soon came to be used for denture bases. They were technique sensitive and had wide variations in color, dimensional stability and strength. They become discolored and unesthetic and being thermosetting it is difficult to repair.

POLYMERS

Denture base and other resins used in dentistry are made up of polymers. Therefore an understanding of the nature and chemistry of polymers is essential. Although work on synthetic polymers were started in the 18th century the nature of these unique materials were not clearly understood. In 1922 Hermann Staudinger (Germany) was the first to propose that polymers consisted of long chains of atoms held together by covalent bonds. He also proposed to name these compounds macromolecules. Before that, scientists believed that polymers were clusters of small molecules (called colloids), without definite molecular weights, held together by an unknown force.

NATURE OF POLYMERS

POLYMER

A polymer is large and often complex macromolecule that is made from smaller molecules. A macromolecule is any chemical possessing a molecular weight greater than 5000. Some polymers have weights in excess of 50 million. The *mer* ending represents the simplest repeating chemical structural unit from which the polymer is composed, e.g. poly (methyl methacrylate) is a polymer having chemical structural units derived from methyl methacrylate.

MONOMER

The molecules from which the polymer is constructed are called monomers (one part). Polymer molecules may be prepared from a mixture of different types of monomers and they are called copolymers.

MOLECULAR WEIGHT

The molecular weight of the polymer molecule equals the molecular weight of the various *mers* multiplied by the number of mer units. They may range from thousands to millions of units depending on preparation conditions. The molecular weight of polymers plays an important role in determining its physical properties. The average molecular weight for various denture polymers range from 8000 to 39000. Cross-linked resin teeth may have weights in excess of 600,000.

DEGREE OF POLYMERIZATION

Defined as total number of mers in a polymer.

❍ The higher the molecular weight of the polymer made from a single monomer, the higher the degree of polymerization.

❍ The strength of the resin increases with increase in the degree of polymerization until a certain molecular weight is reached. Above this there is no change.

MOLECULAR WEIGHT DISTRIBUTION

A narrow molecular weight distribution gives the most useful polymers. However most polymers have a wide range of molecular weights and so vary widely in their properties, e.g. the higher the molecular weight, the higher the softening and melting points and the stiffer the plastic.

STRUCTURE OF POLYMERS (SPATIAL STRUCTURE)

The physical structure of the polymer molecule is also important in determining the properties of the polymer. There are three basic structures.

LINEAR

Here the 'mer' units are connected to each other in a linear sequence *(Fig. 29.8)*. They can be further divided into

Linear homopolymer   It has mer units of the same type.

$$...- M - M - M - M - M - M - M - ...$$

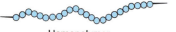 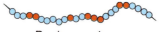 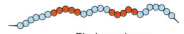

| Homopolymer | Random copolymer | Block copolymer |

FIGURE 29.8 Structure of linear polymers.

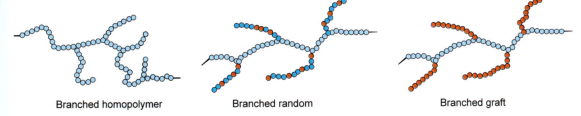

Branched homopolymer   Branched random   Branched graft

FIGURE 29.9 Structure of branched polymers.

Random copolymer of linear type It has two types of mer units, randomly distributed along the chain.

$$...– M – M – M – Y – M – Y – M – M – Y – Y – M – M –...$$

Block copolymer   It has two types of mers distributed in segments or blocks.

$$... – M – M – M –...– M – M – Y – Y –...– Y – Y – M – M – ...$$

Branched

Linear molecules are rarely realized. In practice the mer units are arranged in a branched fashion or cross-linked *(Fig. 29.9)*.

Branched homopolymer   The mer units are of the same type.

$$... – M – M – M – M – M – ... – M – M – M – M – M – ...$$

$$\qquad\qquad M \qquad\qquad\qquad\qquad\qquad M$$

$$\qquad\qquad M \qquad\qquad\qquad\qquad\qquad M$$

Random copolymer of branched type   It has two types of mer distributed randomly.

$$... – M – M – M – M – M – ... – M – M – M – M – M – ...$$

$$\qquad\qquad\vdots\qquad\qquad\qquad\qquad\qquad\vdots$$
$$\qquad\qquad M\qquad\qquad\qquad\qquad\qquad Y$$
$$\qquad\qquad\vdots\qquad\qquad\qquad\qquad\qquad\vdots$$
$$\qquad\qquad M\qquad\qquad\qquad\qquad\qquad M$$
$$\qquad\qquad\vdots\qquad\qquad\qquad\qquad\qquad\vdots$$
$$\qquad\qquad Y\qquad\qquad\qquad\qquad\qquad Y$$

Graft copolymer of branched type It has one type of mer unit on the main chain and another mer for the branches.

$$... – M – M – M – M – M – ... – M – M – M – M – M – ...$$

$$\qquad\qquad\vdots\qquad\qquad\qquad\qquad\qquad\vdots$$
$$\qquad\qquad Y\qquad\qquad\qquad\qquad\qquad Y$$
$$\qquad\qquad\vdots\qquad\qquad\qquad\qquad\qquad\vdots$$
$$\qquad\qquad Y\qquad\qquad\qquad\qquad\qquad Y$$

CROSS LINKED POLYMER

It is made up of a homopolymer cross linked with a single cross-linking agent. It is a network structure *(Fig. 29.10)*.

POLYMERIZATION—CHEMISTRY

The term polymerization refers to a series of chain reactions by which a macromolecule or polymer is formed from a group of smaller single molecules known as 'monomer'. These

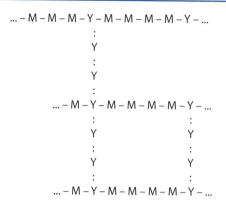

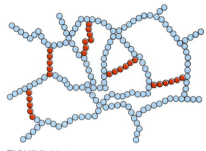

FIGURE 29.10 Cross-linked polymer.

structural units are connected to each other within the polymer molecules by bonds. Polymerization is a repetitive intermolecular reaction that is capable of proceeding indefinitely.

TYPES

Most polymerization reactions fall into two basic types.

Condensation polymerization (step growth)

Condensation resins are divided into two groups

1. Those in which polymerization is accompanied by repeated elimination of small molecules, i.e. the primary compounds react with the formation of byproducts such as water, halogen acids, and ammonia. The process can repeat itself and form macromolecules.
2. Those in which functional groups are repeated in the polymer chains. The mers are joined by functional groups (like amide, urethane, ester or sulfide linkages). Formation of a by-product is not necessary, e.g. polyurethane.

In the past several condensation resins have been used to make denture bases. At present, condensation resins are not widely used in dentistry.

Addition polymerization

Most resins employed extensively in dental procedures are produced by addition polymerization. Here, there is no change in chemical composition and no by-products are formed. In this type of polymer, the structure of the monomer is repeated many times in the polymer.

Starting from an active center, one molecule at a time is added and a chain rapidly builds up, which can grow almost indefinitely as long as the supply of building blocks is available.

CHEMICAL STAGES OF POLYMERIZATION

This occurs in four stages

Induction

Induction or initiation period is the time during which the molecules of the initiator becomes energized or activated and start to transfer the energy to the monomer. Any impurity present increases the length of this period. The higher the temperature, the shorter is the length of the induction period. The initiation energy for activation of each monomer molecular unit is 16000-29000 calories per mol in the liquid phase.

There are three induction systems for dental resins

- *Heat activation* Most denture base resins are polymerized by this method, e.g. the free radicals liberated by heating benzoyl peroxide will initiate the polymerization of methyl methacrylate monomer.
- *Chemical activation* This system consists of at least two reactants, when mixed they undergo chemical reaction and liberate free radicals, e.g. the use of benzoyl peroxide and an aromatic amine (dimethyl-p-toluidine) in self-cured dental resins.
- *Light activation* In this system, photons of light energy activate the initiator to generate free radicals, e.g. camphorquinone and an amine will react to form free radicals, when they are irradiated with visible light.

Propagation

Once the growth has started only 5000 to 8000 calories per mole are required, the process continues rapidly and is accompanied by evolution of heat.

Theoretically, the chain reactions should continue with evolution of heat until all the monomer has been changed to polymer. In reality however, the polymerization is never complete.

Termination

The chain reactions can be terminated either by direct coupling of two chain ends or by exchange of a hydrogen atom from one growing chain to another.

Chain transfer

The chain termination can also result from chain transfer. Here the active state is transferred from an activated radical to an inactive molecule and a new nucleus of growth is created. An already terminated chain can be reactivated by chain transfer resulting in continued growth.

INHIBITION OF POLYMERIZATION

Such reactions are inhibited by

- *Inhibitors* These react with the activated initiator or any activated nucleus, or with an activated growing chain to prevent further growth, e.g. hydroquinone (0.006%) is added to prevent polymerization of the monomer during storage.
- *Oxygen* Presence of oxygen (air) also inhibit polymerization.

COPOLYMERIZATION

The macromolecule may be formed by polymerization of a single type of structural unit. However, in order to improve the physical properties, it is often advantageous to use two or more *chemically different* monomers as starting materials. The polymers thus formed may contain units of these monomers. Such a polymer is called a copolymer and its process of formation is known as copolymerization.

TYPES OF COPOLYMERS

There are three different types of copolymers *(Fig. 29.11)*

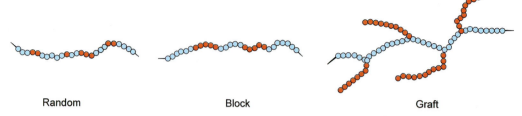

Random   Block   Graft

FIGURE 29.11 Types of copolymers.

Random type

In random type of copolymer the different *mers* are randomly distributed along the chain, such as

– M – M – M – M – Y – M – Y – M – Y – Y – M – M –

Block type

In a block copolymer, identical monomer units occur in relatively long sequences along the main polymer chain.

... – M – M – M – M – ... – M – M – Y – Y – Y – ... – Y – Y – M – M – ...

Graft type

In graft copolymers, sequence of one of the monomers are grafted onto the 'backbone' of the second monomer species.

```
– M – M – M – M – M – ... – M – M – M – M
        ⋮                       ⋮
        Y                       Y
        ⋮                       ⋮
        Y                       Y
```

IMPORTANCE OF COPOLYMERIZATION

Copolymerization is used to improve the physical properties of resins. Many useful resins are manufactured by copolymerization.

❍ Small amounts of ethyl acrylate may be copolymerized with methyl methacrylate to alter the flexibility.

❍ Block and graft polymers show improved impact strength. In small amounts they modify the adhesive properties of resins as well as their surface characteristics.

CROSS-LINKING

The formation of chemical bonds or bridges between the polymer chains is referred to as cross-linking. It forms a three-dimensional network.

```
... – M – M – M – Y – M – M – M – Y – ...
              ⋮
              Y
              ⋮
... – M – M – M – Y – M – M – Y – M – Y – M – ...
              ⋮               ⋮
              Y               Y
              ⋮               ⋮
... – M – M – M – Y – M – M – M – M – Y – M – ...
```

APPLICATIONS

1. The more recent acrylic resins are of cross-linked variety. Cross-linking increases rigidity and decreases solubility and water sorption.
2. Acrylic teeth are highly cross-linked to improve its resistance to solvents, crazing and surface stresses.

PLASTICIZERS

These are substances added to resins

1. To increase the solubility of the polymer in the monomer.
2. To decrease the brittleness of the polymer.

However, it also decreases strength, hardness, and softening point.

TYPES

They are of two types

1. *External*   It penetrates between the macromolecules and neutralizes the secondary bonds or intermolecular forces. It is an insoluble high boiling compound. It is not so widely used as it may evaporate or leach out during normal use of the resin.
2. *Internal*   Here, the plasticizing agent is part of the polymer. It is done by copolymerization with a suitable comonomer.

CLASSIFICATION OF DENTURE BASE MATERIALS

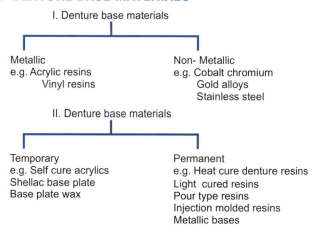

III. ISO 20795-1:2013 Classification

Type I – Heat-polymerizable polymers

Class 1 – Powder and liquid

Class 2 – Plastic cake

Type 2 – Autopolymerizable polymers

Class 1 – Powder and liquid

Class 2 – Powder and liquid for pour-type resins

Type 3 – Thermoplastic blank or powder

Type 4 – Light-activated materials

Type 5 – Microwave cured materials

SYNTHETIC RESINS

Modern living has been greatly influenced by synthetic plastics. Originally they were laboratory nuisances - waxy, sticky residues left after certain organic reactions. These resinous materials composed of giant molecules attracted the attention of chemists giving rise to the field of plastics. Synthetic plastics are nonmetallic compounds which are molded into various forms and then hardened for commercial use (e.g. clothing, electronic equipment, building materials and household appliances). These materials are composed of polymers or complex molecules of high molecular weight.

A variety of resins are used in dentistry. These include acrylics, polycarbonates, vinyl resins, polyurethanes, styrene, cyanoacrylates, epoxy resins, etc.

CLASSIFICATION OF RESINS

Due to their heterogeneous structure and complex nature they are difficult to classify. *Based on the thermal behavior,* they are classified as

○ Thermoplastic
○ Thermosetting

Thermoplastic

These are resins that *can be repeatedly* softened and molded under heat and pressure without any chemical change occurring. They are fusible and are usually soluble in organic solvents. Most resins used in dentistry belong to this group, e.g. polymethyl methacrylate, polyvinyl acrylics and polystyrene.

Thermosetting

This category refers to resins which can be molded only once. They set when heated. These cannot be softened by reheating like the thermoplastic resins. They are generally infusible and insoluble.

IDEAL REQUIREMENTS OF DENTAL RESINS

Dental resins, both restorative and denture base should

1. Be tasteless, odorless, nontoxic and nonirritant to the oral tissues.
2. Be esthetically satisfactory, i.e. should be transparent or translucent and easily tinted. The color should be permanent.
3. Be dimensionally stable. It should not expand, contract or warp during processing and subsequent use by the patient.
4. Have enough strength, resilience and abrasion resistance.
5. Be insoluble and impermeable to oral fluids.
6. Have a low specific gravity (light in weight).
7. Tolerate temperatures well above the temperature of any hot foods or liquids taken in the mouth without undue softening or distortion.

8. Be easy to fabricate and repair.
9. Have good thermal conductivity.
10. Be radiopaque (so that denture/ fragments can be detected by X-rays if accidentally aspirated or swallowed and also to examine the extensions of the resin restoration in a tooth).
11. When used as a filling material it should bond chemically with the tooth.
12. Have coefficient of thermal expansion which match that of tooth structure.
13. Be economical.

USES OF RESINS IN DENTISTRY

1. Fabrication of dentures (denture base resins) *(Figs. 29.12A to D).*
2. Artificial teeth (cross-linked acrylic resins) *(Fig. 29.12E).*
3. Tooth restoration, e.g. fillings, inlays and laminates (composite resins).
4. Cementation of orthodontic brackets, crowns and fixed dental prostheses (FDPs) (resin cements).
5. Orthodontic and pedodontic appliances *(Fig. 29.12B).*
6. Crown and FDP facings (tooth colored acrylic or composite resins).
7. Maxillofacial prostheses (e.g. obturators for cleft palates).
8. Inlay and post-core patterns (pattern resins).
9. Dies (epoxy resins).
10. Provisional restorations *(Fig. 29.12F)* in fixed prosthodontics (tooth colored resins, provisional composites) and polycarbonate crowns *(Fig. 29.12G).*
11. Endodontic obturating materials sealers.
12. Core filling material.

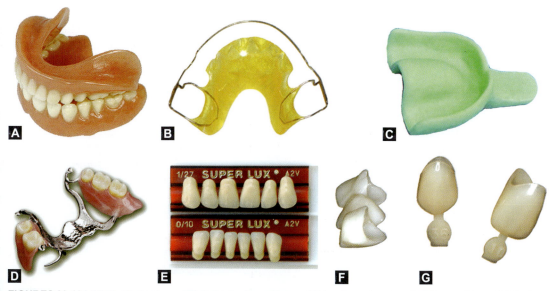

FIGURES 29.12A TO G (A) Dentures. **(B)** Orthodontic appliance. **(C)** Acrylic custom tray. **(D)** Removable partial denture. **(E)** Resin artificial denture teeth. **(F)** Temporary bridge. **(G)** Polycarbonate crowns.

13. Athletic mouth protectors.
14. Custom impression trays *(Fig. 29.12C).*
15. Splints and stents.
16. Models.

ACRYLIC RESINS

The acrylic resins are derivatives of ethylene and contain a vinyl group in their structural formula. The acrylic resins used in dentistry are the esters of

1. Acrylic acid, $CH_2 = CHCOOH$
2. Methacrylic acid, $CH_2 = C(CH_3)COOH$

The acrylic resins were so well received by the dental profession that by 1946, it largely replaced the earlier denture base materials like vulcanite.

POLY (METHYL METHACRYLATE) RESINS

These are widely used in dentistry to fabricate various appliances. One of the reasons for its wide popularity is the ease with which it can be processed. Although, it is a thermoplastic resin, in dentistry it is not usually molded by thermoplastic means. Rather, the liquid (monomer) methylmethacrylate is mixed with the polymer (powder). The monomer plasticizes the polymer to a dough-like consistency which is easily molded.

TYPES

Based on the method used for its activation

○ Heat activated resins
○ Chemically activated resins
○ Light activated resins

HEAT ACTIVATED DENTURE BASE ACRYLIC RESINS

Heat activated polymethyl methacrylate resins are the most widely used resins for the fabrication of complete dentures.

Available as

(1) Powder and liquid *(Fig. 29.13).*
(2) Gels—sheets and cakes.

The powder may be transparent or tooth colored or pink colored (to simulate the gums, some even contain red fibers to duplicate blood vessels). The liquid (monomer) is supplied in tightly sealed amber colored bottles (to prevent premature polymerization by light or ultraviolet radiation on storage).

Commercial names Stellon (DPI), Lucitone (Bayer), Trevelon (Dentsply).

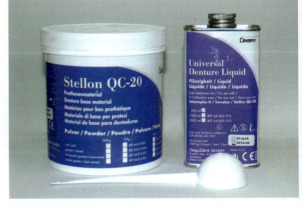

FIGURE 29.13 Heat cured denture base acrylic.

COMPOSITION

Powder

Ingredient	Function
Poly (methyl methacrylate)	Major component
Ethyl or butyl methacrylate (5%)	Copolymers - improves properties
Benzoyl peroxide	Initiator
Compounds of mercuric sulfide, cadmium sulfide, etc.	Dyes
Zinc or titanium oxide	Opacifiers
Dibutyl phthalate	Plasticizer
Inorganic fillers like glass fibers, zirconium silicate, alumina, etc.	Improves physical properties like stiffness etc.
Dyed synthetic nylon or acrylic fibers	To simulate small capillaries

Liquid

Ingredient	Function
Methyl methacrylate	Plasticizes the polymer
Dibutyl phthalate	Plasticizer
Glycol dimethacrylate (1–2%)	Cross-linking agent (reduces crazing)
Hydroquinone (0.006%)	Inhibitor-prevents premature polymerization

POLYMERIZATION REACTION

Polymerization is achieved by application of heat and pressure. The simplified reaction is

Powder + Liquid + Heat $\longrightarrow$ Polymer + Heat

(Polymer)   (Monomer) (External)   (Reaction)

TECHNICAL CONSIDERATIONS

Dentures are usually fabricated by one of the following techniques

1. Compression molding technique (usually heat activated resins).
2. Injection molding technique (heat activated resins).
3. Fluid resin technique (chemically activated resins).
4. Visible light curing technique (VLC resins).

COMPRESSION MOLDING TECHNIQUE

This is the commonly used technique in the fabrication of acrylic resin dentures.

Resin used   Usually heat activated acrylic resin.

Steps

1. Preparation of the waxed denture pattern.
2. Preparation of the split mold.
3. Application of separating medium.

4. Mixing of powder and liquid.
5. Packing.
6. Curing.
7. Cooling.
8. Divesting, finishing and polishing.

Preparation of a Waxed Denture Pattern

Many structures in dentistry are constructed using a *wax pattern*. The structure to be created (in this case a denture) is first constructed in wax. The wax portions will be replaced later with acrylic.

Preparation of the split mold

The waxed denture is *invested* in a dental flask with dental stone or plaster (also called flasking) using a 3 pour technique *(Fig. 29.14)*. After the stone or plaster sets, it is dewaxed by placing the flask in boiling water for not more than 5 minutes. After dewaxing the two halves of the flask are separated and the molten wax is flushed out with clean hot water. Removal of the wax leaves us with an empty space or mold into which soft acrylic is packed *(Figs. 29.15A and B)*. Acrylic replaces the wax, assuming the shape of the final denture.

Application of separating medium

The resin must not contact the gypsum surface while curing.

1. To prevent water from the mold entering into the acrylic resin. This may affect the rate of polymerization and color. It can also result in crazing.
2. To prevent monomer penetrating into the mold material, causing plaster to adhere to the acrylic resin and producing a rough surface.
3. Helps in easier retrieval of the denture from the mold.

Types of separating media
Various separating media used are
○ Tinfoil

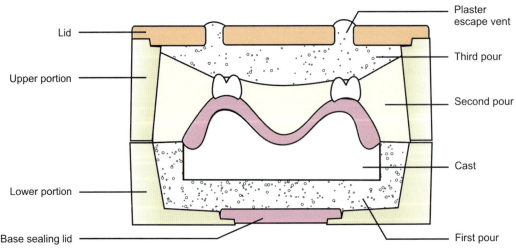

FIGURE 29.14 Schematic diagram of a fully assembled Hanau denture flask. The three pour technique of dental stone helps in easier retrieval of the denture, minimizing the risk of fracture of the prosthesis.

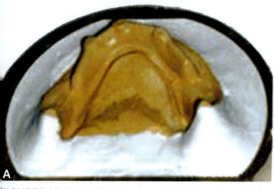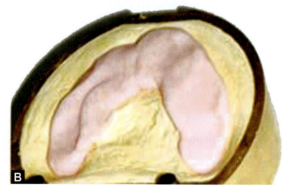

FIGURES 29.15A AND B (A) Lower half of flask containing invested cast. (B) Upper half of flask containing packed acrylic dough.

- Cellulose lacquers
- Solution of alginate compounds
- Calcium oleate
- Soft soaps
- Sodium silicate
- Starches

Tin foil
Tin foil was the material used earlier and was very effective. However, its manipulation is time consuming and difficult. It has been largely replaced by other separating media known as 'tin foil substitutes'.

Sodium alginate solution (Fig. 29.16)
This is the most popular separating medium. It is water soluble. It reacts with the calcium of the plaster or stone to form a film of insoluble calcium alginate.

Composition
2% sodium alginate in water, glycerine, alcohol, sodium phosphate and preservatives.

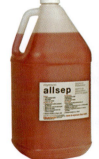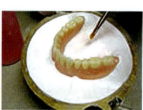

FIGURE 29.16 Sodium alginate is a popular separating media.

Precautions to be taken
1. Waxes or oils remaining on the mold surface will interfere with the action of the separating medium.
2. Mold should be warm, not hot. Continuity of the film will break if the mold is steaming hot.
3. Avoid coating the teeth as it will prevent bonding of teeth with denture base.

Application
Separating media is applied using a brush, coating only the plaster surfaces, and not the acrylic teeth. One or two coats may be applied.

Mixing of powder and liquid
Polymer—monomer proportion = 3:1 by volume or 2:1 by weight.

The measured liquid is poured into a clean, dry mixing jar. Powder is slowly added allowing each powder particle to become wetted by monomer. The mixture is then stirred and allowed to stand in a closed container.

If too much monomer is used (Lower polymer/monomer ratio)

❍   There will be greater curing or polymerization shrinkage.

❍   More time is needed to reach the packing consistency.

❍   Porosity can occur in the denture.

If too little monomer is used (Higher polymer/monomer ratio)

❍   Not all the polymer beads will be wetted by monomer and the cured acrylic will be granular.

❍   Dough will be difficult to manage and it may not fuse into a continuous unit of plastic during processing.

Physical stages

After mixing the material goes through various physical stages. No polymerization reaction takes place during these stages. A plastic dough is formed by a partial solution of the polymer in the monomer.

Stage I: Wet sand stage

The polymer gradually settles into the monomer forming a fluid, incoherent mass.

Stage II: Sticky stage

The monomer attacks the polymer by penetrating into the polymer. The mass is sticky and stringy (cobweb like) when touched or pulled apart.

Stage III: Dough or gel stage

As the monomer diffuses into the polymer, it becomes smooth and dough like. It does not adhere to the walls of the jar. It consists of undissolved polymer particles suspended in a plastic matrix of monomer and dissolved polymer. The mass is plastic and homogenous and can be *packed* into the mold at this stage *(Fig. 29.15B)*.

Stage IV: Rubbery stage

The monomer disappears by further penetration into the polymer and/or evaporation. The mass is rubberlike, non-plastic and cannot be molded.

Stage V: Stiff stage

The mass is totally unworkable and is discarded.

Working time

The working time is the time elapsing between stage II and the beginning of stage IV, i.e. the time the material remains in the dough stage (according to ADA Sp. No. 12, the dough should be moldable for at least 5 minutes).

The working time is affected by temperature. In warm weather when the working time is insufficient, the mixing jar is chilled to prolong the working time. Care is taken to avoid moisture.

Packing

The powder-liquid mixture should be packed into the flask at the dough consistency for several reasons.

○ If it is packed at the sandy or stringy stages, too much monomer will be present between the polymer particles, and the material will be of too low a viscosity to pack well and will flow out of the flask too easily. Packing too early may also result in porosity in the final denture base.

○ If packed at the rubbery to the stiff stage, the material will be too viscous to flow and metal to metal contact of the flask halves will not be obtained. Delayed packing may result in movement or fracture of the teeth, loss of detail and increase in the vertical height of the denture.

Trial closure

The acrylic dough is packed into the flask in slight excess. The excess is removed during trial packing with a damp cellophane or polyethylene film used as a separator for the upper half of the flask. A *hydraulic or mechanical press* may be used to apply pressure *(Fig. 29.17)*. The closing force is applied slowly during the trial packing to allow the excess dough, known as 'flash' *(Fig. 29.18)* to flow out between the halves of the flask. The flask is opened and the flash is trimmed away. Before final closure, the separating film is removed and discarded. The final closure of the flask or metal to metal contact of the flask halves is then completed in the press. The flasks are then transferred to a holding clamp *(Fig. 29.18)* which maintains the pressure throughout the curing process.

Curing (polymerization)

After final closure the flasks, are kept at room temperature for 30 to 60 minutes (sometimes called *'bench curing'*).

Purpose of bench curing

1. Permits an equalization of pressures throughout the mold.
2. It allows time for a more uniform dispersion of monomer throughout the mass of dough.
3. It provides a longer exposure of resin teeth to the monomer in the dough, producing a better bond of the teeth with the base material.

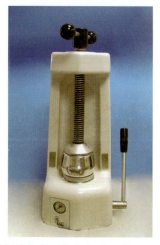

FIGURE 29.17 A hydraulic press (Kavo) is useful for trial and final closure of the flask. The pressure indicator dial indicates the pressure that is applied.

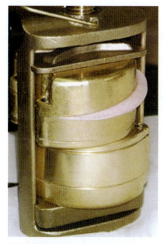

FIGURE 29.18 Assembled flasks after final closure in a holding clamp (Excess acrylic called flash is evident in the picture).

Curing cycle

The curing or polymerization cycle is the technical name for the heating process used to initiate, control and complete the polymerization of the resin in the mold. The curing cycle selected depends on the thickness of the resin. Long curing cycles are recommended for thicker resins to avoid internal porosity. The processing is done in a time-temperature controlled water bath *(Fig. 29.19)*.

Recommended curing cycles*

1. Long cycle a. 74 °C for 8 hours

    b. 74 °C for 8 hours, then boil for 1 hour

2. Short cycle - 74 °C for 2 hours, then boil for 1 hour of the thinner portions (short cycle).

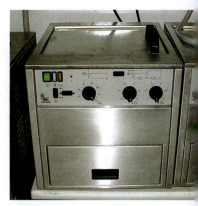

FIGURE 29.19 An automated curing bath (Kavo). The time and temperature of the curing cycle can be preset and regulated for optimum cure.

Cooling

The flask should be cooled slowly, i.e. bench cooled. Fast cooling can result in warpage of the denture due to differential thermal contraction of the resin and gypsum mold. Cooling *overnight* is ideal. However, bench cooling it for 30 minutes and then placing it in cold tap water for 15 minutes is satisfactory.

Deflasking

The cured acrylic denture is retrieved from the flask. This is called deflasking. The flask is opened and the mold is retrieved. The mold separates quickly, because the surrounding plaster was poured in layers (3 pour technique). Plaster cutting forceps may be used to break-up the plaster. Deflasking has to be done with great care to avoid flexing and breaking of the acrylic denture.

Finishing and polishing

The denture is smoothened using progressive grades of sandpaper. Finely ground pumice in water is commonly used for final polishing (refer chapter on abrasives).

INJECTION MOLDING TECHNIQUE

Resin used A special thermoplastic resin (Ivocap - Ivoclar Vivadent) *(Fig. 29.21A)* is used.

BOX 29.1 | **Sources of heat**

Apart from the heated water bath, there are other methods of supplying heat.
- Steam
- Dry air oven
- Dry heat (electrical)
- Infrared heating
- Induction or dielectric heating
- Microwave radiation

Microwave Energy Polymerization
Advantages
- It is cleaner and faster than the conventional hot water.
- The fit of the denture is comparable or superior.

---

* Phillips' Science of Dental Materials; ed. 12.

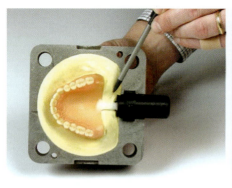
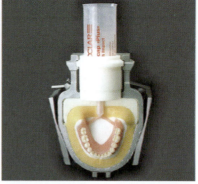

FIGURE 29.20 Injection molded denture resin technique. The picture shows the dentures invested in a special flask. The lower denture utilizes a Y-shaped sprue as shown by the operator.

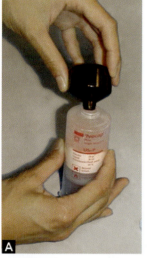
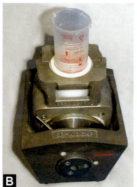
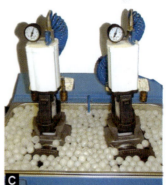

FIGURES 29.21A TO C Injection molded denture resin technique **(A)** Mixing monomer and polymer. **(B)** Assembled flask in clamp. **(C)** Curing water bath.

Equipment   This technique uses special equipment including a special bath for curing *(Fig. 29.21C)*. A sprue hole and a vent hole are formed in the gypsum mold with the help of sprue formers *(Fig. 29.20)*. The soft resin is contained in the injector and is forced into the mold space as needed. It is kept under pressure until it has hardened. Continuous feeding of the material under pressure compensates for shrinkage *(Fig. 29.22)*.

There is no difference in accuracy or physical properties as compared to compression molding technique.

Advantages

1. Dimensional accuracy (low shrinkage).
2. No increase in vertical dimension.
3. Homogeneous denture base.

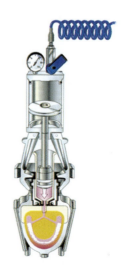

FIGURE 29.22 Schematic representation of the Injection molding process (Ivocap).

TABLE 29.1 Comparison of self cured and heat cured acrylic resin

Self cured	Heat cured
Heat is not necessary for curing	Heat is necessary for curing
Porosity is greater	Porosity of material is less
Has lower average mol. wt.	Higher molecular weights
Higher residual monomer content	Lower residual monomer content
Material is weaker (because of their lower molecular weights)	Material is comparatively stronger
Rheological properties • Shows greater distortion • More initial deformation • Increased creep and slow recovery	• Shows less distortion • Less initial deformation • Less creep and quicker recovery
Poor color stability	Color stability is good
Easy to deflask	Difficult to deflask
Lower rate of monomer diffusion	Increased rate of monomer diffusion at higher temperature

4. Low free monomer content.
5. Good impact strength.

Disadvantages

1. Higher cost of equipment.
2. Mold design problems.
3. Less craze resistance.
4. Special flask is required.

CHEMICALLY ACTIVATED DENTURE BASE ACRYLIC RESINS

The chemically activated acrylic resins polymerize at room temperature. They are also known as 'self-curing', 'cold-cure' or 'auto-polymerizing' resins.

In cold cured acrylic resins, the chemical initiator benzoyl peroxide is activated by another chemical (dimethyl-para toluidine which is present in the monomer), instead of heat as in heat cure resins. Thus, unlike heat activated resins, polymerization is achieved at room temperature *(Table 29.1)*.

AVAILABLE AS

Like the heat activated resins, chemically activated resins are supplied as powder and liquid *(Fig. 29.23)*. The powder may be clear, pink, veined or tooth colored.

USES

1. For making temporary crowns and FDPs.
2. Construction of special trays (this type contains more fillers) *(Fig. 29.12C)*.
3. For denture repair, relining and rebasing.
4. For making removable orthodontic appliances *(Fig. 29.24)*.
5. For adding a post-dam to an adjusted upper denture.

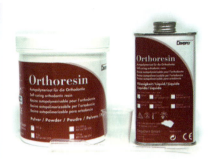

FIGURE 29.23 An example of self curing or autopolymerizing polymethylmethacrylate resin.

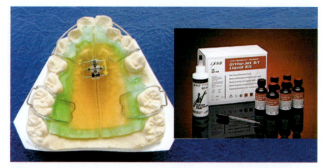

FIGURE 29.24 Orthodontic appliances are sometimes constructed in different colors to make it more attractive to younger patients. Special kits are available for this purpose (inset).

6. For making temporary and permanent denture bases.
7. For making inlay and post core patterns (specialized material is available).

COMPOSITION

Liquid

Ingredient	Action
Methyl methacrylate monomer	Dissolves/plasticizes polymer
Dimethyl-p-toluidine	Activator
Dibutyl phthalate	Plasticizer
Glycol dimethacrylate 1 to 2%	Cross linking agent
Hydroquinone 0.006%	Inhibitor

Powder

Ingredient	Action
Poly (methyl methacrylate) and other copolymers	Forms the resin matrix
Benzoyl peroxide	Initiator
Compounds of mercuric sulfide, cadmium sulfide	Dyes
Zinc or titanium oxide	Opacifiers
Dibutyl phthalate	Plasticizer
Dyed organic fillers and inorganic particles like glass fibers or beads	Esthetics

POLYMERIZATION REACTION

The simplified reaction is outlined

Polymer (Powder) + Monomer (Liquid) ⟶ Polymer + Heat
(Peroxide initiator) (Amine accelerator) (reaction)

ADVANTAGES AND DISADVANTAGES

1. Better initial fit, which is because the curing is carried out at room temperature. Thus there is less thermal contraction.
2. Color stability is inferior to that of heat cure resin, due to subsequent oxidation of the tertiary amine.

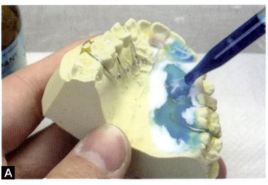 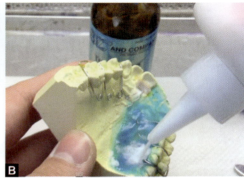

FIGURES 29.25A AND B Salt and pepper technique.

3. Slightly inferior properties because the degree of polymerization of self curing acrylics is less than that of heat cured ones.

4. For repairing dentures, self curing resins are preferable to heat cured resins as heat curing causes warpage.

MANIPULATION OF AUTOPOLYMERIZING RESINS

1. Sprinkle on technique
2. Adapting technique
3. Fluid resin technique (special material is available for this)
4. Compression molding technique*.

FIGURE 29.26 A pressure pot for further curing of chemically activated resins. It has a pressure dial (some models have a temperature indicator). Pressure is increased in the chamber using compressed air.

Sprinkle on technique

Synonym Also known as salt and pepper technique.

Separating media is applied first on the cast. Powder and liquid is applied alternatively from droppers *(Figs. 29.25A and B)*. Powder is sprinkled on the cast and then wet with monomer. The appliance or prosthesis is constructed section by section until completion. To improve the strength, the appliance is further cured in hot water under pressure for around 20 minutes using a *pressure pot (Fig. 29.26)*.

Adapting technique

Powder and monomer liquid is proportioned and mixed in a glass or porcelain jar. When it reaches the dough stage, it is quickly removed and adapted on to the cast and manually molded quickly to the desired shape. An alternative technique uses a *template*. The resin is pre-shaped using a roller and template before adapting it to the cast. Curing is completed in a pressure pot.

Fluid resin technique (pour-type acrylic resins)

A special resin (Castdon by Dreve) is available for this technique.

The chemical composition of the pour-type of denture resin is similar to the poly (methyl methacrylate) materials. The principal difference is that the pour-type of denture resins have

---

* Compression molding technique is similar to the one described for heat cured resins. However because of the reduced working time, trial closure should be kept to a minimum. Although it hardens in 30 minutes. It should remain under pressure for a further 3 hours to ensure completion of polymerization.

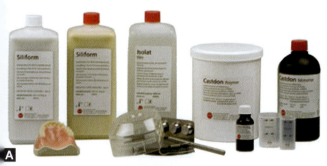

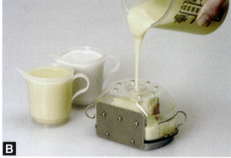

Materials for the fluid resin technique   Silicone mold fabrication

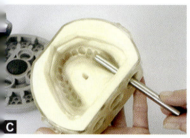

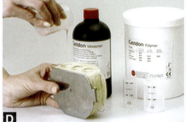

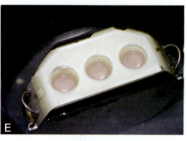

Creating pour channels   Pouring acrylic into the mold   Completion of pour

FIGURES 29.27A TO E Fluid resin technique.

high molecular weight powder particles that are much smaller and when they are mixed with monomer, the resulting mix is very *fluid*. Therefore, they are referred as 'fluid resins'. They are used with significantly lower powder-liquid ratio, i.e. it ranges from 2:1 to 2.5:1. This makes it easier to mix and pour.

Method of flasking and curing
Agar hydrocolloid or silicone is used for the mold preparation in place of the usual gypsum. A special flask and resin *(Fig. 29.27A)* is used for the fluid resin technique. The technique involves preparing the mold with silicone *(Fig. 29.27B)*, creation of channels for pouring and venting *(Fig. 29.27C)* and pouring the fluid resin through one channel in a thin stream *(Fig. 29.27D)* till excess is seen through the vent *(Fig. 29.27E)*. Polymerization is done under pressure at 0.14 MPa (20 psi) at a temperature of 45 °C for 25 minutes.

Composition

Polymer	Monomer
Polymethyl methacrylate copolymer	Methyl methacrylate
Barbiturate acid derivatives	Quaternary sal ammoniac (ammonium chloride)
Color pigments	Stabilizers
	Catalyst
	Vulcaniser

Advantages of fluid resin technique
1. Better tissue fit.
2. Fewer open bites.
3. Less fracture of porcelain teeth during deflasking.
4. Reduced material cost.

5. Simple laboratory procedure for flasking (no trial closure), deflasking and finishing of the dentures.

Disadvantages
1. Air inclusion (bubbles).
2. Shifting of teeth during processing.
3. Infraocclusion (closed bites).
4. Occlusal imbalance due to shifting of teeth.
5. Incomplete flow of denture base material over neck of anterior teeth.
6. Formation of films of denture material over cervical portions of plastic teeth that had not been previously covered with wax.
7. Poor bonding to plastic teeth.
8. Technique sensitivity.

In general, these types of resins have some what lower mechanical properties than the conventional heat cured resins. Clinically acceptable dentures can be obtained when using any of the techniques, provided proper precautions are exercised.

LIGHT ACTIVATED DENTURE BASE RESINS

It consists of a *urethane dimethacrylate* matrix with an acrylic copolymer, microfine silica fillers, and a camphoroquinone-amine photoinitiator system.

Commercial name   VLC triad *(Fig. 29.28A)*

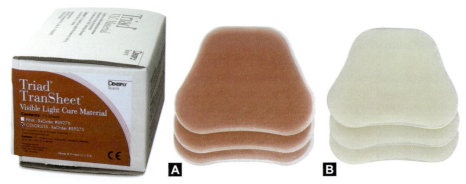

A	B
VLC Triad pink sheet for dentures	Pink denture base sheets

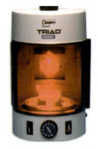

C

Light curing chamber (Dentsply)

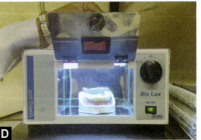

D

Light curing device Blu Lux
(*Courtesy* Yohan and Lippy, The Dental Center, Chennai)

FIGURES 29.28A TO D Light curing acrylic system.

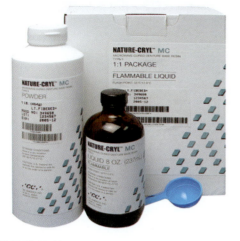

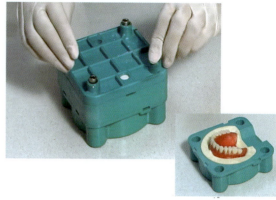

FIGURE 29.29 Microwave cured resins - Nature-Cryl by GC.   **FIGURE 29.30** Special flask for microwave resin technique.

Mode of supply

Triad products are available for various uses including denture base, custom tray, orthodontic appliances and temporary crowns and bridges. It is supplied in premixed sheets of having a clay like consistency *(Figs. 29.28A and B)*. It is supplied in various colors including pink transparent depending on its intended use. It is provided in opaque light tight packages to avoid premature polymerization.

Manipulation

The denture base material is adapted to the cast while it is in a plastic state. The denture base can be polymerized without teeth and used as baseplate. The teeth are added to the base with additional material and the anatomy is sculptured while the material is still soft. It is polymerized in a light chamber (curing unit) with blue light of 400-500 nm from high intensity quartz -halogen bulbs *(Figs. 29.28C and D)*. The denture is rotated continuously in the chamber to provide uniform exposure to the light source.

MICROWAVE CURED DENTURE RESINS

Microwave cured resins are available (Nature-Cryl by GC) *(Fig. 29.29)*. The material should comply with the requirements of ISO 20795-1:2013 type 5 denture base. The denture is invested and cured in a unique plastic flask *(Fig. 29.30)*. Dewaxing is done in a microwave for 1.5 minutes. Following Curing time is 3 to 4 minutes (depending on the product) in a standard household microwave oven.

SPECIALIZED POLY (METHYL METHACRYLATE) MATERIALS

Several modified poly (methyl methacrylate) materials have been used as denture resins. These include hydrophilic polyacrylates, high impact strength resins rapid heat polymerized acrylic, light-activated denture base material (described earlier) and pour type acrylic resins (described earlier).

HIGH IMPACT STRENGTH MATERIALS

These materials are butadiene-styrene rubber-reinforced poly (methyl methacrylate) *(Fig. 29.31)*. The rubber particles are grafted to methylmethacrylate so that they will bond well

TABLE 29.2 Comparison of resin and porcelain denture teeth

Resin	Porcelain
High fracture toughness	Brittle, may chip
Crazing if not cross-linked	Susceptible to crazing by thermal shock
Clinically significant wear	Insignificant wear
Easily ground and polished	Grinding difficult
Silent on contact	Clicking sound on impact
Dimensional change with water sorption	Dimensionally stable
Cold flow under stress	No permanent deformation
Loss of vertical dimension	Stable
Self-adjusting	Difficult to fit in diminished interarch space
Chemical bond to denture	Mechanical retention
Minimal abrasion of opposing dentition	Abrades opposing dentition
Easy to deflask	Difficult to deflask
Lower rate of monomer diffusion	Increased rate of monomer diffusion at higher temperature

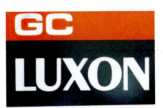

ACRYLIC DENTURE BASE RESIN
WITH HIGH IMPACT RESISTANCE

LIQUID 250g

FIGURE 29.31 Butadiene-styrene rubber-reinforced poly (methyl methacrylate).

to the heat polymerized acrylic matrix. These materials are supplied in a powder-liquid form and are processed in the same way as other heat-accelerated methyl methacrylate materials. These materials have twice the impact strength of conventional acrylic resins. They are indicated for patients who risk dropping their dentures repeatedly, e.g. senility, parkinsonism.

RAPID HEAT-POLYMERIZED RESINS

These are hybrid acrylics (e.g. QC 20) that are polymerized in boiling water immediately after being packed into a denture flask. After being placed into the boiling water, the water is brought back to a full boil for 20 minutes (reverse cure). After the usual bench cooling to room temperature, the denture is deflasked, trimmed and polished in the usual manner. The initiator is formulated to allow for rapid polymerization without the porosity that one might expect.

RESIN TEETH

The composition of resin teeth (*Fig. 29.12E*) is essentially poly (methyl methacrylate) copolymerized with a cross-linking agent. A greater amount of the cross-linking agent is used in resin teeth in order to reduce the tendency of the teeth to craze upon contact with the monomer-polymer dough during construction. The gingival *ridge-lap area* may not be as highly cross-linked as the incisal in order to facilitate chemical bonding to the denture base. Various pigments are utilized to produce a natural esthetic appearance.

The bond between the resin teeth and denture base resin is chemical in nature unlike porcelain teeth which requires mechanical locking. A comparison of resin and porcelain teeth is presented in *Table 29.2.* Failure may occur if the ridge lap area is *contaminated* with residual wax or separating media. The mold should be flushed well with a detergent solution in order to remove the wax completely.

Use of a flame for smoothing of the wax during teeth setting should be done carefully since the teeth surfaces may melt or burn. The resultant stresses induced during cooling may contribute to crazing in service.

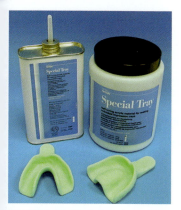

FIGURE 29.32 Autopolymerizing special tray acrylic resin.

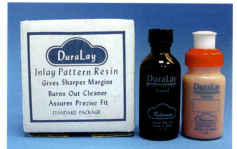

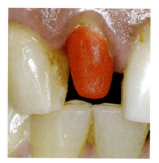

FIGURE 29.33 Duralay (above) is used for making direct patterns of inlays and posts (right). It is colored red to aid visual demarcation.

SPECIAL TRAY ACRYLIC RESINS

These are specialized chemically activated resins and are available as powder and liquid form *(Fig. 29.32)*. Some are available as light activated materials. They contain a high amount of inorganic fillers (e.g. French chalk) which increases the plasticity and workability of the material. They come in colors like green and blue. They are used to fabricate custom trays for making final impressions using zinc oxide eugenol, elastomeric materials and alginate, etc.

The custom-made acrylic resin trays may not be dimensionally stable until 20 to 24 hours after fabrication. Therefore it is advisable to use the tray after this period.

PATTERN RESINS

Commercial Name Duralay *(Fig. 29.33).*

It is a specialized resin intended for making patterns of inlays, posts *(Fig. 23.33)* and other structures in the mouth. Like wax, these materials burn off completely before casting. But unlike wax, they are dimensionally very stable after setting and are not affected by small temperature variations. The inlay cavity is lubricated. The powder and liquid are mixed and inserted into the cavity. It is shaped quickly into the desired form. Further shaping is done after it sets using a bur. The pattern is removed, invested and reproduced in metal.

PROPERTIES OF METHYLMETHACRYLATE DENTURE RESINS

Dentures are subjected to large stresses in the mouth. Acceptable denture resins must meet or exceed the standards specified in ISO 20795-1:2013 *(Table 29.3)*.

TABLE 29.3 Minimum specifications for denture base polymers (ISO 20795-1:2013)

Requirements	Flexural properties		Residual methyl methacrylate monomer	Sorption	Solubility
	Ultimate flexural strength	Flexural modulus			
	σ	E		w_{sp}	w_{sl}
	MPa	MPa	Percent mass fraction	$\mu g/mm^3$	$\mu g/mm^3$
	min.	min.	max.	max.	max.
Types 1, 3, 4, 5	65	2000	2,2	32	1,6
Type 2	60	1500	4,5	32	8,0

METHYL METHACRYLATE MONOMER

It is a clear, transparent, volatile liquid at room temperature. It has a characteristic sweetish odor. The physical properties of monomer are

Melting point	– 48 °C
Boiling point	100 °C
Density	0.945 gm/ml at 20 °C
Heat of polymerization	12.9 Kcal/mol
Volume shrinkage during polymerization	21%

POLY (METHYL METHACRYLATE)

Taste and odor

Completely polymerized acrylic resin is tasteless and odorless. On the other hand poorly made dentures with a high amount of porosity can absorb food and bacteria, resulting in an unpleasant taste and odor.

Esthetics

It is a clear transparent resin which can be pigmented (colored) easily to duplicate oral tissue. It is compatible with dyed synthetic fibers. Thus esthetics is acceptable.

Density

The polymer has a density of 1.19 gm/cm³.

Strength

These materials are typically low in strength. However they have adequate compressive and tensile strength for complete or partial denture applications.

Compressive strength	75 MPa
Tensile strength	48–62 MPa

Self cured resins generally have lower strength values.

The strength is affected by

1. Composition of the resin
2. Technique of processing
3. Degree of polymerization
4. Water sorption
5. Subsequent environment of the denture.

Impact strength

It is a measure of energy absorbed by a material when it is broken by a sudden blow. Ideally denture resins should have high impact strength to prevent breakage when accidentally dropped. Unmodified acrylic resins are generally brittle. Plasticizers increase the impact strength. However, the significant improvement in impact strength is observed when the resin is modified with rubber. The Izod test values* are shown below.

Chemically activated resin	– 13 (J/m)
Conventional heat-cured acrylic resin	– 15 (J/m)

*Values are useful for comparison only, as values vary with test methods, specimen dimensions and presence of surface defects.

Rubber modified acrylic resin	– 31 (J/m)
Polyvinyl resins	– 30 (J/m)

Fatigue strength

Fatigue strength refers to the ability of the denture to withstand large number of small cyclic loading such as during mastication over a period of time. Most current dental plastics have sufficient fatigue strength.

Hardness and wear resistance

Acrylic resins are materials having low hardness. They can be easily scratched and abraded. Polyvinyl acrylics have the best wear resistance and pour type acrylics has the least.

Heat cured acrylic resin	18 KHN
Self cured acrylic resin	16 KHN
Rubber modified acrylic resin	14 KHN
Light cured resin	18 KHN

Modulus of elasticity

They have sufficient stiffness for use in complete and partial dentures.

Self-cured acrylic resins have slightly lower values.

Creep

Denture resins exhibit creep. When a load is applied an initial deflection is observed. If the load is sustained additional deformation is observed over time. The additional deformation is called creep. Chemically activated resins have higher creep rates.

Dimensional stability

A well-processed acrylic resin denture has good dimensional stability. The processing shrinkage is balanced by the expansion due to water sorption.

Polymerization shrinkage

Acrylic resins shrink during processing due to

- Thermal shrinkage on cooling
- Polymerization shrinkage

During polymerization, the density of the monomer changes from 0.94 gm/cc to 1.19 gm/cc. This results in shrinkage in the volume of monomer-polymer dough.

However, in spite of the high shrinkage, the fit of the denture is not affected because the shrinkage is uniformly distributed over all surfaces of the denture. Thus, the actual linear shrinkage observed is low.

Volume shrinkage	8%
Linear shrinkage	0.53%

Self-cured type has a lower shrinkage (linear shrinkage— 0.26%).

Water sorption

Acrylic resins absorb water (0.7 mg/cm^2) and expand. This partially compensates for its processing shrinkage. This process is reversible. Thus on drying they lose water and shrink. However, repeated wetting and drying should be avoided as it may cause warpage of the denture.

Solubility

Acrylic is virtually insoluble in water and oral fluids. They are soluble in ketones, esters and aromatic and chlorinated hydrocarbons, e.g. chloroform and acetone. Alcohol causes crazing in some resins. ISO stipulates solubility should not exceed $1.6 \mu g/mm^3$ for type 1 (heat-cured) and $8.0 \mu g/mm^3$ for type 2 (self-cured).

Thermal properties

Stability to heat Poly (methyl methacrylate) is chemically stable to heat up to a point. It softens at 125 °C. However, above this temperature, i.e. between 125 °C and 200 °C it begins to depolymerize. At 450 °C, 90% of the polymer will depolymerize to monomer.

Thermal conductivity They are poor conductors of heat and electricity. This is undesirable because patients wearing acrylic complete dentures often complain that they cannot feel the temperature of food or liquids they ingest, thus reducing the pleasure. Replacing the palatal portion with metal is one solution, because the metal is a better conductor of heat. Inclusion of sapphire whiskers improves conductivity.

Thermal conductivity for acrylic resin is 5.7×10^{-4} cal/sec/cm^2) (°C/cm).

Coefficient of thermal expansion These materials have a high coefficient of thermal expansion (CTE). The CTE for poly(methylmethacrylate) resin is $81 \times 10^{-6}/$ °C. Addition of fillers reduces the CTE.

Heat distortion temperature This is the measure of the ability of a plastic to resist dimensional change when loaded under heat. It is measured by observing the temperature at which a specimen under a 1.8 MPa load deflects 0.25 mm.

Heat distortion temperature for PMMA   –   71 to 91 °C.

Heat distortion temperature for vinyl resin   –   54 to 77 °C.

Distortion is of concern during procedures like repair or polishing of dentures. Temperatures should be kept low to avoid distortion.

Color stability

Heat-cured acrylic resins have good color stability. The color stability of self-cure resins is slightly lower (yellows very slightly).

Biocompatibility

Completely polymerized acrylic resins are biocompatible.

True allergic reactions to acrylic resins are rarely seen in the oral cavity. The residual monomer (approximately 0.4% in a well-processed denture) is the usual component singled out as an irritant. A true allergy to acrylic resin can be recognized by a patch test.

Direct contact of the monomer over a period of time may provoke dermatitis. The high concentration of monomer in the dough may produce a local irritation and a serious sensitization of the fingers. Inhalation of monomer vapor is avoided.

Precautions to be taken are

1. Minimize residual monomer content by using proper processing techniques.
2. Avoid direct handling of acrylic dough with bare hands.
3. Work in well ventilated areas to avoid inhalation of the monomer vapor.

Residual monomer

During the polymerization process the amount of residual monomer decreases rapidly initially and then later more slowly.

The highest residual monomer level is observed with chemically activated denture base resins at 1 - 4% shortly after processing. When they are processed for less than one hour in boiling water the residual monomer is 1 - 3%. If it is processed for 7 hours at 70 °C and then boiled for 3 hours the residual monomer content may be less than 0.4%.

In heat cured acrylic before the start of curing the residual monomer is 26.2%. In 1 hour at 70 °C it decreases to 6.6% and at 100 °C it is 0.29%.

To reduce the residual monomer in heat cured dentures it should be processed for a longer time in boiling water. The temperature should be raised to boiling only after most of the polymerization is completed otherwise porosity may result.

Adhesion

The adhesion of acrylic to metal and porcelain is poor and mechanical retention is required. Adhesion to plastic denture teeth is good (chemical adhesion). Adhesion to metal or ceramic can be improved by treating with silane coupling agents.

Radiopacity

There have been instances of broken pieces of dentures being aspirated or swallowed. Radiopacity is a desirable property to enable easy location of the fragments. Most denture base materials are radiolucent. However a few radiopaque materials are being manufactured. Radiopacity is obtained by the inclusion of heavy metal salts like bismuth or uranyl at concentrations of 10 to 15%.

Shelf life

Acrylic resins dispensed as powder/liquid have the best shelf life. The gel type has a lower shelf life and has to be stored in a refrigerator.

PROCESSING ERRORS

POROSITY

Porosity presents many problems

1. It makes the appearance of denture base unsightly.
2. Proper cleaning of the denture is not possible, so the denture hygiene and thus, the oral hygiene suffers.
3. It weakens the denture base and the pores are areas of stress concentration, thus the denture warps as the stresses relax.

Porosity may be

A. Internal porosity
B. External porosity.

Internal porosity

Internal porosity appears as voids or bubbles within the mass of the polymerized acrylic. It is usually not present on the surface of the denture. It is confined to the thick portions of the denture base and it may not occur uniformly.

Cause   Internal porosity is due to the vaporization of monomer when the temperature of the resin increases above the boiling point of monomer (100.8 °C) or very low molecular weight polymers. Exothermic heat of the surface resin dissipates easily into the investing plaster. However, in the center of the thick portion the heat cannot be conducted away. Therefore, the temperature in the thick portions may rise above the boiling point of monomer causing porosity.

Avoided by Dentures with excessive thickness should be cured using a long, low temperature curing cycle.

External porosity

It can occur due to two reasons

○ *Lack of homogeneity* If the dough is not homogenous at the time of polymerization, the portions containing more monomer will shrink more. This localized shrinkage results in voids. The resin appears white.

  – *Avoided by* Using proper powder/liquid ratio and mixing it well. The mix is more homogenous in the dough stage, so packing should be done in the dough stage.

○ *Lack of adequate pressure* Lack of pressure during polymerization or inadequate amount of dough in the mold during final closure causes bubbles which are not spherical. The resin is lighter in color *(Fig. 29.34)*.

  – *Avoided by* Using the required amount of dough. Check for excess or flash during trail closure. Flash indicates adequate material.

CRAZING

Crazing is formation of surface cracks on the denture base resin *(Fig. 29.35)*. The cracks may be microscopic or macroscopic in size. In some cases it has a hazy or foggy appearance rather than cracks. Crazing weakens the resin and reduces the esthetic qualities. The cracks formed can cause fracture.

Causes

Crazing is due to

1. Mechanical stresses
2. Attack by a solvent
3. Incorporation of water

In poly (methyl methacrylate) crazing occurs when tensile stresses are present. The cracks are at right angles to the direction of tensile stress. Crazing is a mechanical separation of the polymer chains or groups under tensile stress.

Crazing is visible around the porcelain teeth in the denture and is due to the contraction of the resin around the porcelain teeth during cooling after processing. Weak solvents like alcohol result in randomly placed cracks.

Water incorporation during processing will form stresses due to evaporation of water after processing, causing crazing.

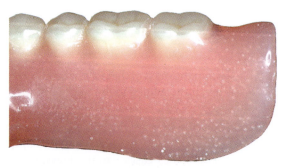

FIGURE 29.34 Surface and subsurface porosity from lack of insufficient pressure during curing.

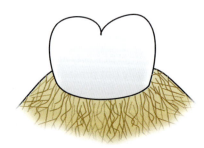

FIGURE 29.35 Representation of crazing in resins.

Avoided by

1. Using cross linked acrylics
2. Tin foil separating medium
3. Metal molds

DENTURE WARPAGE

Denture warpage is the deformity or change of shape of the denture which can affect the fit of the denture *(Fig. 29.36)*. Warpage can occur during processing as well as at other times.

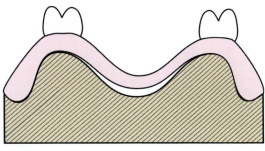

FIGURE 29.36 Denture warpage has resulted in a space between the palatal surface and the cast. Obviously this would affect the fit.

It is caused by a release of stresses incorporated during processing. Some of the stresses are incorporated as a result of the curing shrinkage while other stresses may be a result of the uneven or rapid cooling. Packing of the resin during the rubbery stage can also induce stresses. Some stresses may be incorporated during improper deflasking. These stresses are released subsequently

○ During polishing, a rise in temperature can cause warpage
○ Immersion of the denture in hot water can cause warpage
○ Re-curing of the denture after addition of relining material, etc.

REPAIR OF ACRYLIC RESIN DENTURES

An acrylic denture fractured in service can be repaired. Repair resins may be

○ Heat cured, or
○ Self cured.

Heat cured resin

These resins are cured at 74 °C for 8 hours or more. The use of a heat cured resin will tend to warp the denture during processing.

Self cured resin

Although the repair with a self-cured resin invariably has a lower transverse strength than that of the original heat-cured denture base resin, self-cured resins are usually preferred because warpage is insignificant as curing is done at room temperature.

INFECTION CONTROL FOR DENTURES

Care should be taken to prevent cross-contamination between patients and dental personnel. New appliances should be disinfected after construction.

Items such as rag wheels often can be steam-autoclaved. Appliances can be sprayed with disinfectants before they leave the operatory. Since the polymeric materials can absorb liquids, toxic agents such as phenol or glutaraldehyde are avoided. Ethylene oxide gas is a suitable method.

CARE OF ACRYLIC DENTURES

Denture treatment is time consuming and labor intensive, besides being expensive. Therefore proper care and maintenance of the denture is important.

○ Dentures should be stored in water when not in use, since dimensional changes can occur on drying.

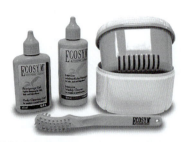

FIGURE 29.37 A commercially available denture cleansing kit. It includes a brush and container for storage.

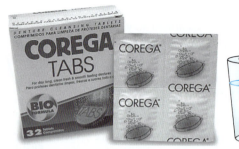

FIGURE 29.38 Immersion type denture cleaning tablets.

- ❍ Acrylic dentures should not be cleaned in *hot water*, since processing stresses can be released and can result in distortion.
- ❍ Abrasive dentifrices (regular toothpastes) should not be used, since the plastic is soft and can be easily scratched and abraded. The *tissue surface* should be brushed carefully with a soft brush *(Fig. 29.37)*, since any material removed alters the fit of the denture.

Besides physical brushing various cleaning agents are commercially available (see denture cleansers).

DENTURE CLEANSERS

A wide variety of agents are used by patients for cleaning artificial dentures. They include dentifrices, proprietary denture cleansers, soap and water, salt and soda, household cleansers, bleaches and vinegar.

Dentures are cleaned by either

1. Immersion in an agent or
2. By brushing with the cleanser.

The most common commercial denture cleansers are the immersion type *(Fig. 29.38)*, which are available as a powder or tablet.

Their composition usually includes

- ❍ Alkaline compounds
- ❍ Detergents
- ❍ Flavoring agents
- ❍ Sodium perborate

When the powder is dissolved in water, the perborate decomposes to form an alkaline peroxide solution, which in turn decomposes to liberate *oxygen*. The oxygen bubbles then acts mechanically to loosen the debris.

Vinegar is effective in dissolving calculus. The household cleansers are contraindicated, as they affect the fit of the denture and produce rough surface on prolonged use.

CAD/CAM DENTURES

Computer Aided Design – Computer Aided Manufacturing (CAD/CAM) technology has already made significant strides in the field of dentistry, especially in the field of ceramic crowns and bridges. Recently, CAD/CAM technology has become commercially available for fabrication of complete dentures *(Fig. 29.39)*. It is a system by which impressions, interocclusal records

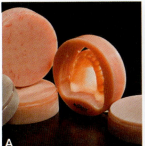

A CAD/CAM blanks

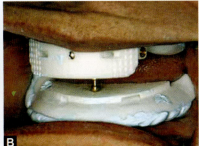

B Anatomical measuring device

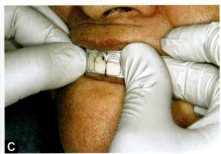

C Teeth selection using mold tabs

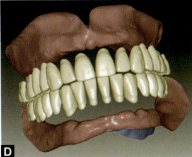

D Virtual designing

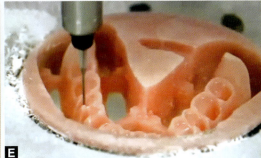

E Milling operation

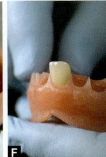

F Teeth arrangement

FIGURES 29.39A TO F CAD/CAM system (AvaDent).

and tooth selection can be completed in one appointment. The dentures are then fabricated using CAD/ CAM technology and placed in the second appointment.

Commercial names AvaDent digital dentures (Global Dental Science, LLC), Dentca CAD/CAM, Nobilium CAD/CAM.

TECHNIQUE

The denture is fabricated in 2 visits.

First visit   Impressions, jaw relation records, occlusal plane orientation, tooth mold and shade selection, and maxillary anterior tooth positioning record.

Second visit   Placement of dentures.

The Avadent denture system involves proprietary equipment which makes it possible to fabricate the dentures in 2 visits. One of this includes the anatomical measuring device (AMD) *(Fig. 29.39B)* which helps to establish maxillomandibular relationship, perform gothic arch tracing, establish lip fullness and assist in teeth selection. Mold tabs *(Fig. 29.39C)* are used for teeth selection. The impressions together with the customized AMD and the selected mold are sent to the specialized labs where they are digitized and a virtual denture designed *(Fig. 29.39D)*. The denture base without teeth is milled *(Fig. 29.39E)* from blanks *(Fig. 29.39A)* and the teeth are bonded subsequently using a proprietary glue *(Fig. 29.39F).*

ADVANTAGES

1. Less number of appointments.
2. Less chairtime.
3. Less waiting period for final denture.
4. Low shrinkage as no polymerization process is involved.
5. Duplicate dentures easy to make as records are stored digitally.

DENTURE RELINERS

Reliners may be classified as

1. Hard or soft (resilient)
2. Heat cured or self cured
3. Short term or long term
4. Resin based or silicone based.

HEAT CURED ACRYLIC RESIN (HARD LINER)

New resin is cured against the old denture by compression molding technique. A low curing temperature is necessary for the relining process to avoid distortion of the denture.

Disadvantages

There is a tendency for it to warp toward the relined side due to

○ Diffusion of the monomer from the reliner before curing, and

○ Processing shrinkage of the liner. For this reason the rebasing is preferred to relining.

CHAIRSIDE RELINERS (HARD SHORT-TERM LINER)

These materials are used for relining resin dentures directly in the mouth *(Fig. 29.40)*. Some of them generate enough heat to injure oral tissues. According to ADA Sp. No. 17, peak temperature reached during curing should not be more than 75 °C. Generally the specifications are far less demanding for these materials than for the regular denture base resins. On the whole their properties are inferior to laboratory processed acrylic resins. They have higher porosity and water sorption. They often contain low molecular weight polymers, plasticizers or

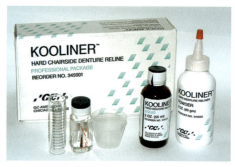

FIGURE 29.40 Hard setting chairside denture liner.

solvents to increase their fluidity while seating the denture. They tend to discolor, become foul smelling and may even separate from the denture base. Thus, these materials have many disadvantages and are therefore considered as short-term materials.

Light-activated resins are also available for relining.

SOFT OR RESILIENT DENTURE LINERS

International standards organization describes two categories of soft liners.

1. Short-term soft liners (also known as tissue conditioners) (ISO 10139 Part 1).
2. Long-term soft liners (ISO 10139 Part 2).

LONG-TERM SOFT LINERS

The purpose of the 'permanent' soft liner *(Fig. 29.41)* is to protect the soft tissue by acting as a cushion. They are used when there is irritation of the mucosa, in areas of severe undercut and congenital or acquired defects of palate.

Requirements

1. Good bonding to the denture base.

2. Should be biocompatible.
3. Should be hygienic and not become foul smelling.
4. Should maintain its resilience for a long period.
5. Should have good dimensional stability.
6. Should inhibit bacterial growth.
7. Low water sorption (max. 20 µg/mm^3).
8. Easy to process.

Classification (ISO 10139-2:2009)

1. Based on depth of penetration

   Type A—soft

   Type B—extra soft

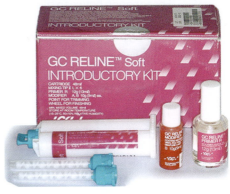

FIGURE 29.41 Soft denture liner.

2. Based on their method of processing they are further divided into
   - Mouth cured or chairside soft liners – does not last beyond a few weeks.
   - Processed soft liners – lasts up to a year.

Types

Several soft lining materials are available commercially

- Plasticized acrylic resin
- Plasticized vinyl resins
- Silicone rubbers
- Polyphosphazine

PLASTICIZED ACRYLIC RESIN

This is most commonly used. It may be self-cured or heat-cured. In self-cured type, poly (ethyl methacrylate), poly (methyl methacrylate) or an acrylate copolymer is mixed with an aromatic ester-ethanol liquid containing 30–60% plasticizer, such as dibutyl phthalate.

The heat-cured resin may be supplied in a sheet form or powder-liquid form. The powder is composed of selected acrylic resin polymers and copolymers, so that when they are mixed with the appropriate monomer and plasticizer liquid, the glass transition (softening) temperature of the cured resin will be below mouth temperature.

Disadvantages   They lose plasticizers and harden with use.

VINYL RESINS

The plasticized poly (vinyl chloride) and poly (vinyl acetate) resins, like the plasticized acrylic resins, lose plasticizer and harden during use.

SILICONE RUBBERS

These materials retain their elastic properties but may loose adhesion to the denture base.

Room temperature curing   chairside silicone.

Heat-cured silicones   They are generally a one-component system. They are supplied as a paste or gel containing an oxygen catalyst. It is heat polymerized against acrylic resin using compression molding technique.

For adhesion between silicones and the denture base, a rubber poly (methyl methacrylate) graft polymer solution cement may be used (one brand does not requires adhesive as it contains a copolymer of silicone and a second polymer that achieves adhesion to the acrylic resin).

Other polymers   Polyurethane and polyphosphazine rubber.

Problems associated with soft liners

1. Inadequate bonding to denture, especially silicone liners.
2. Some silicone liners and the hydrophilic acrylics undergo a high volume change (up to 40%) with gain and loss of water.
3. The heat cured soft acrylics bond well to the hard denture base but loose their softness as plasticizer is leached from the liner.
4. It reduces the denture base strength, not only because of reduced base thickness but also by solvent action of the silicone adhesive and the monomer.
5. Trimming, cutting, adjusting and polishing of a soft liner is difficult. The silicone surface is abrasive and irritating to the oral mucosa when compared to that of hard acrylic resin.
6. The greatest disadvantage of the permanent soft liner, as well as the tissue conditioner (temporary soft liner) is that they often have a characteristic disagreeable taste and odor and they cannot be cleaned as effectively.
7. The debris that accumulate in pores in the silicone liner can promote fungal growth (*Candida albicans*).

None of the soft denture reliners can be considered entirely satisfactory. It is necessary to review the patients periodically and if necessary change the material.

TISSUE CONDITIONERS (SHORT-TERM SOFT LINER)

Unlike the soft liners previously mentioned, tissue conditioners are soft elastomers used to treat irritated mucosa. Their useful function is very short, generally a matter of a few days. They are replaced every 3-5 days. Their hardness ranges from 14–49 Shore A hardness units 24 hours after mixing. They lose alcohol over time resulting in a weight loss of 5–9%. These materials show both viscous and viscoelastic behavior which help in both adaptation to tissue and cushioning of masticatory forces.

Uses

1. Ill-fitting dentures can cause inflammation and distortion of the oral tissues. Relining an ill-fitting denture with tissue conditioner allows the tissues to return to 'normal' at which point a new denture can be made.
2. As an impression material (this material is used in a special impression technique known as *functional impression*).

Composition

These are highly plasticized acrylic resins, supplied as a powder and a liquid.

Powder   Poly (ethyl methacrylate) or one of its copolymers.

Liquid   Aromatic ester (butyl phthalate butyl glycolate) in ethanol or an alcohol of high molecular weight.

Manipulation

The denture base is relieved on the tissue surface. Powder and liquid are mixed together to form a gel and it is placed on the tissue surface of the denture and inserted in the mouth. The gel flows readily to fill the space between the denture base and the oral tissue.

The properties that make tissue conditioners effective are

1. Viscous properties, which allow excellent adaptation to the irritated denture-bearing mucosa over a period of several days and brings it back to health.
2. Elastic behavior which cushions the tissues from the forces of mastication and bruxism.

DENTURE ADHESIVES

Denture adhesives are highly viscous aqueous solutions which are often used to improve the retention of complete dentures.

SUPPLIED AS

Powders or Paste *(Figs. 29.42 and 29.43)*.

COMPOSITION

Keraya gum

Tragacanth

Sodium carboxy methyl cellulose

Polyethylene oxide

Flavoring agents

Some also contain antimicrobial agents and plasticizers.

PROPERTIES

When applied to the denture base and inserted, the polymer portion absorbs water and swells. They improve the retention of the denture base through adhesion. It fills up the spaces between the denture and the tissue. The high viscosity also prevents displacement. They usually have a pleasant smell.

Biological considerations

Most of the components are permitted food additives and are generally safe. However, if ingested in excess, they can cause gastrointestinal disorders. Keraya gum can cause allergic reaction to some patients. It is also acidic (pH 4.7-5) and can cause caries if natural teeth are present. Therefore, its use is contraindicated in partially edentulous patients.

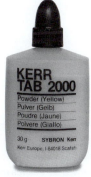

FIGURE 29.42 Denture adhesive powder.

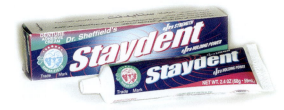

FIGURE 29.43 Denture adhesive paste.

Disadvantages

It has an unpleasant feel, is difficult to clean and is diluted easily by saliva.

Indications

Considering its properties, its use should be limited to

1. Temporary retention of poorly fitting dentures.
2. Patients having poor neuromuscular control.

REBASING OF DENTURES

Because of soft tissue changes that occur during wearing of the denture, it is often necessary to *change the tissue surface* of the denture. Such a readaptation of the denture is done by either rebasing or relining the denture.

DIFFERENCE BETWEEN REBASING AND RELINING

In rebasing, the *original teeth are retained* and a new denture bearing area is constructed with heat-cure acrylic resin. In other words, the entire denture base is replaced with new material.

In relining, only a part of the tissue surface of the denture is removed and replaced with new material.

PROVISIONAL CROWN AND FDP MATERIALS

The fabrication of a crown or fixed partial denture (FDP) is a laboratory procedure, and several weeks may lapse between the preparation of the teeth and the cementation of the final restoration. A provisional restoration *(Fig. 29.44)* provides protection to the pulp from thermal and chemical irritation caused by food and liquids, maintains positional stability, aids mastication and maintains esthetics during this interim period.

Required properties

1. A temporary restoration must be nonirritating to soft tissues and pulp.
2. They should have adequate strength to withstand forces of mastication for the interim period.
3. They should be esthetic especially for the anterior teeth.
4. Low thermal conductivity.
5. Low dimensional change and low exothermic reaction.
6. Easy to manipulate.

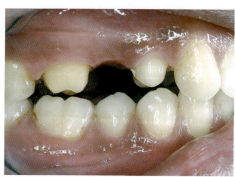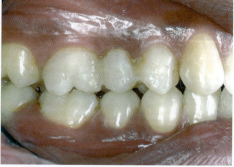

FIGURE 29.44 A provisional fixed partial denture protects the abutment teeth as well as restores esthetics and function during the interim period. The provisional bridge in the picture was constructed with Protemp 2.

Functions of provisional restorations

1. Maintenance of esthetics and function.
2. Protection of prepared dentine from thermal and chemical trauma.
3. Maintenance of gingival position, contour and health.
4. Maintenance of good oral hygiene.
5. Maintenance of occlusal stability and prevention of supraeruption.
6. Prevention of drifting or tilting of adjacent teeth.
7. Allows the dentist to check that sufficient interocclusal reduction has been prepared.
8. Assists the clinician in diagnosis and treatment planning.
9. Assists the clinician in the construction of a new occlusal scheme.
10. Allows the esthetic evaluation of replacements.

Materials

Provisional crown and FDP materials may be preformed or custom-fabricated.

PREFORMED CROWNS

Synonym Anatomic crowns.

A preformed crown forms the external contour of the crown. These crowns can be luted directly to the prepared teeth after adjustment or they may be relined with a resin prior to cementation. The various preformed materials include

- Polycarbonate
- Cellulose acetate
- Aluminum *(Fig. 29.45)*
- Nickel-chrome
- Tin-silver.

Polycarbonate

This is a polymer of high impact resistance *(Fig. 29.45)*. It has an esthetic natural appearance. It is available only in a single shade. They are supplied in incisor, canine and premolar shapes.

Cellulose acetate crown formers

Cellulose acetate is a thin transparent matrix available in all tooth shapes and a range of sizes *(Fig. 29.45)*. It is used in combination with a tooth colored resin. It primarily acts as

Polycarbonate   Cellulose acetate   Aluminum shell

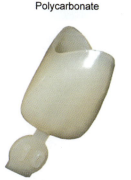 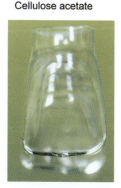 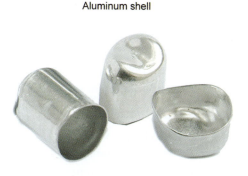

FIGURE 29.45 Different types of provisional preformed crowns.

a template within which the provisional material is filled and placed over the prepared tooth. After the acrylic resin sets, the cellulose acetate is peeled off and discarded and the crown is trimmed and cemented.

CUSTOM-FABRICATED PROVISIONAL RESTORATIONS

Temporary or provisional crowns and FDPs *(Fig. 29.44)* can also be custom-made from various types of resin. The materials used are

- Polymethyl methacrylate resins (Gel)
- Polyethyl (isobutyl) methacrylate resins (Trim, Snap)
- Epimine resins
- Resin based composite provisionals *(Fig. 29.44)* (refer chapter on Resin Based Composites).

Polymethyl methacrylate

These resins are generally self cured.

Commercial name   Gel.

Advantages

1. Acceptable mechanical properties.
2. Color stability is better than that of poly ethylmethacrylate resins.

Disadvantages

1. High polymerization shrinkage.
2. High heat liberation during setting.
3. High irritation to gingival tissues.

Polyethyl (isobutyl) methacrylate resins

These are available as a two component powder-monomer system. The two components are mixed to form a dough and inserted into a template which is placed over the prepared tooth/teeth. When set the material assumes the shape of the crown or FDP. Heat accelerates the setting. The excess material is trimmed and the restoration smoothened and polished. The restoration is tried intraorally and cemented with a suitable temporary cement.

Commercial name   Trim, Snap *(Fig. 29.46)*.

Advantages

1. Less polymerization shrinkage and heat liberation.
2. Flow better during adaptation.
3. Less irritation to soft tissues.

Disadvantages

1. Less tensile strength.
2. Poor color stability.
3. Clogs bur if trimmed with high speed turbines.

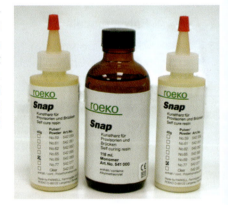

FIGURE 29.46 Snap is a self-curing polyethyl methacrylate resin used for making provisional restorations.

Epimines

The epimines are supplied as a two-component system. A paste containing a high-molecular weight epimine monomer combined with a polyamide (nylon) filler and a liquid containing a benzene sulfonate catalyst.

Advantages

1. Less polymerization shrinkage.
2. Less exothermic heat.
3. Good flow properties.

Disadvantages

1. Tissue irritation (caused by catalyst).
2. Poor impact strength.
3. Poor resistance to abrasion.
4. Expensive.

Maxillofacial Prosthetic Materials

IDEAL REQUIREMENTS

Maxillofacial materials are used to correct facial defects or deformities resulting from cancer surgery, accidents or congenital deformities. Nose, ears, eyes or any other part of the head and neck may be reconstructed by these prostheses *(Figs. 30.1 and 30.2)*. They are also used in the movie industry for special effects. Ancient Chinese and Egyptians used waxes and resins to reconstruct missing portions of the face and head.

Since the 1500 CE when facial prostheses were described by French surgeon Ambrose Pare (1575), they have evolved from prosthesis made from gold, silver, paper, cloth, leather, wrought metals, ceramics and vulcanite. Modern maxillofacial prosthetics saw a resurgence after world war due to severe nature of the war related injuries. In spite of the advances in techniques and materials there is still a lot of scope for further development in this field.

Ideal requirements

1. These materials must be biocompatible, easy and inexpensive to fabricate, strong and durable.
2. The prosthesis must be skin-like in appearance and texture.

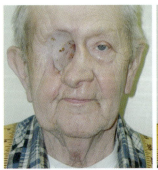 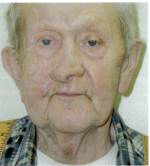

FIGURE 30.1 Pre- and post-treatment photos of an orbital prosthesis.

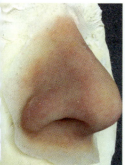
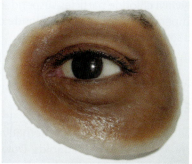
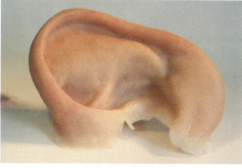

| Nasal prosthesis | Orbital prosthesis | Auricular prosthesis |

FIGURE 30.2 Different types of maxillofacial prostheses. Notice the transparent feathered edges that aid in blending the prosthesis to the face.

3. It must be color stable as it is subjected to sunlight (including ultraviolet light) heat, and cold.
4. It must be easy to clean and manage by the patient.
5. Facial prostheses are often constructed with thin margins to enable blending to the skin. This is then attached to the skin with adhesives. On removing at night, the thin edges can tear. It must be resilient enough to prevent tearing.
6. The water absorption of the prosthetic material is important since facial prostheses may absorb saliva or sweat from surrounding facial tissue. During washing, the prosthesis can absorb water. Any absorbed water may affect the physical properties and also affect the perception of color matching to the surrounding facial tissue.
7. It should be hygienic and prevent growth of microorganisms.
8. It should have translucent properties of the part it is replacing.

No material so far has all of these characteristics.

EVOLUTION OF MAXILLOFACIAL MATERIALS

POLY (METHYL METHACRYLATE) (1940–1960)

It was once commonly used for maxillofacial prosthesis. It is readily available, easy to manipulate, strong, color, stable, hygienic and durable. Its usefulness in extra-oral prosthesis is limited because acrylic is hard and heavy, does not move when the face moves and does not have the feel of skin. Particularly used in cases where there is least movement of tissue bed during function.

LATEXES

Latexes are soft, inexpensive and easy to manipulate. They are realistic and form lifelike prostheses. However, the finished product is weak, degenerates rapidly with age and changes color. Latex is no longer a major facial prosthetic material.

PLASTICIZED POLYVINYL CHLORIDE

Polyvinyl chloride is a rigid plastic and is made more flexible by adding a plasticizer. Other ingredients added to polyvinyl chloride include cross-linking against (for strength) and ultraviolet stabilizers (for color stability). Color pigments can be incorporated to match individual skin tones.

It is supplied as finely divided polyvinyl chloride particles suspended in a solvent. When the fluid is heated above a critical temperature, the polyvinyl chloride dissolves in the solvent. When the mix is cooled, an elastic solid is formed.

The prosthesis becomes hard with age because the plasticizers are lost from the surface of the prosthesis.

CHLORINATED POLYETHYLENE

This material was introduced in the 1970s and 1980s as an alternative to silicone. Processing involves high heat curing pigmented sheets in metal molds. Dow chemicals' chlorinated polyethylene elastomer is an industrial grade thermoplastic elastomer. It is less irritating to the mucosa than silicone, less toxic than thermosetting silicone materials and noncarcinogenic. Chlorinated polyethylene elastomer appears to be a suitable substitute for silicones for the fabrication of extraoral maxillofacial prosthesis in situations where cost of silicone is prohibitive.

Advantages   Higher edge strength, permanent elasticity and lower fungus growth

POLYURETHANE POLYMERS

It is the most recent addition. One of its components is acrylate, which needs careful handling to prevent a toxic reaction to the operator. Although the material is cured at room temperature, it requires accurate temperature control because a slight change in temperature can alter the chemical reaction. A metal mold is used to avoid moisture in the air affecting the processing.

It has lifelike feel and appearance and the color stability is better than that of polyvinyl chloride. But it is susceptible to deterioration with time.

SILICONE RUBBER

Silicones were introduced as a maxillofacial material in the 1950s. Currently silicone based maxillofacial materials are the most widely used. Based on curing mechanism, two types of silicone rubber are available. Both types are widely used.

○ RTV – Room Temperature Vulcanized
○ HTV – Heat Vulcanized Silicones

Supplied as

Both HTV and RTV silicones are available as fluid, semisolid, gel-like or putty-like material. They are generally supplied as clear or translucent materials though occasionally they may be supplied pre-pigmented (e.g. flesh colored - 2009 by Factor II).

They are usually provided as base and catalyst where the base-catalyst ratio is 10:1. However base-catalyst ratio of 1:1 is also available.

Room temperature vulcanized (RTV) silicones

Room vulcanizing silicones \ are available as fluid, semisolid or putty-like material. They may be transparent or translucent. The prosthesis can be easily fabricated in the dental laboratory with little special equipment using RTV silicones *(Fig. 30.3)*. However, such silicones are not as strong as the heat-vulcanized silicones and the intrinsic color is monochromatic.

Types   1. Both condensation (tin catalyzed), and

2. Addition types (platinum catalyzed) are available.

Working time   Ranges from 10 min to 2 hours depending on the product.

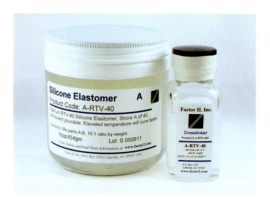

FIGURE 30.3 Room temperature vulcanized (RTV) silicones showing base and catalyst.

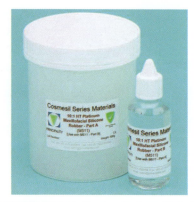

FIGURE 30.4 Heat vulcanized maxillofacial silicone with catalyst (Cosmesil M511).

Curing   Curing time varies with products and can range from 25 minutes to 24 hours depending on the product. Optimal room temperature for curing is around 25 °C. Very high temperatures and humidity reduce working time. Lower temperatures also not recommended (below 20 °C) as it can cause retardation of setting and affect the properties.

Heat vulcanized silicones

Heat vulcanizing silicone is available as semisolid or putty-like material. They are supplied as a two-component system—a base (vinyl and hydride containing siloxanes) and catalyst (chloroplatinic acid catalyst) *(Fig. 30.4)*.

Commercial examples   Cosmesil M511, Nusil, Factor II, TechSil S25, etc.

Fabrication involves milling, packing under pressure and curing. Pigments are milled into the material for intrinsic coloring. This is the material of choice, particularly in terms of strength and color stability. The coloring procedure is faster. Both intrinsic and extrinsic stains *(Figs. 30.5A to C)* can be used making it polychromatic.

Curing   One current silicone (Cosmesil M511) has a working time of approximately 1 hour and curing time approximately 1 hour at 100 °C.

Advantages   Better strength and color stability.

Disadvantages   Milling machine and press is required. A metal mold is normally used and the fabrication of the mold is a lengthy procedure.

Coloring pigments and effects

To simulate natural skin and body appearance, various cosmetic grade pigments both intrinsic *(Fig. 30.5C)* and extrinsic *(Figs. 30.5A and B)* may be applied. They include a range of colors as well as basic skin shades. Pigments and fibers are available as

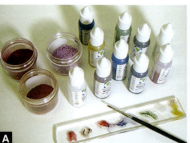
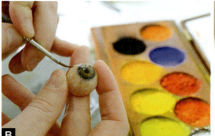
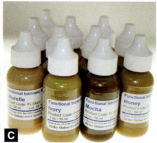

FIGURES 30.5A TO C (A) Extrinsic stains. **(B)** Extrinsic staining of ocular prosthesis. **(C)** Skin tones for intrinsic haracterization.

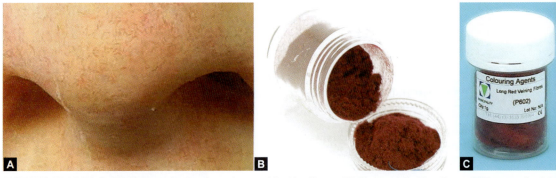

FIGURES 30.6A TO C (A) Characterization through use of flocking fibers. **(B)** Short red flocking fibers. **(C)** Long red veining fibers.

○ Dry powder

○ Liquid stains

○ Flocking microfibers are added to silicones to provide increased appearance of depth and light scattering **(Figs. 30.6A to C)**

○ Short veining fibers

○ Longer fibers for creating appearance of more complex veining structures **(Fig. 30.6C)**

Skin adhesives

Adhesives are often used to attach the prosthesis to the skin **(Figs. 30.7A and B)**. Various forms of adhesives used are water-based gels, creams, liquids or silicone-based pastes. Water-based adhesives are easily washed off with soap and warm water.

PROPERTIES OF SILICONES

Shore hardness

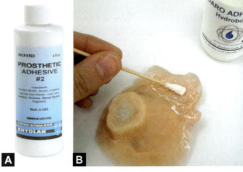

FIGURES 30.7A AND B (A) Skin adhesive. **(B)** Skin adhesive is applied to blend and secure an orbital prosthesis.

In order to achieve a lifelike feel, the material must be soft and compressible like flesh. Most materials have a shore hardness value ranging from 15 to 40. Hardness can be controlled through the use of softening agents supplied by the manufacturer. Depending on the tissue be replaced, tissue consistency may be soft (Shore A:10), medium (Shore A:30) or hard (Shore A:40).

Elongation

Elongation ranges from 340 to 630%.

Bonding to acrylic

Bonding to acrylic is required on occasion to attach dentures an other acrylic prostheses to the silicone prostheses. Bonding may be achieved by the use of a special primer/bonding agent.

Tear strength

Tear strength ranges from 84 to 120 ppi.

ADVANTAGES OF MAXILLOFACIAL SILICONES OVER OTHER MATERIALS

Polyvinyl siloxane is the most successful maxillofacial prosthetic material till date and new advances are being made to this material to overcome their weaknesses.

Silicones became more popular over other materials for the following reasons.

1. They have a range of good physical properties (such as excellent tear and tensile strength) over a greater range temperature range.
2. Easier to manipulate.
3. High degree of chemical inertness.
4. Low degree of toxicity.
5. High degree of thermal and oxidative stability.
6. They can be stained intrinsically and/or extrinsically to give them more life-like natural appearance.
7. When adequately cured, silicones elastomers resist absorbing organic materials that lead to bacterial growth and so with simple cleaning these materials are relatively safe and sanitary compared to other materials.

DISADVANTAGES OF MAXILLOFACIAL SILICONES

1. Susceptible to fungus growth.
2. Susceptible to fraying at the edges.

3D PRINTED MAXILLOFACIAL PROSTHESES

Conventional maxillofacial prostheses are incredibly laborious and expensive to produce can take up to 10 weeks to complete. The process involves taking an impression from the area of trauma, casting a plaster positive, then making a mould, carving the desired form in wax, and finally casting in silicone. The end-result of this handmade process is normally expensive ranging between £1,500 to £3,000.

Among others, Sheffield-based Fripp Design has developed a system for fast and low-cost manufacture of facial prostheses such as nose and ear replacements for accident victims.

Working with researchers at the University of Sheffield, the company developed a process that can print a customised nose or ear within 48 hours. First the patient's face is 3D-scanned, then the specific contours are added to a digital model of the new prosthetic part for a perfect fit. These features are either taken from the scan of the patients' relatives or the patient's own file, for example, one ear can be scanned and mirrored to replicate another.

Work is also in progress on 3D-printed eyes. A handmade eye can cost between $ 1800 to 8300, but a 3D printed one will only cost around $160. The parts are printed in full color in starch powder using a Z Corp Z510 color 3D printer. The lightweight model is then vacuum-infiltrated with medical grade silicone, binding it together *(Fig. 30.8)*. The cost of making such a part is almost the same as a handmade prosthetic, but Fripp says once the file is created, it can be used infinitely and the cost can be lowered to £150.

The main barrier is the high cost of 3D scanning technology as well as getting approval from the health authority.

3D BIOPRINTING

A natural evolution of artificial prostheses would ultimately be the ultimate goal of creating replacements of missing facial parts using living substitutes. The technology of 3D

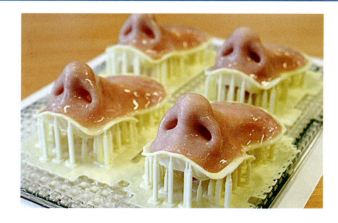

FIGURE 30.8 3D printed nasal prostheses.

bioprinting—the medical application of 3D printing to produce living tissue and organs is rapidly advancing.

In August 2013, the Hangzhou Dianzi University in China announced it had invented the biomaterial 3D printer Regenovo, which printed living cells that survived for up to four months. San Diego medical research company Organovo announced last year it had created slices of functioning, long-lasting human liver which can survive for 40 days, using a 3D printer. Dr Faiz Y Bhora, Director of Thoracic Surgical Oncology at the St Luke's-Roosevelt Hospital Center in New York, focuses his work on producing 3D printed tracheas from completely biologic materials primed with stem cells for growth.

Bioengineering involves the creation of scaffolds on which the tissues can grow. The scaffolds must meet some specific requirements. A high porosity and an adequate pore size are necessary to facilitate cell seeding and diffusion throughout the whole structure of both cells and nutrients. Biodegradability is often an essential factor since scaffolds should preferably be absorbed by the surrounding tissues without the necessity of a surgical removal.

A commonly used synthetic material is polylactic acid (PLA). This is a polyester which degrades within the human body to form lactic acid, a naturally occurring chemical which is easily removed from the body. Other materials are polyglycolic acid (PGA) and polycaprolactone (PCL).

Scaffolds may also be constructed from natural materials. Derivatives of the extracellular matrix have been studied to evaluate their ability to support cell growth. Proteic materials such as collagen or fibrin and polysaccharides like chitosan or glycosaminoglycans (GAGs), have all proved suitable in terms of cell compatibility, but some issues with potential immunogenicity still remain. Among GAGs hyaluronic acid, possibly in combination with cross-linking agents (e.g. glutaraldehyde, water soluble carbodiimide, etc.) is one of the possible choices as scaffold material. Another form of scaffold under investigation is decellularised tissue extracts whereby, the remaining cellular remnants/extracellular matrices act as the scaffold.

Problems to overcome in the field of bioengineering remain problems with revascularization and debate on the ethical ramifications (see also chapter on additive manufacturing).

Appendices

Appendix 1
ADA/ANSI Specifications

ADA Sp.	ISO	Product
No. 1	ISO 1559/24234:2004	Alloy for dental amalgam
No. 2	ISO 7490:2000	Dental gypsum-bonded casting investments
No. 6	ISO 1560/24234:2004	Dental mercury
No. 12	ISO 1567:1999/Amd 1:2003	Denture base polymers
No. 15	ISO 3336:1993	Synthetic polymer teeth
No. 16		Dental impression paste—zinc oxide-eugenol type
No. 17	ISO 10139-1:2005/Cor 1:2006	Denture base temporary relining resins
No. 18	ISO 1563:1990	Alginate impression materials
No. 19	ISO 4823:2000	Dental elastomeric impression material
No. 23		Dental excavating bur
No. 25	ISO 6873:1998	Dental gypsum products
No. 27	2005	Resin-based filling materials
No. 28		Root canal files and reamers, type K for hand use
No. 30	ISO 3107:2004/Cor 1:2006	Dental zinc oxide - eugenol and zinc oxide - noneugenol cements
No. 32		Orthodontic wires
No. 33		Dental product standards development vocabulary
No. 34		Dental aspirating syringes
No. 37		Dental abrasive powders
No. 38	ISO 22674:2006	Metal-ceramic dental restorative systems (ISO 9693:1999/Amd 1:2005 replaced by ISO 22674:2006)
No. 39	ISO 6874:2005	Pit and fissure sealants
No. 41		Biological evaluation of dental materials
No. 39	ISO 6874:2005	Pit and fissure sealants
No. 41		Biological evaluation of dental materials
No. 42	ISO 9694–1998	Dental phosphate-bonded casting investments
No. 43		Electrically powered dental amalgamators
No. 46		Dental chairs
No. 47		Dental units
No. 48		Visible light curing units`

ADA Sp.	ISO	Product
No. 53	ISO 10477:2004	Polymer-based crowns and bridge resins
No. 54		Double-pointed, parenteral, single use needles for dentistry
No. 57	ISO 6876:2001	Endodontic sealing material
No. 58		Root canal files, type H (Hedstrom)
No. 62		Dental abrasive pastes
No. 63		Root canal barbed broaches and rasps
No. 69	ISO 6872:1995/Amd 1:1997	Dental ceramic
No. 70		Dental X-ray protective aprons and accessory devices
No. 71	ISO 3630–3:1994,	Root canal filling condensers (pluggers and spreaders)
No. 73	ISO 7551:1991	Dental absorbent points
No. 74	ISO7493:1997	Dental operator's stool
No. 75	ISO 10139-1:2005/Cor 1:2006	Resilient lining materials for removable dentures - Part 1: Short-term materials
No. 76		Non-sterile natural rubber latex gloves for dentistry
No. 78	ISO 6877:2006	Endodontic obturating cones
No. 80	ISO 7491:2000	Dental Materials—determination of color stability
No. 82	ISO 13716:1999	Dental reversible/irreversible hydrocolloid impression material systems (syringeable materials).
No. 85		Part 1—disposable prophy angles
No. 87		Dental impression trays
No. 88	ISO 9333:1990	Dental brazing alloys
No. 89	ISO 9680	Dental operating lights
No. 91	ISO 11246:1996	Dental ethyl silicate bonded casting investment
No. 92	ISO 11245:1999	Dental phosphate-bonded refractory die materials
No. 93	ISO 11244:1998	Dental brazing investments
No. 94		Dental compressed air quality
No. 95		Root canal enlargers
No. 96	ISO 9917-1:2003	Dental water-based cements
No. 97	ISO 10271:2001/Cor 1:2005	Corrosion test methods
No. 99		Athletic mouth protectors and materials
No. 100		Orthodontic brackets and tubes
No. 101		Root canal instruments: general requirements
No. 102		Non-sterile nitrile gloves
No. 103		Non-sterile polyvinyl chloride gloves for dentistry
No. 109		Procedures for storing dental amalgam waste and requirements for amalgam waste storage/shipment containers: 2006
No. 110		Technical report—dental lasers *NEW!*
No. 113		Periodontal curettes—gracey type *NEW!*
No. 119		Manual toothbrushes *NEW!*
No. 122	ISO 15854:2005	Dental casting and baseplate waxes *NEW!*
No. 3950	ISO 3950–1984	Dentistry—designation system for teeth and areas of the oral cavity
	ISO 22674:2006	Dentistry—Metallic materials for fixed and removable restorations and appliances

Appendix 2
ISO Standards
11.060.10: Dental Materials

ISO 3107:2011	Dentistry - Zinc oxide/eugenol and zinc oxide/non-eugenol cements
ISO 4049:2009	Dentistry - Polymer-based restorative materials
ISO 4823/Amd 1:2007	Elastomeric impression materials
ISO 6872:2015	Dentistry - Ceramic materials
ISO 6873:2013	Dentistry - Gypsum products
ISO 6874:2005	Polymer-based pit and fissure sealants
ISO 6876:2012	Dentistry - Root canal sealing materials
ISO 6877:2006	Root-canal obturating points
ISO 7405:2008/Amd 1:2013	Dentistry— Evaluation of biocompatibility of medical devices used in dentistry AMD 1: Positive control material
ISO 7491:2000	Dental materials - Determination of color stability
ISO 7551:1996	Dental absorbent points
ISO 9333:2006	Dentistry - Brazing materials
ISO 9693-1:2012	Dentistry - Compatibility testing - Part 1: Metal-ceramic systems
ISO/DIS 9693-2	Dentistry - Compatibility testing - Part 2: Ceramic-ceramic systems
ISO 9917-1:2007	Dentistry - Water-based cements - Part 1: Powder/liquid acid-base cements
ISO 9917-2:2010	Dentistry - Water-based cements -- Part 2: Resin-modified cements
ISO 10139-1:Cor 1:2006	Dentistry -- Soft lining materials for removable dentures -- Part 1: Materials for short-term use
ISO 10139-2:2009	Dentistry - Soft lining materials for removable dentures -- Part 2: Materials for long-term use
ISO 10271:2011	Dentistry - Corrosion test methods for metallic materials
ISO 10477:2004	Dentistry - Polymer-based crown and bridge materials
ISO/TS 11405:2015	Dentistry - Testing of adhesion to tooth structure
ISO 13017:2012/ FDAmd 1	Dentistry - Magnetic attachments
ISO 13116:2014	Dentistry - Test Method for Determining Radio-Opacity of Materials
ISO 13897:2003/Cor 1:2003	Dentistry - Amalgam capsules
ISO 14233:2003	Dentistry - Polymer-based die materials
ISO 14356:2003	Dentistry - Duplicating material
ISO/TS 14569-1:2007	Dental materials - Guidance on testing of wear - Part 1: Wear by toothbrushing
ISO/TS 14569-2:2001	Dental materials - Guidance on testing of wear — Part 2: Wear by two - and/or three body contact
ISO 15841:2014	Dentistry - Wires for use in orthodontics
ISO 15854:2005	Dentistry - Casting and baseplate waxes
ISO 15912:2006/Amd 1:2011	Dentistry - Casting investments and refractory die materials
ISO/DTS 16506	Dentistry - Polymer-based luting materials containing adhesive components
ISO 16744:2003	Base metal materials for fixed dental restorations

Cor: Correction; Amd: Amendment; TR: Technical report. TS: Technical specification

ISO/DIS 17254	Dentistry - Coiled springs for use in orthodontics
ISO 17304:2013	Dentistry - Polymerization shrinkage: Method for determination of polymerization shrinkage of polymer-based restorative materials
ISO/TS 17988:2014	Dentistry - Corrosion test methods for dental amalgam
ISO 20795-1:2013	Dentistry - Base polymers - Part 1: Denture base polymers
ISO 20795-2:2013	Dentistry - Base polymers - Part 2: Orthodontic base polymers
ISO 21563:2013	Dentistry - Hydrocolloid impression materials
ISO 21606:2007	Dentistry - Elastomeric auxiliaries for use in orthodontics
ISO 22112:2005	Dentistry - Artificial teeth for dental prostheses
ISO 22674:2006	Dentistry - Metallic materials for fixed and removable restorations and appliances
ISO 24234:2015	Dentistry - Dental amalgam
ISO 27020:2010	Dentistry - Brackets and tubes for use in orthodontics
ISO 28319:2010	Dentistry - Laser welding
ISO/TR 28642:2011	Dentistry - Guidance on color measurement
ISO 29022:2013	Dentistry - Adhesion - Notched-edge shear bond strength test

Appendix 3
ISO Standards
11.060.01: Dentistry in General

ISO 1942:2009	Dentistry - Vocabulary
ISO 3950:2009	Dentistry - Designation system for teeth and areas of the oral cavity
ISO/DIS 3950	Dentistry - Designation system for teeth and areas of the oral cavity
ISO 12836:2015	Dentistry - Digitizing devices for CAD/CAM systems for indirect dental restorations -- Test methods for assessing accuracy
ISO/DIS 13078-2	Dentistry - Dental furnace - Part 2: Test method for evaluation of furnace programme via firing glaze
ISO/TR 15300:2001	Dentistry - Application of OSI clinical codification to the classification and coding of dental products
ISO/TR 15599:2002	Digital codification of dental laboratory procedures
ISO 16059:2007	Dentistry - Required elements for codification used in data exchange
ISO 16443:2014	Dentistry - Vocabulary for dental implants systems and related procedure
ISO/FDIS 17937	Dentistry - Osteotome
ISO/DIS 18618	Dentistry - Interoperability of CAD/CAM Systems
ISO/CD 18675	Dental CAD/CAM Machinable Zirconia Blanks
ISO/DIS 18739	Dentistry - Vocabulary of process chain for CAD/CAM systems
ISO/CD 18845	Dentistry - CAD/CAM systems - Accuracy of machined indirect restorations -- Test methods and marking
ISO 21531:2009	Dentistry - Graphical symbols for dental instruments

Appendix 4
ISO Standards
11.060.15: Dental Implants

ISO 10451:2010	Dentistry - Contents of technical file for dental implant systems
ISO/TR 11175:1993	Dental implants - Guidelines for developing dental implants
ISO 11953:2010	Dentistry - Implants - Clinical performance of hand torque instruments
ISO/TS 13498:2011	Dentistry - Torsion test of implant body/connecting part joints of endosseous dental implant systems
ISO 14801:2007	Dentistry - Implants - Dynamic fatigue test for endosseous dental implants
ISO 16498:2013	Dentistry - Minimal dental implant data set for clinical use
ISO/DTS 18130	Dentistry - Torsional fatigue test of implant body/implant abutment joint of endosseous dental implants
ISO/PRF 19429	Dentistry - Designation system for dental implants
ISO 22794:2007	Dentistry - Implantable materials for bone filling and augmentation in oral and maxillofacial surgery - Contents of a technical file
ISO 22803:2004	Dentistry - Membrane materials for guided tissue regeneration in oral and maxillofacial surgery - Contents of a technical file
ISO/TS 22911:2005	Dentistry - Preclinical evaluation of dental implant systems -- Animal test methods

Appendix 5
ISO Standards
11.060.10: Dental Materials

ISO/DIS 1797	Dentistry - Shanks for rotary, oscillating and reciprocating instruments
ISO 1797-1:2011	Dentistry - Shanks for rotary instruments - Part 1: Shanks made of metals
ISO 1797-2:1992	Dental rotary instruments - Shanks - Part 2: Shanks made of plastics
ISO 1797-3:2013	Dentistry - Shanks for rotary instruments - Part 3: Shanks made of ceramics
ISO/DIS 2157	Dentistry - Nominal diameters and designation code numbers for rotary instruments
ISO 2157:1992	Dental rotary instruments - Nominal diameters and designation code number
ISO/CD 3630-1	Dentistry - Endodontic instruments - Part 1: General requirements
ISO 3630-1:2008	Dentistry - Root-canal instruments - Part 1: General requirements and test methods
ISO 3630-2:2013	Dentistry - Endodontic instruments - Part 2: Enlargers
ISO/FDIS 3630-3	Dentistry - Endodontic instruments - Part 3: Compactors: pluggers and spreaders
ISO 3630-3:1994	Dental root-canal instruments - Part 3: Condensers, pluggers and spreaders
ISO 3630-4:2009	Dentistry - Root canal instruments - Part 4: Auxiliary instruments
ISO 3630-5:2011	Dentistry - Endodontic instruments - Part 5: Shaping and cleaning instruments
ISO 3823-1:1997	Dental rotary instruments - Burs - Part 1: Steel and carbide burs
ISO 3823-2:2003/Amd 1:2008	Dentistry - Rotary bur instruments - Part 2: Finishing burs

ISO/DIS 3964	Dentistry - Coupling dimensions for handpiece connectors
ISO 3964:1982	Dental handpieces - Coupling dimensions
ISO 4073:2009	Dentistry - Information system on the location of dental equipment in the working area of the oral health care provider
ISO 6875:2011	Dentistry - Patient chair
ISO 7488:1991	Dental amalgamators
ISO 7492:1997	Dental explorers
ISO/CD 7492	Dental explorers
ISO 7493:2006	Dentistry - Operator's stool
ISO 7494-1:2011	Dentistry - Dental units - Part 1: General requirements and test methods
ISO 7494-2:2015	Dentistry - Dental units - Part 2: Air, water, suction and wastewater systems
ISO 7711-1:1997/Amd 1:2009	Dental rotary instruments - Diamond instruments - Part 1: Dimensions, requirements, marking and packaging
ISO 7711-2:2011	Dentistry - Rotary diamond instruments - Part 2: Discs
ISO 7711-3:2004	Dentistry - Diamond rotary instruments - Part 3: Grit sizes, designation and colour code
ISO 7786:2001	Dental rotary instruments - Laboratory abrasive instruments
ISO/DIS 7787-1	Dentistry - Laboratory cutters - Part 1: Steel laboratory cutters
ISO 7787-1:1984	Dental rotary instruments - Cutters - Part 1: Steel laboratory cutters
ISO 7787-2:2000	Dental rotary instruments - Cutters - Part 2: Carbide laboratory cutters
ISO 7787-3:1991	Dental rotary instruments - Cutters - Part 3: Carbide laboratory cutters for milling machines
ISO/CD 7787-3	Dental rotary instruments - Cutters - Part 3: Carbide laboratory cutters for milling machines
ISO 7787-4:2002	Dental rotary instruments - Cutters - Part 4: Miniature carbide laboratory cutters
ISO 7885:2010	Dentistry - Sterile injection needles for single use
ISO 8282:1994	Dental equipment -- Mercury and alloy mixers and dispensers
ISO 8325:2004	Dentistry - Test methods for rotary instruments
ISO 9168:2009	Dentistry - Hose connectors for air driven dental handpieces
ISO 9173-1:2006	Dentistry - Extraction forceps -- Part 1: General requirements and test methods
ISO/DIS 9173-1	Dentistry - Extraction forceps - Part 1: General requirements
ISO 9173-2:2010	Dentistry - Extraction forceps - Part 2: Designation
ISO 9173-3:2014	Dentistry - Extraction forceps - Part 3: Design
ISO 9680:2014	Dentistry - Operating lights
ISO 9687:2015	Dentistry - Graphical symbols for dental equipment
ISO 9873:1998	Dental hand instruments -- Reusable mirrors and handles
ISO/CD 9873/Cor 1:2000	Dental hand instruments - Reusable mirrors and handles
ISO 9997:1999	Dental cartridge syringes
ISO 10323:2013	Dentistry -- Bore diameters for rotary instruments such as discs and wheels
ISO 10637:1999	Dental equipment - High- and medium-volume suction systems
ISO/AWI 10637	Dentistry - High and medium volume suction systems for dental equipment
ISO/FDIS 10650	Dentistry - Powered polymerization activators
ISO 10650-1:2004	Dentistry - Powered polymerization activators - Part 1: Quartz tungsten halogen lamps
ISO 10650-2:2007	Dentistry - Powered polymerization activators - Part 2: Light-emitting diode (LED) lamps

ISO 11040-1:1992	Prefilled syringes - Part 1: Glass cylinders for dental local anaesthetic cartridges
ISO/DIS 11040-1	Prefilled syringes - Part 1: Glass cylinders for dental local anaesthetic cartridges
ISO 11040-2:2011	Prefilled syringes - Part 2: Plunger stoppers for dental local anaesthetic cartridges
ISO 11040-3:2012	Prefilled syringes - Part 3: Seals for dental local anaesthetic cartridges
ISO 11143:2008	Dentistry - Amalgam separators
ISO 11499:2014	Dentistry - Single-use cartridges for local anaesthetics
ISO 13078:2013	Dentistry - Dental furnace - Test method for temperature measurement with separate thermocouple
ISO 13295:2007	Dentistry - Mandrels for rotary instruments
ISO 13397-1:1995	Periodontal curettes, dental scalers and excavators - Part 1: General requirements
ISO 13397-2:2005/Amd 1:2012	Dentistry -- Periodontal curettes, dental scalers and excavators - Part 2: Periodontal curettes of Gr-type
ISO 13397-3:1996	Periodontal curettes, dental scalers and excavators - Part 3: Dental scalers - H-type
ISO 13397-4:1997	Periodontal curettes, dental scalers and excavators - Part 4: Dental excavators - Discoid-type
ISO 13397-5	Dentistry - Periodontal curettes, dental scalers and excavators - Part 5: Jacquette scalers
ISO 13402:1995	Surgical and dental hand instruments - Determination of resistance against autoclaving, corrosion and thermal exposure
ISO 15087-1:1999	Dental elevators - Part 1: General requirements
ISO 15087-2:2000	Dental elevators - Part 2: Warwick James elevators
ISO 15087-3:2000	Dental elevators - Part 3: Cryer elevators
ISO 15087-4:2000	Dental elevators - Part 4: Coupland elevators
ISO 15087-5:2000	Dental elevators - Part 5: Bein elevators
ISO 15087-6:2000	Dental elevators - Part 6: Flohr elevators
ISO 15098-1:1999	Dental tweezers - Part 1: General requirements
ISO 15098-2:2000	Dental tweezers - Part 2: Meriam types
ISO 15098-3:2000	Dental tweezers - Part 3: College types
ISO 15606:1999	Dental handpieces - Air-powered scalers and scaler tips
ISO 16635-1:2013	Dentistry - Dental rubber dam technique - Part 1: Hole punch
ISO 16635-2:2014	Dentistry - Dental rubber dam instruments - Part 2: Clamp forceps
ISO 16954:2015	Dentistry - Test methods for dental unit waterline biofilm treatment
ISO/DIS 17509	Dentistry - Torque transmitter for handpieces used for implantation
ISO/DIS 18556	Dentistry - Intraoral spatulas
ISO/DIS 18559	Dentistry - Extraoral spatulas for mixing dental cements
ISO/CD 19715	Dentistry - Filling instruments with contra set
ISO 21530:2004	Dentistry - Materials used for dental equipment surfaces - Determination of resistance to chemical disinfectants
ISO 21533:2003/Cor 1:2009	Dentistry - Reusable cartridge syringes intended for intraligamentary injections
ISO 21671:2006/Amd 1:2011	Dentistry - Rotary polishers
ISO/TS 22595-1:2006	Dentistry - Plant area equipment - Part 1: Suction systems
ISO/TS 22595-2:2008	Dentistry - Plant area equipment - Part 2: Compressor systems
IEC 80601-2-60:2012	Medical electrical equipment - Part 2-60: Particular requirements for basic safety and essential performance of dental equipment

Appendix 6
ISO Standards
11.060.25: Dental Instruments

ISO 6360-1:2004/Cor 1:2007	Dentistry - Number coding system for rotary instruments - Part 1: General characteristics
ISO 6360-2:2004/Amd 1:2011	Dentistry - Number coding system for rotary instruments - Part 2: Shapes
ISO 6360-3:2005	Dentistry - Number coding system for rotary instruments - Part 3: Specific characteristics of burs and cutters
ISO 6360-4:2004	Dentistry - Number coding system for rotary instruments - Part 4: Specific characteristics of diamond instruments
ISO 6360-5:2007	Dentistry - Number coding system for rotary instruments - Part 5: Specific characteristics of root-canal instruments
ISO 6360-6:2004	Dentistry - Number coding system for rotary instruments - Part 6: Specific characteristics of abrasive instruments
ISO 6360-7:2006	Dentistry - Number coding system for rotary instruments - Part 7: Specific characteristics of mandrels and special instruments
ISO 13504:2012	Dentistry - General requirements for instruments and related accessories used in dental implant placement and treatment
ISO 14457:2012	Dentistry - Handpieces and motors
ISO/FDIS 18397	Dentistry - Powered scaler
ISO/CD 19490	Dentistry - Sinus elevator
ISO 21672-1:2012	Dentistry - Periodontal probes - Part 1: General requirements
ISO 21672-2:2012	Dentistry - Periodontal probes - Part 2: Designation
ISO 22374:2005	Dentistry - Dental handpieces - Electrical-powered scalers and scaler tips

Appendix 7

To convert from	To	Multiply by
kilograms force	pounds	2.2046
kilograms force	Newtons	9.807
pounds	kilograms force	0.4536
pounds	Newtons	4.448
Newtons	kilograms force	0.1020
Newtons	pounds	0.2248
Force per unit urea		
psi	MPa (MN/m^2)	0.006895
psi	Kg/cm^2	0.0703
Kg/cm^2	MPa (MN/m^2)	0.09807
Kg/cm^2	psi	14.2233
MN/m^2	psi	145.0
MN/m^2	Kg/cm^2	10.1968

Appendix 8
ISO Specification 3107: For Zoe Cement—Sample

International Standard   **ISO 3107:2004(E)**

DENTISTRY - ZINC OXIDE/EUGENOL AND ZINC OXIDE/NONEUGENOL CEMENTS

1. Scope

This International Standard specifies the requirements and performance test methods for non-water-based zinc oxide/eugenol cements suitable for use in restorative dentistry for temporary cementation, for permanent cementation, for cavity liners and bases and as temporary restorations.

This International Standard is also applicable to noneugenol cements containing zinc oxide and aromatic oils suitable for temporary cementation.

2. Normative References

The following referenced documents are indispensable for the application of this document. For dated references, only the edition cited applies. For undated references, the latest edition of the referenced document (including any amendments) applies.

ISO 2590, *General method for the determination of arsenic—Silver diethyldithiocarbamate photometric method*

ISO 3696:1987, *Water for analytical laboratory use—Specification and test methods*

ISO 8601, Data *elements* and *interchange* formats—*Information interchange—Representation of dates and times.*

3. Classification

For the purposes of this document, the following classification for cements is used, based on their intended use:

a.   Type I: for temporary cementation;

       1. Class 1: setting cement;

       2. Class 2: non-setting cement.

b.   Type II: for permanent cementation;

c.   Type III: for bases and temporary restorations;

d.   Type IV: for cavity liners.

Appendix 8.
ISO Specification 3107: For Zoe Cement—Sample

International Standard ISO 3107:2004(E)

DENTISTRY - ZINC OXIDE/EUGENOL AND ZINC OXIDE/NON-EUGENOL CEMENTS

1. Scope

Further Reading

1. Abdullah MA. Surface detail, compressive strength, and dimensional accuracy of gypsum casts after repeated immersion in hypochlorite solution. J Prosthet Dent. 2006;95:462-8.

2. Adabo GE, Zanarotti E, Fonseca RG, Cruz CA. Effect of disinfectant agents on dimensional stability of elastomeric impression materials. J Prosthet Dent. 1999;81:621-4.

3. Amit P, Hegde M. Dental composites: past present and future. Nat J Comm Med. 212;3:754.

4. Andreasen GF, Morrow RE. Laboratory and clinical analyses of Nitinol wire. Am J Orthod. 1978;73:143.

5. Anusavice, Sehn Rawls. Phillips' Science of Dental Materials. 12th ed. St. Louis. Saunders, 2013.

6. Anusavice KJ, Shen C, Vermost B, Chow B. Strengthening of porcelain by ion exchange subsequent to thermal tempering. Dent Mater. 1992;8:149.

7. Asmuseen E, Munksgaard EC. Bonding of restorative resins to dentine: Status of dentine adhesives and impact on cavity design and filling techniques. Int Dent J. 1988;38:97.

8. Association Report: Classification System for Cast Alloys. J Am Dent Assoc. 1984;109:838.

9. Bailey JH, Donovan TE, Preston JD. The dimensional accuracy of improved dental stone, silver-plated, and epoxy resin die materials. J Prosthet Dent. 1988;59:307.

10. Ballard GT, Leinfelder KF, Taylor DF. Permeability and porosity of dental casting investments. J Prosthet Dent. 1975;34:170-8.

11. Barrett NVJ, Brukl CE. Compatibility of agar hydrocolloid duplicating materials with dental stones. J Prosthet Dent. 1985;54:586-91.

12. Barron T. Mercury in our Environment. CDA Journal. 2004;32(7):556-63.

13. Bayne SC, Heymann HO, Swift Jr EJ. Update on dental composite restorations. Am J Dent Assoc. 1994;125:687-701.

14. Bertassoni LE, et al. Biomechanical perspective on the remineralization of dentin. Caries research. 2009;43:70-7.

15. Bertassoni LE, et al. Direct-write bioprinting of cell-laden methacrylated gelatin hydrogels. Biofabrication. 2014;6:24.

16. Brien WJ. Dental materials and their selection. 4th edition, Quintessence, 2008.

17. Brune D, Beltesbrekke H. Dust in dental laboratories. Part I: Types and levels in specific operations. J Prosthet Dent. 1980;43:687-92.

18. Buonocore MG. A simple method of increasing the adhesion of acrylic filling materials to enamel surfaces. J Dent Res. 1955;34:849-53.

19. Burke FJT, Watts DC. Fracture resistance of teeth restored with dentine-bonded crowns. Quintessence Int. 1994;25:335-40.

20. Burstone CJ, Goldberg AJ. Beta titanium: A new orthodontic alloy. Am J Orthod. 1980;77:121.

21. Butta R, Tredwin CJ, Nesbit M, Moles DR. Type IV gypsum compatibility with five addition-reaction silicone impression materials. J Prosthet Dent. 2005;93:540-4.

22. Chai JY, Yeung TC. Wettability of nonaqueous elastomeric impression materials. Int J Prosthodont. 1991;4:555.

23. Chaing BKP. Polymers in the service of prosthetic dentistry. J Dent. 1984;12:203.

24. Chaturvedi TP, Upadhayay SN. An overview of orthodontic material degradation in oral cavity. Indian J Dent Res. 2010;21(2):275-84.

25. Chaturvedi TP. Allergy related to dental implant and its clinical significance. Clin Cosmet Investig Dent. 2013;5:57-61.

26. Chaturvedi TP. An overview of the corrosion aspect of dental implants (titanium and its alloys). Indian J Dent Res. 2009;20:91-8.

27. Chee WWL, Donovan TE. Polyvinyl siloxane impression materials: A review of properties and techniques. J Prosthet Dent. 1992;68:728.

28. Chen MH. Update on dental nanocomposites. J Dent Res. 2010;9:549-60.

29. Cheung GS, Lai SC, Ng RP. Fate of vital pulps beneath a metal-ceramic crown or a bridge retainer. Int Endod J. 2005;38:521-30.

30. Collins CJ, Bryant RW, Hodge KLV. A clinical evaluation of posterior composite resin restorations: 8-year finding. J Dent. 1998;26:311-7.

31. Council on dental materials, instruments, and equipment: Infection control recommendations for the dental office and the dental laboratory. J Am Dent Assoc. 1988;116:148.

32. Council on Dental Materials, Instruments, and Equipment: Report on base metal alloys for crown and bridge applications: Benefits and risks. J Am Dent Assoc. 1985;111:479.

33. Davis DR. Effect of wet and dry cellulose ring liners on setting expansion and compressive strength of a gypsum-bonded investment. J Prosthet Dent. 1996;76:519-23.

34. Davis DR. Limiting wax pattern distortion caused by setting expansion. J Prosthet Dent. 1987;58:229-34.

35. Derrien G, Sturtz G. Comparison of transverse strength and dimensional variations between die stone, die epoxy resin, and die polyurethane resin. J Prosthet Dent. 1995;74:569-74.

36. Dong JK, et al. Heat-pressed ceramics: Technology and strength. Int J Prosthodon. 1992;5:9.

37. Douglas WH. Clinical status of dentine bonding agents. J Dent. 1989;17:209.

38. Drennon DG, Johnson GH. The effect of immersion disinfection of elastomeric impressions on the surface detail reproduction of improved gypsum casts. J Prosthet Dent. 1990;63:233-41.

39. Duke P, Moore BK, Haug SP, Andres CJ. Study of the physical properties of type IV gypsum, resin-containing, and epoxy die materials. J Prosthet Dent. 2000;83:466-73.

40. Duret F, Blouin JL, Duret B. CAD-CAM in dentistry. JADA. 1998;117:715-20.

41. Eames WB, O'Neal SJ, Monteiro J, et al. Techniques to improve the seating of castings. J Am Dent Assoc. 1978;96:432.

42. Earnshaw R. The effect of casting ring liners on the potential expansion of a gypsum-bonded. J Dent Res. 1988;67:1366-70.

43. Emmer TJ, et al. Bond strength of permanent soft denture liners bonded to denture liners bonded to denture base. J Prosthet Dent. 1995;74:595-600.

44. Finger W, Ohsawa M. Accuracy of cast restorations produced by a refractory die-investing technique. J Prosthet Dent. 1984;52:800.

45. Fusayama T, et al. Non-pressure adhesion of a new adhesive restorative system. J Dent Res. 1979;58:1364.

46. Fusayama T, Kurosaki N, Node H, Nakamura M. A laminated hydrocolloid impression for indirect inlays. J Prosthet Dent. 1982;47:171.

47. Fusayama T. Factors and prevention of pulp irritation by adhesive composite resin restorations. Quintessence Int. 1987;18:633-41.

48. Gallegos LI, Nicholls JI. In vitro two-body wear of three veneering resins. J Prosthet Dent. 1988;60:172-8.

49. Garhammer P, et al. Patients with local adverse effects from dental alloys: frequency, complaints, symptoms, allergy. Clin Oral Investig. 2001;5(4):240-9.

50. Gauthier MA, Stangel I, Ellis TH, Zhu XX. Oxygen inhibition in dental resins. J Dent Res. 2005;8:725-9.

51. Giordano R. Zirconia: A proven, durable ceramic for esthetic restorations. Compend Contin Educ Dent. 2012;33:46-9.

52. Guess PC, Kuliša A, Witkowskia S, Wolkewitzb M, Zhangc Y, Struba JR. Shear bond strengths between different zirconia cores and veneering ceramics and their susceptibility to thermocycling. Dent Mater J. 2008;24:1556-67.

53. Guilin Y, Nan L, Yousheng L, Yining W. The effects of different types of investments on the alpha-case layer of titanium castings. J Prosthet Dent. 2007;97:157-64.

54. Harper RH, Schnell RJ, Swartz ML, Phillips RW. In vivo measurements of thermal diffusion through restorations of various materials. J Prosthet Dent. 1980;43:180.

55. Harrison A, Huggett R, Azouka A. Some physical and mechanical properties of shellac dental baseplate material. J Oral Rehabil. 1995;22(7):509-13.

56. Hicks J, Garcia-Godoy F, Donly K, Flaitz C. Fluoride-releasing restorative materials and secondary caries. Dent Clin North Am. 2002;46:247-76.

57. Hinoura K, Moore BK, Phillips RW. Tensile bond strength between glass ionomer cement and composite resin. J Am Dent Assoc. 1987;114:167.

58. Hiyasat A. The abrasive effect of glazed, unglazed, and polished porcelain on the wear of human enamel, and the influence of carbonated soft drinks on the rate of wear. Int J Prosthodont. 1997;10:269-82.

59. Hondrum SO, Fernandez R (Jr). Effects of long-term storage on properties of an alginate impression material. J Prosthet Dent. 1997;77:601-6.

60. Hondrum SO. A review of strength properties of dental ceramics. J Prosthet Dent. 1992;67:859-64.

61. Hung SH, Purk JH, Tira DE, Eick JD. Comparison of the dimensional accuracy of one- and two-step techniques with the use of putty/wash addition silicone impression materials. J Prosthet Dent. 1995;74:535-41.

62. Isidor F, Brondum K. A clinical evaluation of porcelain inlays. J Prosthet Dent. 1995;74:40-4.

63. Islam I, Chang HK, Yap HU. Comparison of physical and mechanical properties of MTA and Portland cement. J Endod. 2006;32(3):193-7.

64. Johnson GH, Bales DJ, Gordon GE, Powell LV. Clinical performance of posterior composite resin restorations. Quintessence Int. 1992;23(10):705-11.

65. Johnson GH, Craig RG. Accuracy and bond strength of combination agar/alginate hydrocolloid impression materials. J Prosthet Dent. 1986;55:1-6.

66. Johnson GH, Lepe X, Aw TC. The effect of surface moisture on detail reproduction of elastomeric impressions. J Prosthet Dent. 2003;90:354-64.

67. Jo LJ. Spark erosion process: An overview. J Dent Implant. 2011;1:2-6.

68. Jones DE. Effects of topical fluoride preparations on glazed porcelain surfaces. J Prosthet Dent. 1985;53:483.

69. Juntavee N, Giordano R, Nathanson D. Porcelain shear bond strength to a new ceramo-metal system. J Dent Res. 1995;74:159.

70. Kahn RC, Lancaster MV, Kate Jr W. The microbiologic cross-contamination of dental prostheses. J Prosthet Dent. 1982;47:556-9.

71. Kanca J III. Resin bonding to wet substrate I. Bonding to dentin. Quintessence Int. 1992;23:39-41.

72. Kaylakie WG, Brukl CE. Comparative tensile strengths of non-noble dental alloy solders. J Prosthet Dent. 1985;53:455.

73. Kelly JR, Nishimura I, Campbell SD. Ceramics in dentistry: Historical roots and current perspectives. J Prosthet Dent. 1996;75:18-32.

74. Kelly R. Ceramics in Dentistry: Historical roots and current perspectives. J Prosthet Dent. 1996;75:18-29.

75. Khoroushi M, Keshani F. A review of glass-ionomers: From conventional glass-ionomer to bioactive glass-ionomer. Dent Res J. 2013;10: 411-20.

76. Klineberg I, Earnshaw R. Physical properties of shellac baseplate materials. Aust Dent J. 1967;12:468-45.

77. Klooster J, Logan GI, Tjan AHL. Effects of strain rate on the behavior of elastomeric impressions. J Prosthet Dent. 1991;66:292.

78. Kusy RP, Greenberg AR. Effects of composition and cross section on the elastic properties of orthodontic archwires. Angle Orthop. 1981;51:325.

79. Lambrechts P, Braem M, Vanherle G. Evaluation of clinical performance for posterior composite resins and dentin adhesives. J Oper Dent. 1987;12:53.

80. Larsson KS. Potential teratogenic and carcinogenic effects of dental materials. Int Dent J. 1991;41:206-11.

81. Leinfelder KF, Bayne SC, Swift EJ (Jr). Packable composites: overview and technical considerations. J Esthet Dent. 1999;11(5):234-49.

82. Letzel H. Survival rates and reasons for failure of posterior composite restorations in multicentre clinical trial. J Dent. 1989;17:S10-7.

83. Leung RL, Schonfeld SE. Gypsum casts as a potential source of microbial cross-contamination. J Prosthet Dent. 1983;49:210-1.

84. Lim KC, Chong YH, Soh G. Effect of operator variability on void formation in impressions made with an automixed addition silicone. Aust Dent J. 1992;37:35.

85. Lin A, McIntyre NS, Davidson RD. Studies on the adhesion of glass ionomer cements to dentin. J Dent Res. 1992;71:1836-41.

86. Lind PO. Oral lichenoid reactions related to composite restorations: Preliminary report. Acta Odontol Scand. 1988;46:63-5.

87. Lindquist TJ, Stanford CM, Knox E. Influence of surface hardener on gypsum abrasion resistance and water sorption. J Prosthet Dent. 2003;90:441-6.

88. Lineham AD, Windeler AS. Passive fit of implant-retained prosthetic super-structures improved by electric discharge machining. J Prosthodont. 1994;3:88-95.

89. Luk HW, Darvell BW. Effect of burnout temperatures on strength of phosphate-bonded investments-Part II: Effect of metal temperature. J Dent. 1997;25: 423-30.

90. Lutz F, Phillips RW. A classification and evaluation of composite resin systems. J Prosthet Dent. 1983;50:480.

91. MacCulloch WT. Advances in dental ceramics. Br Dent J. 1968;124:361.

92. Machado CE1, Guedes CG. Effects of sulfur-based hemostatic agents and gingival retraction cords handled with latex gloves on the polymerization of polyvinyl siloxane impression materials. J Appl Oral Sci. 2011;19(6):628-33.

93. Mackert JR (Jr), Ringle RD, Parry EE, et al. The relationship between oxide adherence and porcelain-metal bonding. J Dent Res. 1988;67:474.

94. Mahalaxmi S. Materials used in dentistry. 1st Ed. Wulters Kluwer health (India), New Delhi. 2013.

95. Mahler DB, Ady AB. Explanation for the hydroscopic setting expansion of dental gypsum products. J Dent Res. 1960;39:578.

96. Maldonado A, Swartz M, Phillips RW. An in vitro study of certain properties of a glass ionomer cement. J Am Dent Assoc. 1978;96:785.

97. Maldupa I, et. al. Evidence-based toothpaste classification, according to certain characteristics of their chemical composition. Stomatologija, Baltic Dental and Maxillofacial Journal. 2012;14:12-22.

98. Matsuya S, Yamane M. Decomposition of gypsum-bonded investments. J Dent Res. 1981;60:1418.

99. Matthew I, Frame JW. Allergic responses to titanium. J Oral Maxillofac Surg. 1998;56(12):1466-7.

100. McCabe JF, Walls AWG. Applied dental materials. 8th ed. Blackwell. 1998.

101. McKinney JE, Antonucci JM, Rupp NW. Wear and microhardness of a silver-sintered glass ionomer cement. J Dent Res. 1988;67:831.

102. McLaren EA, Sorensen JA. High-strength alumina crowns and fixed partial dentures generated by

copy-milling technology. Quint Dent Technol. 1995;18:310.

103. McLean JW, Nicholson JW, Wilson AD. Proposed nomenclature for glass ionomer dental cements and related materials. Quintessence Int. 1994;25:587-9.

104. McLean JW, Sced IR. The bonded alumina crown. The bonding of platinum to aluminous dental porcelain using tin-oxide coatings. Aust Dent J. 1976;21:119.

105. McLean JW. The science and art of dental ceramics. Quintessence, Volume I and II. 1979;1980.

106. Mc Manus KR, Fan PL, et al. Purchasing installing and operating dental amalgam separators : Practical issues. J Am Dent Assoc. 2003;134(8):1054-65.

107. Miller MB. Self-etching adhesives: solving the sensitivity conundrum. Pract Proced Aesthet Dent. 2002;14:406.

108. Mitra A, et al. Maxillofacial prosthetic materials— An inclination toward silicones. J Clin Diagn Res. 2014;8:8-13.

109. Miura R, Masakuni M, Ohura Y, et al. The superelastic property of the Japanese Ni-Ti alloy wire for use in orthodontics. Am J Ortho Dent Orthoped. 1986;90:1.

110. Mjör IA, Jokstad A. Five-year study of class II restorations in permanent teeth using amalgam, glass polyalkenoate (ionomer) cement and resin-based composite materials. J Dent. 1993;21(6): 338-43.

111. Mjör IA. Glass-ionomer cement restorations and secondary caries: A preliminary report. Quintessence Int. 1996;27:171-4.

112. Moffa JP, Jenkins WA, Ellison JA, Hamilton JC. A clinical evaluation of two base metal alloys and a gold alloy for use in fixed prosthodontics: A five-year study. J Prosthet Dent. 1984;52:491.

113. Mori T. Titanium—A review of investments for high temperature casting. Aust Prosthodont J. 1993;7:31-4.

114. Morrow RM, Brown CE (Jr), Stansbury BE, DeLorimier JA, Powell JM, Rudd KD. Compatibility of alginate impression materials and dental stones. J Prosthet Dent. 1971;25:556-66.

115. Mount GJ. An Atlas of Glass Ionomer Cements. 3rd ed. Martin Dumitz, London. 2002.

116. Nakabayashi N. Resin reinforced dentin due to infiltration of monomers into the dentin at the adhesive interface. J Jpn Dent Mat Devices. 1982;1:78-81.

117. Neiman R, Sarma AC. Setting and thermal reactions of phosphate investments. J Dent Res. 1980;59: 1478-85.

118. Nomura GT, Reisbick MH, Preston JD. An investigation of epoxy resin dies. J Prosthet Dent. 1980;44:45.

119. Noort RV. Introduction to dental materials. 2nd Ed. Mosby; 2002.

120. Norman RD, Rydberg RJ, Felkner LL. A 5-year study comparing a posterior composite resin and an amalgam. J Prosthet Dent. 1990;64:523-9.

121. Parekh RB, Shetty O, Tabassum R. Surface modifications for endosseous dental implants. Int J Oral Implantol Clin Res. 2012;3(3):116-21.

122. Parr GR, Gardner LK, Toth RW. Titanium: The mystery metal of implant dentistry-dental materials aspects. J Prosthet Dent. 1985;54:410-4.

123. Phillips RW, Swartz ML, Lund MS, et al. In vivo disintegration of luting agents. J Am Dent Assoc. 1987;114:489.

124. Powers, Sakaguchi. Craig's Restorative Dental Materials 12th edition, Mosby, 1993.

125. Powers JM, Wataha JC. Dental materials, properties and manipulation. 9th ed. Mosby, 1992.

126. Powis DR, Folleras T, Merson SA, Wilson AD. Improved adhesion of a glass ionomer cement to dentin and enamel. J Dent Res. 1982;61:1416.

127. Prakash R, Gopalkrishna V, Kandaswamy D. Gutta-Percha—An untold story. Endodontology. 2005;17(2):32-6.

128. Pratten DH, Novetsky M. Detail reproduction of soft tissue: A comparison of impression materials. J Prosthet Dent. 1991;65:188-91.

129. Prithviraj DR, Regish KM, Deeksha S, Shruthi DP. Extraction and immediate placement of root analogue zirconia implants: an overview. J Clin Exp Dent. 2011;3:240-5.

130. Qualtrough A, Piddock V. Recent Advances in ceramic materials and systems for dental restorations. March Dental Update. 1999;65-72 .

131. Qvist V, Qvist J, Mjör IA. Placement and longevity of tooth-coloured restorations in Denmark. Acta Odontol Scand. 1990;48:305-11.

132. Rao A, Shenoy R. Mineral trioxide aggregate—A review. J Clin Pediatr Dent. 2009;34(1):1-7

133. Rasmussen EJ, Goodkind RJ, Gerberich WW. An investigation of tensile strength of dental solder joints. J Prosthet Dent. 1979;41:418.

134. Reed HV. Reversible agar-agar hydrocolloid. Quintessence Int. 1990;21:225.

135. Rekow D. Computer-aided design and manufacturing in dentistry: A review of the state of the art. J Prosthet Dent. 1987;58:512-6.

136. Richter WA, Cantwell KR. A study of cohesive gold. J Prosthet Dent. 1965;15:722.

137. Roberto S, Massimiliano L. Reliability of antagonistic arch in dental prosthesis: Clinical evaluation of different preimpression preparation procedures. J Prosthet Dent. 1995;74:127-32.

138. Roberts HW, et al. Mineral trioxide aggregate material use in endodontic treatment: A review of the literature. Dent Mater. 2008;24(2):149-64.

139. Roekel V. Electrical discharge machining in dentistry. Int J Prosthodont. 1992;5(2):114-21.

140. Rosen M, Touyz LZ. Influence of mixing disinfectant solutions into alginate on working time and accuracy. J Dent. 1991;19:186.

141. Roulet JF. The problems associated with substituting composite resins for amalgam: a status report on posterior composites. J Dent. 1988;16:101-13.

142. Rueggeberg FA, et al. Sodium hypochlorite disinfection of irreversible hydrocolloid impression material. J Prosthet Dent. 1992;67:628-31.

143. Rübeling G. New techniques in spark erosion: The solution to an accurately fitting screw-retained implant restoration. Quintessence Int. 1999;30:38-48.

144. Santos JFF, Ballester RY. Delayed hygroscopic expansion of gypsum products. J Prosthet Dent. 1984;52:366-70.

145. Schelb E, Mazzocco CV, Jones JD, Prihoda T. Compatibility of type IV dental stones with polyvinyl siloxane impression materials. J Prosthet Dent. 1987;58:19-22.

146. Schnitman PA, Shulman LB. Vitreous carbon implants. Dent Clin North Am. 1980;24:441-63.

147. Schutt RW. Bactericidal effect of a disinfectant dental stone on irreversible hydrocolloid impressions and stone casts. J Prosthet Dent. 1989;62:605-7.

148. Schwedhelm ER, Lepe X. Fracture strength of Type IV and Type V die stone as a function of time. J Prosthet Dent. 1997;78(6):554-9.

149. Seghi RR, Crispin BC, Mito W. The effect of ion exchange on flexural strength of feldspathic porcelains. Int J Prosthodont. 1990;4:130-4.

150. Seghi RR, Denry IL, Rosentiel SF. Relative Fracture toughness and hardness of new dental ceramics. J Prosthet Dent. 1995;74:145-50.

151. Seha MM, Pamuk S, Balkaya MC, Akgüngör G. Effect of Tuf-Coat on Feldspathic porcelain materials. J Oral Rehabil. 2005;32:39-45.

152. Sehgal A, Rao YM, Joshua M, Narayanan LL. Evaluation of the effects of the oxygen-inhibited layer on shear bond strength of two resin composites. J Conserv Dent. 2008;11(4):159-61.

153. Shah S. Evaluation of electric discharge machining to achieve passive fit of implant superstructure—An in vitro study. World J Dent. 2012;3:32-6.

154. Shalak R. Biomechanical considerations in osseointegrated prostheses. J Prosthet Dent. 1983;49:843-8.

155. Shoher I, Whiteman A. Captek—A new capillary casting technology for ceramometal restorations. Quintessence of Dental Technology. 1995;18:9

156. Shoher I, Whiteman A. Reinforced porcelain system: A new concept in ceramo-metal restorations. J Prosthet Dent. 1983;50:489-96.

157. Shoher I. Reinforced porcelain system. Dent Clin North Am. 1985;29:805-18.

158. Siervo S, Parnpalone A, Siervo P, Siervo R. Where is the gap? Machinable ceramic systems and conventional laboratory restorations at a glance. Quintessence Int. 1994;25:773-9.

159. Simonsen R, Thompson VP, Barrack G. Etched cast restorations: Clinical and Laboratory Techniques. Chicago: Quintessence. 1983.

160. Simonsen RJ. Retention and effectiveness of dental sealant after 15 years. J Am Dent Assoc. 1991;122:34.

161. Smith, Wright, Brown. The clinical handling of dental materials. 2nd ed. Butterworth-Heinemann; 1994.

162. Smith DC, Ruse ND. Acidity of glass ionomer cements during setting and its relation to pulp sensitivity. J Am Dent Assoc. 1986;112:654.

163. Sowygh ZA. The effect of various interim fixed prosthodontic materials on the polymerization of elastomeric impression materials. J Prosthet Dent. 2014;112:176-81.

164. Stackhouse JA (Jr). Electrodeposition in dentistry. A review of the literature. J Prosthet Dent. 1980;44:259-63.

165. Stackhouse JA (Jr). The accuracy of stone dies made from rubber impression materials. J Prosthet Dent. 1970;24:377.

166. Stanley HR. Local and systemic responses to dental composites and glass ionomers. Adv Dent Res. 1992;6:55-64.

167. Suzuki S. Does the wear resistance of packable composite equal that of dental amalgam? J Esthet Restor Dent. 2004;16(6):355-65; discussion 365-7.

168. Swartz ML, Phillips RW, Rhodes B. Visible light-activated resins: Depth of cure. J Am Dent Assoc. 1983;106:634.

169. Söderholm KJ, Mariotti A. Bis-GMA-based resins in dentistry: are they safe? JADA. 1999;130:201-8.

170. Takamata T, Setcos JC, Phillips RW, Boone ME. Adaptation of acrylic resin dentures influenced by the activation mode of polymerization. J Am Dent Assoc. 1989;118:271.

171. Takamata T, Setcos JC. Resin denture bases: Review of accuracy and methods of polymerization. Int J Prosthodont. 1989;2:555.

172. Thouati A. Dimensional stability of seven elastomeric impression materials immersed in disinfectants. J Prosthet Dent. 1996;76:8-15.

173. Torabinejad M, Hong CU, McDonald F, Pitt Ford TR. Physical and chemical properties of a new root-end filling material. J Endod. 1995(7);21:349-353.

174. Torabinejad M, Parirokh M. Mineral trioxide aggregate: a comprehensive literature review—Part I: chemical, physical, and antibacterial properties. J Endod. 2010;36(1):16.

175. Torabinejad M, Parirokh M. Mineral trioxide aggregate: a comprehensive literature review—part II: leakage and biocompatibility investigations. J Endod. 2010;36(2):190-202.

176. Tuncer N, Tufekçioglu HB, Alikkocaoglu SC. Investigation on the compressive strength of several gypsum products dried by microwave oven with different programs. J Prosthet Dent. 1993;69:333-9.

177. Van Meerbeek B, Inoue S, Perdigao J, et al. In: Carol Stream (Ed). Fundamentals of Operative Dentistry. 2nd Ed. Ill Quintessence. Publishing Co, Inc. 2001;194-214.

178. Wagner WC. Biaxial flexural strength and indentation fracture toughness of three new dental core ceramics. J Prosthet Dent. 1996;76:140-4.

179. Wakefield CW. Laboratory contamination of dental prostheses. J Prosthet Dent. 1980;44:143-6.

180. Walter M, Boenig K, Reppel PD. Clinical performance of machined titanium restorations. J Dent. 1994;22:346-8.

181. Wee AG. Comparison of impression materials for direct multi-implant impressions. J Prosthet Dent. 2000; 83:323-31.

182. Weinmann W, Thalacker C, Guggenberger R. Siloranes in dental composites. Dent mater. 2005;21:68-74.

183. Weiss PA, Munyon RE. Repairs, corrections, and additions to ceramo-metal frameworks. II. Quint Dent Technol. 1980;7:45.

184. Willems G, Lambrechts P, Braem M, Celis J, vanherle G. A classification of dental composites according to their morphological and mechanical characteristics. Dent Mater. 1992;8:310-9

185. Williams HN, Falkler WA (Jr), Hasler JF. Acinetobacter contamination of laboratory dental pumice. J Dent Res. 1983;62:1073-5.

186. Wilson HJ. Impression materials. Br Dent J. 1988;164:221.

187. Winkler MM, Monaghan P, Gilbert JL, Lautenschlager EP. Comparison of four techniques for monitoring the setting kinetics of gypsum. J Prosthet Dent. 1998;79:532-6.

188. Wolff MS, Barretto MT, Gale EN, et al. The effect of the powder-liquid ratio on in vivo solubility of zinc phosphate and polycarboxylate cements. J Dent Res. 1985;64:316.

189. Wunderlich R, Yaman P. In vitro effect of topical fluoride on dental porcelain. J Prosthet Dent. 1986;55:385.

190. Xavier Lepe, Johnson GH. Accuracy of polyether and addition silicone after long-term immersion disinfection. J Prosthet Dent. 1997;78:245-9.

191. Yen TW, Blackman RB, Baez FJ. Effect of acid etching on the flexure strength of a feldspathic porcelain and a castable glass ceramic. J Prosthet Dent. 1993;70:224-33.

Index

Page numbers followed by *f* refer to figure, *b* refer to box and *t* refer to table.